A Practical Guide to the Evaluation of Child Physical Abuse and Neglect

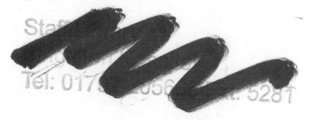

A Practical Guide to the Evaluation of Child Physical Abuse and Neglect

Second Edition

Edited by

Angelo P. Giardino, MD, PhD, MPH

Texas Children's Health Plan, Houston, TX, USA
Baylor College of Medicine

Michelle A. Lyn, MD

Baylor College of Medicine, Houston, TX, USA
Texas Children's Hospital

Eileen R. Giardino, RN, PhD, FNP-BC

The University of Texas Health Science Center at Houston — School of Nursing,
Houston, TX, USA

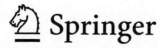 Springer

Editors
Angelo P. Giardino
Texas Children's Health Plan, Inc.
Baylor College of Medicine
2450 Holcombe Blvd.
Houston TX 77021
Suite 34L
USA
apgiardi@texaschildrens.org

Michelle A. Lyn
Baylor College of Medicine
Texas Children's Hospital
Children's Assessment Center
6621 Fannin St.
Houston TX 77030-2399
A210/MC1-1481
USA
malyn@texaschildrens.org

Eileen R. Giardino
Department of Acute & Integrative Care
School of Nursing at Houston
University of Texas
6901 Bertner
Houston TX 77030
USA
eileen.r.giardino@uth.tmc.edu

ISBN 978-1-4419-0701-1   e-ISBN 978-1-4419-0702-8
DOI 10.1007/978-1-4419-0702-8
Springer New York Dordrecht Heidelberg London

Library of Congress Control Number: 2010921596

To our senior institutional leaders who create the academic and clinical environment that permits us to advocate for vulnerable children and families by writing books such as this. These visionary leaders consistently encourage us and our colleagues to embrace the responsibility to challenge our professional beliefs by constantly reviewing our work and making changes to our practices and approaches as the evidence emerges and calls for such changes to be made:

Christopher M. Born
President, Texas Children's Health Plan

Joan E. Shook, MD
Professor and Director of Pediatric Emergency Medicine,
Baylor College of Medicine/Texas Children's Hospital
Chief Patient Safety Officer, Texas Children's Hospital

Patricia L. Stark, DSN, RN, FAAN
Dean, School of Nursing and John P. McGovern Distinguished Professor,
University of Texas Health Science Center at Houston School of Nursing

Mark A. Wallace
President and Chief Executive Officer, Texas Children's Hospital

APG
MAL
ERG

Foreword

As we near the 50th anniversary of the landmark article by C. Henry Kempe and his colleagues entitled "The Battered Child Syndrome", which ushered in the modern era of professional attention by pediatricians and other child health professionals, we have reason for both celebration and concern. We can take heart that over the recent five decades, a great deal of professional attention focused on the problem of child abuse and neglect. In every state of the country, there are mandatory reporting laws that require nurses, physicians, and social workers to report suspicions of maltreatment to the appropriate authorities for investigation. The act of reporting provides legal immunity to the reporter except when performed in bad faith. Progress in understanding the factors that place children at risk for harm from physical abuse and neglect now permits prevention and intervention. The peer-reviewed literature dealing with child abuse and neglect has proliferated with high quality work being done and reported on the many dimensions related to the epidemiology, mechanism, treatment, and prognosis of child maltreatment. Efforts are being directed toward developing an evidence-based approach to the prevention of child abuse and neglect. These are some of the positives. However, negatives exist and remain reasons for concern. Despite a tremendous amount of attention to the problem of maltreatment, there are at least 3 million reports of suspected child abuse and neglect made annually, with nearly 1 million cases being substantiated. While the incidence has been declining recently, it still remains at an unacceptable level. A single case is one too many. There is increased awareness among both the professional and lay members of our society. Underreporting continues to be a problem. There is a different standard for health professionals reporting suspected child abuse and a layperson reporting the same. The work of Jenny and colleagues documented that victims of abuse are often missed on initial evaluations by physicians. This group of patients presents on subsequent visits with more serious signs of abuse. This book represents a valuable and current resource for health professionals who can use it to guide the evaluation of children suspected of abuse or neglect.

On the international scene, there may be even more reason for concern about all forms of violence toward children, including in large part, the risk for child abuse and neglect by the child's own caregivers. In 2006, the "World Report on Violence against Children" presented to the Secretary General of the United Nations, began with: "The central message of the study is that no violence against children can be justified; all violence against children can and must be prevented. Every society, no matter its cultural, economic or social background can and must stop every form of violence. A multidimensional approach, grounded in human rights principles and guided by evidence-based research is urgently needed to prevent and respond to violence in all circumstances." Quantifying the actual number of child maltreatment victims globally is difficult because of variations in definitions from nation to nation, limited data collection efforts and the tragic realization that some forms of violence against children are socially acceptable in some parts of the world and indeed may be legal and occasionally State-sponsored.

In critical care we often provide care to child abuse victims and families who suffer from the more extreme effects of inflicted injuries. Rigorous work in the field of outcome measures determines that victims of child abuse have longer hospital length of stay, more complications and difficulties in discharge planning on average when compared to children with non-inflicted injuries. They are also more likely to be readmitted to hospitals. Each year, at least 1,500 children are known to die as a result of child abuse and neglect. Recent estimates show that 90% of the fatal cases of child abuse and neglect are in children under three years of age and more than 60% are in children under one year of age. At Texas Children's Hospital, the Chair of Pediatrics in 2004, Dr. Ralph D. Feigin, addressed the fact that more children died as a result of abuse than malignancy. Texas Children's responded by building a well-organized and strong child protection team to assist our community in evaluating suspected cases, training large numbers of health care professionals and child advocates in how best to recognize child maltreatment and then to comply with the mandated reporting responsibility. Additionally, the team has an academic component to engage in further work in our understanding of the multiplicity of aspects of this social problem.

We have traveled a long journey toward dealing with child abuse and neglect. This book represents a practical contribution to the understanding and evaluation of child maltreatment.

Houston, TX   Fernando Stein, MD
July 2009

Foreword for First Edition, 1997

The study of the condition we label child abuse and neglect is the study of all parents' struggle to raise their children and, in particular, the study of those who went wrong in some way. Parenting is a complex and sometimes frustrating role. It is a job for which there is no single charted pathway; there are many unexpected twists and turns, often few external supports, and always high societal expectation for competence. It is no wonder that some parents go astray and end up hurting their offspring rather than nurturing them. In fact, recent statistics indicate that more than 1 million children were abused or neglected in 1994, and more than 1,100 died as the result of abuse.

In 1969, as a medical student, I attended a grand rounds given at St. Christopher's Hospital for Children in Philadelphia. The speaker was Ray Helfer, MD. The topic was child abuse. Dr. Helfer described his formulation of the etiology and pathophysiology of child abuse. There were three required elements: a vulnerable child, an abuse-prone parent, and a family stressor. It was described so simply, and it was analogous to the fuel, oxygen, and spark triad of the elements of fire. It was a captivating lecture, and one that stayed with me as I left medical school and went on to pediatric residency. Dr. Helfer had passed down a parcel of information and understanding in the best tradition of the great medical educators (of which he was a part).

In my 25 years of pediatric practice since that time, I have found that simple paradigm both true and untrue. It is true at its core, and the concepts have held up over time. But the study of child abuse and neglect has proven to be so much more. It has been more complex, more intricate, and more enigmatic than I ever imagined. The parents I have met along the way have been varied beyond description, from homeless unemployed to wealthy professionals. The children have presented every imaginable form of injury, from mild cutaneous trauma to traumatic death. They have varied in age from newborns to adolescents. Their stories have been remarkable in many ways and often tragic in that they could have been avoided. The family stresses have also been many, and they also have changed over the course of time, including economic stress, substance abuse, and relationship problems. As background to the triad of abuse, there has been a societal factor: constant violence. Violence is woven through the entire cloth of our culture. Violence is so much a part of our daily lives that it is no wonder that our children are also its victims.

Throughout my career as physician and teacher, I have tried to impart an interest in and respect for the phenomenon that we recognize as child abuse. It is a study that has proven worth-while for me, and although it is not at as global a level as that of the late Dr. Helfer, I have been pleased to see some younger colleagues pick up the banner.

Such is the case of the book that follows. It is an excellent work of several young and dedicated authors who have them-selves studied child abuse and now stand ready to help others. The book stresses the recognition and initial management of child abuse. It is written clearly and succinctly. It follows a logical pattern that helps the practitioner in what is often a difficult and emotionally charged clinical situation. Although it is a compact reference, it is comprehensive and meticulous in its attention to detail. It is a book that will help the reader, just as that simple formulation of Ray Helfer's helped me so many times.

I congratulate the authors on their outstanding accomplishment and the publisher on its continued dedication to helping the helping professionals deal with the complex and challenging field of practice. All have helped children and their parents—there can be no more noble or important goal.

Philadelphia, PA   Stephen Ludwig, MD

Preface

... something I learned in 1968 when I walked into the University of Colorado School of Medicine as a pediatric intern. I learned then, from [C.] Henry Kemp, that child abuse and neglect is not just a medical problem, a social problem, or a legal problem. It is ultimately a child's and a family's problem, and solving it requires each of us in medicine, social work, law enforcement, the judiciary, mental health, and all related fields to work together for that child and family.

Krugman (1991, p. 101)

Child abuse and neglect is a major threat to the health and well-being of children throughout the world. Maltreatment has long been know to occur primarily in the family setting and is a problem firmly rooted in the pattern of caregiving provided to the child (Ludwig & Rostain, 1992). Historical review and cultural studies indicate that caregivers have maltreated children in all cultures and nations of origin (Hobbs, Hanks, & Wynne, 1993; Korbin, 1987; Lazoritz, 1992; Levinson, 1989; Radbill, 1987; Solomon, 1973). Over the past decade, we have seen growth of the child protection movement, a steady increase in the professional literature dealing with child abuse and neglect, increased public awareness of the issues surrounding child maltreatment, and the promulgation and enactment of model legislation. Despite a greater focus on the issues of abuse, child abuse and neglect remain a major problem facing children and families today (CM, 2008).

The revised manual, *A Practical Guide to the Evaluation of Child Physical Abuse and Neglect (2nd edition),* is intended as an updated resource for health care professionals. Many of the new photographs that have been included in this revision came from the teaching archive at Texas Children's Hospital and we recognize the dedication and commitment of medical photographer, Jim deLeon, who tirelessly sought to serve children and families during his quarter century of service at the hospital. It is the purpose of the text to help increase knowledge of abuse and provide easy access to basic information concerning the health care evaluation of a child suspected of having been physically abused or neglected. The manual provides a framework from which to comprehensively evaluate the child and draws upon the most up to date literature for the available evidence to support best practices. The intended audience for the manual includes health care providers and related professionals who work with abused children, including physicians, nurses, nurse practitioners, clinical social workers, mental health professionals, and child protection workers. Law enforcement personnel and attorneys may use the manual as a resource when working with children and families. The text provides practical information with a balance between the areas of content and the comprehensiveness of material included. The authors include clinically relevant information to guide the initial interview, examination, and the ac-curate documentation of the evaluation of a child who may have been physically maltreated. Toward that end, the ultimate goal of this manual is to assist the professional in performing and documenting a complete and accurate evaluation.

The text uses the terms *health care professional* and *health care provider* interchangeably in recognition that many disciplines provide care to abused and neglected children and their families. The term *parenting* is often subsumed in the term *caregiving* to indicate the practices and actions to which the child is subject.

. . .a short historical reflection on professional attention to child abuse and neglect:

In undertaking the revision process to produce the second edition, we had the opportunity to reflect upon the professional journey that our field has been traveling upon. This is most clearly illustrated by the trajectory of our peer-reviewed literature regarding child abuse and neglect.

Although child abuse is as old as recorded history, it has become an issue for pediatricians only in the mid-20th century. John Caffey first described the association between subdural hemorrhage and long bone fractures in 1946 (Caffey, 1946). He recognized that both were traumatic in origin but did not recognize the causal mechanism. Caffey thought that trauma leading to these injuries was either unobserved or denied because of negligence. In one reported case, Caffey (1946) raised the possibility of inflicted trauma but stated that the "evidence was inadequate to prove or disprove [intentional mistreatment]" (p. 172). In the early 1950s, Frederic Silverman (1953) emphasized the repeated, inflicted nature of the trauma, despite denial by caregivers. Subsequent medical literature contained reports of abuse, but little attention was given to the issue. It was not until C. Henry Kempe and his colleagues coined the term "battered child" in 1962 that the medical and legal communities took action (Kempe, Silverman, Steele, Droegemueller, & Silver, 1962).

Within a few years, most states in the US had adopted abuse-reporting statutes (Heins, 1984). By 1967, all fifty states had some form of legislation regarding child maltreatment (Fontana & Besharov, 1979; Heins, 1984). Legislative efforts culminated in a 1974 federal statute called the Child Abuse Prevention and Treatment Act (PL 93-247). This law focused national concern on the prevention, diagnosis, and treatment of child abuse. Model legislation was part of this effort, and states were encouraged to evaluate their statutes and adequately address the issues of child abuse and neglect.

Of historical interest, Kempe first used the term battered child in a 1961 address to the American Academy of Pediatrics to describe young children who were victims of serious physical abuse. Subsequently, he and his colleagues published a study by the same name in 1962 (Heins, 1984; Kempe et al., 1962). The first description was of children generally younger than 3 years old, often with evidence of malnutrition and multiple soft tissue injuries. Subdural hemorrhages and multiple fractures were commonly found. Kempe et al. (1962) also included children with less severe or isolated injuries in their description of the battered child. Although any child with an inflicted injury has been battered, the term battered child is typically used to describe a child with repeated injuries to multiple organ systems. Health care providers who treat children should be able to identify those who are severely abused and injured and should know how to respond accordingly as well.

Fontana, Donovan, and Wong (1963) extended the early conceptualization of child abuse to include forms beyond physical injury by introducing the term maltreatment syndrome. Maltreatment included both battered children and children who were poorly fed and inadequately supervised. Fontana et al. (1963) added neglect to the evolving description of child abuse.

The original articles by Caffey (1946), Silverman (1953), Kempe et al. (1962), and Fontana et al. (1963) provide the modern medical history of child abuse. Their insight and persistence set the stage for the recognition of child abuse as a pediatric problem and resulted in an outpouring of medical, social, and psychological literature dealing with abuse and neglect.

Thirty years after the Kempe et al. (1962) article, Dr. Richard Krugman (1992), then the director of the C. Henry Kempe National Center for Prevention of Child Abuse and Neglect, observed how far the child protection movement had come in a short time. He compared the 1962 figure of 447 reported victims of battering to the 1991 estimate of 2.7 million reports of abuse (Krugman, 1992). Krugman stressed the staggering disparity between 447 cases and 2.7 million reports, even if not all reports of abuse result in a determination of maltreatment. In addition, Krugman (1992) observed that the 1991 estimate of 2.7 million reports of abuse did not account for the number of unreported cases that were either not suspected, misdiagnosed, or simply not reported. Figure 1 shows the exponential growth of the professional literature moving from occasional articles to and evidence base of hundreds and now thousands of peer-reviewed articles currently available.

Child abuse and neglect is now regarded as a public health problem throughout the globe. It is recognized as part of continuum of violence and victimization against the vulnerable that includes other forms of family violence as well. Paolo Sergio Pinheiro in his August, 2006 report to the UN General Secretary made clear that there can be no compromise in challenging violence against children: "Children's uniqueness—their potential and vulnerability, their dependence on adults—makes it imperative that they have more, not less, protection from violence." (The United Nations Secretary General's Study on Violence Against Children, 2006, p. 5)

It is the responsibility of the health care professional to conduct the health care evaluation of the child suspected of having been abused or neglected, to consider a broad differential diagnosis, and to accurately identify the child's condition based

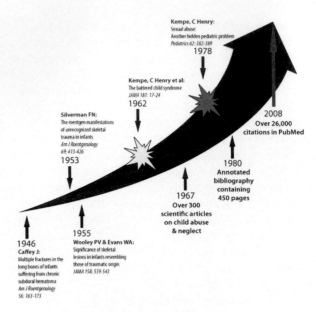

on the information available. Working in the context of a multidisciplinary team, the health care provider then participates in the investigation and works to ensure proper medical and community action involves treating the child's existing injuries and ensuring protection from future injury.

... how the the book is organized:

The manual is organized into four main sections, as follows. Part I contains Chapters 1 and 2 which provide an overview on the phenomenon of child abuse and neglect and offer a general approach to the evaluation of the maltreated child. The need for a systematic and comprehensive approach in the evaluation of suspected child maltreatment cases is highlighted. In addition, the authors support an interdisciplinary evaluation to enhance attention to both physical and psychosocial aspects and to facilitate the development of comprehensive treatment plans that build upon each discipline's different skills and perspectives.

Part II, composed of Chapters 3, 4, 5, 6, 7, 8, and 9 address specific forms of maltreatment such as skin injury, abusive head trauma and neglect. Each of these chapters addresses mechanisms of the specific type of injury, characteristic findings, clinical approach, differential diagnosis, and proposed treatments where applicable. Some information is repeated in several chapters to allow for those providers who may need to use a specific chapter as a reference when working with a child with a given symptom or finding. When more detailed information is available in a related chapter, the reader is referred there as well. In addition, Chapter 9 concludes with current information on the evaluation of child fatalities including information on the postmortem examination.

Part III, includes Chapters 10, 11 and 12 and addresses the relationship of child maltreatment to children with special needs, the overlap of intimate partner violence with child maltreatment and on approaches to the prevention of child abuse and neglect. Finally, Part IV comprised of Chapters 13, 14, 15, and 16 covers a number of the issues related to the teamwork so essential to the evaluation and investigation of child abuse and neglect. Overarching team issues as well as specifics related to psychosocial assessment and interaction with the child protection system are addressed as well as, legal issues, and the important interface with mental health professionals that may occur in cases of suspected and substantiated abuse and neglect. These chapters are intended to give more detail regarding these critically important issues.

In conclusion, this manual is written to assist the health care provider in performing a systematic evaluation of the child suspected of abuse or neglect. It is our hope that as the clinician develops greater expertise in the evaluation of the maltreated child, he or she will recognize patterns suggestive of physical abuse and neglect more easily, be better able to complete the appropriate medical and psychosocial evaluations of the child, and become more cognizant of the ultimate responsibility to work with other professionals and agencies to ensure the safety and recovery of the victimized child. We believe that the needs of the child and family are best served by knowledgeable health care professionals who clearly understand their role as health care provider and child advocate. We agree with Dr. Krugman that in the final analysis, child abuse and neglect is a "child's and a family's" problem and we hope that this book helps health care professionals assist children and families as they confront this challenge.

Houston, TX

Angelo P. Giardino, MD, PhD, MPH
Michelle A. Lyn, MD
Eileen R. Giardino, RN, PhD, FNP-BC

References

Caffey, J. (1946). Multiple fractures in the long bones of infants suffering from chronic subdural hematoma. *American Journal of Roentgenology, 56*, 163–173.

Fontana, V. J., & Besharov, D. J. (1979). The maltreated child: The maltreatment syndrome in children—a medical, legal, and social guide (4th ed.). Springfield, IL: Charles C Thomas.

Fontana, V. J., Donovan, D., & Wong, R. J. (1963). The maltreatment syndrome in children. *New England Journal of Medicine, 269*, 1389–1394.

Heins, M. (1984). The battered child revisited. *Journal of the American Medical Association, 251*, 3295–3300.

Hobbs, C. J., Hanks, H. G. I., & Wynne, J. M. (1993). *Child abuse and neglect: A clinician's handbook.* New York: Churchill Livingstone.

Kempe, R. S., Silverman, F. N., Steele, B. F., Droegmueller, W., & Silver, H. K. (1962). The battered child syndrome. *Journal of the American Medical Association, 181*, 17–24.

Korbin, J. E. (1987). Child abuse and neglect: The cultural context. In R. E. Helfer & R. S. Kempe (Eds.), *The battered child* (4th ed., pp. 23–41). Chicago: University of Chicago Press.

Krugman, R. D. (1991). Closing remarks. In R. D. Krugman & J. M. Leventhal (Eds.), *Child sexual abuse: The twenty-second Ross roundtable on critical approaches to common pediatric problems* (pp. 100–101). Columbus, OH: Ross Laboratories.

Krugman, R. D. (1992). Commentary on child abuse and neglect. *Pediatric Annals, 21*, 475–476.

Lazoritz, S. (1992). Child abuse: An historical perspective. In S. Ludwig & A. E. Kornberg (Eds.), *Child abuse: A medical reference* (2nd ed., pp. 85–90). New York: Churchill Livingstone

Levinson, D. (1989). *Family violence in cross-cultural perspective* (Vol. 1). Newbury Park, CA: Sage.

Ludwig, S., & Rostain, A. (1992). Family function and dysfunction. In M. D. Levine, W. B.
Carey, & A. C. Crocker (Eds.), *Developmental behavioral pediatrics* (2nd ed., pp. 147–159). Philadelphia, PA: W. B. Saunders

Radbill, S. X. (1987). Children in a world of violence: A history of child abuse. In R. E. Helfer & R. S. Kempe (Eds.), *The battered child* (4th ed., pp. 3–22). Chicago: University of Chicago Press.

Silverman, F. N. (1953). The roentgen manifestations of unrecognized skeletal trauma in infants. *American Journal of Roentgenology, 69*, 413–426.

Solomon, T. (1973). History and demography of child abuse. *Pediatrics, 51*, 773–776.

The United Nations Secretary General's Study on Violence Against Children (2006) http://www.violencestudy.org/IMG/pdf/English.pdf

US Department of Health and Human Services. Administration on Children, Youth and Families (2008) Child Maltreatment 2006. Washington, DC: US Government Printing Office.

Authors' Note

Every effort has been made to ensure that information concerning the recommended ordering of laboratory and diagnostic tests, the interpretation of laboratory values, and suggested drug dosages and usages stated in this manual are accurate and conform to the accepted standards at the time of publication. However, the reader is advised to consult printed information on each test or drug prior to ordering a study or administering any medication, especially when ordering unfamiliar tests or using infrequently used drugs.

Contents

Author Biographies

Eleanor J. Ashford, BA, received her Bachelor's degree in Journalism and Communications from Creighton University. She studied journalism abroad at New York University in London and then received her Masters in Global Communications from the American University of Paris.

Tal Ben-Galim, MD, is an Israeli board certified pediatrician and currently doing her second year of fellowship in Academic General Pediatrics in Baylor College of Medicine.

She was born and raised in Israel. After completing her military service as medical instructor she turned to medicine studies in Hadassah medical school in Jerusalem. She did her internship and residency in pediatrics in Sheba medical center, and practiced for over two years in two private practices after her graduation. In 2005, Dr Ben-Galim moved to US with her family. She started her fellowship in Academic General Pediatrics in July 2007. Dr Ben-Galim is in her second year of studies for Master in Public Health in University of Texas as part of her fellowship and taking Health Promotion as her major.

Her main interest is pediatric nutrition including childhood obesity and Failure to Thrive, and she intends to complete her thesis in this area.

Kelli Connell-Carrick, PhD, MSW, is an Assistant Professor at the University of Houston Graduate College of Social Work. Dr. Connell-Carrick has devoted her career to the children and families affected by child maltreatment. She has over 60 competitively selected publications and presentations in the areas of child maltreatment, neglect of infants and toddlers, substance abuse, foster care and aging out, and professional development of child welfare staff. She has also co-authored a two books, *Understanding Child Maltreatment: An Ecological and Developmental Perspective* published by Oxford University Press (with M. Scannapieco) and *Methamphetamine: What You Need to Know* (with Sallee, Liebe, Myers and Sallee) published by Eddie Bowers in 2007. She is published in such journal as *Child Welfare,*

Child and Adolescent Social Work, and *The Journal of Interpersonal Violence.* Dr. Connell-Carrick was the PI on a large federal grant from 2005 to 2008 that involved developing, delivering, evaluating and disseminating a training curriculum to CPS supervisors throughout the state of Texas on the needs of youth aging out of foster care. In 2004, Dr. Connell-Carrick won the Humanitate Award for Outstanding Literary Achievement from the North American Resource Center for Child Welfare. She is a faculty associate of the Office of Community Projects at the University of Houston Graduate College of Social Work and the University of Texas at Arlington Center for Child Welfare, and is involved in a statewide evaluation of retention and job training of CPS and adult protection workers.

Allan DeJong, MD, Clinical Professor of Pediatrics at Jefferson Medical College, has been managing suspected child physical and sexual abuse cases for over 30 years. He became the Director of the CARE Program (Child At Risk Evaluation) at the Nemours—Alfred I. duPont Hospital for Children in Wilmington, Delaware in 1994. Dr De Jong has been the Medical Director for the Children's Advocacy Center of Delaware (CACD) since it opened in 1996, and helped establish CACD sites in each of Delaware's three counties by 2003. Over the past twelve years these positions have evolved into a full time clinical practice for the evaluation of suspected abuse cases from Delaware, southeastern Pennsylvania, southwestern New Jersey and northeastern Maryland. Dr. De Jong has 32 publications in the field of child abuse. He is a member of the Ray Helfer Society, the Pennsylvania Attorney General's Medical/Legal Advisory Board for Child Abuse, and the Delaware Child Protection Accountability Commission.

Erin E. Endom, MD, is an Assistant Professor in the Department of Pediatrics, Baylor College of Medicine, and is a member of the section of Pediatric Emergency Medicine. In addition to her other clinical and academic responsibilities, Dr. Endom serves as an attending physician in the busy Texas Children's Hospital Emergency Center, where approximately 80,000 children are seen and cared for annually.

Dr. Endom received her M.D. degree in 1988 from the University of Texas Medical School in Houston, Texas and subsequently completed a 3-year pediatric residency in 1991 from Baylor College of Medicine affiliated hospitals. She is a subboard-certified pediatric emergency physician.

Her special interests include child abuse and neglect, and emergency and disaster preparedness. From 1998 to 2007, she served as the Pediatric Emergency Medicine section editor for the online medical textbook UpToDate (www.uptodate.com).

Angelo P. Giardino, MD, PhD, MPH, is the medical director of Texas Children's Health Plan, a clinical associate professor of pediatrics at Baylor College of Medicine, and an attending physician on both the Texas Children's Hospital Child Protection Team and the forensic pediatrics service at the Children's Assessment Center in Houston, Texas. In addition, Dr. Giardino serves as the physician advisor to the Texas Children's Hospital Center for Childhood Injury Prevention. Dr. Giardino earned his MD and PhD at the University of Pennsylvania and his MPH from the University of Massachusetts. Dr. Giardino completed his pediatric residency and child maltreatment fellowship training at The Children's Hospital of Philadelphia (CHOP) and also completed training in secondary data analysis related to child maltreatment from the National Data Archive on Child Abuse and Neglect's Summer Research Institute at Cornell University.

Dr. Giardino's clinical work focuses on child maltreatment and in 1995 he collaborated with a multidisciplinary team to develop and lead the Abuse Referral Center for Children with Special Health Care Needs at the Children's Seashore House which was funded by a 3-year grant from a local philanthropy in Philadelphia. This program was designed to provide medical evaluations to children with developmental disabilities who were suspected of having been abused or neglected. In 1998, he was appointed associate chair for clinical operations in the Department of Pediatrics at CHOP and also served on the hospital's child abuse evaluation service. In 2002, Dr. Giardino joined the Department of Pediatrics at Drexel College of Medicine as the associate chair for clinical affairs and was appointed associate physician-in-chief at St. Christopher's Hospital for Children where he also served as the medical director for the hospital's Suspected Child Abuse and Neglect program. This program collaborated with the Institute for Safe Families and Lutheran Settlement House to secure a Pennsylvania Children's Trust Fund grant which supported a community-based Intimate Partner Violence Screening program at St. Christopher's aimed at identifying at risk families and working to prevent child maltreatment. Additionally, while at St. Christopher's, Dr. Giardino collaborated with colleagues at the Drexel University School of Public Health to launch the Philadelphia Grow Project which provided clinical care to children with the diagnosis of Failure to Thrive and which also conducted policy research on the issues surrounding food insecurity and childhood hunger. Dr. Giardino is board certified in pediatrics, is a fellow of the American Academy of Pediatrics, and a member of both the Texas Pediatric Society, and the Harris County Medical Society. He is a member of the Helfer Society, the American College of Physician Executives, and the American College of Medical Quality. Dr. Giardino is a certified physician executive and is also certified in medical quality. Prior to relocating to Houston, Dr. Giardino served as chair of the Philadelphia Branch Board of the Southeastern Chapter of the American Red Cross, president of the board for Bethany Christian Services in Fort Washington, PA, and a two term member of the board for the Support Center for Child Advocates, where he was named a 2005 Champion for Children. His academic accomplishments include publishing articles and several textbooks on child abuse and neglect, contributing to several national curricula on the evaluation of child maltreatment, presenting on a variety of pediatric topics at both national and regional conferences, and, most recently, he completed a three-year term on the National Review Board (NRB) for the US Conference of Catholic Bishops, providing advice on how best to protect children from sexual abuse. While on the NRB, Dr. Giardino served as the chair for its Research Committee. Currently, Dr. Giardino serves on the national board of directors for Justice for Children (an advocacy organization providing assistance for children and families involved with the Court system around issues related to child abuse and neglect), the national advisory board for the Institute for Safe Families (an advocacy organization that seeks to train professionals in screening and prevention around issues related to Intimate Partner Violence), and the national board of directors for Prevent Child Abuse America.

Eileen R. Giardino RN, PhD, FNP-BC, is an Associate Professor at the School of Nursing at the University of Texas Health Science Center (UTHSC) at Houston. Dr Giardino received her BSN and PhD from the University of Pennsylvania, her MSN from Widener University, and her NP certification in adult and family from LaSalle University. Clinically, Dr. Giardino works as a nurse practitioner at a university student health service. Her academic accomplishments include co-editing several text books in the areas of child maltreatment and intimate partner violence and she presents at professional meetings on issues related to physical assessment and conducting a differential diagnosis. Prior to moving to Houston, Dr. Giardino served on the board of directors for Bethany Christian Services in Fort Washington, PA, was on the advisory board for the LaSalle University Nursing Center in Philadelphia and completed two terms on the board of directors for the Philadelphia Children's Alliance where she also chaired the xxx committee. Finally, Dr. Giardino teaches on a variety of topics in the adult and family nurse practitioner tracks at UTHSC at Houston and is involved in supervising a number of clinical preceptorships within the nurse practitioner training program.

Rebecca G. Girardet, MD, was awarded a Bachelor's of Arts degree in Human Biology with honors from Stanford University in 1987 and her Doctorate of Medicine from the University of Arizona in 1992.

She completed her residency in pediatrics at Baylor College of Medicine in 1995. Dr. Girardet was in private practice and later worked as an instructor in the Baylor College of Medicine division of pediatric emergency medicine.

Dr. Girardet joined the division of community and general pediatrics at The University of Texas-Houston Medical School in 1998, where her work has focused on child maltreatment. She is a nationally recognized expert in child abuse.

Dr. Girardet has conducted several medical research projects, including clinical research funded by The Centers for Disease Control and Prevention. Dr. Girardet is Director of the UT-Child Abuse Research and Education Center, and she is the Medical Director of the Texas Forensic Assessment Center Network.

Her professional associations include: The American Academy of Pediatrics, the Pediatric Academic Societies, and the Ray Helfer Society. She is also a co-chair of the Child Abuse and Neglect Committee of the Texas Pediatric Society.

Dr. Girardet is fluent in English, French and Spanish. She is married and has 3 children.

Arne H. Graff, MD, was specialty trained in Family Medicine and subspecialty trained in Child Abuse Pediatrics, having completed the Pediatric fellowship at Hasbro Children's Hospital under the direction of Dr Carole Jenny and Dr. Christine Barron. I am currently the medical director for the Child and Adolescent Maltreatment Services Department with MeritCare Health Systems, in Fargo ND.

Dr. Graff is also the medical consultant for the Dakota Children's Advocacy Center (Bismarck ND) and the Red River Children's Advocacy Center (Fargo ND).

As an Clinical Associate Professor of Pediatrics, for the University of North Dakota School of Medicine, he is involved in the teaching of medical students and residents. He is also on the APSAC board of directors.

Christopher S. Greeley, MD, was received his undergraduate degree from Hobart College in Geneva New York where he majored in Biology and Religious Studies. He received his medical degree from the University of Virginia in 1992 and complete internship and residency in pediatrics at Vanderbilt University. He spent three years in private pediatric practice in Franklin Tennessee before returning to Vanderbilt University in the Division of General Pediatrics in 1998. In 2007, Dr. Greeley moved to the University of Texas Health Sciences Center at Houston. He is board certified in pediatrics and is a member of the AMA and the AAP. He is a member of the AAP Section on Child Abuse and Neglect and Section on International Child Health.

Dr. Greeley was the 2006 Ray E Helfer Award winner. The Ray E Helfer Award is an annual award jointly presented by The American Academy of Pediatrics and The National Alliance of Children's Trust and Prevention Funds "to a distinguished pediatrician for his or her contribution to the prevention of child abuse and neglect."

Dr. Greeley currently is Vice Chair for Academic Affairs in the Department of Pediatrics at the University of Texas health Sciences Center at Houston. He is Associate Professor of Pediatrics in the Division of Community and General Pediatrics.

He is also on the national Board of Director for Prevent Child Abuse America. He is the Chair of the Prevent Child Abuse America's Committee on Research and was the chair of the ad hoc Committee on Healthy Families America.

Dr. Greeley has published on various areas of child abuse and is on the editorial board for The Quarterly Update, a prominent child abuse publication. He has written book chapters on Child Abuse Prevention as well as Mimics of Child Abuse. He is also a contributing editor for the AAP publication, Grand Rounds.

Pamela W. Hammel, DDS, DABFO, is a Board Certified Forensic Odontologist, and is the Forensic Dental Consultant to Children's Hospital of Michigan, Detroit, Michigan, and a consultant to the Macomb and Oakland County Medical Examiner's offices. She was also a consultant to Wayne County Medical Examiner's Office from 1985 to 2000, and is an advisor to the Medical Advisory Board to the state of Michigan's Family Independence Agency. She served on the Michigan State Board of Dentistry from 1992 to 2000, and has been Assistant Team Leader to the Michigan Forensic Dental Identification Team since its inception in 1985. She has participated in three aviation disasters, the World Trade Center Identification Unit in New York, 2001, and Hurricanes Katrina and Rita in New Orleans, 2005

Dr. Hammel also is a member of DMORT (Disaster Mortuary Operational Response Team) and NDMS (National Disaster Medical System.) She has served on the Board of Trustees to the American Society of Forensic Odontology (1991–1994), and the Board of Directors to the American Board of Forensic Odontology, 2001–2006. She was elected to Program Chair for the Odontology Section of the American Academy of Forensic Sciences 1998–2000, to Section Secretary 2000–2002, and to Section Chair 2002–2004.

Her publications include Journal of the Michigan Dental Association (cover story), "The Dentist's Role in Recognizing Domestic Violence", April/May 1995; Archives of Pediatric and Adolescent Medicine (cover story) "Human Bite Marks" April, 1996; New England Journal of Medicine "Human Bites versus Dog Bites", September, 2003. She was a member of the policy planning committee of the American Dental Association to explore "Does Dentistry Have a Role in the Event of a Bioterrorist Attack?" June, 2002.

Dr. Hammel is a Fellow of the American Academy of Forensic Sciences, a Fellow of American College of Dentists, a Fellow of the International College of Dentists, and a Fellow of the Pierre Fauchard Academy.

Nancy S. Harper, MD, is the Medical Director for the CARE (Child Abuse Resource & Evaluation) Team at Driscoll Children's Hospital in Corpus Christi, TX. She graduated from Dartmouth Medical School in 1995, and completed her pediatric residency in 1998 at Naval Medical Center Portsmouth in Virginia. After graduation, Dr. Harper served as a staff pediatrician and Child Abuse Consultant for Naval Medical Center Portsmouth, and then moved overseas to US Naval Hospital Okinawa in Japan where she continued as a Child Abuse Consultant and chair of the medical staff. In 2004, Dr. Harper resigned from the US Navy and entered into fellowship training in Forensic Pediatrics at Brown University in RI, graduating in January 2007. Dr. Harper serves as a consultant on the medical advisory committee for Superior Health Plan for foster care. Special interests include the proper use and interpretation of skeletal surveys and urine drug screens as well as drug-facilitated sexual assault.

Toi B. Harris, MD, received her undergraduate and graduate degrees from the University of Missouri-Kansas City. She completed her Psychiatry Residency and Child and Adolescent Psychiatry Fellowship at Baylor College of Medicine (BCM). Since 2005, Dr. Harris has been on the faculty at BCM and served as the director of the child psychiatry consultation and liaison service at Texas Children's Hospital.

She has received national awards from the American Psychiatric Association (APA) and the American Medical Association (AMA) and been an active member on committees such as the APA's National Committee of Family Violence and Sexual Abuse, APA's corresponding committee for poverty and homelessness, a board member of the All Healers Mental Health Alliance.

In addition to her academic interests and responsibilities, Dr. Harris is the community liaison of Missouri City Baptist Church's Total Person Ministry. This group provides community-based psychoeducational programs targeting the areas of grief, loss, trauma and gang-prevention.

Reena Isaac, MD, is a child abuse pediatrician with the Child Protection Section of the Emergency Center of Texas Children's Hospital in Houston, TX. She is an Assistant Professor of Pediatrics at Baylor College of Medicine. Dr. Isaac completed her pediatrics training at Jacobi Medical Center in New York City and a forensic pediatrics fellowship at Brown Medical Center in Providence, RI. At Texas Children's Hospital in Houston, Texas, she assists in the Child Protection medical consultation service in identifying, evaluating, and diagnosing suspected child Mal-treatment cases. She is also staff physician at the Children's Assessment Center's medical clinic. She has conducted numerous medical investigations involving sus-pected medical child abuse and has testified in both family and criminal court in such cases.

John F. Knutson, PhD, is a professor of psychology at the University of Iowa. He received his PhD in Clinical Psychology from Washington State University. After completing a post-doctoral fellowship in Medical Psychology at the University of Oregon Medical School, he joined the faculty at Iowa. He has held editorial posi-tions at the Journal of Abnormal Psychology and the Journal of Clinical Psychology. He is a fellow of the American Psychological Association and the American Psy-chological Society. He has had more than 100 journal articles published and book chapters on aggression, physical child abuse, neglect, the association between abuse and disabilities, cochlear implants and methodology pertaining to the assessment of child maltreatment.

Penelope T. Louis, MD, is a pediatrician in Houston, Texas. She is part of the Academic Service at Texas Children's Hospital (TCH) and is board certified by the American Board of Pediatrics and a member of the American College of Emer-gency Physicians, the American Academy of Pediatrics and the Society of Criti-cal Care Medicine. She is an Associate Professor Pediatrics in Academic General Medicine at Baylor College of Medicine (BCM) in Houston. Her specialties are pediatric critical care, pediatric emergency medicine, and physical medicine and rehabilitation. In addition to being in clinical practice, Dr. Louis' academic work includes co-authoring journal articles on pediatric care with a number of colleagues from BCM/TCH/

Michelle A. Lyn, MD, is an Associate Professor of Pediatrics at Baylor College of Medicine, Chief of Child Protection Section of Emergency Medicine at Texas Chil-dren's Hospital and serves as the Medical Director of The Children's Assessment Center. Dr. Lyn earned her M.D. degree from State University of New York at Buf-falo School of Medicine, completed her residency in Pediatrics at Albert Einstein College of Medicine-Montefiore Medical Center in Bronx, New York, where she served as the Pediatric Chief Resident as well as completed a fellowship in Pediatric Emergency Medicine at Baylor College of Medicine in Houston, Texas. Her aca-demic, clinical, research and community outreach work focuses largely on children in crisis. She teaches medical students, interns, residents and fellows of emergency medicine and family practice about child maltreatment and she educates community medical professionals, teachers, law enforcement officers, military personnel and first responders through SCAN (Suspect Child Abuse & Neglect) community out-reach program. Dr. Lyn is a board certified pediatrician who is also certified in pedi-atric emergency medicine. She is a fellow of the American Academy of Pediatrics. Her community board memberships include St. Luke's Episcopal Health Charities and Healthy Family Initiatives, both in Houston Texas. She has presented numer-ous lectures, television, and radio appearances on topics of pediatric and adolescent physical and sexual abuse. Dr. Lyn's work to help children in crisis and to teach medical professionals about the field of child maltreatment and pediatric emergency medicine has been recognized by her receiving Baylor College of Medicine's (BCM) Department of Pediatrics Award of General Excellence in Teaching as well as BCM's Fulbright and Jaworski Excellence Teaching award. Additionally, community recognition has manifested itself as the Texas Executive Women's Women on the Move honoree, Martin Luther King Foundation's Keeping the Dream Alive recipient and the Wesleyan College Alumni Recognition award. Prior to leading the Child Protection Team at Texas Children's Hospital, Dr. Lyn served as the Medical Director for the Pediatric Emergency Medicine at Ben Taub General Hospital in Houston which is dedicated to serving the under and uninsured population in Harris County Texas.

Maria D. McColgan, MD, is a board certified Pediatrician and the Director of the Child Protection Program at St. Christopher's Hospital for Children. After graduating from Temple University College of Medicine, Dr. McColgan completed her pediatric residency at St. Christopher's Hospital for Children in June 2003, where she then practiced as an Urgent Care Physician in the Emergency Department. Currently, in addition to her work as the Director of the Child Protection Program, Dr. McColgan is the site director for the Pediatric Clerkship at Drexel University. Dr. McColgan completed the Pennsylvania Chapter of the American Academy of Pediatrics Preceptorship in Child Abuse and the Michigan State University Primary Care Development Fellowship. Dr. McColgan developed a child abuse curriculum for pediatric residents, as well as a successful domestic violence screening project in the pediatric setting.

Donna Mendez, MD, is a board certified Pediatrician as well as Pediatric Emergency Medicine physician. She completed her pediatric residency at University of Texas Health Science Center in Houston, and a fellowship in Pediatric Emergency Medicine at University of Texas Southwestern. She is currently an attending at Baylor College of Medicine/Texas Children's Hospital Emergency Department and is a member of the Texas Children's Hospital Child Protection Team. Her research focus is on head injury. Dr. Mendez is currently investigating retinal hemorrhages in children suspected of having abusive head injury. Dr. Mendez is a co-investigator on two NIH studies looking at neuropsychological outcomes in children who have sustained head injury. Dr. Mendez is also involved in 3 research projects involving physical abuse in children, in which she is the principal investigator.

Vincent J. Palusci, MD, MS, graduated with honors in Chemistry from the University of Pennsylvania. He received his medical degree from the University of Medicine and Dentistry of New Jersey and completed his internship and residency in pediatrics at New York University/Bellevue Hospital Center in New York. He entered private practice and later joined the faculty of the College of Human Medicine at Michigan State University where he was also a TRECOS scholar and earned a M.S. in Epidemiology. He recently returned to NYU School of Medicine and Bellevue Hospital's Frances L. Loeb Child Protection and Development Center.

Dr. Palusci's work has focused on epidemiologic and health services issues for child abuse victims, and the educational needs of general and specialist pediatricians. He received the Ray E. Helfer Award for child abuse prevention in 2004. He has edited *Shaken Baby Syndrome: A Multidisciplinary Response* with Dr. Steven Lazoritz and *A Colour Atlas of Child Abuse and Neglect*, due out in 2009.

Thomas A. Roesler, MD, is associate professor of psychiatry and human behavior at Warren Alpert Medical School at Brown University and co-director of the Hasbro Children's Hospital Partial Hospital Program for children with both medical and emotional illness. He received his undergraduate degree in Philosophy from Whitman College and a medical degree from the University of Washington School of Medicine. He completed training in psychiatry and child psychiatry at the Hospital of the University of Pennsylvania and Philadelphia Child Guidance Clinic. His research interests include the psychological effects of childhood sexual abuse, medical child abuse, and the delivery of medical and psychiatric services in a collaborative day hospital environment. He recently published, along with his co-author, Carole Jenny, MD, MBA, a book entitled "Medical Child Abuse: Beyond Munchausen Syndrome by Proxy."

Albert J. Sargent, MD, is the Director of Child and Adolescent Psychiatry at Tufts Medical Center and Professor of Psychiatry and Pediatrics at Tufts University School of Medicine. Prior to assuming that position he was Professor of Psychiatry and Pediatrics at the Baylor College of Medicine and Director of Child and Adolescent Psychiatry at Ben Taub General Hospital in Houston, Texas. He also served as the Clinical Director of the System of Hope, a community system of care for seriously emotionally disturbed children in Houston. He is currently a member of the Massachusetts Children's Behavioral Health Advisory Council which is responsible for monitoring and improving children's behavioral health throughout the state. He has experience in all aspects of clinical child and adolescent psychiatry and special interest in developing clinical systems of care for poor and underserved children and adolescents with mental health problems. His other special interests include child and family responses to trauma and violence, eating disorders, adolescent suicide, family therapy and international child mental health program development. He has published over 70 articles and books on these topics. Dr. Sargent is a nationally known family therapist and has training and certification in general psychiatry, child and adolescent psychiatry and pediatrics. Dr. Sargent is also President of the American Family Therapy Academy. Before joining the Baylor College of Medicine faculty in 2001, Dr. Sargent had been Director of Education and Research at the Menninger Clinic in Topeka, Kansas and previously was Director of General and Child and Adolescent Psychiatry Training at the University of Pennsylvania in Philadelphia, Pennsylvania. He also has served as Deputy Director of the Eastern European Child Abuse and Child Mental Health Project and has extensive experience in training mental health professionals throughout the world.

Maria Scannapieco, PhD, MSW, is Professor at the School of Social Work, University of Texas at Arlington and Director of the Center for Child Welfare. She is the

Director of Certification for the Texas Protective Services Institute, which certifies all Texas Department of Family and Protective Services workers and supervisors across all for programs; child protective services, adult protective services, child care licensing, and statewide intake. The certification program covers more than 4,000 state employees.

Dr. Maria Scannapieco has worked in the public child welfare arena for over 25 years as an educator and researcher, with direct child protection and foster care administrative experience. She has received over a million dollars a year since 1996 from state and federal grants for training programs and research. She has extensive experience in grant development, implementation, management, and dissemination. As PI on a current Children's Bureau grant on curriculum development for CPS Supervisors on issues concerning youth aging out of foster care, Dr. Scannapieco has successfully managed the development, delivery, evaluation, and dissemination of a statewide training initiative.

Dr. Scannapieco has over 100 publications and presentations competitively selected many in the areas of child maltreatment, out-of-home placement, preparation for adult living programs, and training and retention of child welfare workers. She has been published in such professional journals as *Child Welfare, Social Service Review, Children and Youth Services Review*, and *Social Work*. Dr. Maria Scannapieco has two books with Oxford University Press, the first titled (with Rebecca L. Hegar) *Kinship Foster Care: Practice, Policy, & Research (1999)*, and another with *Understanding Child Maltreatment: An Ecological and Developmental Perspective (2005) (with Kelli Connell-Carrick).*

Carl J. Schmidt, MD, MPH, grew up in Latin America where he graduated from medical school at the Universidad Anahuac. After 2 years of general surgery training and 2 years of graduate school in neurobiology, he trained in pathology at the Medical College of Ohio in Toledo, Ohio, now the University of Toledo Medical Center. He did his fellowship in forensic pathology at the Wayne County Medical Examiner's Office in Detroit, where he became the Chief Medical Examiner in 2003. His main interests are pediatric trauma, forensic toxicology and the neurobiology of addiction. He is Clinical Assistant Professor in the Department of Pathology at the Wayne State University School of Medicine. He has participated in a program sponsored by the U.S. Department of Justice since 1998 that provides assistance for forensic issues in Latin America.

Philip V. Scribano, DO, MSCE, graduated from Rutgers University, and The University of Medicine and Dentistry of New Jersey–School of Osteopathic Medicine. He also received a Master of Science degree in Clinical Epidemiology at the University of Pennsylvania.

He is the Medical Director of the Center for Child and Family Advocacy at Nationwide Children's Hospital, Chief of the Division of Child and Family Advocacy, and Associate Professor of Pediatrics at The Ohio State University College of Medicine. He is the recipient of multiple research and program grants including awards from the Administration on Children and Families, Agency for Healthcare Research and Quality, and the Centers for Disease Control.

He is active with the American Academy of Pediatrics, and is chair of the Ohio AAP Committee on Child Abuse and Neglect. He is a board member of the Academy on Violence and Abuse, and co-chair of the Helfer Society's Fellowship Program Directors Committee.

Rohit Shenoi, MD, is an assistant professor of pediatrics at the Baylor College of Medicine, Houston and an attending physician in the emergency center at Texas Children's Hospital, Houston.

Dr Shenoi is also the coordinator of Houston Trauma Link, a coalition formed in 2000 to reduce the morbidity and mortality of childhood injuries in Houston/Harris County, Texas. The coalition comprises entities from the public and private health sectors, City and County Health Departments, Texas Department of Transportation, educational institutions, City Police, Fire and EMS, Houston Independent School District and the Regional Poison Control Center. The coalition integrates existing data sources to provide a local pediatric injury data system that supports injury prevention and control activities of the community.

Patricia M. Sullivan, PhD, is a licensed psychologist who obtained her Ph.D. degree in pediatric psychology from the University of Iowa. Dr. Sullivan is a Professor of Psychiatry and Psychology at Creighton University. She has extensive experience with children and families and has conducted several forensic evaluations for use in both district court and juvenile court proceedings. She has provided numerous presentations to guardians ad litem, county attorneys and to juvenile, county and district court judges on psychological evaluations. She is an NIH funded researcher and currently involved in the study of the long-term effects of violence exposure, including child abuse, domestic and community violence, in childhood.

Suzanna Tiapula, JD, is the Director of the National District Attorneys Association's National Center for Prosecution of Child Abuse. Ms. Tiapula manages the Center's outreach to 2,400 prosecutor's offices, approximately 37,000 prosecutors and thousands of allied child abuse professionals. Ms. Tiapula trains child abuse professionals across the country on a range of child maltreatment issues. In 2004/2005 Ms. Tiapula coordinated the development of two advanced trial advocacy courses for prosecution of online crimes against children (Unsafe Havens I and II) as part of NCPCA's Child Sexual Exploitation program. Ms. Tiapula has also developed materials and authored publications on a range of child maltreatment issues.

Ms. Tiapula began her legal career as a deputy prosecuting attorney for the City and County of Honolulu. As an Assistant Attorney General in American Samoa (1999–2001), Ms. Tiapula was responsible for all family violence, sexual assaults and institutional violence cases prosecuted in the territory. During this period, Ms. Tiapula worked with a criminal code that codified traditional Samoan practice. Ms. Tiapula is currently working with advocates and agency officials in American Samoa to establish a child abuse commission in Samoa and develop a regional network focusing on child protection in the south Pacific/Pacific Rim.

In addition to criminal prosecution, Ms. Tiapula has professional experience in the Pacific Rim working with diverse populations and legal systems. Early in her professional career, Ms. Tiapula developed quantitative and qualitative evaluation techniques for program evaluation in immigrant/refugee communities in Hawaii. Ms. Tiapula also studied law at the National University of Singapore's Faculty of Law and worked for a corporate law firm in Bangkok, Thailand. Ms. Tiapula has taught for Hawaii Pacific University, Chaminade University, George Mason University and Pennsylvania State University. As Associate Director of the Rhetoric Program at P.S.U. in 2002 and 2003, she designed curriculum, taught honors courses for the Schreyers Honors College, evaluated pedagogy and mentored new instructors.

Jennifer J. Tscholl, MD, completed her undergraduate education at Bowling Green State University and medical education at the Medical College of Ohio (currently renamed University of Toledo College of Medicine). She completed her residency in Pediatrics at the Johns Hopkins Hospital in Baltimore, MD. She is currently amidst subspecialty fellowship training in Child Abuse Pediatrics at Nationwide Children's Hospital in Columbus, OH.

Dr. Tscholl is a member of the American Academy of Pediatrics and its associated Section on Child Abuse and Neglect. Her research interests include child physical abuse, with particular focus on abusive head trauma.

Part I

Child Abuse as a Health Problem

Chapter 1

Introduction: Child Abuse and Neglect

Angelo P. Giardino, Michelle A. Lyn, and Eileen R. Giardino

Definition

Child Abuse

Child abuse and neglect, child maltreatment, and *child victimization* are interchangeable terms that refer to a major public health problem confronting children and families. Abuse manifests when the child or adolescent's caregiver fails to provide for the youth's health and well-being either by causing an injury or, as in neglect, by not meeting a basic need. Because of the multifaceted nature of abuse, a comprehensive definition of child abuse and neglect draws upon information from a number of disciplines and a variety of professionals. The phenomenon of child maltreatment has diverse medical, developmental, psychosocial, and legal consequences. Child abuse and neglect, along with its synonyms, describes a wide range of situations. It involves caregiver acts of commission or omission that had or are likely to have injurious effects on the child's physical, developmental, and psychosocial well-being. Child maltreatment is broadly categorized into (a) physical abuse, (b) sexual abuse, (c) emotional/psychological abuse, and (d) neglect. Neglect is further subcategorized into specific areas, such as physical, supervisional, educational, and emotional/psychological (see Chapter 7).

Physicians and nurses commonly focus on definitions that highlight the medical aspects of injury, while clinical social workers tend to focus on family and caregiving systems that gave rise to abuse. Law enforcement officers and attorneys may concentrate on the evidence that determines guilt or innocence of the suspected perpetrator of the abuse. Definitions are purposely broad to encompass the many different etiologies, presentations, and clinical manifestations of abuse or neglect cases (Azar, 1991; Bourne, 1979; Helfer & Kempe,

A.P. Giardino et al. (eds.), *A Practical Guide to the Evaluation of Child Physical Abuse and Neglect*, DOI 10.1007/978-1-4419-0702-8_1, © Springer Science+Business Media, LLC 1997, 2010

1987; Hobbs, Hanks, & Wynne, 1993; Ludwig, 1992; Wissow, 1990). Clinical situations may vary widely, ranging from the relatively rare case of a child who is tortured to death by a psychotic caregiver to the more commonly seen case of a toddler who sustains a bruise to his or her buttocks during the application of corporal punishment. The unifying theme in all definitions of child maltreatment is that abuse and neglect occur in the context of either active or passive caregiving behavior that is destructive to the normal growth, development, and well-being of the child (Ludwig, 1993).

Regardless of personal or professional preference for a specific definition, it is important that health care providers both (1) understand the definition of child abuse and (2) comply with the required actions contained in the state laws governing the geographical area in which they practice. In the United States, health care professionals such as nurses, physicians, and social workers are considered mandated reporters and are required to report suspected cases of child abuse and neglect to the appropriate authorities. According to the U.S. Department of Health and Human Services' Administration on Children and Families (2008b), the Federal Child Abuse Prevention and Treatment Act (CAPTA) which was amended by the Keeping Children and Families Safe Act of 2003 child abuse and neglect is defined as occurring at a minimum when

- any recent act or failure to act on the part of a parent or caretaker, which results in death, serious physical or emotional harm, sexual abuse or exploitation,
- or an act or failure to act which presents an imminent risk of serious harm (Section 111, 2).

State and Federal laws on child abuse refer to cases of harm caused by caregivers, either parents or those in caregiving roles (DHHS, 2008a). Cases of harm to children and adolescents caused or perpetrated by non-caregivers are also seen as crimes (e.g., assault) but are not viewed as child maltreatment owing to the lack of a caregiving relationship between perpetrator and victim.

Physical Abuse and Neglect

Physical abuse occurs when a child has suffered injury due to the actions of his or her caregiver. *Neglect* describes inadequate parenting or caregiving where there is potential for injury resulting from omissions on the part of the caregivers in meeting the child's basic needs. Neglect is present when a child experiences poor hygiene, exposure to the elements, lack of compliance with medical therapy, inadequate supervision, and forms of malnutrition related to parental control over feeding (see Chapter 7).

Corporal Punishment

Corporal punishment is a discipline method that uses physical force or the threat thereof as a behavior modifier (Hobbs et al., 1993). Its use is widespread, is nearly universal, and has been practiced for generations (American Humane Association,

1994). It stems from cultural, religious, and societal views of how children should be disciplined. Forms of corporal punishment include pinching, spanking, shoving, shaking, choking, excessive exercise, confinement in closed spaces, and denial of bathroom privileges (Grossman, Rauh, & Rivara, 1995). In the United States, forms of corporal punishment such as slapping, spanking, paddling, and general hitting of children by adult caregivers are widely accepted (Hyman, 1990; American Academy of Pediatrics, 1998a; Zolotor, Theodore, Chang, Berkoff, & Runyan, 2008).

Proponents of corporal punishment claim that it is a valid approach to discipline that leads the family "to live in harmony and love toward each other" (Nelson, 1991, p. 17). However, in situations where the child's undesired behaviors are repeated after the application of corporal punishment, the caregiver may become angry and frustrated and reapply the punishment in this more emotionally charged state of mind. There is increased potential to lose control while angry and engage in violent behavior toward the child. "For the child's own good," well-meaning parents may apply physical forms of punishment which may get out hand and cause injury to the child. Such an action is defined by law as child abuse. The American Academy of Pediatrics' (AAP) Committee on Psychosocial Aspects of Child and Family Health (1998b) calls attention to the "limited effectiveness" of corporal punishment and its potential deleterious side effects. It recommends that pediatricians "use a comprehensive approach that includes consideration of the parent–child relationship, reinforcement of desired behaviors and the consequences for negative behaviors" (p. 723) when offering guidance to families on effective discipline.

Child discipline aims for limit setting, helping the child learn right from wrong, assisting in appropriate decision making, and assisting the child's development of self-control (Crittenden, 1992). Therefore, opponents of corporal punishment believe that discipline is necessary and best achieved through consistent, nonviolent discipline techniques such as time out, loss of privileges, parental disappointment, and grounding, which are not associated with significant potential for physical harm (American Humane Association, 1994; AAP, 1998a). There is little to support the effectiveness of corporal punishment over non-physical forms of discipline, and in fact, there are potential deleterious effects from promoting violence as a problem-solving strategy (Gershoff, 2008; McCormick, 1992).

Caregiver reliance on corporal punishment is long recognized as a significant risk factor for physical abuse (Berger, Knutson, Mehm, & Perkins, 1988; Straus, 1987). Punishment becomes child abuse when the correction causes bodily harm. Clinical findings such as hematomas, ecchymoses, fractures, muscle injury, intracranial bleeds, and death may result from punishment that becomes uncontrolled. When a child manifests signs of abuse, the health care provider is legally mandated to report the caregiver for physical abuse regardless of his or her initial intention (Straus, Gelles, & Steinmetz, 1980).

Despite negative outcomes, corporal punishment remains a socially acceptable form of punishment (Socolar & Stein, 1995). In a 1990 publication, 93% of college students studied reported being spanked at some time in their childhood, with 64% reporting the effects of spankings as being helpful to very helpful (Graziano & Namaste, 1990). In more recent work, Theodore and colleagues summarize reported data that suggest at most a modest decline in the use of spanking or slapping as a form of corporal punishment. Data drawn from surveys in North and South Carolina found an overall use of spanking at 45%, with children between 3 and 10 years of age being spanked most frequently, and rates peaking at 80–90% for children between 3 and 5 years old (Theodore et al., 2005; Zolotor et al., 2008). A 2002 telephone survey determined the association between corporal punishment using spanking with an index of harsh physical punishment defined as behaviors that included beating, burning, kicking, hitting with an object somewhere other than the buttocks, or shaking a child less than 2 years old. Zolotor et al. (2008) found that parents who reported spanking with an object or who spanked frequently were more likely to report other harsh punishments consistent with definitions of physical abuse.

Hyman (1996) addressed the use of research to change policy regarding corporal punishment. He stated that corporal punishment persists despite a lack of evidence for its superiority or effectiveness in managing misbehavior. He called attention to "get tough" political rhetoric toward youth misbehavior and fear rooted in the public's perception of high crime rates as creating the social environment that maintains impassioned adherence to corporal punishment as a solution that distracts from the growing body of work that shows other, more positive forms of discipline as effective. Hyman asked the question, "what is the worst thing that would happen if all Americans stopped hitting children in any setting?" (p. 820). His response was that "most parents and teachers would discover what behavioral scientists already know. A combination of reward, positive motivational techniques, and appropriate, nonphysical punishments would prevent most misbehavior" (p. 820). Hyman further stated that "...in the next generation, rates of childhood aggression and child abuse would drop dramatically, since corporal punishment would not be considered a viable and automatic reaction to misbehavior" (Hyman, 1996, pp. 820–821). Hyman concluded with a call for continued informed dialogue and policy change stating: "Not a bad result for giving up something that has never been supported by the majority of those who study discipline in homes and schools. This is the message researchers and practitioners should actively convey to parents, policy makers and the media" (p. 821).

The AAP concludes its guidance on effective discipline with an equally reasoned and evidence-based approach to spanking:

Because of the negative consequences of spanking and because it has been demonstrated to be no more effective than other approaches for managing undesired behavior in children, the American Academy of Pediatrics recommends that parents be encouraged and assisted in developing methods other than spanking in response to undesired behavior. (AAP, 1998b, p. 726)

Reporting

The health care professional uses clinical skills and judgment to decide if a child's injuries are due to abuse and/or neglect. They are mandated reporters of suspected child abuse and neglect and are obligated in all jurisdictions to comply with the law (see Chapter 15). Clinical social workers are an excellent resource for helping health care professionals understand specific child abuse reporting laws and guidelines.

Scope of the Problem

Epidemiology

The incidence of child maltreatment (the number of new cases identified in a 1-year period of time) is often determined through research using data sources from reports of abuse and neglect. The data sources represent those cases known to social service or law enforcement agencies. The flaw in determining incidence by this method is that not all abuse is reported, and not all reports are considered to be actual abuse or neglect after investigation. Aggregation and comparisons among studies are problematic because reports often originate from reporting standards that vary. For example, a legal standard that holds up to rules of evidence governing an adversarial courtroom situation would likely yield different results than a social services' standard for abuse, which is less strict and allows the investigator's judgment as well as physical evidence to be used.

In 2006, approximately 3.3 million reports involving 6 million children were made to Child Protective Services (CPS) agencies (U.S. Department of Health and Human Services, 2008a). Of these, 61.7% were accepted as needing further investigation, and, once evaluated, the investigations concluded that child abuse and neglect had affected approximately 905,000 children, with 16% of this total representing cases of substantiated physical abuse (U.S. Department of Health and Human Services, 2008). A child abuse report is considered to be substantiated if investigation yields a determination that the child has been abused or is at significant risk of being abused or neglected. Substantiation implies a degree of certainty on the part of the child protective services (CPS) agency that the abuse occurred or that the child is at significant risk of such. The most common form of substantiated abuse in 2006 was child neglect, which accounted for 64.1% of cases, followed by physical abuse at 16%, then child sexual abuse at 8.8% of cases, and, finally, emotional maltreatment which accounted for 6.6% of cases (U.S. Department of Health and Human Services). See Figure 1.1.

Finkelhor and Jones (2008) analyzed trends in reporting and substantiation rates for child abuse and neglect from the 1990s through 2006. They identified a decline in the number of substantiated cases of physical abuse (Finkelhor & Jones, 2008). According to their most recent analysis, the incidence of substantiated physical abuse cases declined 48% from 1992 to 2006. Between 2005 and 2006, incidence declined by 3%. Cases of child sexual abuse have also declined substantially, with a 53% decrease in the number of substantiated cases of sexual abuse observed from 1992 to 2006. However, child neglect which is the most common form of child maltreatment has not declined. Substantiated cases of child neglect increased by 2% from 2005 to 2006. See Figure 1.2.

The Fourth National Incidence Study (NIS-4) is currently underway and is mandated by the US Congress in the Keeping Children and Families Safe Act of 2003

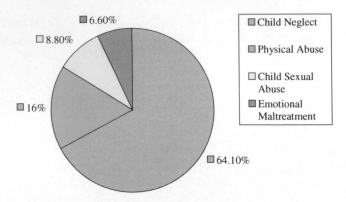

Figure 1.1 Most common forms of sustained abuse in 2006 (Child Maltreatment, 2006). Adapted from U.S. Department of Health and Human Services. Administration for Children and Families. Child Maltreatment 2006.

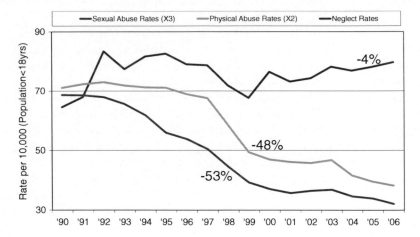

Figure 1.2 Child maltreatment trends.
Finkelhor and Jones (2008), used with permission.

(P.L. 108-36). Once completed, NIS-4 will provide the most up-to-date epidemiologic incidence data (U.S. Department of Health and Human Services, 2009). The NIS methodology views maltreated children who are investigated by CPS agencies as representing only the "tip of the iceberg." Children investigated by CPS are included along with maltreated children who are identified by professionals in a wide range of agencies in representative communities (see Figure 1.3). The NIS-4 uses data gathered from a nationally representative sample of 122 counties. CPS agencies in these counties provide data about all children in cases they accept for investigation during one of two reference periods (September 4, 2005

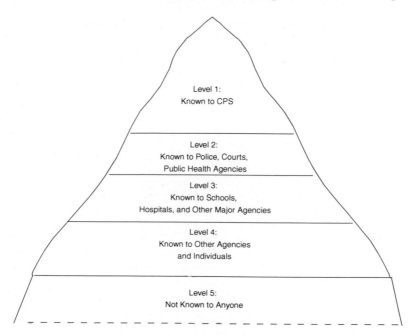

Figure 1.3 Levels of recognition of child abuse and neglect.
U.S. Department of Health and Human Services. Children's Bureau, Administration for Children, Youth and Families, Administration for Children and Families. (2001). A history of the National Incidence Study of Child Abuse and Neglect (p. 9). Accessed February 14, 2008, https://www.nis4.org/NIS_History.pdf.

through December 3, 2005, or February 4, 2006 through May 3, 2006). Additionally, professionals in these same counties serve as NIS-4 sentinels and report data about maltreated children identified by the following organizations: elementary and secondary public schools; public health departments; public housing authorities; short-stay general and children's hospitals; state, county, and municipal police/sheriff departments; licensed daycare centers; juvenile probation departments; voluntary social services and mental health agencies; shelters for runaway and homeless youth; and shelters for victims of domestic violence. The final report for the NIS-4 is expected to be available in 2010 at http://www.nis4.org/nishome.asp.

Fatal Child Abuse

According to the 1993 NIS-3 study, an estimated 1,500 children were known to have died as a result of maltreatment (Sedlak & Boradhurst, 1996). According to a report by Prevent Child Abuse America's National Center on Child Abuse Prevention Research, in 2006 an estimated 1,530 were known to have died as a result of child maltreatment, which is an average of four children each day of the year (Child Welfare Information Gateway, 2008; National Center on Child Abuse Prevention Research, 2006). Children aged 0–3 years accounted for 78% of the child abuse and neglect fatalities, with infants younger than 1 year accounting for 44.2% of these maltreatment-related fatalities. Child abuse and neglect fatalities include those caused by neglect only 41.1% and medical neglect 1.9%. Multiple forms of maltreatment account for 31.4% of fatalities, physical abuse 22.4%, child sexual abuse 0.3%, and psychological abuse 2.9% which includes unknown other cases. See Figure 1.4. The estimated death rate for child abuse and neglect in the United States is 2.04 per 100,000 children.

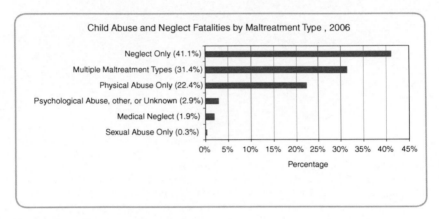

Figure 1.4 How do deaths occur?
U.S. Department of Health and Human Services. Child Welfare Information Gateway (2008).

Inflicted vs. Non-inflicted Injuries

Different forms of injury have different risks. For example, CNS injury in younger children is particularly serious. Bruises may be superficial or harbingers of more serious deeper injury. Burns observed in child maltreatment cases tend to be highly severe. Finally, skeletal injuries may be isolated or multiple in nature and may be associated with other injuries. DiScala, Sege, Guohua, and Reece (2000) conducted a 10-year retrospective of medical records in the National Pediatric Trauma Registry (NPTR) from 1988 to 1997 that compared hospitalized, injured children younger than 5 years to determine differences between inflicted ($n = 1,997$) and accidental injuries ($n = 16,831$) (DiScala et al., 2000).

The study compared children who had accidental injury with children who were abused and found that abused children tended to be younger (12.8 months vs. 25.5 months) and were mainly injured by battering (53%) and shaking (10.3%), and were more likely to have a preinjury medical history of a medical problem or condition.

Table 1.1 Outcomes by group, NPTR, 1988–1997[a].

	Unintentional injury, No. (%)	Child abuse, No. (%)
Total	16,831 (100)	1,997 (100)
Length of stay, d[b] Mean (SD) [median]	3.8 (8.0) [2.0]	9.3 (14.1) [5.0]
Survival[c]		
Alive	16,393 (97.4)	1,744 (87.3)
Dead	438 (2.6)	253 (12.7)
Functional limitations[c]		
0	11,295 (68.9)	1,063 (60.9)
1–3	4,388 (26.8)	418 (24.0)
4 or more	448 (2.7)	152 (8.7)
NA	261 (1.6)	111 (6.4)
Disposition[c]		
Home	15,761 (96.1)	624 (35.8)
Foster/custodial care/CPS	205 (1.2)	988 (56.6)
Other medical	348 (2.1)	101 (5.8)
Other	79 (0.5)	31 (1.8)

[a]NPTR, National Pediatric Trauma Registry; CPS, Child protective Services; NA, not applicable/not available.
[b]$P < 0.001$ by t test.
[c]$P < 0.001$ by χ^2 test.
Source: DiScala et al. (2000) (used with permission).

The unintentionally injured children were mainly injured by falls (58.4%) and motor vehicles (37.1%). See Table 1.1.

Etiology of Physical Abuse and Neglect

Models for Abuse

There is no single cause of physical abuse and neglect. Therefore, theoretical approaches and conceptual models help to organize the complex issues involved with child abuse and neglect. A jigsaw puzzle approach captures the multifactorial nature of child abuse and helps to explain causes (Hobbs et al., 1993). This approach incorporates diverse knowledge and understanding from a variety of sources including anthropology, child advocacy, criminology, education, history, law, medicine, political science, psychology, and sociology.

Early theories and models based on the existence of psycho-pathology in the parent (usually the mother) have evolved into more holistic cognitive and ecological models that try to account for factors involved in child maltreatment (Gil, 1975; Newberger & Newberger, 1981; Steele, 1987). At present, cognitive and ecological models are most accepted and focus more on what the abuser has learned and experienced and how these forces may predispose him or her to function in a family context (Zuravin, 1989). Models describe the cause of abuse as multilevel and interactive involving the individual, the caregivers, the community, and the global sociocultural context (Gil, 1975; Newberger & Newberger, 1981).

The ecological approach is associated with the seminal work of psychologist Urie Bronfenbrenner (1977). It defines child development in the context of an interacting, dynamic system. The ecology for child development includes family (microsystem), the community in which the family exists, forces applied to the system (exosystem), and sociocultural values that overlay the community and its families (macrosystem) (Bronfenbrenner, 1977). Garbarino (1977) applied ecological principles to the study of abuse and neglect, thus introducing the interactional nature of the roles of the parent and child, family, social stress, and social and cultural values (Belsky, 1980; Justice, Calvert, & Justice, 1985). The human ecology or socioecological model is a useful paradigm from which to address the factors that place people at risk for a variety of forms of violence, including child abuse and neglect. See Figure 1.5.

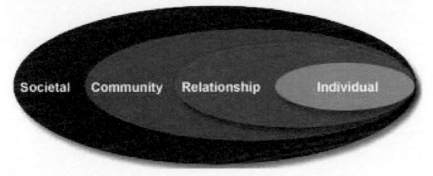

Figure 1.5 Ecological model for understanding violence.
Center for Disease Control (2009).
Note: This Socio-ecological Model considers the complex interplay between individual, relationship, community, and societal factors. It allows us to address the factors that put people at risk for experiencing or perpetrating violence.

Clinically Useful Approaches

Helfer (1973, 1987) provides a clinical and developmental perspective to the application of the ecological model to understanding child abuse and neglect. He states that the caregiver and child interact around an event or in an environment where the end result is that the child is injured or put at significant risk of injury or neglect. Helfer's (1987) approach accounts for the caregiver, the child, and triggers and stressors of the event or environment.

The Helfer (1973, 1987) model uses caution in defining the child's contribution to an abusive interaction. A child needs parenting, and nothing a child does, says, or thinks is reason to inflict injury on that child. However, personality or physical characteristics can be predisposing factors to child abuse or neglect. Characteristics of the child associated with risk for abuse or neglect include such conditions as prematurity and disability (Breslau, Staruch, & Mortimer, 1982; White, Benedict, Wulff, & Kelly, 1987; Garbarino, Brookhouser, &, Authier, 1987). Proposed reasons why premature infants are at higher risk for abuse and neglect include decreased bonding between child and parent, medical fragility of the child, and stress associated with the level of medical care that prematurity requires (Sameroff & Abbe, 1978). Proposed reasons that physically and mentally challenged children are at increased risk center around the high demand that special needs place on the caregiver (Frisch & Rhodes, 1982). The health care provider can identify child factors that may place the child at risk for injury and provide to the caregiver ongoing anticipatory guidance related to these stressors.

The Child Abuse and Prevention, Adoption, and Family Services Act of 1988 commissioned the study of the incidence of child maltreatment among children with disabilities. This study provided data on the incidence of abuse among children with disabilities (U.S. Department of Health and Human Services, 1993):

- The incidence of maltreatment (number of children maltreated annually per 1,000 children) among children with disabilities was 1.7 times higher than the incidence of maltreatment for children without disabilities.
- For 47% of the maltreated children with disabilities, Child Protective Service (CPS) caseworkers reported that the disabilities led to or contributed to child maltreatment.
- CPS caseworkers reported that a disability led to or contributed to maltreatment for 67% of the maltreated children with a serious emotional disturbance, 76% of those with a physical health problem, and 59% of those who were hyperactive.
- The incidence of physical abuse among maltreated children with disabilities was 9 per 1,000, a rate 2.1 times the rate for maltreated children without disabilities.
- Among maltreated children with disabilities, the incidence of physical neglect was 12 per 1,000, a rate 1.6 times the rate for maltreated children without disabilities.
- The incidence of emotional neglect among maltreated children with disabilities was 2.8 times as great as for maltreated children without disabilities.

Sullivan and Knutson (1998) designed a more rigorous study that used medical–professional determinations of disability.

This hospital-based epidemiological study provided further evidence that a disability rate among maltreated children was approximately twice the disability rate among non-maltreated children. Sullivan and Knutson (2000) later studied a school-based population and reported that children with disabilities were 3.4 times more likely to be maltreated than their nondisabled peers. Additionally, these researchers showed that while the risk for physical abuse among children with a physical disability was approximately 1.2 times that of nondisabled children, the risk for physical abuse among children with other disabilities ranged from 2 to 7.3 times that of nondisabled children (Sullivan & Knuston, 1998, 2000; Westat, 1993).

Among the 905,000 victims of substantiated child maltreatment in 2006, 7.7% had a reported disability. Specific disabilities included global cognitive problems, emotional disturbances, visual or hearing difficulties, a variety of learning disabilities, physical challenges, behavioral problems, or some other disabling condition (U.S. Department of Health and Human Services, 2008).

Stress defined as internal anxiety related to a perception of an inability to meet external demands is often cited as a factor in abusive interactions (Selye, 1956). Because stress is a subjective phenomenon, what is stressful to one individual may or may not be stressful to another. Coping strategies may mitigate the amount of stress experienced in a given situation. Subsequently, caregiver stress and frustration figure prominently in the occurrence of child abuse (Straus & Kantor, 1987). Stressors most often related to child abuse are those associated with poverty, significant life events, caregiver–child interaction patterns, and caregiver role conflicts (Justice & Justice, 1976; Straus & Kantor, 1987).

Helfer (1973) cites the following as factors associated with potential abuse or neglect:

Caregiver Factors

- Personal history
- Personality style
- Psychological functioning
- Expectations of the child
- Ability to nurture and assist the child's developmental progress
- Rearing practices modeled during the parents' own upbringing
- Degree of social isolation characteristic of the parent
  His or her ability to ask for and receive help from other individuals in the social network
- Support of the caregiver's partner in assisting with the parenting role
- Ability to deal with internal and external difficulty and coping strategies

Child Factors

- Prematurity and disability
- Poor bonding with caregiver
- Medical fragility
- Level of medical care of premature children
- Special needs of physically and mentally disabled children
- Child perceived as "difficult"

Environmental Factors

- Poverty
- Significant life events
- Caregiver–child interaction patterns
- Caregiver role conflicts

The relationship of domestic violence or intimate partner violence (IPV) and child maltreatment is receiving increasing attention. The American Academy of Pediatrics (AAP) recommends that pediatricians assess for the presence of domestic violence and intimate partner violence in the child's family and observes that intervening on behalf of the victimized parent (typically the child's mother) may be an effective child-abuse prevention strategy (AAP, 1998a) (Figure 1.6).

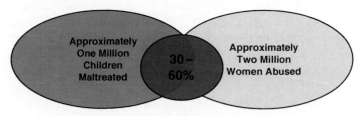

Figure 1.6 Overlap of child maltreatment and domestic violence.
DHHS (1998) and Tjaden and Thoennes (1998), In Harm's Way: Domestic Violence and Child Maltreatment.

The National Violence Against Women (NVAW) Survey is a telephone survey on a nationally representative sample of 8,000 women and 8,000 men conducted between November 1995 and May 1996. The study found that nearly 25% of women and 8% of men reported they had been sexually and/or physically assaulted by an intimate partner at some point in their lives. At least 1.5 million women and 835,000 men had been assaulted by an intimate partner in the previous 12 months. Publicly reported IPV statistics are thought to underreport the incidence of IPV because of the stigma and perceived sense of shame surrounding the problem (Tjaden, 2000).

Child maltreatment and IPV are intricately related. Studies show that within groups of children with suspected abuse or neglect, 45–59% of their mothers have been battered (Stark & Flitcraft, 1988). Children of battered mothers are 6–15 times more likely to be abused than children who do not live in violent homes. Child abuse occurs in 33–77% of families in which there is abuse of an adult (Straus & Gelles, 1990).

Over time, professionals have come to realize that witnessing violence in the home may be as psychologically and developmentally traumatic to children as being directly abused (Kitzmann, Gaylord, Hold, & Kelly, 2003). Children's exposure to violence in the form of witnesses far outnumbers those who are the direct recipients of violence. In the United States, it is estimated that between 3.3 and 10 million children yearly witness physical assaults between their parents (Carlson, 2000). Children who witness violence can be anxious, socially withdrawn, depressed, have fewer interests and social activities, and be preoccupied with physical aggression. Their behavioral problems have been reported to include aggressiveness, hyperactivity, conduct disorders, reduced social competence, school problems, truancy, bullying, excessive screaming, clinging behaviors, and speech disorders (Kitzmann et al., 2003). They can also have physical symptoms such as headaches, bed-wetting, disturbed sleep, failure to thrive, vomiting, and diarrhea. Post-traumatic stress disorder

(PTSD)-type symptoms can include recurrent images of the battering, sleep disturbances, excessive worry about the mother's safety, and avoidance of certain activities and thoughts. Witnessing violence as children may predispose them to be violent in their own intimate relationships in adulthood. Males raised in a household where the mother was beaten by her partner are more likely to be abusive to their own female partner in the future. Of note, in a comprehensive literature review that examined relevant peer reviewed literature spanning the 11 years between 1995 and 2006, Holt, Buckley, and Whelan (2008) found substantial empiric evidence to support the observation that children may be significantly affected by living situations in which they are exposed to IPV. The impact of such exposure to IPV may endure even after the steps are taken to ensure the safety to the child and family. Additionally, this comprehensive review could find to direct causal pathway to a particular outcome and thus concluded that children construct their own social worlds and the ultimate impact is highly variable and its manifestation depends on many factors related to the child and their own unique environmental situation (Holt et al., 2008). Optimistically, the review identified a range of protective factors that helped mitigate against negative consequences and which clinically appeared as resilience in the face of a difficult situation. The final conclusion from the review focused on providing timely interventions that were individually tailored to each child and his or her circumstances in order to "build on the resilient blocks in the child's life" (p. 797) (Holt et al., 2008).

Effects

The physically abused or neglected child may sustain physical, emotional, and developmental effects. Injured or neglected children experience physical consequences that vary in severity depending on the type of injury, organ systems involved, and extent of tissue damage inflicted. Physical effects of abuse are discussed separately in subsequent chapters.

Maltreatment also may have negative effects on the child's behavior, development, and psychosocial functioning. Studies using "clinical" populations of seriously disturbed individuals found a high correlation between maltreatment and poor behavioral, psychosocial, and developmental outcomes (Lamphear, 1985; Oates, 1982; Parish, Myers, Brandner, & Templin, 1985). However, reliable, consistent predictions concerning the effects of maltreatment are difficult to make, and this remains an active area of research interest. Well-designed, longitudinal studies of the long-term effects of physical abuse and neglect point toward a complex relationship between child maltreatment and subsequent development. The impact of victimization on development hinges on "mediating" factors that mitigate against the negative effects of abuse and neglect on the child (Augoustinos, 1987; Crittenden, 1992; Martin & Elmer, 1992). Possible mediating variables identified are the child's personality characteristics and coping strategies, available resources in the environment, the child's perception of how responsive people are to his or her plight, and the modeled adult behavior that the child observes during the aftermath of the abuse (Augoustinos, 1987).

Felitti et al. (1998) looked at potential long-term impacts of childhood abuse on health and well-being. They explored the connection between exposure to childhood abuse and the connection between household dysfunction to subsequent health risks and the development of illness in adulthood. They developed a series of studies referred to as the Adverse Childhood Experiences (ACE) studies (Felitti et al., 1998). Of 13,494 adults who completed a standard medical evaluation in 1995–1996, 9,508 completed a survey questionnaire that asked about their own childhood abuse and exposure to household dysfunction; the investigators then made correlations to risk factors and disease conditions.

In order to assess exposure to child abuse and neglect, the ACE questionnaire asked about categories of child maltreatment, specifically psychological, physical, and sexual maltreatment. When asking about physical abuse, the questionnaire asked the patients if a parent or other adult in the household had (1) often or very often pushed, grabbed, shoved, or slapped them or (2) often or very often hit them so hard that marks or other injuries resulted.

In order to assess exposure to household dysfunction, the ACE questionnaire explored categories of dysfunction, such as having a household member who had problems with substance abuse (e.g., problem drinker, drug user), mental illness (e.g., psychiatric problem), criminal behavior in household (e.g., incarceration), or having a mother who was treated violently. In assessing if the respondent's mother was treated violently when the patient was a child, the survey asked if their mother or stepmother was (1) sometimes or very often pushed, grabbed, slapped, bitten, hit with a fist, or with something hard or had something thrown at her, or (2) was ever repeatedly hit for at least a few minutes or threatened with or hurt by a knife or gun.

In addition to the questionnaire information, the standardized medical examination of the adults assessed risk factors and actual disease conditions. The risk factors included smoking, severe obesity, physical inactivity, depressed mood, suicide attempts, alcoholism, any drug abuse, a high lifetime number of sexual partners, and a history of sexually transmitted disease (STD). The disease conditions included ischemic heart disease, cancer, stroke, chronic bronchitis, emphysema, diabetes, hepatitis, and skeletal fractures. The ACE study found that the most prevalent adverse childhood experience (ACE) was substance abuse (25.6%), the least prevalent adverse experience was criminal behavior (3.4%), and the prevalence of physical abuse was 10.8% and the prevalence of the mother being treated violently was 12.5%.

Overall, 52% of the respondents had one or more adverse childhood experience and 6.2% had four or more adverse experiences. The following were findings in respondents who experienced four or more ACEs compared with those who had none:

- Risk of alcoholism, drug abuse, depression, and suicide attempt increased 4- to 12-fold.
- Rates of smoking, poor self-rated health, and high number of sexual partners and STDs increased 2- to 4-fold.
- Physical inactivity and severe obesity increased 1.4- to 1.6-fold.

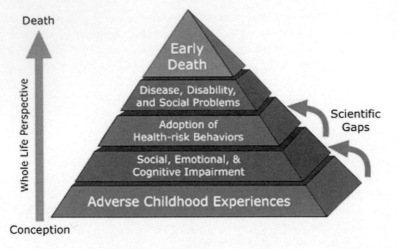

Figure 1.7 Adverse child experiences pyramid.
Felitti et al. (1998) and The Center for Disease Control from http://www.cdc.gov/nccdphp/ace/pyramid.htm.

The major finding of the ACE studies was a graded relationship between the number of exposures to maltreatment and household dysfunction during childhood to the presence in later life of multiple risk factors and several disease conditions associated with death in adulthood (see Figure 1.7).

Researchers, policy makers, and clinicians have long been intrigued by the question of whether or not a "cycle of violence" exists wherein exposure to child abuse and neglect might be seen as leading to adult criminal behavior. Widom and Maxfield (2001) report on a longitudinal study of 908 substantiated cases of child maltreatment drawn from a metropolitan area in the Midwestern United States and processed by the courts from 1967 to 1971. Substantiated cases of abuse are compared to a group of 667 non-maltreated children who were matched according to gender, age, ethnicity, and family socioeconomic status. Analyzing arrest records from 1994 when the average age of the subjects was 32.5 (the peak years for committing violent offenses is 20–25 years of age), the study found that while many individuals in both groups had no juvenile or adult criminal record, those who were maltreated had an increased likelihood of arrest as a juvenile by 59% and as an adult by 28%. Additional key findings included the following (Widom & Maxfield, 2001):

- Maltreated children were younger at the time of their first arrest.
- Maltreated children committed nearly twice as many offenses and were arrested more frequently.
- Physically abused and neglected (versus sexually abused) children were the most likely to be arrested later for a violent crime.
- New results indicate that abused and neglected females were also at increased risk of arrest for violence as juveniles and adults.

- White abused and neglected children were no more likely to be arrested for a violent crime than their nonabused and non-neglected white counterparts.
- Black abused and neglected children showed significantly increased rates of violent arrests compared with black children who were not maltreated.

Widom and Maxfield (2001) observed that while exposure to physical abuse had the highest percentage of arrests for violent crimes at 21.1%, those exposed to neglect were not far behind at 20.2% and those exposed to sexual abuse had the lowest percentage of arrests for violent crimes at 8.8%. See Figure 1.8. Thus, exposure to child abuse and neglect must be seen as a significant problem that has the potential for widespread and serious social consequences that includes childhood delinquency, adult criminality, and the potential for violent criminal behavior with almost half of the abused and neglected individuals having had an arrest for a nontraffic offense (i.e., 49% overall). Widom and colleagues (2008) conducted a later analysis focused on the risk for revictimization in which the study participants, both maltreated and non-maltreated, were interviewed in the time period between 2000 and 2002 when these participants had a mean age of 39.5 years of age). They found that abused and neglected individuals reported a higher number of victimization experiences than did non-maltreated controls and that all types of maltreatment including physical abuse, sexual abuse, and neglect were associated with an increased risk for lifetime revictimization (Widom et al., 2009). Furthermore, childhood victimization increased the risk for the following: physical and sexual assault, kidnapping, being stalked, having a family friend murdered, or having a family friend commit suicide.

Early work in the field of child abuse and neglect estimated that approximately 25–35% of children subjected to all forms of child abuse will go on to abuse their own children as compared to controls who were not abused (Kaufman & Ziegler, 1987). Although abusive parenting occurs in some cases, abused children do not inevitably become abusive parents. Martin and Elmer (1992) found that although some abused children are at risk of becoming abusive toward their own children, the majority of such survivors do not go on to abuse their children.

Exhibit 5. **Does only violence beget violence?**

Abuse Group	Number of subjects	Percentage Arrested for Violent Offense
Physical Abuse Only	76	21.1
Neglect Only	609	20.2
Sexual Abuse Only	125	8.8
Mixed	98	14.3
Control	667	13.9

Figure 1.8 Association of type of abuse with arrest for violent crimes.
Widom and Maxfield (2001) from http://www.ncjrs.gov/pdffiles1/nij/184894.pdf.

It is important that the health care professionals appreciate that children who are abused are not "doomed" and that the child needs to be nurtured and supported in a safe environment for healing and normal development to occur. One of Widom's final recommendations addressed the need for early intervention to help children who have been maltreated avoid a myriad of problems that in addition to delinquency and criminality include poor educational performance, mental health problems, and generally low levels of achievement.

These updated findings reinforce the need for police, teachers, and health care workers to recognize the signs of abuse and neglect and make serious efforts to intervene as early as possible. The later the intervention, the more difficult the change process becomes. It is suggested that special attention be paid to abused and neglected children with early behavior problems. These children show the highest risk of later juvenile and adult arrest, as well as violent criminal behavior. (Widom & Maxfield, 2001, p. 7)

The AAP's Committee on Child Abuse and Neglect (2008) issued a clinical report that called attention to the ongoing challenge of understanding the behavioral and emotional consequences from exposure to child maltreatment (American Academy of Pediatrics, 2008). The AAP report issued in collaboration with the American Academy of Child and Adolescent Psychiatry and the National Center for Child Traumatic Stress reminds practitioners that children who experience child abuse and neglect may later manifest significant mental and behavioral problems including emotional instability, depression, and a tendency to be aggressive or violent with others (Stirling et al., 2008). The pervasive effects of maltreatment on adult functioning have come to light and Briere (1992) developed a framework from which to view the mental health implications of abuse and neglect. He describes three stages of potential impact that maltreatment may have on the child: (a) initial reactions that include post-traumatic stress, alterations in normal development, painful affect, and cognitive distortions; (b) accommodation to ongoing abuse, including coping behaviors intended to increase safety and/or decrease pain; and (c) long-term effects and ongoing accommodation that reflect on the initial reactions and accommodations and that are rooted in the ongoing coping responses (Briere, 1992). Briere (1992) describes a number of serious mental health problems found in abuse survivors that, at the extreme, include post-traumatic stress disorder (PTSD) and dissociative disorders. Although the majority of survivors of abuse will not experience the most extreme impairment, Briere (1992) contends that a large number of victims experience some level of dysfunction.

The mental health consequences from exposure to maltreatment appear to occur along a continuum from passivity and withdrawal to aggression and violence. The continuum depends on the tendency of the child or adolescent toward internalizing or externalizing emotions and behaviors (Goldman, Salus, Wolcott, & Kennedy, 2003). Children and adolescents who have been maltreated may demonstrate a myriad of symptoms and conditions including: low self-esteem, depression, anxiety, PTSD, attachment difficulties, eating disorders, sleep disturbances, poor peer relations, and various self-destructive behaviors including substance abuse and suicide attempts (Goldman, Salus, Wolcott, & Kennedy, 2003). However, not all children who experience maltreatment go on to manifest significant behavioral or emotional disorders (Giardino & Harris, 2006). Such capacity for "resilence" relates to the presence of various protective factors that mitigate and buffer the child from developing the severe negative consequences (Heller, Larrieu, D'Imperio, and Boris, 1993). Among the protective factors are (1) personal characteristics inherent in the child or adolescent, including a sense of optimism, high self-esteem, high intelligence, and a general hopeful outlook and perspective, and (2) environmental characteristics such as a supportive social network that includes supportive caregivers, interested relatives and professionals, and social supports that are accessible and available (Goodman et al., 2003).

Therapeutic efforts that are focused on the coping strategies of the child or adult can help the survivor's healing process (Briere, 1992). The AAP's report calls upon health care professionals to assist in the recovery of the maltreated child by helping those responsible for their care to recognize the abused or neglected child's likely altered responses to environmental stimuli, to assist them in formulating more effective coping strategies and in mobilizing all available community resources to the end of supporting the child and effectively responding to their immediate and ongoing needs (Stirling et al., 2008)

In summary, physical abuse and neglect may have far-reaching implications for the child victim. Research describing outcomes from abuse and neglect shows that deleterious effects from exposure to child abuse can be mitigated if supportive, responsive people and systems respond to the child victim in a substantive manner.

Costs

In addition to the impact on the child and family, child abuse and neglect also impacts the community and society as well. At the most basic level, societal impacts can be quantified in terms of direct and indirect costs (Wang & Holton, 2007). Prevent Child Abuse America estimated the costs related to child abuse and neglect using 2007 dollar values. Direct costs are defined as those associated with the immediate needs of the maltreated children and include such items as hospitalizations, mental health services, child protection, and law enforcement. Direct costs were estimated to be over 33 billion dollars. Indirect costs are those associated with the long-term needs of the maltreated children. Indirect costs include those related to special education, juvenile justice, physical health care, mental health care, adult criminal justice, and the lost productivity to the society and were estimated to be over 70 billion. Thus, a conservative estimate for the total societal costs of child abuse and neglect in 2007 dollar value would be in excess of 103 billion and this estimate is conservative and could be much higher if all costs were also included: (1) outpatient medical evaluations that did not lead to hospitalization, (2) substance abuse treatment services, as well as treatment services for high-risk behaviors leading to sexually transmitted diseases in those victims who manifest these problems, and (3) the intervention and treatment services for the victims' families as well as for the perpetrators. See Table 1.2.

Table 1.2 Total annual cost of child abuse and neglect in the United States.

	Estimated annual cost (in 2007 dollars)
Direct costs	
Hospitalization	$6,625,959,263
Rationale: 565,000 maltreated children suffered seriously in 1993.[a] Assume that 50% of seriously injured victims require hospitalization.[b] The average cost of treating one hospitalized victim of abuse and neglect was $19,266 in 1993[c]	
Calculation: 565,000 × 0.50 × $19,266 = $5,442,645,000	
Mental health care system	$1,080,706,049
Rationale: 25–50% of child maltreatment victims need some form of mental health treatment.[d] For a conservative estimate, 25% is used. Mental health care cost per victim by type of maltreatment is physical abuse ($2,700); sexual abuse ($5,800); emotional abuse ($2,700); and educational neglect ($910).[d] Cross-referenced against NIS-3 statistics on number of each incident occurring in 1993[a]	
Calculations: Physical abuse – 381,700 × 0.25 × $2,700 = $257,647,500 = sexual abuse – 217,700 × 0.25 × $5,800 = $315,665,000; emotional abuse – 204,500 × 0.25 × $2,700 = $138,037,500; and educational neglect – 397,300 × 0.25 ×$910; Total = $801,735,750	
Child welfare services system	$25,361,329,051
Rationale: The Urban Institute conducted a study estimating the child welfare expenditures associated with child abuse and neglect by state and local public child welfare agencies to be $23.3 billion in 2004[e]	
Law enforcement	$33,307,770
Rationale: The National Institute of Justice estimated the following costs of police services for each of the following interventions: physical abuse ($20); sexual abuse ($56); emotional abuse ($20); and education neglect ($2).[d] Cross-referenced against NIS-3 statistics on number of each incident occurring in 1993[a]	
Calculations: Physical abuse – 381,700 × $20 = $7,634,000; sexual abuse – 217,700 × $56 = $12,191,200; emotional abuse –204,500 × $20 = $4,090,000; and educational neglect –397,000 × $2 = $794,000; total = $24,709,800	
Total direct costs	$33,101,302,133

Table 1.2 (continued)

	Estimated annual cost (in 2007 dollars)
Indirect costs	
Special education Rationale: 1,553,800 children experienced some form of maltreatment in 1993.[a] 22% of maltreated children have learning disorders requiring special education.[f] The additional expenditure attributable to special education services for students with disabilities was $5,918 per pupil in 2000[g] Calculation: 1,553,800 × 0.22 × $5,918 = $2,022,985,448	$2,410,306,242
Juvenile delinquency Rationale: 1,553,800 children experienced some form of maltreatment in 1993.[a] 27% of children who are abused or neglected become delinquents, compared to 17% of children in the general population,[h] for a difference of 10%. The annual cost of caring for a juvenile offender in a residential facility was $30,450 in 1989[i] Calculation: 1,553,800 × 0.10 × $30,450 = $4,731,321,000	$7,174,814,134
Mental health and health care Rationale: 1,553,800 children experienced some form of maltreatment in 1993.[a] 27% of children who are abused or neglected become delinquents, compared to 17% of children in the general population,[h] for a difference of 10%. The annual cost of caring for a juvenile offender in a residential facility was $30,450 in 1989[i] Calculation: 1,553,800 × 0.10 × $30,450 = $4,731,321,000	$7,174,814,134
Mental health and health care Rationale: 1,553,800 children experienced some form of maltreatment in 1993.[a] 30% of maltreated children suffer chronic health problems.[f] Increased mental health and health care costs for women with a history of childhood abuse and neglect, compared to women without childhood maltreatment histories, were estimated to be $8,175,816 for a population of 163,844 women, of whom 42.8% experienced childhood abuse and neglect.[j] This is equivalent to $117 ($8,175,816)/(163,844 × 0.428) additional health care costs associated with child maltreatment per woman per year. Assume that the additional health care costs attributable to childhood maltreatment are similar for men who experienced maltreatment as a child Calculation: 1,553,800 × 0.30 × $117 = $54,346,699	$67,863,457

Table 1.2 (continued)

	Estimated annual cost (in 2007 dollars)
Adult criminal justice system Rationale: The direct expenditure for operating the nation's criminal justice system (including police protection, judicial and legal services, and corrections) was $204,136,015,000 in 2005.[k] According to the National Institute of Justice, 13% of all violence can be linked to earlier child maltreatment[d] Calculations: $204,136,015,000 × 0.13 = $26,537,681,950	$27,979,811,982
Lost productivity to society Rationale: The median annual earning for a full-time worker was $33,634 in 2006.[l] Assume that only children who suffer serious injuries due to maltreatment (565,000[a]) experience losses in potential lifetime earnings and that such impairments are limited to 5% of the child's total potential earnings.[b] The average length of participation in the labor force is 39.1 years for men and 29.3 years for women[m]; the overall average 34 years is used Calculation: $33,634 × 565,000 × 0.05 × 34 = $32,305,457,000	$33,019,919,544
Total indirect costs	$70,652,715,359
Total cost	$103,754,017,492

[a]Sedlak and Broadhurst (1996);
[b]Daro (1988);
[c]Rovi, Chen, and Johnson (2004);
[d]Miller, Cohen, and Wiersema (1996);
[e]Scarcella, Bess, Zielewski, and Geen (2006);
[f]Hammerle (1992);
[g]Chambers, Parrish, and Harr (2004);
[h]Widom and Maxfield (2001);
[i]U.S. Bureau of the Census (1993);
[j]Walker et al. (1999);
[k]U.S. Department of Justice (2007);
[l]U.S. Department of Labor (2007);
[m]Smith (1985);
Wang and Holton (2007) (used with permission from Prevent Child Abuse America).

In Brief

- Child maltreatment is categorized into (a) physical abuse, (b) sexual abuse, (c) emotional/psychological abuse, and (d) neglect.
- There is no single cause of physical abuse and neglect.
- The result of abuse and neglect is a child who either sustains injury or is at risk for injury, and whose growth and development may be impeded.
- Maltreatment primarily occurs in the family setting and is a problem firmly rooted in the caregiving environment.
- Corporal punishment ends and child abuse begins when the punishment inflicted by the parent causes bodily harm.
- When a child manifests the signs of abuse, the health care provider is legally mandated to report the caregiver for physical abuse regardless of the caregiver's intention.
- Health care professionals are mandated reporters of suspected child abuse and neglect and are obligated in all jurisdictions to comply with the law.
- Health care providers must understand and comply with the definition of child abuse in the state laws governing the geographical area in which they practice.
- Health care providers understand that children who are abused need to be nurtured and supported in a safe environment for healing and normal development to occur.
- Injured or neglected children experience physical consequences that vary in severity depending on the type of injury, tissues involved, and extent of damage.
- Therapeutic efforts focused on the child's and/or adult's coping strategies can help the survivor live in a satisfying and productive manner.
- Prevent Child Abuse America conservatively estimates that child abuse and neglect has a societal cost in excess of 103 billion dollars per year.

References

American Academy of Pediatrics. Committee on Child Abuse and Neglect. (1998a). The role of the pediatrician in recognizing and intervening on behalf of abused women. *Pediatrics, 101*, 1091–1092.

American Academy of Pediatrics. Committee on Psychosocial Aspects of Child and Family Health. (1998b). Guidance for effective discipline. *Pediatrics, 101*(4), 723–728.

American Academy of Pediatrics, Stirling, J., et al. (2008). Understanding the behavioral and emotional consequences of child abuse. *Pediatrics, 122*, 667–673.

American Humane Association. (1994). *AHA fact sheet #12: The use of physical discipline*. Englewood, CO: Author.

Augoustinos, M. (1987). Developmental effects of child abuse: Recent findings. *Child Abuse and Neglect, 11*, 15–27.

Azar, S. T. (1991). Models of child abuse: A metatheoretical analysis. *Criminal Justice and Behavior, 18*, 30–46.

Belsky, J. (1980). Child maltreatment: An ecological integration. *American Psychologist, 35*, 320–335.

Berger, A. M., Knutson, J. F., Mehm, J. G., & Perkins, K. A. (1988). *Child Abuse and Neglect*, *12*, 251–262.

Bourne, R. (1979). Child abuse and neglect: An overview. In R. Bourne and E. H. Newberger (Eds.), *Critical perspectives on child abuse*. Lexington, MA: Lexington Books.

Breslau, N., Staruch, K. S., & Mortimer, E. A. (1982). Psychological distress in mothers of disabled children. *American Journal of Disabilities of Children*, *136*, 682–686.

Briere, J. N. (1992). *Child abuse trauma: Theory and treatment of the lasting effects*. Newbury Park, CA: Sage.

Bronfenbrenner, U. (1977). Toward an experimental ecology of human development. *American Psychologist*, *32*, 513–531.

Carlson, B. E. (2000). Children exposed to intimate partner violence: Research findings and implications for intervention. *Trauma, Violence, and Abuse*, *1*(4), 321–340.

Center for Disease Control. Adverse childhood experiences study. http://www.cdc.gov/nccdphp/ace/pyramid.htm

Center for Disease Control. Violence protection. The social-ecological model: A framework for prevention. Accessed March 30, 2009, http://www.cdc.gov/ncipc/dvp/Social-Ecological-Model_DVP.htm

Chambers, J. G., Parrish, T. B., & Harr, J. J. (2004). *What are we spending on special education services in the United States, 1999–2000?* Palo Alto, CA: American Institutes for Research. Retrieved August 28, 2007 from http://www.csef-air.org/publications/seep/national/AdvRpt1.PDF

Child Welfare Information Gateway. (2008). *Child abuse and neglect fatalities: Statistics and interventions*. Washington, DC: U.S. Department of Health and Human Services. Accessed April 14, 2009, http://www.childwelfare.gov/pubs/factsheets/fatality.cfm

Crittenden, P. M. (1992). Children's strategies for coping with adverse home environments: An interpretation using attachment theory. *Child Abuse and Neglect*, *16*, 329–343.

Daro, D. (1988). *Confronting child abuse: Research for effective program design*. New York: Free Press.

DiScala, C., Sege, R., Guohua, L., & Reece, R. M. (2000, January). Chile abuse and unintentional injuries. *Pediatric Adolescent Medicine*, *154*, 20.

Felitti, V. J., Anda, R. F., Nordenberg, D., Williamson, D. F., Spitz, A. M., Edwards, V., et al. (1998). Relationship of childhood abuse and household dysfunction to many of the leading causes of death in adults – The Adverse Childhood Experiences (ACE) Study. *American Journal of Preventive Medicine*, *14*, 245–258.

Finkelhor, D., & Jones, L. (2008) Crimes against children research center. Updated trends in child maltreatment. Accessed March 30, 2009, http://cyber.law.harvard.edu/sites/cyber.law.harvard.edu/files/Trends%20in%20Child%20Maltreatment.pdf

Frisch, L., & Rhodes, F. (1982). Child abuse and neglect in children referred for learning evaluations. *Journal of Learning Disabilities*, *15*, 583–586.

Garbarino, J. (1977). The human ecology of child maltreatment: A conceptual model for research. *Journal of Marriage and the Family*, *39*, 721–727.

Garbarino, J., Brookhouser, P., & Authier, K. J. (Eds.). (1987). *Special children, special risks: The maltreatment of children with disabilities*. New York: Aldine.

Gershoff, E. T. (2008). *Report on physical punishment in the United States: What research tells us about its effects on children*. Columbus, OH: Center for Effective Discipline.

Giardino, A. P., & Harris, T. B. (2006) Child abuse & neglect: Posttraumatic stress disorder. eMedicine. Accessed April 15, 2009, http://emedicine.medscape.com/article/916007-overview

Gil, D. G. (1975). Unraveling child abuse. *American Journal of Orthopsychiatry, 45*, 346–358.

Goldman, J., Salus, M., Wolcott, D., & Kennedy, K. (2003). A coordinated response to child abuse and neglect: The foundation for practice. National Clearinghouse on Child Abuse and Neglect Information. Department of Health and Human Services, Administration for Children and Families, Children's Bureau Office on Child Abuse and Neglect. http://www.childwelfare.gov/pubs/usermanuals/foundation/foundation.pdf

Graziano, A. M., & Namaste, K. A. (1990). Parental use of physical force in child discipline: A survey of 679 college students. *Journal of Interpersonal Violence, 5*, 449–463.

Grossman, D. C., Rauh, M. J., & Rivara, F. P. (1995). Prevalence of corporal punishment among students in Washington State schools. *Archives of Pediatrics & Adolescent Medicine, 149*, 529–536.

Hammerle, N. (1992). *Private choices, social costs, and public policy: An economic analysis of public health issues.* Westport, CT: Greenwood, Praeger.

Helfer, R. E. (1973). The etiology of child abuse. *Pediatrics, 51*, 777–779.

Helfer, R. E. (1987). The developmental basis of child abuse and neglect: An epidemiological approach. In R. E. Helfer & R. S. Kempe (Eds.), *The battered child* (4th ed., pp. 60–80). Chicago: University of Chicago Press.

Helfer, R. E., & Kempe, R. S. (1987). *The battered child* (4th ed.). Chicago: University of Chicago Press.

Heller, S. S., Larrieu, J. A., D'Imperio, R., & Boris, N. W. (1993). Research on resilience to child maltreatment: Empirical considerations. *Child Abuse and Neglect, 23*, 32–338.

Hobbs, C. J., Hanks, H. G. I., & Wynne, J. M. (1993). *Child abuse and neglect: A clinician's handbook.* New York: Churchill Livingstone.

Holt, S., Buckley, H., & Whelan, S. (2008). The impact of exposure to domestic violence on children and young people: A review of the literature. *Child Abuse and Neglect, 32*, 797–810.

Hyman, I. (1990). *Reading, writing, and the hickory stick: The appalling story of physical and psychological abuse in American schools.* Lexington, MA: Lexington Books.

Hyman, U. A. (1996). Using research to change public policy: Reflections on 20 years of effort to eliminate corporal punishment in schools. *Pediatrics, 98*, 818–821.

Justice, B., Calvert, A., & Justice, R. (1985). Factors mediating child abuse as a response to stress. *Child Abuse and Neglect, 9*, 359–363.

Justice, B., & Justice, R. (1976). *The abusing family.* New York: Human Sciences Press.

Kaufman, J., & Ziegler, E. (1987). Do abused children become abusive parents? *American Journal of Orthopsychiatry, 57*, 186-192.

Kitzmann, K., Gaylord, N., Hold, A., & Kelly, E. (2003). Child witness to domestic violence: a meta-analytic review. *Journal of Consulting and Clinical Psychology, 71*, 339–352.

Lamphear, V. S. (1985). The impact of maltreatment on children's psychosocial adjustment: A review of the research. *Child Abuse and Neglect, 9*, 251–263.

Ludwig, S. (1992). Defining child abuse. In S. Ludwig & A. E. Kornberg (Eds.), *Child abuse: A medical reference* (2nd ed., pp. 1–12). New York: Churchill Livingstone.

Ludwig, S. (1993). Psychosocial emergencies: Child abuse. In G. R. Fleisher & S. Ludwig (Eds.), *Textbook of pediatric emergency medicine* (3rd ed., pp. 1429–1463). Baltimore: Williams and Wilkins.

Martin, J. A., & Elmer, E. (1992). Battered children grow up: A follow-up study of individuals severely maltreated as children. *Child Abuse and Neglect, 16*, 75–87.

McCormick, K. F. (1992). Attitudes of primary care physicians toward corporal punishment. *Journal of the American Medical Association*, 267, 3161–3165.

Miller, T. R., Cohen, M. A., & Wiersema, B. (1996). *Victim costs and consequences: A new look.* The National Institute of Justice. Retrieved August 27, 2007 from http://www.ncirs.gov/pdffiles/victcost.pdf.

National Center on Child Abuse Prevention Research. (2006). National child maltreatment statistics. Prevent child abuse America. Chicago, IL. Accessed April 15, 2009, http://member.preventchildabuse.org/site/DocServer/Child_Maltreatment_Fact_Sheet_2005.pdf?docID=221

National Clearing House on Child Abuse and Neglect Information. In Harm's Way: Domestic Violence and Child Maltreatment. Accessed March 30, 2009, http://www.calib.com/dvcps/facts/harmway.doc

Nelson, F. P. (1991). Corporal punishment versus child abuse. *AAP News*, 17.

Newberger, C. M., & Newberger, E. H. (1981). The etiology of child abuse. In N. S. Ellerstein (Ed.), *Child abuse and neglect* (pp. 11–20). New York: Wiley.

Oates, K. (1982). *Child abuse—A community concern.* New York: Brunner/Mazel.

Parish, R. A., Myers, P. A., Brandner, A., & Templin, K. H. (1985). Developmental milestones in abused children, and their improvement with a family-oriented approach to the treatment of child abuse. *Child Abuse and Neglect*, 9, 245–250.

Rovi, S., Chen, P. H., & Johnson, M.S. (2004). The economic burden of hospitalizations associated with child abuse and neglect. *American Journal of Public Health*, 94, 586–590. Retrieved September 7, 2007 form http://www.ajph.org/cgi/reprint/94/4/586?ck=nck

Sameroff, A., & Abbe, L. (1978). The consequences of prematurity: Understanding and therapy. In H. Pick (Ed.), *Psychology: From research to practice*. New York: Plenum.

Scarcella, C. A., Bess, R., Zielewski, E. H., & Geen, R. (2006). *The cost of protecting vulnerable children V: Understanding state variation in child welfare financing.* The Urban Institute. Retrieved August 27, 2007 from http://www.urban.org/UploadedPDF/311314_vulnerable_children.pdf

Sedlak, A. J., & Broadhurst, D. D. (1996). *Third incidence study of child abuse and neglect (NIS-3).* Washington, DC: U.S. Department of Health and Human Services.

Selye, H. (1956). *The stress of life.* New York: McGraw-Hill.

Smith, S. J. (1985). Revised worklife tables reflect 1979–80 experience. *Monthly Labor Review*, August 1985, 23–30. Retrieved September 4, 2007 from http://www.bls.gov/opub/mlr/1985/08/art3full.pdf

Socolar, R. R. S., & Stein, R. E. K. (1995). Spanking infants and toddlers: Maternal belief and practice. *Pediatrics*, 95, 105–111.

Stark, E., & Flitcraft, A. H. (1988). Women and children at risk: A feminist perspective on child abuse. *International Journal of Health Services*, 18, 97–118.

Steele, B. (1987). Psychodynamic factors in child abuse. In R. E. Helfer & R. S. Kempe (Eds.), *The battered child* (4th ed., pp. 81–114). Chicago: University of Chicago Press.

Straus, M. A. (1987). Is violence toward children increasing? A comparison of 1975 and 1985 national survey rates. In R. J. Gelles (Ed.), *Family violence* (2nd ed., pp. 78–88). Newbury Park, CA: Sage.

Straus, M., & Gelles, R. J. (1990). How violent are American families? Estimates from the national family violence resurvey and other studies. In M. A. Straus & R. J. Gelles (Eds.), *Physical violence in American families: Risk factors and adaptations to violence in 8145 families*. New Brunswick, NJ: Transaction.

Straus, M. A., Gelles, R. J., & Steinmetz, S. K. (1980). *Behind closed doors: Violence in American families*. Garden City, NY: Anchor.

Straus, M. A., & Kantor, G. K. (1987). Stress & child abuse. In R. E. Helfer & R. S. Kempe (Eds.), *The battered child*. Chicago: University of Chicago Press.

Sullivan, P. M., & Knutson, J. F. (1998). The association between child maltreatment and disabilities in a hospital-based epidemiological study. *Child Abuse and Neglect, 22,* 271–288.

Sullivan, P. M., & Knutson, J. F. (2000). Maltreatment and disabilities: A population-based epidemiological study. *Child Abuse and Neglect, 24,* 1257–1274.

Theodore, A. D., Chang, J. J., Runyan, D. K., Hunter, W. M., Bangdiwala, S. I., & Agans, R. (2005). Epidemiologic features of the physical and sexual maltreatment of children in the Carolinas. *Pediatrics, 115,* e331–e337.

Tjaden, T. N. (2000). *Extent, nature, and consequences of intimate partner violence: Findings from the National Violence against Women Survey*. Washington, DC: Department of Justice (US), Publication No. NCJ 181867.

U.S. Bureau of the Census (1993). *Statistical abstract of the United States, 1993* (113th ed.). Washington, DC: Government Printing Office. Retrieved September 6, 2007 from http://www2.census.gov/prod2/statcomp/documents/1993-03.pdf

U.S. Department of Health and Human Services. (1993). *A report on the maltreatment of children with disabilities*, James Bell Associates, Inc., No. 105-89-16300. Washington, DC: Westat, Inc.

U.S. Department of Justice. (2007). Key facts at a glance: Direct expenditures by criminal justice function, 1982–2005. Bureau of Justice Statistics. Retrieved September 5, 2007 from http://www.ojp.usdoj.gov/gis/glance/tables/exptyptab.htm

U.S. Department of Labor. (2007). National compensation survey: Occupational wages in the United States, June 2006. U.S. Bureau of Justice Statistics. Retrieved September 5, 2007 from http://www.ojp.usdoj.gov/bis/glance/tables/exptyptab.htm

U.S. Department of Health and Human Services. Administration for Children and Families. (2008a). Child maltreatment 2006. Accessed April 15, 2009, http://www.acf.hhs.gov/programs/cb/pubs/cm06/cm06.pdf

U.S. Department of Health and Human Services. Administration for Children and Families. (2008b). Child abuse prevention and treatment act. Accessed March 30, 2009, http://www.acf.hhs.gov/programs/cb/laws_policies/cblaws/capta/capta1.htm#101.

U.S. Department of Health and Human Services. Administration for Children and Families. (2008c). Child Welfare Information Gateway. Child abuse and neglect fatalities: Statistics and intervention. Accessed March 27, 2009, http://www.childwelfare.gov/pubs/factsheets/fatality.pdf

U.S. Department of Health and Human Services. Administration for Children and Families. (2009). National incidence study of child abuse and neglect (NIS-4) https://www.nis4.org/nishome.asp

U.S. Department of Health and Human Services. Children's Bureau, Administration on Children, Youth, Families. Administration for Children and Families. National Clearing House on Child Abuse and Neglect Information. In Harm's Way: Domestic Violence and Child Maltreatment. Accessed May 11, 2009, http://www.calib.com/dvcps/facts/harmway.doc

Walker, E. A., Unutzer, J., Rutter, C. Gelfand, A., Saunders, K., VonKorff, M., et al. (1999). Costs of health care use by women HMO members with a history of childhood abuse and neglect. Archives of General Psychiatry, 56, 609613. Retrieved August 22, 2007 from http://archpsyc.ama-assn.org/cgi/reprint/56/7/609?ck=nck

Wang, C.-T., & Holton, J. (2007) Total estimated cost of child abuse and neglect in the United States. Economic Impact Study. Prevent Child Abuse America. Chicago, IL.   http://www.preventchildabuse.org/about_us/media_releases/pcaa_pew_economic_impact_study_final.pdf

Westat, I. (1993). *A report on the maltreatment of children with disabilities*. Washington, DC: National Center on Child Abuse and Neglect.

White, R., Benedict, M. I., Wulff, L., & Kelly, M. (1987). Physical disabilities as risk factors for child maltreatment: A selected review. *Physical Disabilities, 57*, 93–101.

Widom, C. S., Czaja, S. J., & Dutton, M. A. (2008). Childhood victimization and lifetime revictimization. *Child Abuse and Neglect, 32,* 785–796.

Widom, C. S., & Maxfield, M. G. (2001, Feburary). An Update on the "Cycle of Violence". National Institute of Justice. Research in Brief. U.S. Department of Justice. Office of Justice Programs. National Institute of Justice. http://www.ncjrs.gov/pdffiles1/nij/184894.pdf

Wissow, L. S. (1990). Child maltreatment. In F. A. Oski, C. D. DeAngelis, R. D. Feigin, & J. B. Warshaw (Eds.), *Principles & practice of pediatrics* (pp. 589–605). Philadelphia: J. B. Lippincott.

Zolotor, A. J., Theodore, A. D., Chang, J. J., Berkoff, M. C., & Runyan, D. K. (2008). Speak softly – Forget the stick: Corporal punishment and child physical abuse. *American Journal of Preventive Medicine, 35*(4), 364–369.

Zuravin, S. J. (1989). The ecology of child abuse and neglect: Review of literature and presentation of data. *Violence and Victims, 4*(2), 101–120.

Chapter 2

Evaluation of Physical Abuse and Neglect

Rebecca G. Girardet and Angelo P. Giardino

Approach to the Medical Evaluation

It may be difficult to identify children who are victims of physical abuse. Many injuries are not pathognomonic, and the diagnosis may not be obvious (Kellogg et al., 2007). The history given by the caregiver may be misleading or incomplete, causing a delay or mistake in diagnosis. In addition, victims of abuse often are too young to provide a history. Although only a small percentage of injuries seen by health care professionals are the result of abuse, there are a number of historical and physical findings that should raise the suspicion of nonaccidental trauma.

Diagnosing child abuse requires knowledge of child development, the epidemiology of trauma, mechanisms of injury in children, and the differential diagnosis of various forms of injury. The medical evaluation includes a history, physical examination, indicated laboratory and diagnostic studies, and observation of the caregiver–child interaction. Careful attention to the possibility of child maltreatment in the differential diagnosis generated when evaluating children for injuries is essential. There is a growing body of evidence highlighting the devastating consequences of cases in which an initial evaluation fails to diagnose abuse only to present again for care later with additional injuries. These later injuries could have been prevented had the child been accurately diagnosed as having been maltreated when they first presented on the initial or previous evaluations (Jenny, Hymel, Ritzen, Reinert, & Hay, 1999; Skellern, Wood, & Crawford, 2000). Of note, Jenny and colleagues (1999) retrospectively reviewed medical records from a 5-year period of time of children presenting with head trauma and of 173 abused children, 54 (31.2%) has

31

A.P. Giardino et al. (eds.), *A Practical Guide to the Evaluation of Child Physical Abuse and Neglect*, DOI 10.1007/978-1-4419-0702-8_2, © Springer Science+Business Media, LLC 1997, 2010

been seen by a physician after the abusive head trauma injury and the diagnosis was
not recognized (Jenny et al., 1999). Fifteen of the children (27.8%) sustained additional injury after the diagnosis was missed and 22 (40.7%) experienced medical
complications related to the failure to diagnose the abuse. The authors conclude that
4 of 5 deaths in the group of unrecognized abusive head trauma might have been
prevented had the maltreatment been recognized upon earlier presentation (Jenny
et al., 1999). The recognition of abuse stems from the "building block" approach,
which synthesizes data from each part of the clinical evaluation to develop and confirm a suspicion of abuse (Ludwig, 2005) (see Figure 2.1, 2.2, and 2.3). Completing
a detailed history and physical examination is paramount because many cases of
abuse are first detected by identifying discrepancies between the history and physical findings. It is ideal for two health care providers, such as a physician and nurse
or social worker, to obtain a history together. The likelihood that important questions will be missed decreases if more than one person is present to interview the
family. In addition, information can be recorded by one person while the other asks
questions. After the interview, the questioners can review information for accuracy.

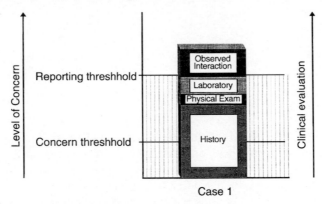

Case 1

Figure 2.1 Building block approach to diagnosis of child maltreatment. Each component
of the clinical evaluation is viewed as a building block that, as they are stacked during the
process of the evaluation, can lead to higher and higher levels of concern. At a certain point,
the stack of blocks may lead to a reporting threshold for the clinician.
Source: (Ludwig, 2005) used with permission.

The History and Interview

A complete history elicited by the health care provider helps determine whether an
injury is the result of abuse or an accident. Professionals who evaluate injured children and their families consider the possibility of abuse when evaluating all pediatric
injuries. Although the majority of childhood injuries seen by medical personnel are
accidental, missing a case of child abuse puts the patient at great risk for future
injury (Kellogg et al., 2007). In a comprehensive review of injury biomechanics
research, Pierce and Bertocci call attention to child maltreatment being the leading
cause of trauma-related death in children under 4 years of age and specifically state:
"...many of these children present for medical care with earlier warning signs of

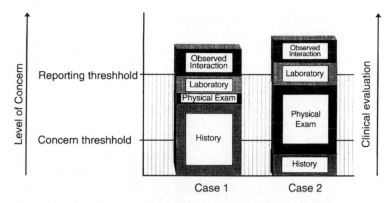

Figure 2.2 Building block approach to diagnosis of child maltreatment. The blocks may be of different sizes depending on how much of a concern the information is that is uncovered during that component of the evaluation. In Case 1, the history is very much of a concern for abuse and contributes a great deal toward reaching the clinician's reporting threshold. In Case 2, the history is of minimal concern, but the physical examination contributes a great deal toward reaching the clinician's reporting threshold.
Source: (Ludwig, 2005) used with permission.

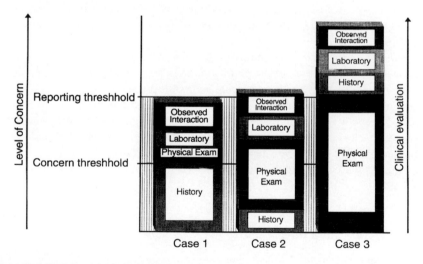

Figure 2.3 Building block approach to diagnosis of child maltreatment. Case 3 demonstrates how one component can be so much of a concern that it alone causes the clinician to reach a reporting threshold (e.g., the physical findings of loop marks on a child's skin).
Source: (Ludwig, 2005) used with permission.

maltreatment where the diagnosis of abuse was missed or the significance of the injury was not recognized" (Jenny et al., 1999; Pierce & Bertocci, 2008; Skellern et al., 2000).

It is important to be thorough yet nonaccusatory during the evaluation (Kellogg et al., 2007). Health care providers conduct a health care evaluation and as such are not investigators and do not apportion blame. The health care history or interview is conducted professionally, without displays of anger or reproach that would serve only to alienate the caregiver and not improve the condition of the child.

Documentation

It is essential to complete a detailed medical record in cases of suspected physical abuse. A standardized form can be used to document the evaluation (see Appendix). Health care providers are asked to justify the medical diagnosis more commonly in child abuse cases than for almost any other pediatric condition. County social workers, law enforcement officials, and attorneys often become involved in cases of child abuse, and details regarding the medical findings are necessary for their investigations. Health care professionals are often asked to testify in criminal or civil court regarding the child's injuries and the basis for the diagnosis of abuse (see Chapter 15).

A complete and thorough medical record is essential because court proceedings may occur 1–2 years after the child is injured. Although the health care professional may have some independent memory of the case, it may be difficult to recall details months or years after the examination was completed. A health care provider who has had the painful experience of reviewing a record in court that is incomplete or substandard recognizes the need for meticulously documented information as it relates to the abused child.

The details of the history and interview are documented in the record using quotes to indicate exact responses of the child whenever possible. Because the record is a legal document that may be used in legal and court proceedings, it is necessary that statements reflect the nonleading and unbiased nature of the questions asked in the history, interview, and examination. The record is written clearly to document all significant history related to past and present occurrences of abuse or neglect. The record should contain the date and time of injury, the identity of the caregivers who bring the child for care, and any reasons offered for or denials of any known trauma to the child.

The Caregiver–Child Interaction

An essential component of the child abuse evaluation is the observation of how the caregiver and child interact with one another (Schmitt, Grosz, & Carroll, 1976). Of great concern to the health care provider are caregivers who seem unaware of the seriousness of the child's injuries, are indifferent to the child's needs, or appear unsupportive of the child. Additional concern arises when the caregiver belittles the child, is overly directive in his or her communication, and is inattentive to the child's requests. Children who interact with their caregiver in an unusual manner and do not look to their caregiver for emotional support are also of concern. Caregivers and children vary in their response to stress and trauma and may not be behaving normally in an emergency setting. Caution is taken to avoid overgeneralizing and attributing meaning or blame to these observations in the acute clinical setting.

History Related to Injuries

The history is integral in establishing the diagnosis of child abuse. A thorough approach to history taking in all cases of trauma identifies injuries that may have been inflicted. A standard format for gathering medical data is used that includes chief complaint, history of present illness, review of symptoms, and past medical and psychosocial history. Family history related to bleeding disorders, osteogenesis imperfecta, or other injury-related disorders is important to include. Children who are verbal often can provide a history of injury, unless they are developmentally impaired, in a great deal of pain, or frightened. As a general rule, separating the caregivers and verbal child helps to obtain a more reliable history from the child. For injured infants and young children, it is common for the caregiver to provide the history. The improvement of verbal abilities in children as they reach school age is reflected in the details that the child describes regarding an injury. A school-aged child would be expected to know some of the details surrounding the circumstances around a significant injury unless a clinical reason exists for lack of memory such as a head injury.

Regardless of who provides information, the history begins by asking for a narrative of the injury. The interviewer then asks questions to clarify confusing statements and fill in missing details in the story. It is important to ask open-ended, nonleading questions. The following are questions that should be explored in all evaluations (see Table 2.1).

Table 2.1 Central questions related to the injury.

What was the date and time of the injury?
Where did the injury occur?
Who was caring for the child at the time of the injury? Did the caregiver witness the injury?
What events preceded the injury?
What was the child's reaction to the injury?
What did the caregiver do after the injury occurred?

1. *What was the date and approximate time that the injury occurred?* In some cases, a history of injury cannot be provided, either because the adult with the child was not present at the time of the injury or because there was no known trauma to the child. In this situation, it is important to know when the child last seemed perfectly well. For example, an infant who sustained a femur fracture may have been injured by a parent prior to being dropped off at the babysitter, only to be recognized by late morning, when the caregiver noted swelling of the leg. A history of irritability throughout the morning would support this scenario, whereas a history of playfulness and well-being all morning would not.
2. *Where did the injury occur?* Abusive injuries are most commonly sustained in the privacy of the home rather than in public places. Accidental injuries that occur in public often have been witnessed by unrelated adults who may provide

information to police or emergency medical technicians (EMTs). This information can corroborate an accidental mechanism of injury.

3. *Did the caregiver witness the injury?* In an attempt to provide a history of trauma, caregivers sometimes provide a likely scenario for an injury they did not actually witness. Determine whether the injury was witnessed or unwitnessed. Both can be accidental. Ask detailed questions regarding the injury, such as approximate distance the child fell, the surface onto which the child fell, the position in which the child landed, parts of the body that appeared to be injured, and whether there were any objects in the path of the fall.

4. *What events preceded the injury?* What were the child and caregiver doing just before the injury? Search for signs of chaos or stress, which maybe related to abusive injuries. For example, an infant who sustains abusive head injury may have kept a tired caregiver up all night and then refused a bottle that was meant to quiet the baby. Beware of claims that a child with major injury went for hours or days without pathology or changes in behavior.

5. *What was the child's reaction to the injury?* Determine whether the child's reported behavior after the injury is compatible with the disability or pain caused by the injury.

6. *What did the caregiver do after the injury?* Determine when the caregiver first noted the injuries and what treatment was given to the child prior to being seen by a health care provider.

7. *How much time elapsed between the injury and the time the child arrived for medical care?* If significant time elapsed, determine what occurred during that time and the reason for the delay. If there was a delay in seeking care, determine why the caregiver chose this time to bring the child for evaluation.

Past Medical History

The past medical history of the child may help to identify suspicious injuries and medical conditions that can be mistaken for abuse. In evaluating suspicious injuries, the interviewer asks about the child's health to reassure the caregiver that he or she is interested in the child's well-being and not merely trying to apportion blame for an injury. The interviewer explores the child's general health, previous hospitalizations, operations, and any past significant trauma. Document what the caregiver states in the initial history about trauma and the child and if the caregiver denies any recent or past trauma to the child. It is essential to obtain phone numbers and addresses of the caretakers and family members for future reference.

It is important to determine former injuries that the child sustained and where the child was treated. In abuse, there may be evidence of old and unexplained injury. This is accomplished by asking the caregiver and by checking past records within the same hospital, at other hospitals, and at facilities or offices where the child has been treated. The history uncovers whether the child receives regular health care with a single provider or has been to multiple physicians. Abusive caregivers often bring children with inflicted injuries to multiple medical care providers in an attempt to avoid the recognition of abuse. Although seeking care with multiple health care providers may indicate abuse, it is not a definite indicator. The interviewer explores reasons for using multiple health care providers and then reviews old records.

The past medical history reflects information about the mother's pregnancy and the child's birth. Family history explores the health of family members and inheritable diseases that may affect the diagnosis of the child such as osteogenesis imperfecta, bleeding and bone disorders, and Ehlers-Danlos syndrome.

A developmental history of the child is obtained that includes the child's present level of abilities and the age at which the child reached standard developmental milestones. For school-aged children, it is important to know if the child requires any special education and how the child functions in school. An understanding of normal child development is essential in evaluating injuries that are said to be self-inflicted. In addition, a child's slow development may be a source of frustration and stress for a caregiver, thereby increasing the risk for abuse in some situations (see Table 2.2).

Table 2.2 Developmental milestones.

Age	Physical characteristics	Social-emotional intellectual characteristics
0–3 months	Raises head and chest when lying on stomach Supports upper body with arms when lying on stomach Stretches legs out and kicks when lying on stomach or back Opens and shuts hands Pushes down on legs when feet are placed on a firm surface Brings hand to mouth Takes swipes at dangling objects with hands Grasps and shakes hand toys *Vision* Watches faces intently Follows moving objects Recognizes familiar objects and people at a distance Starts using hands and eyes in coordination *Hearing and speech* Smiles at the sound of your voice Begins to babble Begins to imitate some sounds Turns head toward direction of sound	Begins to develop a social smile Enjoys playing with other people and may cry when playing stops Becomes more expressive and communicates more with face and body Imitates some movements and facial expressions

Table 2.2 (continued)

Age	Physical characteristics	Social-emotional intellectual characteristics
3–7 months	*Movement* Rolls both ways (front to back, back to front) Sits with, and then without, support on hand Supports whole weight on legs Reaches with one hand Transfers object from hand to hand Uses hand to rake objects *Vision* Develops full color vision Distance vision matures Ability to track moving objects improves *Cognitive* Finds partially hidden object Explores with hands and mouth Struggles to get objects that are out of reach *Language* Responds to own name Begins to respond to "no" Can tell emotions by tone of voice Responds to sound by making sounds Uses voice to express joy and displeasure Babbles chains of sounds	Enjoys social play Interested in mirror images Responds to other people's expressions of emotion and appears joyful often
8–12 months	*Movement* Reaches sitting position without assistance Crawls forward on belly Assumes hands-and-knees position Creeps on hands and knees Gets from sitting to crawling or prone (lying on stomach) position Pulls self up to stand Walks holding on to furniture (cruising) Stands momentarily without support May walk two or three steps without support	Shy or anxious with strangers Cries when mother or father leaves Enjoys imitating people in his play Shows specific preferences for certain people and toys Tests parental responses to his actions during feedings Tests parental responses to his behavior May be fearful in some situations Prefers mother and/or regular caregiver over all others Repeats sounds or gestures for attention

Table 2.2 (continued)

Age	Physical characteristics	Social-emotional intellectual characteristics
	Cognitive	Finger-feeds himself
	Explores objects in many different ways (shaking, banging, throwing, dropping)	Extends arm or leg to help when being dressed
	Finds hidden objects easily	
	Looks at correct picture when the image is named	
	Imitates gestures	
	Begins to use objects correctly (drinking from cup, brushing hair, dialing phone, listening to receiver)	
	Language	
	Pays increasing attention to speech	
	Responds to simple verbal requests	
	Responds to "no"	
	Uses simple gestures, such as shaking head for "no"	
	Babbles with inflection (changes in tone)	
	Says "dada" and "mama"	
	Uses exclamations, such as "Oh-oh!"	
	Tries to imitate words	
	Hand and finger skills	
	Uses pincer grasp	
	Bangs two objects together	
	Puts objects into container	
	Takes objects out of container	
	Lets objects go voluntarily	
	Pokes with index finger	
	Tries to imitate scribbling	
13–24 months	*Movement*	Imitates behavior of others, especially adults and other children
	Walks alone	
	Pulls toys behind her while walking	
	Carries large toy or several toys while walking	More aware of herself as separate from others
	Begins to run	More excited about company of other children
	Stands on tiptoes	
	Kicks a ball	Demonstrates increasing independence
	Climbs onto and down from furniture unassisted	Begins to show defiant behavior
	Walks up and down stairs holding on to support	Separation anxiety increases toward midyear then fades

Table 2.2 (continued)

Age	Physical characteristics	Social-emotional intellectual characteristics
	Cognitive Finds objects even when hidden under two or three covers Begins to sort by shapes and colors Begins make-believe play *Language* Points to object or picture when it's named Recognizes names of familiar people, objects and body parts Says several single words (by 15–18 months) Uses simple phrases (by 18–24 months) Uses 2- to 4-word sentences Follows simple instructions Repeats words overheard in conversation *Hand and finger skills* Scribbles on his or her own Turns over container to pour out contents Builds tower of four blocks or more Might use one hand more often than the other	
25–36 months	*Movement* Climbs well Walks up and down stairs, alternating feet (1 ft per stair step) Kicks ball Runs easily Pedals tricycle Bends over easily without falling *Cognitive* Makes mechanical toys work Matches an object in her hand or room to a picture in a book Plays make-believe with dolls, animals, and people Sorts objects by shape and color Completes puzzles with three or four pieces Understands concept of "two" *Language* Follows a two- or three-part command Recognizes and identifies almost all common objects and pictures	Imitates adults and playmates Spontaneously shows affection for familiar playmates Can take turns in games Understands concept of "mine" and "his/hers" Expresses affection openly Expresses a wide range of emotions By 3, separates easily from parents Objects to major changes in routine

Table 2.2 (continued)

Age	Physical characteristics	Social-emotional intellectual characteristics
	Understands most sentences	
	Understands placement in space ("on," "in," "under")	
	Uses 4- to 5-word sentences	
	Can say name, age, and sex	
	Uses pronouns (I, you, me, we, they) and some plurals (cars, dogs, cats)	
	Strangers can understand most of her words	
	Hand and finger skills	
	Makes up-and-down, side-to-side, and circular lines with pencil or crayon	
	Turns book pages one at a time	Imitates adults and playmates
	Builds a tower of more than six blocks	Spontaneously shows affection for familiar playmates
	Holds a pencil in writing position	Can take turns in games
	Screws and unscrews jar lids, nuts, and bolts	Understands concept of "mine" and "his/hers"
	Turns rotating handles	Expresses affection openly
		Expresses a wide range of emotions
		By 3, separates easily from parents
		Objects to major changes in routine
37–48 months	*Movement*	Interested in new experiences
	Hops and stands on 1 ft up to 5 seconds	Cooperates with other children
	Goes upstairs and downstairs without support	Plays "Mom" or "Dad"
	Kicks ball forward	Increasingly inventive in fantasy play
	Throws ball overhand	Dresses and undresses
	Catches bounced ball most of the time	Negotiates solutions to conflicts
	Moves forward and backward with agility	More independent
	Cognitive	Imagines that many unfamiliar images may be "monster"
	Correctly names some colors	Views self as a whole person involving body, mind, and feelings
	Understands the concept of counting and may know a few numbers	Often cannot tell the difference between fantasy and reality
	Tries to solve problems from a single point of view	
	Begins to have a clearer sense of time	
	Follows three-part commands	
	Recalls parts of a story	
	Understands the concepts of "same" and different	
	Engages in fantasy play	

Table 2.2 (continued)

Age	Physical characteristics	Social-emotional intellectual characteristics
	Language Has mastered some basic rules of grammar Speaks in sentences of five to six words Speaks clearly enough for strangers to understand Tells stories	
49–60 months	*Movement* Stands on 1 ft for 10 seconds or longer Hops, somersaults Swings, climbs May be able to skip *Cognitive milestones* Can count 10 or more objects Correctly names at least four colors Better understands the concept of time home (money, food, appliances) *Language* Recalls part of a story Speaks sentences of more than five words Uses future tense Tells longer stories Says name and address Hand and finger skills Copies triangle and other shapes Draws person with body Prints some letters Dresses and undresses without help Uses fork, spoon, and (sometimes) a table knife Usually cares for own toilet needs	Wants to please friends Wants to be like her friends More likely to agree to rules Likes to sing, dance, and act Shows more independence and may even visit a next-door neighbor by herself Aware of gender Able to distinguish fantasy from reality Sometimes demanding, sometimes eagerly cooperative

Finally, the social history of the family is explored, including family composition and individuals living in and outside the home. The social history includes financial and emotional supports for the family and recent or chronic family stresses. Caregivers are screened for alcohol and/or drug abuse and a history of domestic violence (see Chapters 11 and 14).

Histories That Raise the Concern for Abuse

There are a number of historical clues that raise suspicion of abuse (Kellogg et al., 2007). None is used in isolation to diagnose maltreatment. The health care professional considers the complete history when evaluating children with injuries. The following are factors that raise the suspicion for abuse:

- History of trauma that is incongruous, inconsistent, or not plausible with the physical examination
- History of minor trauma with extensive physical injury
- History of no trauma with evidence of injury (magical injuries)
- History of self-inflicted trauma that is incompatible with child's development
- History of the injury changes with time
- Delays in seeking treatment
- Caregiver ascribes blame for serious injuries to a young sibling or playmate

History Incongruous with the Physical Examination

History of Minor Trauma with Extensive Physical Injury

Infants and young children are relatively resistant to injuries from both common household falls and free falls of low–moderate heights. *A history of minor trauma that results in serious or life-threatening injury to a child should be suspect, and an evaluation for possible abuse should be performed.* A number of studies have examined the consequences of minor trauma (Bertocci et al., 2004; Chadwick et al., 2008; Chiaviello, Christoph, and Bond, 1994; Helfer, 1977; Joffe & Ludwig, 1988; Johnson et al., 2005; Lyons & Oates, 1993; Khambalia et al., 2006; Nimityongskul & Anderson, 1987; Tarantino, Dowd, & Murdock, 1999). Joffe and Ludwig (1988) analyzed pediatric stairway injuries. Of 363 consecutive children seen in a pediatric emergency department after falling down stairs, none had life-threatening injuries or required intensive care. A majority of patients sustained minor soft tissue injuries such as abrasions and contusions. Seven percent of the children fractured one bone, most commonly the skull or a distal extremity. Only three children required hospitalization, all for observations after head trauma. Stairway falls did not result in abdominal visceral injuries, multiple fractures, intracranial hemorrhages, or cerebral contusions. Overall, stairway injuries resulted in occasional significant injuries but much less than free falls of the same vertical distance. Severe, truncal, and proximal extremity injuries did not occur in this population. Chiaviello et al. (1994) reviewed 69 children less than 5 years of age who fell down the stairs. The majority of injuries were minor and involved the head and neck. Injuries to more than one body area did not occur. In contrast to Joffe and Ludwig's (1988) findings, a few children sustained significant head injury including one child with a subdural hematoma, one with a C-2 fracture, and two with cerebral contusions. Further evidence for the typical minor nature of common household injuries comes from Warrington, Wright and colleagues who used a large regional data base from the United Kingdom to assess the characteristics of injuries to non-ambulatory infants over their first 6 months of life and based on 11,466 parental responses to a mailed questionnaire. Surprisingly, 22% of infants (2,554 children) had experienced a fall, 53% from a bed and 12% from caregiver's arms. Injuries were infrequent and "generally trivial" (p. 107) with only 14% reporting a visible injury almost always to the head, with 56% suffering a bruise and less than 1% suffering a serious injury described as a concussion or fracture. (Warrington & Wright, 2001).

In one of the largest studies of short falls to date, Chadwick and colleagues reviewed injury databases, peer-reviewed articles, previous literature reviews, and other published materials to calculate the risk of death resulting from falls of less than 1.5 meter among children up to 5 years of age. They arrived at an overall incidence of less than 0.48 deaths per 1 million children and discovered no reliable reports of short fall deaths among children in day care centers (Chadwick et al., 2008). Similarly, a systematic review by Khambalia of risk factors for unintentional injuries due to falls in children 0–6 years of age concluded that it is uncommon for children to suffer serious injury from falls of less than 5 feet (Khambalia et al., 2006).

Tarantino, Dowd, and Murdock studied the medical records for 167 infants and found significant injuries in 25 (15%), which included skull fractures, other skeletal fractures, and 2 children with intracranial bleeds. The children with intracranial bleeds were later determined to have been abused. After excluding these two children, the only risk factor found to be independently associated with injury was being dropped by the caretaker as opposed to rolling off of a bed or other object (Tarantino et al., 1999). In separate studies, Helfer (1977), Lyons and Oates (1993), and Nimityongskul and Anderson (1987) reviewed injuries sustained to children who fell out of bed while in the hospital. Of approximately 450 children who fell out of beds or cribs from a height of less than 4.5 feet, none was seriously injured. Most sustained no identifiable injuries. All injuries were minor such as contusions, small lacerations, or an occasional skull or clavicular fracture.

Whereas falls from single beds result in minimal injury, bunk bed injuries tend to be more severe. Selbst, Baker, and Shames (1990) prospectively studied children seen in a pediatric emergency department after bunk bed injuries. Lacerations (40% of patients) and contusions (28% of patients) were the most common injuries. One percent of patients sustained a concussion and 10% of patients fractured a bone. Although 9% of patients required hospitalization, no life-threatening, internal-abdominal, neck, or genital injuries or deaths resulted from bunk beds in this study.

A number of studies examined the relationship between the height of free falls and injury and death in children. These studies show that the predominant injury in falls from heights occurs to the head and skeleton. Using a test dummy to simulate feet-first free falls of a 3-year-old child, Bertocci and colleagues found a low risk of contact-type head injury for short distance falls, regardless of surface type, and less head acceleration for falls onto playground foam as compared to wood, linoleum, or padded carpet. However, playground foam was associated with a higher incidence of bending of the lower extremities, likely because the dummy foot was more likely to stick to the foam upon landing (as opposed to sliding free) (Bertocci et al., 2004). Musemeche, Barthel, Cosentino, and Reynolds (1991) reviewed the outcomes of children who fell more than 10 ft (or at least one story). Of the 70 records reviewed, the majority of children fell from one to three stories. Head (54%) and skeletal (33%) trauma were common but no deaths occurred. Chadwick, Chin, Salerno, Landsverk, and Kitchen (1991) reviewed the outcome of 317 children with a reported fall who were seen at a pediatric trauma center. Interestingly, 7 of the 100 children who reportedly fell less than 4 ft died of their injuries, whereas no deaths occurred in 65 children who fell between 5 and 9 ft and only one child died who fell between 10 and 45 ft. Further analysis of the data showed that the seven children who died from short falls were victims of abuse whose caretakers falsified their history. In contrast to these reports, Plunkett concluded that it is possible for children to die in falls of less than 3 meter, based on a case series of 18 deaths reported to the National Electronic Injury Surveillance System (NEISS). However, many of the falls in this series were either unwitnessed or supported by unclear histories, and several involved rotational forces such as falls off of swings. One child had a platelet count of 24,000 at the time of hospital admission for his fall (Plunkett, 2001). Estimating the population base for the NEISS sample to be approximately 400,000 for children 0–5 years and determining that among the nine deaths in young children only three appeared to have truly represented short fall deaths, Chadwick and colleagues concluded that the risk of death in the Plunkett sample was 0.625 cases per 1 million young children per year (Chadwick et al., 2008). Williams (1991) studied 106 children younger than 3 years of age who sustained free falls and whose history was corroborated by a person other than the caregiver. Other than three children who sustained depressed skull fractures from falls less than 10 ft, no life-threatening or other serious injuries (intracranial hemorrhage, cerebral edema or contusion, ruptured organ, or compound or comminuted fracture) occurred from falls from this height. Severe injuries occurred in 11 patients who fell between 10 and 40 ft. One child died from a fall of 70 ft. These data again show *that falls of less than 10 ft are unlikely to produce life-threatening injury or death.*

A History of No Trauma with Evidence of Injury (Magical Injury)

In most cases of accidental injury, the history of trauma can be explained by a caregiver or a verbal child. Minor injuries, such as small bruises, minor scrapes, or lacerations, are often unexplained. The trauma associated with these injuries is often minimal and not remembered. It is important to distinguish between unwitnessed and inflicted trauma because not all accidental trauma is witnessed. Children may sustain injuries when they are out of sight of their caregivers. In cases of significant unwitnessed injury to preverbal children, the health care provider obtains historical details related to specific events surrounding the time of the injury. For unwitnessed trauma, determine the child's condition before and after the event. It is important to determine the position in which the child was found and to describe any changes in behavior after the incident, such as refusal to walk. The history also includes the sequence of events from the time of the injury until the child was taken for medical care. For example, a toddler fracture (spiral tibial fracture in a young child) may result from a simple fall (Mellick & Reesor, 1990). The caregiver states that the child ran into the next room and soon screamed. He was found sitting on the floor, crying. After being held, he refused to bear weight on his leg. The caregiver sat him on the couch and gave him juice to calm him down. After an hour, he still refused to bear weight on his leg and was brought for medical evaluation. This scenario is consistent with the finding of a toddler's fracture.

Caregivers describe various scenarios to explain identified injuries. They may provide a false history or deny that the child sustained any trauma. It is the norm that children with significant injury have some history related to a traumatic event. Children with "magical injuries," that seemingly occur spontaneously, are likely to be victims of abuse. *In cases of unexplained injury, the suspicion of abuse generally increases as the age of the child decreases.* Infants in the first 6 months of life are not developmentally capable of self-inflicting significant trauma. Depending on the severity of injury and the age and developmental abilities of the patient, magical injuries may be either pathognomonic of abuse or just one factor to consider in evaluating for the possibility of maltreatment.

A History of Self-Inflicted Trauma Incompatible with the Development of the Child

The possibility of child abuse is considered when the history of trauma is discordant with the child's developmental abilities. Caregivers may claim that injuries to abused children are self-inflicted (or inflicted by peers or siblings). In some cases, the child is developmentally incapable of injuring him- or herself in the manner described. Therefore, knowledge of infant and child development is essential to the evaluation of pediatric injuries.

Children develop increasingly complex motor abilities during the first years of life. Although the acquisition of new skills follows a predictable sequence, the rate and, to some extent, the order in which children reach new developmental milestones vary (see Table 2.2). As infants and young children gain new motor skills, the risk of self-inflicted injury increases as they explore their environment.

Whenever there is a report of a child with a self-inflicted injury, the health care provider considers the compatibility of the child's development and the history of the injury provided. A history of self-inflicted injury requires careful evaluation. Most self-inflicted injuries in young children are minor, although serious and life-threatening injuries can occur. Toddlers, for example, can pull hot liquids off of stove tops or counters and can crawl out of unprotected windows (Barlow, Niemirska, Ghandi, & Leblanc, 1983; Finkelstein, Schwartz, Madden, Marano, & Goodwin, 1992).

A careful and detailed history is obtained to determine whether a child's developmental ability conflicts with the history of trauma. Always ask open-ended, nonleading questions that do not put words or thoughts into the mind of the history giver. The caregiver's ability to provide precise descriptions may vary, causing an erroneous suspicion of abuse. For example, a 1-month-old infant brought for medical care because of irritability after "rolling off the couch" is found to have a linear parietal skull fracture. The history is suspicious because of the apparent discrepancy between the "rolling" and the motor abilities of most 1-month-old infants. Further history reveals that the baby actually squirmed off the couch when the mother left him to answer the phone on the other side of the room. The history is now more reasonable with regard to the child's development and the suspicion of an inflicted injury lessened.

Caregiver Blame for Serious Injuries on a Young Child

Caregivers may falsely ascribe an injury to an incident with a sibling or young child in an attempt to protect themselves. Verbal children are sometimes coerced into blaming a sibling for an injury out of fear of losing a parent or of further injury if the truth is discovered. On occasion, a child may seriously injure a sibling. A decades old case series by Rosenthal and Doherty (1984) reports on 10 preschool children who either seriously injured siblings or attempted to do so. They described skull and leg fractures, extensive bruising, lacerations, and stab wounds. Although siblings do fight and injuries can result, serious or life-threatening injuries are not commonly attributable to young children. Children with multiple or serious injuries are not often injured by another young child, and the possibility of abuse should be raised in this situation.

In some cases, an injury inflicted by a child can be distinguished from that of an adult. For example, bite marks are sometimes abusive injuries that are blamed on young children. The size of the bite arc and the individual teeth can often differentiate adult and pediatric bites (Barsley & Landcaster, 1987; Kemp et al., 2006). (See Chapter 9 for further discussion of bite marks.)

History of Injury Changes with Time

It is common for an abusive caregiver to provide a false history of injury or illness and to expand or change the history. *Documented histories that change over time increase the suspicion of abuse and support the diagnosis.* However, to obtain a complete and detailed history, the health care provider asks for detail and clarification of confusing statements. The caregiver of a seriously injured child initially may be overwhelmed and too upset to provide a coherent, detailed history. More detailed information obtained later during the evaluation may be misinterpreted as a changing history.

Delay in Seeking Treatment

Caregivers who have abused a child sometimes delay a medical visit until the injuries have partially resolved. Some children are brought for immediate medical care by either the abusive caregiver or an unrelated adult, whereas others are brought for care only when an adult uninvolved with the abuse recognizes the injury to the child. Some seriously injured children are never taken for medical care and may die of their injuries. The suspicion of abuse arises when there is a delay in seeking appropriate treatment.

There are a number of factors to consider in determining whether a delay in seeking care is reasonable (Jenny et al., 2007). The more symptomatic the child is, the more of a concern a delay in seeking care becomes. For example, it is inappropriate to delay care in symptomatic children with life-threatening injuries such as severe closed head injury or abdominal visceral injury. Children with bone fractures may be symptomatic at the time of the injury, yet the seriousness of the injury may not always be recognized immediately. Some examples include clavicle fractures and "toddler's fractures," where the initial symptoms may be nonspecific. (See Chapter 4 for further discussion of fractures.)

In evaluating delayed treatment, it is important to ask about the child's behavior from the time of the injury. For example, a child with a broken tibia may refuse to walk on the leg or will limp and be in pain. It is suspicious when the history does not reflect these facts. Caregivers may delay seeking treatment when symptoms are nonspecific, as in young infants with closed head injury. In such cases, the history reflects a change in the behavior of the child and may help to date the injury.

A skull fracture may not be recognized for a number of days. The initial scalp hematoma associated with the fracture may expand so rapidly as to have a bony consistency. It is not until the hematoma softens that the caregiver feels the swelling and brings the child for care (Ludwig, 1993).

Caregivers may delay bringing a child for medical care until a home remedy fails to cure the patient. Burns that require medical attention are occasionally treated at home until they fail to heal or become infected. Not all of these burns are inflicted, although some professionals would categorize this type of care as neglectful. It must be noted that accidents due to neglect or lack of supervision are reportable as neglect on the part of the caregivers.

Finally, some caregivers do not bring an injured child for timely care because of true and/or perceived barriers to care. These include financial constraints, lack of transportation, work obligations, and child care problems (McCullock & Melnyk, 1988). Using an ecological framework, Jenny and the AAP's Committee on Child Abuse and Neglect call attention, especially in cases involving adolescents, to the role of the child's attitudes and behavior as a potential factor affecting adherence to medical regimens, particularly in situations where the child or adolescent is attempting to assert his or her independence by not complying with medications, treatments or special diets (Jenny et al., 2007). Although a delay in seeking care is often a flag for child abuse, each case is evaluated carefully with respect to all identified factors.

See Table 2.3 for an overview of the steps of the history taking/interview process.

Table 2.3 The interview process at a glance.

Introductions

Determine how the caregiver is related to the child

Obtain names, address, phone numbers of history givers and child

Narrative of the child's injury or medical problem (history is dependent on whether there is a history of trauma)

With history of trauma

    Date and time of the injury

    Where did the injury occur?

    Where did the injury occur?

    What were the events leading up to the injury?

    Did the caregiver witness the injury?

    Did anyone else witness the injury?

    What was the child's reaction to the injury?

    What was the caregiver's response to the injury?

With no history of trauma

    When was the last time the child appeared well?

    When did the child become ill? How did the illness begin and progress?

    Who was caring for the child when he or she first developed symptoms?

    Who were the child's caregivers in the days (hours) before the child became ill?

    What are the child's symptoms? How have the symptoms progressed?

    Was the child given any treatment?

***Clarify* any confusing statements/fill *in* missing details upset or confused caregiver may add to or change details of the history**

    Note any discrepancies in the history

Note time between onset of symptoms and arrival for evaluation

    With excessive delay, note amount of time that reportedly has elapsed

    Reasons for the delay

    Caregiver treatment for the child prior to being seen. Child's behavior since the injury (or onset of symptoms)

    Reasons for bringing the child for care at this time

Past medical history

    Child's general health, including prenatal and birth history

    Child's doctor

    Previous hospitalizations

    Previous injuries

    Treatment sites for previous injuries

    Immunization status

Developmental history

    Present developmental level

    Age of developmental milestones

    History of behavior problems

    School history, need for special education

Family/social history

    Family composition

    Health of family members

    Child's caregivers. Include those living both in and outside of the home

    Evidence of family stress

Table 2.3 (continued)

Financial supports of the family
Emotional supports for the caregivers
History of domestic violence
Screen for caregiver drug and alcohol use
Previous involvement with social services

The Physical Examination

The purpose of the examination of the physically abused child is to identify trauma and injuries. It is important to maintain the child's modesty during the examination because it can be embarrassing for the child to be completely undressed. However, the whole body should be inspected with the child wearing an examining gown or by using appropriate draping. The examination proceeds from the least to most invasive procedure, saving the obviously injured areas for last. In severe injury, pediatric life support is instituted first and then followed by a systematic assessment of the trauma.

Documentation of the physical examination includes a general description of the child, followed by plotted growth parameters. Record the location of each injury, and describe each in detail. Even minor injuries are important. Include in the description any appropriate negatives such as "abdomen was not tender," rather than using the phrase "within normal limits." Likewise, do not use the descriptor *normal* when more specific words or terms can be used. Document the color, size and shape of each bruise. Burn descriptions include location, size, patterns, lines of demarcation, and the approximate thickness of the burn. Use accurate terms such as *abrasions*, *lacerations*, *ecchymoses*, *hematomas*, and *scars*. Carefully drawn diagrams are a useful adjunct to written description. Standard forms that contain anterior and posterior line drawings of the body are helpful in documenting injuries (see Appendix).

The abuse evaluation emphasizes the following areas:

1. *Growth.* Measure the child's weight, height or length, and head circumference (when indicated) and record on a standard pediatric growth chart. If available, old growth points are plotted to evaluate the child's growth over time (see Chapter 7 for more detailed discussion).
2. *Skin.* Note bruises, burns, scars, or rashes and describe the injury in detail. Record the following characteristics of bruises: the measured size, location, pattern (if applicable), and color. Note the precise location of burns, including small splash marks, lines of demarcation, or patterns identified.
3. *Head.* Palpate for areas of swelling, bogginess, or cephalohematomas. Note step-offs or depressions overlying fractures. Observe for avulsed hair and bruises. Feel the fontanel to assess for increased intracranial pressure. It is often difficult to see scalp bruising because of the overlying hair. The scalp can be

examined further during hair shampooing if the patient is admitted to the hospital.

4. *Ears*. Note bruises to the outer ear, and check behind the ear for Battle's sign (bleeding in the subcutaneous tissue of the mastoid area due to a basilar skull fracture). Note the presence of foreign bodies and the condition of tympanic membranes. Examine the middle ear for blood (hemotympanum) or infection.

5. *Eyes*. Note evidence of direct trauma such as edema, scleral hemorrhage, hyphema, or bruises. Assess scleral color, because blue sclera is associated with osteogenesis imperfecta (see   Chapter 4). A fundoscopic examination is an essential part of the workup of an infant or young toddler who has sustained a shaking or impact injury, because up to 80% of these patients have retinal hemorrhages (Levin, 1990). It is not always possible to see the fundus well. A complete examination by an ophthalmologist is essential. Indirect ophthalmoscopy by an ophthalmologist is indicated as soon as possible in children suspected of a shaking injury.

6. *Nose*. Examine for edema, nasal bleeding, septal deviation, foreign bodies, and CSF rhinorrhea.

7. *Mouth/pharynx*. Examine for evidence of trauma. Labial or lingular frenulum lacerations (tears of the tissue that connects the gums to the midline of the upper or lower lips or the tongue to the base of the mouth) are pathognomonic of child abuse in young infants. Older infants and young toddlers can sustain these injuries accidentally by falling and hitting their mouths. The patient's teeth should be examined for trauma and caries (see Chapter 8).

8. *Chest/cardiac/lungs*. Feel for signs of healing rib fractures. Assess for tachycardia, murmurs, flow murmurs secondary to anemia, and signs of cardiac instability.

9. *Abdomen*. Listen for bowel sounds. Assess for indications of abdominal trauma, including abdominal tenderness, guarding, and rebound tenderness. Look for bruises, burns, or patterned marks.

10. *Back*. Look for bruises and unusual midline masses (which may represent vertebral injuries).

11. *Genitals/anus/rectum*. Assess for signs of trauma, including erythema, bleeding, bruising, bite marks, lacerations, abnormal anal tone, and signs of infection (see Photo 2.1). Retract labia majora and minora and assess external structures. Note Tanner Stage of development.

12. *Extremities*. Assess for soft tissue swelling, point tenderness, and function.

13. *Neurologic*. For patients with significant trauma, the Glascow Coma Scale provides a quick assessment of neurologic impairment. (Modifications in the scale are made to account for the abilities of infants and children). A neurologic exam to evaluate for focal deficits and to assess for cerebral or spinal injury is indicated in all children with possible head trauma.

14. *Development*. A developmental screening examination is done if the child is clinically stable.

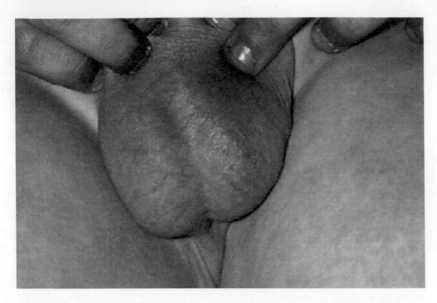

Photo 2.1 Scrotum trauma—punch to the scrotum.

See Table 2.4 for an overview of the physical examination.

Table 2.4 Overview of the Physical Examination

Extremities
Look for bruises
Feel for tenderness, fractures, joint pain
Assess function
Neurologic
Glascow Coma Scale
Neurological examination
Development
Assessment done if child is stable

Indicated Laboratory/Diagnostic Evaluation

The history and examination findings of the physically abused child guide the laboratory evaluation. *Laboratory and diagnostic tests help support or confirm the diagnosis of abuse and evaluate medical problems that can imitate abuse.* In cases of multiple system trauma resulting from abuse, laboratory data provide further evidence against alternative medical diagnoses. Cases of serious physical abuse sometimes will result in criminal prosecution. It is the responsibility of the medical caregivers to rule out illnesses that a jury or judge may believe would result in the injuries. This can be done by considering all of the medical findings and explaining why traumatic injury is the only reasonable explanation. Specific tests to rule out other causes may add credibility to the testimony. In addition, there are medical diagnoses that imitate child abuse, and part of the thorough evaluation of a child who presents with trauma is to evaluate for alternative medical explanations when clinically indicated.

The laboratory and diagnostic evaluation of the abused child varies depending on the age of the patient and the presenting injuries, and it is tailored to the clinical situation. The following tests are commonly performed when indicated in the evaluation of abuse.

Radiographic Skeletal Survey

A skeletal survey is a series of X-rays taken of the injured child to detect occult or healing fractures (AAP, 1991; AAP, 2000; ACR, 2006). Some fractures identified by skeletal survey in infants and young toddlers are specific enough to diagnose child abuse even without a clinical history. *A skeletal survey is indicated in all infants and children less than 2 years of age who are suspected of being physically abused.* Occult or clinically silent fractures are unusual in the older abused child, and therefore the skeletal survey generally is not a useful screening tool for children over the age of 5. For toddlers between the ages of 2 and 5, the decision to do a skeletal survey is based on the clinical findings and suspicion of bony injury. Belfer, Kelin, and Orr (2001) reviewed the medical records of 203 children ages 2 weeks to 16 years of age who were admitted for suspected child maltreatment over a 30-month period of time. Ninety-six skeletal surveys were obtained and 25 were positive for at least one clinically unsuspected fracture and 80% were in children under 1 year of age (Belfer et al., 2001). In addition to the patient's age, the type of suspicious injury was also useful in guiding the decision to obtain a skeletal survey with those presenting with a new fracture or intracranial injury being at higher risk for occult fracture while those with burn injuries had the lowest yield for occult fracture being detected on the skeletal survey (Belfer et al., 2001).

A skeletal survey is the method of choice for imaging the bones in cases of suspected physical abuse. The American College of Radiology (ACR) revised its practice guideline for skeletal surveys in children in 2006 (ACR) (see Table 2.5). All skeletal surveys should consist of a series of X-rays, including specific views of the arms, forearms, hands, femurs, lower legs and feet, as well as views of the axial skeleton and skull, all on separate exposures. The skeletal survey should not consist of a single image of the patient's skeleton (baby-gram) because the detail is not sufficient to recognize subtle injuries. It is essential that the X-rays are read by a physician trained to recognize skeletal manifestations of child abuse. Some of the subtle but specific findings of abuse are missed easily by the untrained eye.

The value of performing follow-up skeletal surveys in children strongly suspected of having been abused based on history, physical examination, or various imaging studies including the initial skeletal survey was explored by Kleinman and colleagues (1996). In a retrospective series of 23 infants and

Table 2.5 Complete skeletal survey table.

Appendicular skeleton
  Humeri (AP)
  Forearms (AP)
  Hands (PA)
  Femurs (AP)
  Lower legs (AP)
  Feet (PA) or (AP)
Axial skeleton
  Thorax (AP and lateral), to include ribs, thoracic and upper
    lumbar spine
  Pelvis (AP), to include the mid lumbar spine
  Lumbosacral spine (lateral)
  Cervical spine (AP and lateral)
  Skull (frontal and lateral)

Reprinted with permission of the American College of Radiology. No other representation of this guideline is authorized without express, written permission from the American College of Radiology.

toddlers strongly suspected of having been maltreated (out of 181 skeletal surveys conducted during a 5 year period) who received a follow-up skeletal survey approximately 2 weeks after the initial evaluation, 14 of the 23 follow-up skeletal surveys (61%) yielded additional information with the number of definite fractures increasing from 70 to 89 (a 27% increase) with most of these being the classic metaphyseal lesion and rib fractures (Kleinman et al., 1996). Specifically, the follow-up skeletal survey either detected a missed finding on the initial study (13/19 or 68%) or confirmed a fractures that was initially suspected but of which there was some question on the initial radiographs (6/19 or 32%) (Kleinman et al., 1996). An additional help to the evaluation from the information obtained on the follow-up skeletal survey was important information surrounding the age of the fractures. A prospective study conducted by Zimmerman and colleagues found similar results. Among 74 children with a mean age of 7.4 months (±10.6 months), 48 infants and toddlers returned for follow-up skeletal surveys which revealed additional information in 22 (46%) and in 3 patients (6%) the outcome of the evaluation changed with 1 child being ruled out for child maltreatment while child abuse was confirmed in the remaining 2 (Zimmerman, Makoroff, Care, Thomas, & Shapiro, 2005). The authors concluded that despite the added time, expense and radiation exposure for follow-up skeletal surveys, routinely ordering this follow-up study is justified in that it identified additional fractures or clarified tentative findings in children where were suspected of having been physically abused. Factors that led to the recommendation for a follow-up survey included (1) multiple fractures present, (2) fractures of varying ages indentified, (3) fracture type or appearance inconsistent with history provided, (4) concerning but not diagnostic initial skeletal survey or imaging study, (5) concerning physical examination, and or (6) a radiologic finding consistent with physical abuse (Zimmerman et al., 2005). Kleimnan and colleagues' (1996), offer a reasoned and cautious recommendation around ordering follow-up skeletal surveys, and in their words: "A follow-up skeletal survey performed approximately 2 weeks after the initial study appears to provide additional information regarding the number, character, and age of injuries inflicted on infants and toddlers. When child abuse is strongly suspected on the basis of the findings of the initial skeletal survey, other imaging studies, history, or physical examination, a follow-up skeletal survey is recommended to provide a thorough and accurate assessment of osseous injuries" (Kleinman et al., 1996, p. 896).

Radionuclide Bone Scan

The skeletal survey is the method of choice for imaging the bones in cases of suspected abuse. The bone scan (bone scintigraphy) is sometimes used as an adjunct to plain films. A bone scan is most often used in cases of suspected abuse of infants in which the skeletal survey is negative and more sensitive evaluation may diagnose the abuse with more certainty. A bone scan uses radioisotopes to identify areas of rapid bone turnover. It is more invasive and costly than a skeletal survey but more sensitive for detecting new (less than 7–10 days old) rib fractures, subtle diaphyseal fractures, and early periosteal elevation. A bone scan is not specific for fractures because a positive scan may indicate bone infection or tumor. Bone scans cannot be used to date fractures and do not identify skull or metaphyseal fractures reliably. In a 10-year retrospective review of 124 medical records for children who had both a skeletal survey and a bone scan from the United Kingdom, Mandelstam, Cook, Fitzgerald, and Ditchfield (2003) found that overall 70% of bony injuries were identified on both tests, 20% of injuries where present on the bone scan alone and 10% were identified on the skeletal survey alone—supporting the complementary nature of skeletal surveys and bone scans in the evaluation of suspected physical abuse in children (Mandelstam et al., 2003) (see Figure 2.4).

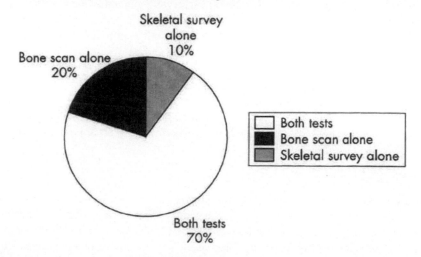

Figure 2.4 Percentage of boney injuries detected. Mandelstam et al. (2003) used with permission.

Computed Tomography

CT scans are often an essential part of the child abuse evaluation. They are a series of radiologic images that provide sliced (CT) Scan views through the area of the body scanned. CT scans of the head can identify manifestations of abusive head trauma, such as subarachnoid hemorrhage, most subdural hemorrhages, and cerebral edema and infarcts. A CT scan of the head is indicated in any infant or child that may have sustained significant head trauma (Le & Gean, 2006; Rubin, Christian, Bilaniuk, Zazyczny, & Durbin, 2003). Unlike plain X-rays of the skull, CT scans provide images of the brain. Plain X-rays are sensitive indicators of skull fractures, are relatively easy and quick to obtain and as such remain the test of choice for evaluating potential skull fractures (Cattaneo et al., 2006; Kleinman, 1998). CT scans of the chest and abdomen are the most sensitive and effective way to document injuries of the lungs and solid abdominal organs, such as the liver. CT scans are done under sedation because movement will cause artifact and potentially destroy the usefulness of the test. Recently, technological advancements permit the use of various computer imaging techniques that permit the generation of three-dimension (3D) digital images that capture the 3D aspects of soft tissue and bone injuries that are useful forensically and scientifically (Thali et al., 2003) (Figures 2.5 and 2.6). These 3D digital images permit further analysis of the suspected injury mechanism and as the equipment and techniques become more available, one can expect that the 3D documentation of injuries may become more commonplace in the evaluation of suspected child maltreatment-related injuries as well as other non-inflicted injuries (Bruschweiler, Braun, Dirnhofer, & Thali, 2003).

Magnetic Resonance Imaging (MRI)

MRI scans provide sliced views through the body using interactions of hydrogen atoms with a magnetic field to provide an image of the scanned body in any plane desired (Le & Gean, 2006). MRI generally is more sensitive than a CT scan and has the added advantage of being better able to identify subdural blood of different ages. MRI can be used instead of CT scans or as an adjunct to the CT scan (Le & Gean, 2006; Chan, Chu, Wong, & Yeung, 2003; Parizel et al., 2003). MRI is not universally available, is an expensive study, and takes longer to perform than does a CT scan. Presently, CT scan is typically the first method of imaging used in the acute setting, followed by MRI to further delineate injury or to evaluate injury that is highly suspected but not identified by CT (Eltermann, Beer, & Hermann, 2007).

Bleeding Evaluation

Children who present with excessive bruising, in whom a hematologic condition is suspected based on history and physical examination, are screened for a bleeding diathesis (Kellogg et al., 2007; Khair & Liesner, 2006; Lee, 2008). Both congenital and acquired bleeding disorders can present with excessive bleeding or bruising that may mimic child abuse (see Chapter 3). The standard screen done on the child

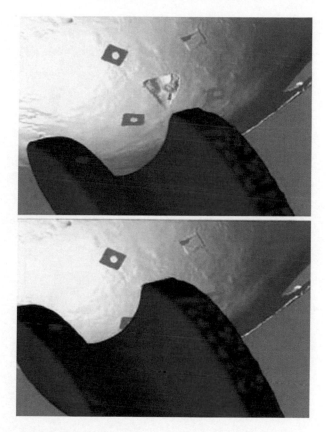

Figure 2.5 3D visualization of the match and the impact angle of the injury-causing tool with the two impression fractures. Thali et al. (2003) used with permission.

with excessive bruising includes a complete blood count (CBC) with platelet count, a prothrombin time (PT), and a partial thromboplastin time (PTT). In the setting of suspected child abuse and neglect, the health care professional conducting the evaluation may consider obtaining a hematology consultation from a skilled pediatric hematologist in order to refine the evaluation and order the appropriate tests based on the clinical suspicions and findings. In the majority of cases, a thorough history and physical examination, along with normal screening blood work, will rule out medical problems that would cause bruising, including hemophilia, leukemia, idiopathic thrombocytopenic purpura, and others. The CBC also evaluates for anemia, which may be due to blood loss, toxins such as lead, or nutritional abnormalities such as iron deficiency. If Von Willebrand's disease, the most common inherited bleeding disorder is suspected, a pediatric hematologist familiar with the laboratory capabilities in one's clinical environment would be ideal. Von Willebrand's disease is a heterogenous condition that has several subtypes resulting from quantitative or qualitative defects in Von Willebrand's factor and presents variably, making the

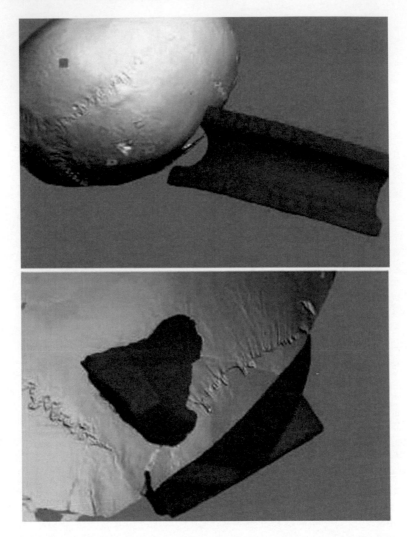

Figure 2.6 3D visualization of the match and the impact angle of the injury-causing tool with the two impression fractures. The picture at the bottom graphically demonstrates a view of the strike from inside the skull. Thali et al. (2003) used with permission.

diagnosis of the more subtle forms challenging (Liesner, Hann, Khair, Hann, & Khair, 2004). Historically a bleeding time was the test recommended but this test is notoriously inaccurate and highly dependent on technician skill and experience (Cariappa, Wilhite, Parvin, & Luchtman-Jones, 2003). More specific tests are available but require access to highly skilled laboratories, typically at referral centers, to obtain accurate results (Liesner et al., 2004). The platelet-function analyzer, PFA-100, is a increasingly recognized method for rapid in-vitro evaluation of primary clotting and is expected to become more readily available and standardized in the pediatric setting and likely to replace the bleeding time in the years to come (Cari-appa et al., 2003; Harrison, 2005; Franchini, 2005).

Toxicology Screens

Childhood ingestion of both legal and illegal substances is a common pediatric problem. Ingestion can be intentional, as with an adolescent drug overdose, or accidental, such as the toddler who ingests iron pills. At times, caregivers poison children knowingly, as in cases of medical child abuse/Munchausen syndrome by proxy (Rosenberg, 1987; Roesler & Jenny, 2009), or inadvertently allow ingestion to occur as seen with poor supervision.

An infant or child with unexplained neurologic symptoms, such as seizures, lethargy, change in mental status, or coma, is evaluated with toxicologic screens and blood alcohol level. Urine, blood, and gastric content are available for screening. Variability exists among laboratories related to the drugs tested for on the standard toxicologic screen. See Chapter 9 for further discussion.

Tests for Abdominal Trauma

Recent studies have shown that abdominal injury as the result of abuse is under-recognized (Coant, Kornberg, Brody, & Edward-Holmes, 1992). Physically abused infants, toddlers, and children who are too ill to give a history of their injuries should be screened for possible abdominal trauma. Elevations in the hepatic transaminases (AST, ALT) suggest liver injury, and an elevated amylase and lipase suggest pancreatic injury. After uncomplicated blunt liver trauma, hepatic transaminase levels are known to rise rapidly in the serum, often within hours and then to decline predicatabally over the ensuing days following the injury (Baxter, Lindberg, Burke, Shults, & Holmes, 2008). The screen for renal injuries includes a urinalysis to identify hematuria by dipstick and RBCs by microscopy. Occasionally, a dipstick will identify children with hematuria, but no RBCs are seen on microscopy. These children have either myoglobinuria or hemoglobinuria, which have both been reported as a result of abuse (Mukerji & Siegel, 1987; Rimer & Roy, 1977). When measured in the acute setting, an elevated serum myoglobin, creatine phosphokinase (CPK), or urine myoglobin confirms the diagnosis of significant muscle injury (Schwengel & Ludwig, 1985). It is essential to order these screening tests immediately in the acute setting because these levels all rapidly return to normal. The tests described serve as a noninvasive, rapid way of identifying possible intra-abdominal injury. More extensive testing will be needed to characterize the extent and type of injuries identified by screening.

The above list represents common screening tests used in the evaluation of the abused child. Of course, each case is evaluated individually, and not all tests are necessary in every case. For some children, the history and physical examination are all that is needed to diagnose abuse (see Figure 2.2). Critically ill or injured children will require extensive testing. The above serves as an introduction to the tests that are often used in the evaluation of suspected inflicted injury. Further information

Table 2.6 Laboratory/diagnostic evaluation of the physically abused child.

Radiographic skeletal survey
   Method of choice for screening abused children for bony injury
   For all children less than 2 years old with suspected physical abuse
   Of limited use in children older than 5
   For children 2–5 years old, use clinical findings
   Follow-up skeletal survey recommended unless radionuclide bone scan performed
Radionuclide bone scan
   Adjunct to skeletal survey
   Most useful if there is high suspicion of bony injury and skeletal survey is negative
Computed tomography (CT) scan
   Provides sliced views through internal organs, such as brain and abdominal organs
   Essential part of the evaluation of seriously injured children
   Initial test used for children with suspected abusive head trauma
Magnetic resonance imaging (MRI)
   More sensitive than CT for many injuries
   Can provide images in multiple planes
   Generally used as an adjunct to CT in the acute setting
Blood tests for easy bruising/bleeding
   Complete blood count (CBC)
   Prothrombin time (PT)
   Partial thromboplastin time (PTT)
Consider hematology consultation for coagulation work-up, if indicated
Screening tests for evidence of abdominal trauma
   Liver
     Alanine aminotransferase (ALT, SGPT)
     Aspartate aminotransferase (AST, SGOT)
   Pancreas
     Amylase
     Lipase
   Kidney
     Urinalysis looking for blood or red cells
Toxicology screens
   For children with unexplained neurological symptoms or symptoms compatible
     with ingestion. Drugs tested for in "tox screen" vary among laboratories
   Urine and/or gastric contents are sent for screening (consider blood for targeted
     substances)
   Consider blood alcohol levels for children with altered mental status

regarding laboratory testing is found in the chapters describing specific patterns of injury. See Table 2.6 for an overview of the laboratory/diagnostic evaluation.

Photographic Documentation

Photographic documentation of findings of abuse is part of the comprehensive evaluation and serves as an accurate record of a child's injuries. Photographs are the only way to preserve physical findings that will undoubtedly disappear as healing occurs. All visible lesions should be photographed. The benefits of photography in the evaluation and description of abuse are multifold. Photographs facilitate review of the findings by multiple people, provide a standard for comparison during other evaluations, and are a valuable tool used in court to describe abusive findings and condition of the abused child (Ricci & Smistek, 2000).

Although photographs are an important documentation tool for injuries, they cannot be used exclusively and cannot replace the written and diagrammed description of the injuries. Cameras and photographers are not foolproof, and the techniques used to photograph the child, including the camera, lighting, and background, will affect the quality of the photograph. Some hospitals have a medical photography department whose employees can take photographs. Law enforcement agencies also have photographers adept at photographing injuries, crime scenes, and so on. However, the replacement of conventional silver-based cameras with digital technology has made it common for medical providers to produce their own images.

Unfortunately, even with relatively "user-friendly" digital cameras, poor-quality images are not uncommon. The photographer needs to be familiar with his or her camera and know how to take pictures that are clear and adequately lighted. Frequently seen errors involve improper placement of measuring devices, such that they cover up part of the injury, are placed at an angle relative to the mark rather than parallel to it, and/or compress the surrounding skin such that distortion is introduced into the image. See Table 2.7 for suggestions regarding photographing suspected victims of child maltreatment. If an American Board of Forensic Odontology (ABFO) 90-degree scale is not available, then a ruler should be photographed

Table 2.7 Photographing child maltreatment: helpful hints.

Photographing suspected victims of physical abuse and neglect
- Take two pictures of every view and angle, one for the file and one for court
- Photograph the injury with an anatomic landmark. The inclusion of an elbow, knee, belly button, or other body part identifies the location of the wound
- Include two pictures of each wound or other injury—one that identifies a landmark and one that provides a closeup (fills the film frame) of the wound
- Position the camera so that the film surface or plane is parallel to or directly facing the injury
- Vary the perspective of the picture by taking various shots from different angles and distances
- Place a measuring device such as an adhesive metric scale directly above or below the injury to ensure accurate representation of the size and depth of the injury. A standardized color bar may be placed in the photographic plane for comparison with the color of the injury
- Ultraviolet light is a method of photography in which a standard, high-speed (ISO 800/1600) color slide film is used in conjunction with a high-powered electronic flash. The result of UV photography is an image that may display healed wounds, bite marks, belt imprints, and old pattern-type injuries

Adapted from Ricci and Smistek (2000, pp. 6–7).

both parallel and perpendicular to the mark in question. Photographs of traumatic injuries should include views with and without the measuring device. In addition to close-up shots, images should be taken that include anatomic landmarks, such as a knee, elbow, or belly button. A whole-body photograph that shows the child's face helps to match the injuries to the child. A marker that includes the child's identifying information (name, date of birth, etc.) should be placed in the photographs or later added to the digital files. Straight-on views of an injury demonstrate its extent, whereas views taken from an angle better show depth and texture. For this reason, pictures of bite marks should include perpendicular views. Angled views can also be helpful when light reflection is a problem, as may occur when edema is present. Because the appearance of acute injuries often changes over time, additional photographs on subsequent days are sometimes needed to document the healing process. This is particularly helpful for acute injuries that may be confused with permanent body marks, e.g. a bruise that may initially resemble a nevus. Ultraviolet light can be helpful for improving visualization of fading marks (Pretty, 2008; Ricci & Smistek, 2000). See Table 2.8 for suggestions regarding specific injuries in child maltreatment.

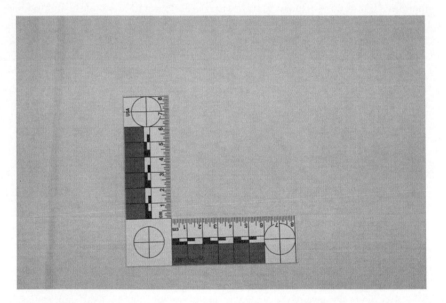

Photo 2.2 An American Board of Forensic Odontology (ABFO) 90-degree scale.

Some processing issues that arise with digital cameras are compression of information, and enhancement and restoration techniques. Many modern cameras automatically compress images into JPEG format, with the unavoidable loss of information. Ideally, the cameras used for forensic photographs remove only redundant and "irrelevant" information. The degree of compression can be lowered prior to storing images when there is a concern that important image content may be lost. Enhancement and restoration techniques are commonly used to improve the appearance of

Table 2.8 Photographing specific injuries.

Injury type	Suggested methods
Amputation	Photograph the dismembered part alone and then in relation to the body. Close-ups should also be taken of the skin's torn edges, which may help verify the method of amputation in court
Bite marks	Best interpreted by a forensic dentist or pathologist. Can be recorded for punctures, and slashes; but size, shape, color, depth of indentations, and three-dimensional contours need to be documented. Parallel or direct views best depict shape and size, while slanted or indirect views and lighting highlight texture
Bruises	Bruising goes through several stages of development—as time goes on, additional photographs will be needed to document the injury. If a child shows evidence of having old and new bruises, repeated abuse may be suspected. Both old and new bruises should be photographed. To help minimize reflections caused by swelling, take photographs from several angles, then do a follow-up series when swelling has gone down
Burns	Take pictures from all angles *before* and *after* treatment. Accidental burns usually exhibit splash marks or indiscriminate patterns of injury. Intentional burns often show distinct lines or well-defined areas of damaged skin
Facial injuries	If injury is to the mouth, use a tongue depressor to keep the mouth open and injury visible. If injury is to the eye, use a flashlight or toy to distract the child's gaze in different directions to show the extent of the damage to the eye area
Neglect	Child's general appearance should be photographed, including any signs (splinters in soles of feet, hair loss, extreme diaper rash, wrinkled or wasted buttocks, prominent ribs, and/or a swollen belly)
Punctures, slashes, rope, and/or pressure injuries	Take photographs straight on (for overall view of the surface and extent of injury) and at a slight angle (provides depth and texture)

Adapted from Ricci and Smistek (2000, pp. 9–10).

an image, and to remove motion or other artifacts, respectively. Specific documentation is usually not required when enhancement techniques involve processes that are comparable to traditional dark-room methods. Traditional enhancement techniques include brightness adjustment, contrast adjustment, color balancing, and cropping. More advanced enhancement techniques need to be documented. Likewise, any restoration efforts applied to an image should always be documented. A copy of the original digital image must be maintained whenever any alteration techniques are used, as all steps in the production of an image are discoverable by a court of law. A digital photography specialist may be consulted to examine images for evidence of manipulation if challenged [International Association for Identification,

Scientific Working Group on Imaging Technologies (SWGIT), Recommendations and Guidelines for the Use of Digital Image Processing in the Criminal Justice System, 2006].

It is a common misconception that the ease with which digital images may be manipulated complicates the process of establishing their authenticity in legal settings. In fact, this is rarely the case when the images are properly identified and supported with adequate documentation. Proper accompanying information must identify the location of injuries depicted in the images, as well as the name of the photographer and the date that the photographs were taken. Another common misconception is that image files should be left on the camera's flash drive and made available to the court if requested. Because flash media is designed as temporary storage and is susceptible to corruption by improper handling and storage over time, it is not recommended that it be used for permanent storage. Duplicate images stored onto a hard drive, CD, or DVD are generally admissible as original images in court proceedings (SWGIT, 2008). Written protocols regarding the process for producing photographic evidence and standardized documentation can help child abuse teams minimize errors that can lead to questions regarding the reliability, reproducibility, and/or security of the images. See Appendix for examples of photos.

In Brief

- The medical evaluation of the abused child includes a history, physical examination, indicated laboratory and diagnostic studies, and observation of the caregiver–child interaction.
- A history of minor trauma that results in serious or life-threatening injury to a child should be suspect, and an evaluation for possible abuse should be performed.
- The recognition of abuse stems from the "building-block" approach, which synthesizes data from each part of the clinical evaluation to develop and confirm a suspicion of abuse.
- Knowledge of child development, mechanisms of injury, and the epidemiology of trauma is needed for proper diagnosis of child abuse.
- The diagnosis of physical abuse rests with the professional's ability to obtain a thorough history from the patient or family and to recognize discrepancies between the history and physical findings.
- The physical examination of the injured child should include careful attention to subtle signs of trauma.
- Laboratory data and radiologic studies are important tools used to support the diagnosis of abuse and evaluate for medical conditions that may mimic abuse.
- Meticulous documentation of the history, physical examination, and laboratory data is an integral part of the evaluation of the abused child.
- If taken properly, photographs serve as an accurate record of a child's injuries.

References

American Academy of Pediatrics, Section on Radiology. (1991). Diagnostic imaging of child abuse. *Pediatrics, 87*, 262–264.

American Academy of Pediatrics, Section on Radiology. (2000) Diagnostic imaging of child abuse. *Pediatrics, 105* (6), 1345–1348.

American College of Radiology (ACR) ACR Practice Guideline for Skeletal Surveys in Children 2006 http://www.acr.org/SecondaryMainMenuCategories/quality_safety/guidelines/pediatric/skeletal_surveys.aspx

Barlow, B., Niemirska, M., Ghandi, R. P., & Leblanc, W. (1983). Ten years' experience of falls from a height in children. *Journal of Pediatric Surgery, 18*, 509–511.

Barsley, R. E., & Landcaster, D. M. (1987). Measurement of arch widths in a human population: Relation of anticipated bite marks. *Journal of Forensic Science, 32*, 975–982.

Baxter, A. L., Lindberg, D. M., Burke, B. L., Shults, J., & Holmes, J. F. (2008). Hepatic enzyme decline after pediatric blunt trauma: A tool for timing child abuse? *Child Abuse and Neglect, 32*, 838–845.

Belfer, R. A., Kelin, B. L., & Orr, L. (2001). Use of the skeletal survey in the evaluation of child maltreatment. *American Journal of Emergency Medicine, 19* (2), 122–124.

Bertocci, G. E., Pierce, M. C., Deemer, E., Aguel, F., Janosky, J. E., & Vogeley, E. (2004). Influence of fall height and impact surface on biomechanics of feet-first free falls in children. *International Journal of the Care of the Injured, 35*, 417–424.

Bruschweiler, W., Braun, M., Dirnhofer, R., & Thali, M. J. (2003). Analysis of patterned injuries and injury-causing instruments with forensic 3D/CAD supported photogrammetry (FPHG): An instruction manual for the documentation process. *Forensic Science International, 132*, 130–138.

Cariappa, R., Wilhite, T. R., Parvin, C. A., & Luchtman-Jones, L. (2003). Comparison of PFA-100 and bleeding time testing in pediatric patients with suspected hemorrhagic problems. *Journal of Pediatric Hematology/Oncology, 25* (6), 474–479.

Cattaneo, C., Marinelli, E., Di Giancamillo, A., Di Giancamillo, M., Travetti, O., Vigano' L., Poppa, P., Porta D., Gentilomo, A., & Grandi, M. (2006). Sensitivity of autopsy and radiological examination in detecting bone fractures animal model: Implications for the assessment of fatal child physical abuse. *Forensic Science International. 164* (2): 131–137.

Chadwick, D. L., Bertocci, G., Castillo, E., Frasier, L., Guenther, E., Hansen, K., et al. (2008). Annual risk of death resulting from short falls among young children: Less than 1 in 1 million. *Pediatrics, 121*, 1213–1224.

Chadwick, D. L., Chin, S., Salerno, C., Landsverk, S., & Kitchen, L. (1991). Deaths from falls in children: How far is fatal? *Journal of Trauma, 31*, 1353–1355.

Chan, Y. L., Chu, W. C. W., Wong, G. W. K., & Yeung, D. K. W. (2003). Diffusion-weighted MRI in shaken baby syndrome. *Pediatric Radiology, 33*, 574–577.

Chiaviello, C. T., Christoph, R. A., & Bond, R. (1994). Stairway-related injuries in children. *Pediatrics, 94*, 679–681.

Coant, P. N., Kornberg, A. E., Brody, A. S., & Edward-Holmes, K. (1992). Markers for occult liver injury in cases of physical abuse in children. *Pediatrics, 89*, 274–278.

Eltermann, T., Beer, M., & Hermann, J. G. (2007). Magnetic resonance imaging in child abuse. *Journal of Child Neurology, 22*, 170–175.

Finkelstein, J. L., Schwartz, S. B., Madden, M. R., Marano, M. A., & Goodwin, C. W. (1992). Pediatric burns. *Pediatric Clinics of North America, 39*, 1145–1163.

Franchini, M. (2005). The platelet-function analyzer (PFA-100). *Hematology, 10* (3), 177–181.

Harrison, P. (2005). The role of PFA-100 testing in the investigation and management of haemostatic defects in children and adults. *British Journal of Haematology, 130* (1), 3–10.

Helfer, R. E. (1977). Injuries resulting when small children fall out of bed. *Pediatrics, 60*, 533–535.

International Association for Identification, Scientific working Group on Imaging Technologies (SWGIT), Recommendations and Guidelines for the Use of Digital Image Processing in the Criminal Justice System, version 2.0, January 2006, available at http://www.theiai.org/guidelines/swgit/index.php, accessed 12/17/2008

International Association for Identification, Scientific working Group on Imaging Technologies SWGIT, Section 17, Digital imaging technology issues for the courts, version 1.0 June 2008, available at http://www.theiai.org/guidelines/swgit/guidelines/section_17_v1-0.pdf, accessed 12/17/2008

Jenny C. and the Committee on Child Abuse and Neglect (2007). American Academy of Pediatrics. *Pediatrics. 120* (6):1385–1389

Jenny, C., Hymel, K. P., Ritzen, A., Reinert, S. E., & Hay, T. C. (1999). Analysis of missed cases of abusive head trauma. *JAMA, 282* (7), 621–626.

Joffe, M., & Ludwig, S. (1988). Stairway injuries in children. *Pediatrics, 82*, 457–461.

Johnson, K., Fischer, T., Chapman, S., & Wilson, B. (2005). Accidental head injuries in children under 5 years of age. *Clinical Radiology, 60*, 464–468.

Kellogg, N. D., the Committee on Child Abuse and Neglect. (2007). Evaluation of suspected child physical abuse. *Pediatrics, 119* (6), 1232–1241.

Kemp, A., Maguire, S. A., Sibert, J., Frost, R., Adams, C., & Mann, M. (2006). Can we identify abusive bites on children? *Archives of Disease in Childhood, 91*, 951.

Khair, K., & Liesner, Ri. (2006). Bruising and bleeding in infants and children – A practical approach. *British Journal of Haematology, 133* (3), 221–231.

Khambalia, A., Joshi, P., Brussoni, M., Raina, P., Morrongiello, B., & Macarthur, C. (2006). Risk factors for unintentional injuries due to falls in children aged 0–6 years: A systematic review. *Injury Prevention, 12*, 378–385.

Kleinman, P. K. (Ed.) (1998). *Diagnostic imaging of child abuse*. Baltimore: Williams and Wilkins.

Kleinman, P. K., Nimkin, K., Spevak, M. R., Rayder, S. M., Madansky, D. L., Shelton, Y. A., et al. (1996). Follow-up skeletal surveys in suspected child abuse. *American Journal of Roentgenology, 167*, 893–896.

Le, T. H., & Gean, A. D. (2006). Imaging of head trauma. *Seminars in Roentgenology, 41* (3), 177–189.

Lee, A. C. W. (2008). Bruises, blood coagulation tests and the battered child syndrome. *Singapore Medical Journal, 49* (6), 445–449.

Levin, A. (1990). Ocular manifestations of child abuse. *Ophthalmology Clinics of North America, 3*, 249–264

Liesner, R., Hann, I., Khair, K., Hann, I., & Khair, K. (2004) Non-accidental injury and the haematologist: The causes and investigation of easy bruising. *Blood Coagulation & Fibrinolysis, 15* (1), S41–S48.

Ludwig, S. (2005). Psychosocial emergencies: Child abuse. In G. R. Fleisher & S. Ludwig (Eds.), *Textbook of pediatric emergency medicine* (5th ed., pp. 1761–1802). Baltimore: Williams and Wilkins.

Lyons, T. J., & Oates, K. (1993). Falling out of bed: A relatively benign occurrence. *Pediatrics, 92*, 125–127.

Mandelstam, S. A., Cook, D., Fitzgerald, M., & Ditchfield, M. R. (2003). Complementary use of radiological skeletal survey and bone scintigraphy in detection of bony injuries in suspected child abuse. *Archives of Disease in Childhood, 88,* 387–390.

Mellick, L. B., & Reesor, K. (1990). Spiral tibial fractures of children: A commonly accidental spiral long bone fracture. *American Journal of Emergency Medicine, 8* (3), 234–237.

McCullock Melnyk, K. A. (1988). Barriers: A critical review of recent literature. *Nursing Research, 37* (4), 196–200.

Mukerji, S. K., & Siegel, M. J. (1987). Rhabdomyolysis and renal failure in child abuse. *American Journal of Radiology, 148,* 1203–1204.

Musemeche, C. A., Barthel, M., Cosentino, C., & Reynolds, M. (1991). Pediatric falls from heights. *Journal of Trauma, 31,* 1347–1349.

Nimityongskul, P., & Anderson, L. D. (1987). The likelihood of injuries when children fall out of bed. *Journal of Pediatric Orthopedics, 7,* 184–186.

Parizel, P. M., Ceulemans, B., Laridon, A., Ozarlak, O., Van Goethem, J. W., & Jorens, P. G. (2003). Cortical hypoxic-ischemic brain damage in shaken-baby (shaken impact) syndrome: Value of diffusion-weighted MRI. *Pediatric Radiology, 33,* 868–871.

Pierce, M. C., & Bertocci, G. (2008). Injury biomechanics and child abuse. *Annual Review of Biomedical Engineering, 10,* 85–106.

Plunkett, J. (2001). Fatal pediatric head injuries caused by short-distance falls. *American Journal of Forensic Medicine and Pathology, 22* (1): 1–12.

Pretty, I. A. (2008). Forensic dentistry: 2. Bitemarks and bite injuries. *Dental Update, 35,* 48–61.

Ricci, L. R., & Smistek, B. S. (2000). Photodocumentation in the Investigation of Child Abuse. National Institute of Justice. http://www.ncjrs.gov/App/publications/abstract.aspx?ID=160939

Rimer, R. L., & Roy, S. (1977). Child abuse and hemoglobinuria. *Journal of American Medical Association, 238,* 2034–2035.

Roesler, T.A. L & Jenny, C. (2009). Medical Child Abuse: Beyond Munchausen Syndrome. American Academy of Pediatrics: USA.

Rosenberg, D. A. (1987). Web of deceit: A literature review of Munchausen syndrome by proxy. *Child Abuse and Neglect, 11,* 547–563.

Rosenthal, P. A., & Doherty, M. D. (1984). Serious sibling abuse by preschool children. *Journal of American Academy of Child Psychiatry, 23,* 186–190.

Rubin, D. M., Christian, C. W., Bilaniuk, L. T., Zazyczny, K. A., & Durbin, D. R. (2003). Occult head injury in high-risk abused children. *Pediatrics, 111* (6), 1382–1386.

Schmitt, B. D., Grosz, C. A., & Carroll, C. A. (1976). The child protection team: A problem oriented approach. In R. E. Helfer & C. H. Kempe (Eds.), *Child abuse and neglect: The family and the community* (pp. 91–113). Cambridge, MA: Ballinger.

Schwengel, D., & Ludwig, S. (1985). Rhabdomyolysis and myoglobinuria as manifestations of child abuse. *Pediatric Emergency Care, 1* (4), 194–197.

Selbst, S. M., Baker, M. D., & Shames, M. (1990). Bunk bed injuries. *American Journal of Diseases of Children, 144,* 721–723.

Shelov, S. P., & Hannemann, R. D. (Eds.) The American Academy of Pediatrics The Complete and Authoritative Guide. (2004). *Caring for your baby and young child: Birth to age 5* (4th ed.). New York: Bantam Books.

Skellern, C. Y., Wood, D. O., & Crawford, M. (2000). Non-accidental fractures in infants: Risk of further abuse. *Journal of Pediatrics and Child Health, 36,* 590–592.

Tarantino, C. A., Dowd, M. D., & Murdock, T. C. (1999). Short vertical falls in infants. *Pediatrics Emergency Care, 15* (1), 5–8.

Thali, M. J., Braun, M., & Dirnhofer, R. (2003). Optical 3D surface digitizing in forensic medicine: 3D documentation of skin and bone injuries. *Forensic Science International, 137*, 203–208.

Warrington, S. A., & Wright, C. N., ALSPAC Study Team. (2001). Accidents and resulting injuries in premobile infants. *Archives of Disease in Childhood, 85*, 104–107.

Williams, R. A. (1991). Injuries in infants and small children resulting from witnessed and corroborated free falls. *Journal of Trauma, 31*, 1350–1352.

Zimmerman, S., Makoroff, K., Care, M., Thomas, A., & Shapiro, R. (2005) Utility of follow-up skeletal surveys in suspected child physical abuse evaluations. *Child Abuse and Neglect, 29*, 1075–1083.

Appendix

Notice the documentation of the injuries, the measuring tape placement and the identification of the side of the body

Series 1: Series of photos showing bruising on a child's thighs. Please take note of the various angles and different distance of the photos and the ruler placement.

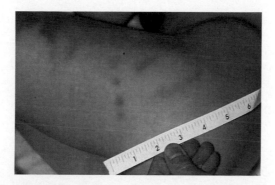

Photo 1a Photo of bruising on a child's left thigh.

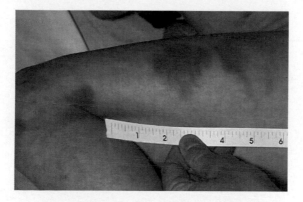

Photo 1b Photo of bruising on child's lower thigh from a different perspective.

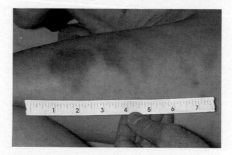

Photo 1c Photo from a different angle and distance.

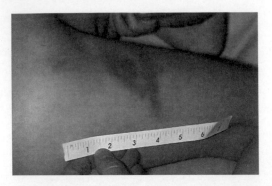

Photo 1d Photo of same child with bruising of right thigh.

Series 2: Child with horizontal bruise and overlying abrasion of left cheek. Notice the various angles and distance of the photos that enhance the description of the injuries.

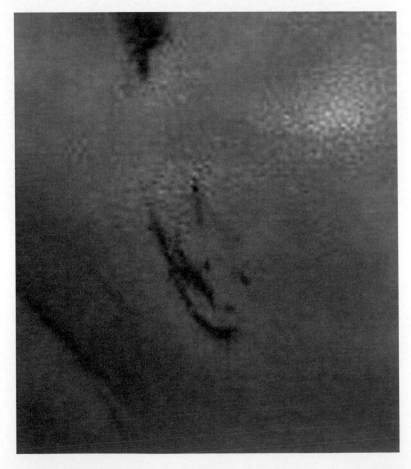

Photo 2a Photo of the child with horizontal bruise and overlying abrasion of left cheek.

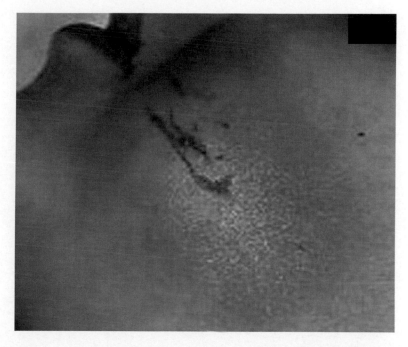

Photo 2b Photo taken straight on of the child with horizontal bruise and overlying abrasion of left cheek.

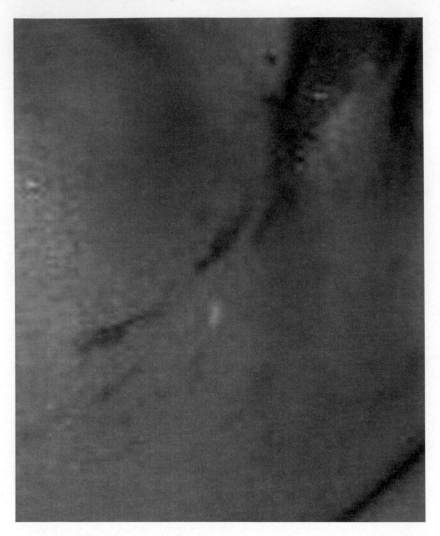

Photo 2c Same patient as in previous image with a similar patterned injury on the right side of the face.

Series 3: Suprapubic and penile bruising.

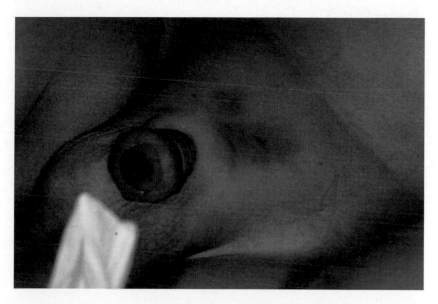

Photo 3a Photo taken at a distance of suprapubic and penile bruising.

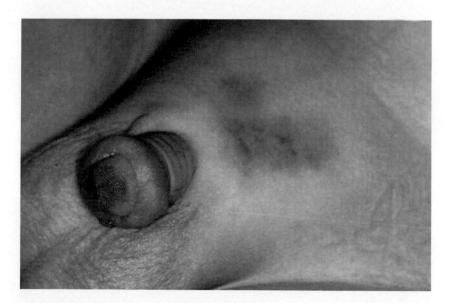

Photo 3b Photo of patient in 3a at a closer distance.

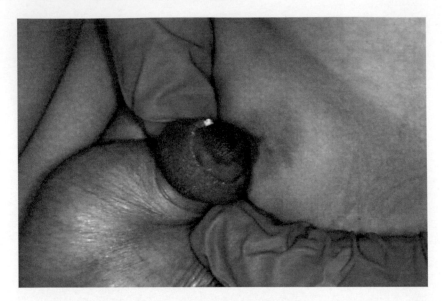

Photo 3c Photo of patient in 3a, with examiner positioning penis to further demonstrate bruise on tip of penis.

Series 4: Photo documentation of injury to left thigh. Notice the varying distances at which the photos were taken.

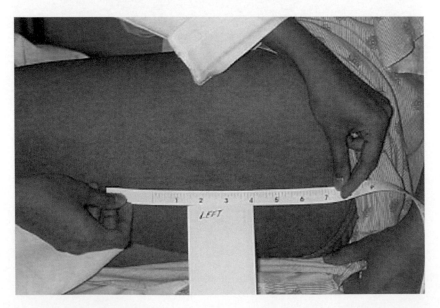

Photo 4a Photo of injury to left thigh. Notice the placement of the ruler with the identification of the side of the body.

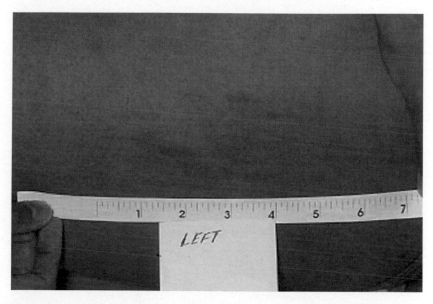

Photo 4b Closer view of the injury to left thigh.

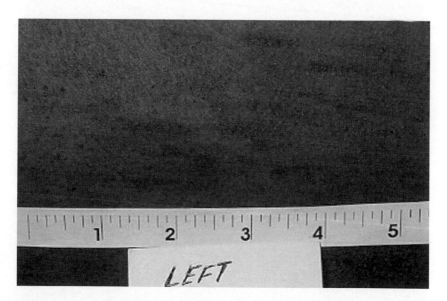

Photo 4c Close up view of the injury to left thigh.

Series 5: Photo documentation of injured shoulders. Notice identification of body part along with ruler placement.

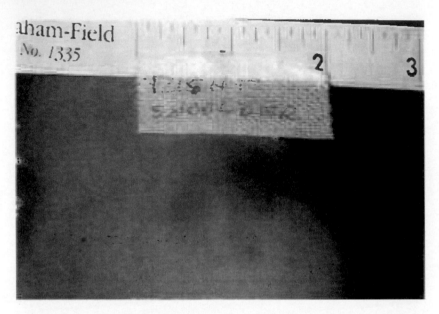

Photo 5a Photo of right shoulder injury.

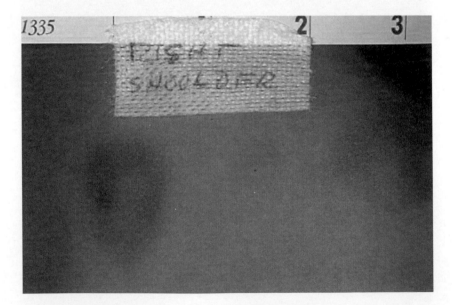

Photo 5b Photo of right shoulder injury taken at a different angle.

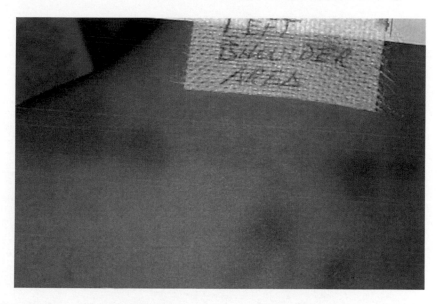

Photo 5c Photo of left shoulder injury.

Series 6: Adolescent female with multiple bruise on the neck. Notice the different angles from which the photos are taken.

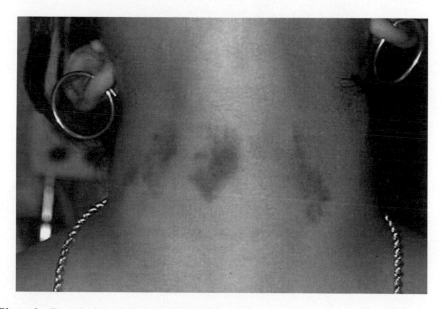

Photo 6a Frontal view of the bruising on the neck.

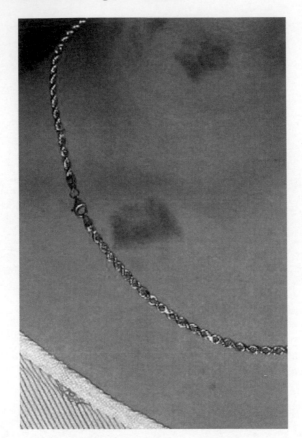

Photo 6b Close up of the bruising on the neck.

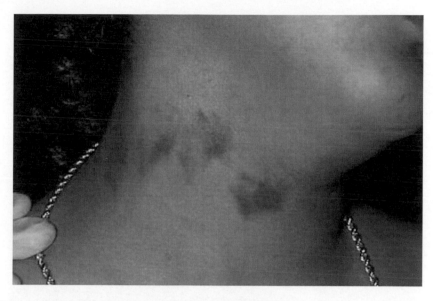

Photo 6c Photo of the right side of the bruising on the neck.

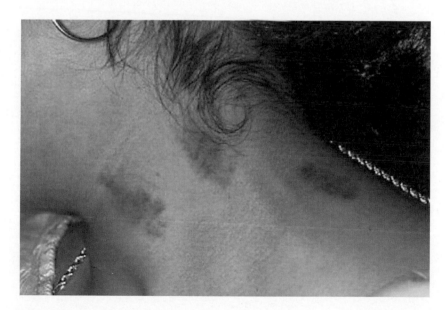

Photo 6d Photo of the left side of the bruising on the neck.

Series 7: Photo documentation of locations of injuries with ruler

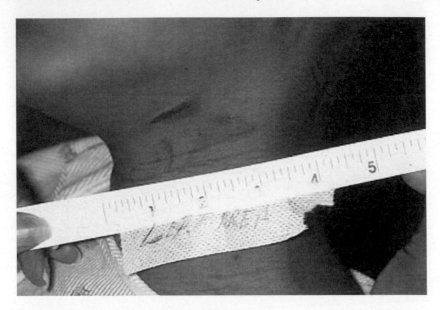

Photo 7a Photo of injury on left side of the neck.

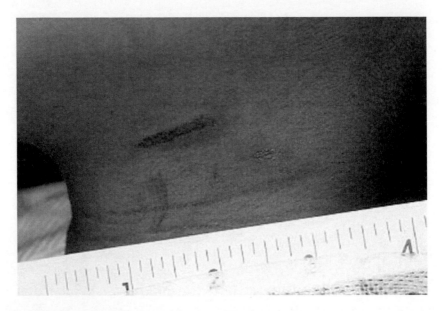

Photo 7b Closer view of the patient in photo 7a.

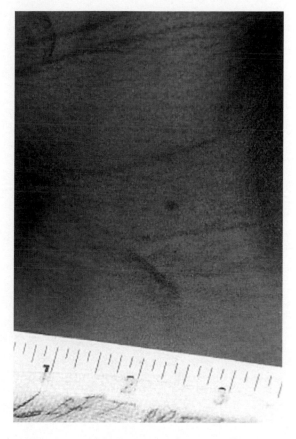

Photo 7c Close up of the injury to patient in photo 7a on the right side of the neck.

Part II

Specific Injuries

Chapter 3

Skin Injury: Bruises and Burns

Erin E. Endom and Angelo P. Giardino

Careful examination of the child's skin is an essential component of the abuse evaluation. Injuries to the skin are common findings in maltreated children and may include (a) contusions (bruises), abrasions, lacerations; (b) burns from scalding, direct contact with flame or hot objects, and electricity; (c) frostbite (O'Neill, Meacham, Griffin, & Sawyers, 1973); and (d) scars resulting from these injuries (Richardson, 1994). In one study examining the injuries of 616 children suspected of having been abused, at least 80% of the 775 primary injuries involved the skin, including (a) bruises/ecchymoses/hematomas (56%); (b) erythema/marks (9%); (c) burns (8%); and (d) abrasions/scratches (7%) (Johnson & Showers, 1985). Ellerstein (1979, 1981) noted the importance of cutaneous findings in maltreated children, because the recognition of these easily observed injuries by the child's relatives, neighbors, and schoolteachers may trigger contact with the health care provider. Health care providers evaluating children with suspicious skin findings need to consider physical abuse and/or neglect as a potential etiology and pursue a thorough evaluation.

O'Neill (1979) documented that soft tissue trauma, essentially skin injuries, is frequently the earliest and most common manifestation of physical maltreatment. He found that many seriously injured children had been evaluated previously for soft tissue injuries such as bruises and burns. Early recognition of minor injuries that may be inflicted may result in intervention and prevention of many serious injuries (O'Neill, 1979). In an epidemiologic study of injury variables, Johnson and Showers (1985) suggest that children with evidence of chronic maltreatment, such as nonhealed injuries of different ages, were at a 50% risk for further abuse and at a 10% risk for fatal injury.

This chapter focuses on the skin findings most commonly seen in both abused and nonabused children, namely, bruises and burns. Specific attention will be placed on the characteristics of these soft tissue injuries that suggest abuse and/or neglect. As

A.P. Giardino et al. (eds.), *A Practical Guide to the Evaluation of Child Physical Abuse and Neglect*, DOI 10.1007/978-1-4419-0702-8_3, © Springer Science+Business Media, LLC 1997, 2010

in all cases of suspected maltreatment, the evaluation consists of a comprehensive history of the injury, a thorough physical examination, directed laboratory assessment, psychosocial assessment, and meticulous documentation.

Bruises

Overview

Bruises are common injuries in childhood, with all children from time to time having minor accidental bruising. Clinicians expect toddlers and young children to sustain minor bruising owing to the rough and tumble play that occurs during normal exploration and activity. A typical accidental bruise involves the skin overlying bony prominences such as the anterior tibia (shins), knees, elbows, forehead, and dorsum of the hands. Carpenter (1999) studied the distribution of bruising in 177 nonabused children aged 6–12 months and found that all bruises occurred (1) on the front of the body and (2) over bony prominences. Bruising, especially on the shins, increased with increase in age and mobility. Caregivers typically provide a history of noting the child's bruise after a bump or fall or of noting the bruise incidentally while bathing or dressing the child. The child's physical examination may reveal other minor bruises in expected areas and no other injuries. Accidental bruising is uncommon on the ears, back, buttocks, hands, forearms, upper arms, face, abdomen, hips, backs of the legs, and feet (Maguire, Mann, Sibert, & Kemp, 2005). Deviation from the typical childhood pattern of accidental bruising, such as to areas on the posterior aspect of the body (buttocks), soft areas (cheeks), or protected areas (genitals, upper legs, axilla pinnae), raises the health care provider's suspicion of possible child maltreatment (see Photo 3.1).

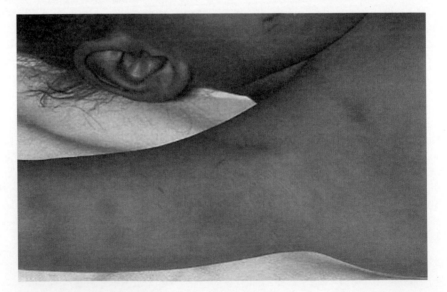

Photo 3.1 Child with old bruises to axilla and body.

Inflicted injuries to the child's skin also may cause bruising. However, patterns of abusive bruising overlap with "expected" patterns found in accidental bruising. Although inflicted bruises may be differentiated from accidental bruises by their location, age, shape, number, and severity, few bruising patterns are pathognomonic for child abuse (Sussman, 1968), with the exception of bruises carrying the clear imprint of the implement used (Maguire et al., 2005). Pascoe, Hildebrandt, Tarrier, and Murphy (1979) found that bruises to the soft, relatively protected skin sites on the cheeks, neck, trunk, genitals, and upper legs were seen significantly more often in children suspected of having been abused or neglected (see Photo 3.2). Other bruising patterns that may raise concern for maltreatment include: bruises in the young (premobile) infant; multiple bruises of different ages; multiple bruises in clusters; multiple bruises of uniform shape; bruises and marks that have geometric shapes suggestive of the object used to strike the child; and/or severe bruising that is not explained by the history provided (Maguire et al., 2005).

Pathophysiology

A bruise or black-and-blue mark generally results from the application of a blunt force to the skin surface that results in the disruption of capillaries (and possibly larger blood vessels, depending on the force applied). As the bruise forms, subcutaneous blood leaks from the disrupted capillaries into the unbroken overlying skin (Wilson, 1977). A multitude of factors account for the size and depth of a bruise. These factors include (a) force of impact, (b) size of the disrupted blood vessels, (c) vascularity and connective tissue density of the injured tissue, and (d) fragility of the blood vessels involved (Ellerstein, 1979; Kornberg, 1992; Richardson, 1994). For example, the periorbital area is a well-vascularized tissue with relatively loosely supported blood vessels that may bruise extensively if subjected to blunt force.

The depth and location of the vessels and the arrangement of fascial planes in the surrounding tissue are also a consideration when assessing the extent and age of a bruise. Injury depth is a factor in when the bruise appears. Relatively deep injuries may not be apparent for hours to days (Johnson, 1990; Langlois & Gresham, 1991). For example, a powerful blow applied to the thigh may result in injury to deep structures and may not be apparent for a day or two until bleeding from the deep vessels tracks toward the more superficial areas and becomes visible through the overlying unbroken skin.

What Is an Inflicted Bruise?

In 2002, the American Academy of Pediatrics Committee on Child Abuse and Neglect released a guideline regarding skin injuries serious enough to be considered abusive (American Academy of Pediatrics Committee on Child Abuse and Neglect, 2002):

1. The injury is inflicted.
2. The injury is nonaccidental.
3. The injury pattern fits a biomechanical model of trauma that is considered abusive (handprint, instrument pattern such as a loop cord injury).

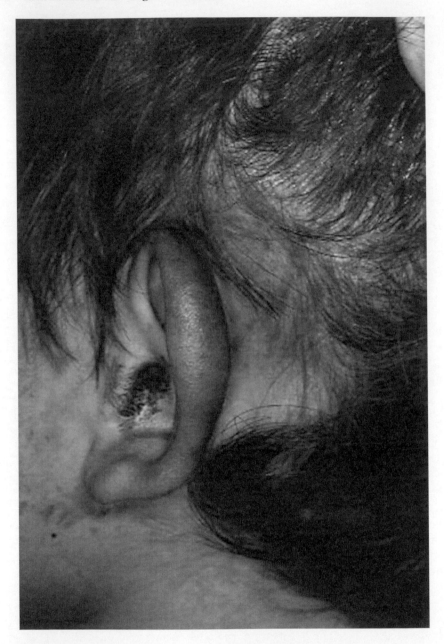

Photo 3.2 Bruises and swelling on ear lobe, behind ear; also notice blood in the canal.

4. The history of injury is inconsistent with the child's developmental stage.
5. The history of injury is inconsistent with the injury itself.
6. The injury is significant if it produces visible tissue damage that lasts more than 24 hr (that is, beyond temporary redness of the skin).

Evaluation for Abuse

History

The evaluation of suspicious bruises begins with a history that includes the explanation of the injury, evaluation for medical conditions associated with easy bruisability or those that mimic bruising, and a history of prior allegations of maltreatment.

A. History of Injury

    1. How and when was the bruising noted? By whom?
    2. What is the explanation for the bruise(s)?
    3. If age appropriate, what is the child's explanation of the bruise?
    4. Was the injury witnessed?
    5. Was the bruise attributed to the child's self-injury or to the actions of a sibling or playmate?
    6. Is the explanation for the bruising implausible because of the age or developmental ability of the child?
    7. Do explanations change over time, or are disparate accounts rendered by different caregivers?
    8. If the injury is serious, is there a delay in seeking treatment after the injury? If so, why?
    9. With a significant injury or suspicious bruising pattern, is there a lack of appropriate concern over the seriousness of the child's condition?

B. Medical and Family History

    1. Does the child have a medical condition associated with easy bruisability or that mimics bruising? Is the child receiving any medications that might interfere with clotting?
    2. Is there a history of unusual bleeding or bruising, such as extensive bleeding with circumcision, deep muscle bleeds with immunizations, recurrent nosebleeds, or excessive gum bleeding with dental care?
    3. Is there a family history of any of the above?

C. History of Prior Maltreatment

    1. Is there a prior history of maltreatment or frequent visits for injury?
    2. Is the family known to social services for previous concerns of maltreatment?

An implausible history to explain the bruising should immediately alert the health care provider to the possibility of abuse. Basic knowledge of child development is essential in determining the plausibility of a history. For example, 6-month-old children are not developmentally able to climb onto furniture, raising the suspicion of abuse when the caregiver explains this as the cause of a baby's bruised back or neck (Kornberg, 1992).

Physical Examination

The physical examination of the bruised child includes a detailed description of each injury, identification of bruising patterns that are suggestive of abuse, and a search for other injuries (see Photo 3.3). Bruises are potentially a subtle manifestation of more severe internal injury, especially in the infant or young toddler. Faint bruises, or those that are not visible to the naked eye, may be enhanced with a Wood lamp, enabling not only detection but digital photographic documentation (Vogeley, Pierce, & Bertocci, 2002).

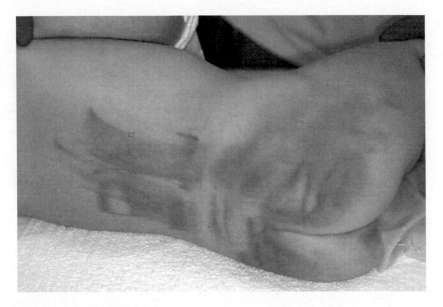

Photo 3.3 Bruises on back and buttock.

A. Describe Each Bruise Carefully

   1. Size of the bruise as measured with a millimeter ruler
   2. Location of the bruise
   3. Shape of the bruise (see below)
   4. Color of the bruise (see below for dating of bruises)

B. Bruising Patterns (note characteristics of the bruises identified)

   1. Do the bruises appear to be of different ages?
   2. Are the bruises in centrally located or protected areas?
   3. Do the bruises appear to be older or younger than disclosed in the history?
   4. Does the pattern of bruising differ from the history provided?

5. Does the pattern of bruising suggest an inflicted mechanism (e.g., handprints, geometric shapes, loop marks)?
6. Are multiple body surfaces bruised from a single episode of trauma?

C. Identification of Other Signs of Inflicted Injury

1. Examine for underlying bone or internal organ injury.
2. Assess for signs of physical neglect.

Shape

The shape of the bruise may help distinguish accidental from nonaccidental injury. A bruise may assume the shape of the object used to injure the child (Johnson, 1990) (see Figure 3.1). Identifiable marks may be left from corporal punishment using instruments, such as a belt, cord, or paddle, depending on how the instrument is held as it is used against the child's skin (Kornberg, 1992). A cord folded over and used to strike a child will customarily leave ecchymotic loop marks which are essentially pathognomonic for physical abuse. A belt produces a broad band of bruising, with a horseshoe shape at one end from the buckle; puncture marks may be present from penetration of the skin by the tongue of the buckle. Restraint of a child's limbs during abuse may cause circumferential ligature marks around the ankles and wrists (Kornberg, 1992); gag marks (bruising at the corners of the mouth) may also be seen. The perpetrator's hand may leave an impression upon the child's skin when

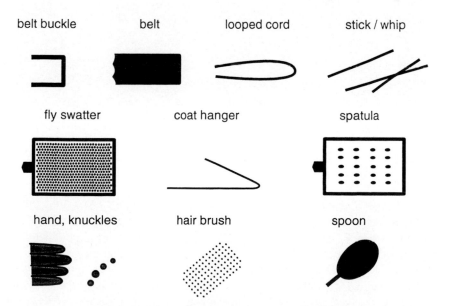

Figure 3.1 Marks left by objects on child's skin. Johnson (1990) used with permission. Pediatrics Clinics of North america. 37:791–817, Copyright © Elsevier 1990.

sufficient force is used to either grab or slap the child (Kessler & Hyden, 1991); the imprint may appear negative (an outline of the hand with bruising between the fingers, rather than at the actual point of impact of the fingers themselves) due to capillary rupture as blood is pushed away from the point of impact (Reece and Ludwig, 2001).

Bite marks produce a characteristic roughly circular or oval shape, consisting of two opposing arches separated by open spaces at their bases; the mandibular teeth are usually more clearly defined than the maxillary teeth (Reece and Ludwig, 2001; American Board of Forensic Odontology, 2000). The distance between the canine teeth can help to differentiate adult bites from bites by other children: an intercanine distance less than 2.5 cm is consistent with the deciduous teeth of a young child, 2.5–3 cm either a child or a small adult, and 3–4.5 cm an adult (Kemp, Maguire, Sibert, Frost, Adams, & Mann, 2006).

Bruises taking on the shape of objects are rarely accidental and require thorough investigation and protection of the child from further harm (Johnson, 1990; Kornberg, 1992; Richardson, 1994) (see Photo 3.4).

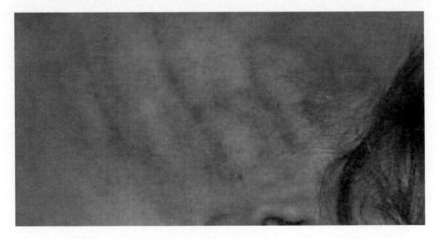

Photo 3.4 Slap on the face with imprint of hand.

Dating of Bruises

Bruises undergo visible color changes as they heal (see Photo 3.5). Although clinicians are frequently asked to "date" injuries based on the progression of color changes seen in bruised skin, current literature cautions the accuracy of the dating criteria (Schwartz & Ricci, 1996). Knowledge of bruise pathology and the basis for color changes helps practitioners understand the pathophysiologic process and provides reason for caution in trying to date the age of a bruise. Detailed color changes occur as a bruise progresses through various stages of healing (Richardson, 1994; Wilson, 1977). However, there may be no clearly predictable order or chronology of color progression in the healing process even though certain patterns seem

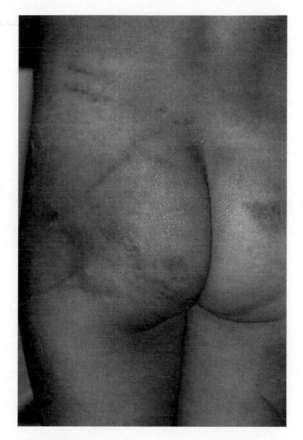

Photo 3.5 Child with multiple bruises in various stages of healing.

to emerge (Schwartz & Ricci, 1996). However, after impact and until resolution, the bruise is a deep red, blue, or purple (Langlois & Gresham, 1991). Swelling is common for approximately 2 days until the serum is reabsorbed (Richardson, 1994). With time, the blood collection separates into serum and a fibrin mass clot, and swelling decreases with the resorption of the serum from the injured area. Pigmented breakdown products of free hemoglobin, deoxygenated hemoglobin, biliverdin, and bilirubin are believed to account for the "play of colors" that the bruise undergoes over the next 2 to 4 weeks, as hemoglobin in the clot degenerates and is reabsorbed (Cotran, Kumar, & Robbins, 1989). The bruise may progress from a deep reddish purple to a more bluish color and then develop a greenish coloring that fades into a yellowish brown coloring prior to full resolution. Bruises with yellow coloring are generally older than 18 hr (Langlois & Gresham, 1991), although yellow coloration may appear "earlier than most forensic charts indicate" (Schwartz & Ricci, 1996, p. 255). The amount of time for each color change to occur depends on the amount of blood involved, distance of the bruise from the skin, and baseline skin pigmentation of the individual. All combine to create the colors seen at the surface. Because of inherent limitation of efforts to estimate the age or date of injuries, Wilson (1977) suggests that clinicians document that the appearance of a bruise is consistent with a given estimated age rather than stating an exact age. Schwartz and Ricci (1996) caution that the bruise literature does not support any certainty in determining the age of a bruise because of the varied factors in bruise development and the healing process.

The Differential Diagnosis of Bruising

The differential diagnosis of a child who appears bruised includes accidental trauma; inflicted trauma (physical abuse); and a variety of dermatologic, hematologic, vasculitic, and infectious conditions, as well as congenital defects in collagen synthesis (Bays, 1994; Coffman, Boyce, & Hansen, 1985; Davis & Carrasco, 1992; Ellerstein, 1979; Johnson, 1990; Kornberg, 1992; Richardson, 1994; Saulsbury & Hayden, 1985; Wissow, 1990a).

Mongolian spots are blue-gray areas of hyperpigmentation, usually located over the lower back and buttocks but also on the upper back and extremities, which are frequently noted in infants of African-American, Asian, or Hispanic descent. They may be mistaken for bruises, but lack associated swelling or tenderness, and do not evolve over days as do bruises.

Disorders of coagulation span a wide range of possible defects in hemostatic function, including (a) congenital and acquired abnormalities of platelet function, such as thrombocytopenia absent radius syndrome (TAR) and idiopathic thrombocytopenia purpura (ITP); (b) congenital and acquired abnormalities of coagulation factors, such as hemophilia (factor VIII deficiency) and vitamin K deficiency; and (c) congenital and acquired vascular abnormalities, such as hereditary hemorrhagic telangiectasia and a variety of vasculitides. Henoch-Schönlein purpura, a self-limited IgA-mediated vasculitic, is the most common vasculitic disorder of childhood; it presents with palpable purpura, which may occur anywhere on the body but are most concentrated on the legs and buttocks; other findings may include joint pain and swelling, abdominal pain, and hematuria (Gedalia , 2004).

In addition, folk-healing practices may cause bruising and raise the concern of possible abuse. Coining (cao gio), also known as quat sha, gua sha, scraping, or spooning, is an East Asian practice which involves rubbing the skin with the edge of a coin or other object in order to relieve symptoms of illness; it produces a characteristic ecchymotic pattern on the skin that may be mistaken for abuse (Nielsen, Knoblauch, Dobos, Michalsen, & Kaptchuk, 2007; Look & Look, 1997) (see Photo 3.6a and Photo 3.6b).

As in all differential diagnoses, the history, physical examination, and laboratory assessment are crucial to the inclusion and exclusion of diagnoses and guide the assessment and workup. Bays (1994) made a comprehensive review of the medical literature on conditions reportedly mistaken for child abuse. Note that children with medical conditions that cause easy bruisability tend to bruise most in com-

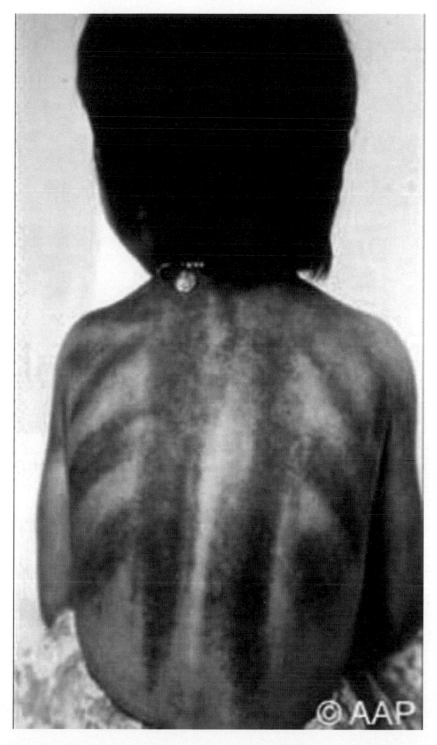

Photo 3.6 (a) Coining. Used with permission. American Academy of Pediatrics. Visual Diagnosis of Child Abuse on CD-ROM. 2nd Edition. Elk Grove Village, Ill. 2003.

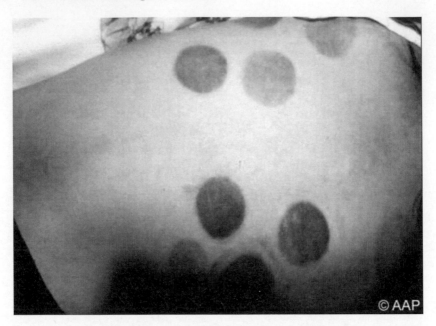

Photo 3.6 (continued) (**b**) Cupping: a cultural practice that may be mistaken for child abuse. Used with permission. American Academy of Pediatrics. Visual Diagnosis of Child Abuse on CD-ROM. 2nd Edition. Elk Grove Village, Ill. 2003.

mon locations. Furthermore, children with hematologic or other medical conditions associated with bruising and bleeding are not immune to maltreatment (Johnson & Coury, 1988). Careful consideration of the possible conditions that mimic abuse serves the child's interests and prevents the misdiagnosis of abuse (see Table 3.1).

Forensic and Laboratory Evaluation

The clinician interprets the plausibility of the injury in conjunction with the past medical history, noted bruises, developmental factors, and laboratory data (Richardson, 1994). A child with bruising may not automatically require laboratory evaluation to assess for a hematologic disorder. However, it is important to focus on a screening history and physical examination for such disorders that guide the selection of indicated laboratory studies (Rapaport, 1983). After eliciting a thorough history and performing a complete physical examination, the health care provider may conclude that (a) the screening information is complete and consistent with normal clotting; no further workup is necessary; (b) the screening information is incomplete (or insufficient); further workup is necessary to ensure normal clotting; or (c) the screening information suggests a medical condition that is associated with easy bruisability or bleeding; further workup is necessary (Casella,1990).

Table 3.1 Differential diagnosis of bruising.

Dermatologic	
Mongolian spots	—Slate blue patches of skin commonly seen in pigmented skin
	—Approximately 90% of African Americans have such spots
	—Congenital, commonly found on the lower back and buttocks (may occur anywhere)
	—Fade early in life (in most cases, completely faded by age 5 years)
	—Do not progress through the 2-week color sequence described for bruise healing (Tunnessen, 1990)
Hemangioma	—Visible vascular malformations
	—Capillary hemangiomas (strawberry marks), composed of capillaries
	—Congenital
	—Characteristic growth pattern: (a) rapid growth for approximately the first 6 months, (b) slowed growth paralleling the child's somatic growth until about age 3 years, and (c) involution with at least partial regression by age 6 years in more than 85% of cases (Pokorny, 1990)
Eczema	—Atopic skin condition
	—Reddened, dry areas on the child's skin
	—Pruritic, frequently associated with a family history for other atopic conditions such as asthma and hayfever, and occur episodically in "flares"
	—Responsive to topical steroids such as hydrocortisone
Erythema multiforme (EM)	—Acute hypersensitivity skin condition whose hallmark is red, target-like lesions
	—Occurs in response to a number of drugs, foods, immunizations, and infections with both bacteria and viral agents (Cohen, 1993)
	—Severity of EM ranges from a minor form that is self-limited to a major form, Stevens-Johnson syndrome, which has serious systemic consequences, involves mucous membranes, and manifests large areas of epidermal necrosis and sloughing
	—Variable in appearance, classically symmetric, may involve the palms and soles, and has variable lesions that typically progress from dusky red to a target-like character occurring in crops and resolving in 1–3 weeks (Cohen, 1993)
Phytophoto dermatitis	—Skin reaction to psoralens, chemical compounds found in citrus fruits such as limes
	—Skin in contact with psoralens upon exposure to sunlight manifests red marks that appear as bruises and, if severe, as burns
	—History contains information related to contact with psoralens followed by exposure to the sun (Coffman et al., 1985)
"Tattooing"	—Dye from fabric such as denim discolors the child's skin, giving the appearance of a bruise; lightens or fades with rigorous washing

Table 3.1 (continued)

	—History should reveal contact with dyed fabric that became wet and "ran" (Tunnessen, 1985)
Hematologic	
Disorders of hemostasis, congenital and acquired hemophilia (Factor VIII & IX deficiency)	—A plasma coagulation disorder
	—In the neonatal period, cord separation or circumcision may result in prolonged bleeding (hemophilia; approximately 50% of affected males having such a bleeding history)
	—Bruising may become more pronounced as the child begins to cruise and walk, owing to falls and bumps
	—Bruising may have a nodular or firm consistency secondary to the deep bleeding into soft tissues seen in hemophilia
	—Hemophilia suggested by prolonged PTT
	—Consultation with a qualified pediatric hematologist necessary (Casella, 1990)
Von Willebrand's disease	—Heterogenous group of disorders that results in decreased platelet adhesiveness, impaired agglutination of platelets in presence of ristocetin, and prolonged bleeding time
	—Patients have mild to moderate bleeding tendency typically involving mucous membranes
	—Easy bruising, nosebleeds, and prolonged bleeding after dental procedures are hallmarks (Casella, 1990)
Vitamin K deficiency	—May be secondary to malabsorption (e.g., cystic fibrosis)
	—Hemorrhagic disease of the newborn might be expected in an infant who failed to receive prophylactic Vitamin K at birth (Pearson, 1983). Breast-fed children born at home are most at risk. Presentation is typically in the first few days of life, and a high percentage occurs with a catastrophic intracerebral bleed (Bays, 1994; Wetzel, Slater, & Dover, 1995).
	—Acute, usually self-limited
Idiopathic thrombocytopenic purpura (ITP)	—Platelets are peripherally consumed via an immunologic mechanism (Pearson, 1983)
	—Follows a viral illness in approximately 70% of cases
	—Petechiae and bruising are noted approximately 2–4 weeks after the minor illness resolves
	—Physical examination reveals petechiae or bruising, and normal lymph node, spleen, and liver size
	—CBC reveals a low platelet count
	—Resolution typically occurs in 8–12 weeks in more than 75% of cases

Table 3.1 (continued)

Leukemia	—Bone marrow becomes progressively infiltrated with neoplastic cells —Systemic signs and symptoms are typically present —CBC is markedly abnormal —Coagulation studies may also be aberrant depending on the stage of the illness —Children may ingest anticoagulants from either medications in the household or those contained in commercial rat poison (Bays, 1994; Johnson & Coury, 1988)
Anticoagulant ingestion	—May be seen in MSBP (see Chapter 8)
Vasculitis	
Henoch-Schönlein purpura (HSP)	—Palpable purpura and petechiae —Notable for (a) a variable purpuric rash that often involves the buttocks and lower extremities; (b) arthralgia/arthritis; (c) abdominal pain; (d) renal disease; and (e) occasionally subcutaneous, scrotal, or periorbital edema (Martin & Walker, 1990) —Tends to develop acutely, is usually self-limited, and runs its course over a 6-week period of time —Most common in children less than 7 years but older than 1 year —Up to 50% of affected children may have recurrences; these tend to be in older children —Purpura without a low platelet count is essential for the diagnosis
Infections	—May be associated with the appearance of petechia and/or purpura (e.g., rickettsial disease) —Severe infections may result in complications such as disseminated intravascular coagulation (DIC) and purpura fulminans —History, physical examination, and laboratory evaluation confirmatory of serious infection
Collagen synthesis defects	
Ehlers-Danlos (ED) Syndrome	—Congenital defect in collagen synthesis, may lead to easy bruising —At least 10 forms are identified —Involves a variety of unique basic defects and inheritance patterns —Basic clinical triad that each variant shares to a greater or lesser extent: (a) skin hyperextensibility, (b) joint hypermobility, and (c) skin fragility —Consultation with an experienced clinical geneticist is recommended for children manifesting this triad (Zinn, 1994)

Table 3.1 (continued)

Osteogenesis imperfecta (OI)	—Congenital abnormality in quantity or quality of type I collagen synthesis
	—Heterogenous disorder with four subtypes
	—OI type I associated with easy bruising. Hallmarks include blue sclera, hearing impairment (35% of children after first decade), osteopenia, fractures, bony deformities, and excessive laxity of joints (Silence, 1983)
	—Punch biopsy of skin for analysis of collagen synthesis in children with repeat fractures when other s/s are not consistent with abuse (Bays, 1994)
	—Consultation with metabolic specialist and geneticist required
Folk-healing practices coining	—Described in Asian cultures as healing method
	—In coining, warmed oil is applied to the child's skin, which is then rubbed with the edge of a coin or a spoon in a linear fashion, usually on the chest or back
	—The repetitive rubbing leads to linear bruises and welts (Yeatman & Dang, 1980)
Cupping	—Described in Asian and Mexican cultures
	—In cupping, a cup is warmed and placed on the skin. A vacuum is created between the cup and the child's skin as the cup cools, which leads to a bruise (Sandler & Haynes, 1978)
	Coining and cupping are not done to injure the child but to comply with cultural beliefs that view them as necessary to help the child heal or recover from minor illnesses. Parental education is needed to assist the parent in understanding the injurious nature of these practices.

Screening for bleeding problems includes platelet count, prothrombin time (PT), partial thromboplastin time (PTT), and bleeding time. Additional tests are indicated for abnormal screens and are best obtained through consultation with a qualified pediatric hematologist. Regardless of how complex the workup becomes, tests are ordered based upon what the history and physical suggest rather than a random effort to exclude unlikely possibilities.

Bite marks may require special analysis, including careful measurement of the vertical and horizontal size, along with the distance between the maxillary canines if this can be determined, and photography of the wound with a distance scale in the frame for forensic matching with the teeth of the perpetrator. The injury may also be swabbed to obtain saliva traces for DNA analysis. Sweet et al. have described a reliable technique for bite wound swabbing, known as the double swab method: the skin is swabbed first with a wet swab, followed by a dry swab; both swabs are air-dried before being submitted for analysis (Sweet, Lorente, Lorente, Valenzuela, & Villanueva, 1997).

Burns

Overview

Burns represent a major public health problem for children. Each year, approximately 30,000 children are hospitalized for serious burns, and a significant number suffer disability, permanent disfigurement, and death (Ahlgren, 1990; Meagher, 1990). The mortality rate for burns ranks second behind automobile deaths and accounts for approximately 3,000 pediatric deaths each year in the United States. For burns involving more than 40% of body surface area, the mortality rate is close to 90% (Hathaway, Hay, Groothuis, & Paisley, 1993). Eighty percent of burn injuries occur in the child's own home, and approximately 10 to 25% of pediatric burns are a result of abuse (O'Neill, 1979; Purdue, Hunt, & Prescott, 1988); 6 to 20% of abusive injuries to children are burns (Peck & Priolo-Kapel, 2002). Mortality for accidental burns is approximately 2%, compared to a mortality rate near 30% for abusive burn injuries (Purdue et al., 1988). The number of children who suffer serious disability from burn injuries is approximately three times higher than the number of those who die from such injuries (O'Neill, 1979).

Burns, whether accidental or inflicted, occur more frequently in children under 5 years of age, with the highest incidence occurring in infants and toddlers under 3 years of age (Feldman, 1987; Johnson & Showers, 1985; Showers & Garrison, 1988). Burn injuries are classified as scalds (hot liquid), flame, contact (hot solid object), electrical, and chemical (Meagher, 1990). Scalding accounts for the majority of childhood burns, including both accidental and inflicted burn injuries, and accounts for 45% of all pediatric burn admissions (Ahlgren, 1990).

Pathophysiology

Human skin sustains injury from contact with heat. Human skin is composed of three layers: epidermis, dermis, and subcutaneous tissue. The deepest cells in the dermis are called the basal layer, and they serve to replenish the skin cells as they are sloughed or injured (see Figure 3.2). Cells that make up the skin contain protein and enzymes that function within limited temperature ranges. Permanent damage to the skin occurs when the proteins are subjected to temperature extremes that cause denaturation and an inability of the cellular mechanism to function.

At the cellular level, burn injuries consist of three concentric zones of affected tissue (Jackson, 1953; Robson & Heggers, 1988) (see Figure 3.3). The first zone consists of skin that has the most direct contact with the heat source. This area, known as the zone of coagulation, undergoes immediate coagulation necrosis with

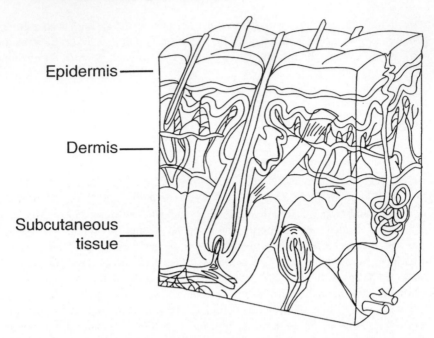

Epidermis—

Dermis—

Subcutaneous
tissue ——

Figure 3.2 Skin layers. The skin is divided into layers. The uppermost or most superfi-cial layer is the epidermis. The dermis is deeper, is composed mainly of structural proteins, and contains skin appendages such as hair follicles, sweat glands, and nerve endings. These appendages contain reserves of skin cells that serve to aid in the healing process after injury. Finally, the subcutaneous tissue layer serves as an underlying support structure composed of fibrous bands and fat.

denaturation of proteins and no potential for cellular repair. Cells in the second zone, the zone of stasis, are exposed to direct injury from the heat source but retain some ability to repair themselves. Tissue in this zone is ischemic, and cells usually necrose in 1 to 2 days after the injury unless the burn is treated properly. Finally, cells in the third zone, called the zone of hyperemia, have sustained minimal direct injury and usually recover from insult over a 7- to 10-day period.

As cells die in the various zones, they release inflammatory mediators that may lead to further progression of injury. Furthermore, necrotic tissue that accumulates within the wound provides an excellent growth medium for microorganisms that have an adverse effect on the healing process.

Burn injuries are classified by the depth of the skin injured. The size of a burn is calculated as a percentage of body surface area involved. The depth of burns has historically been described as first-, second-, third-, and fourth-degree burns. Currently, the terms *superficial, partial,* or *full thickness* are used to describe the depth of the burn. Partial thickness burns are further classified as either superficial partial thickness (not to be confused with the simple "superficial" burn described above) or deep partial thickness.

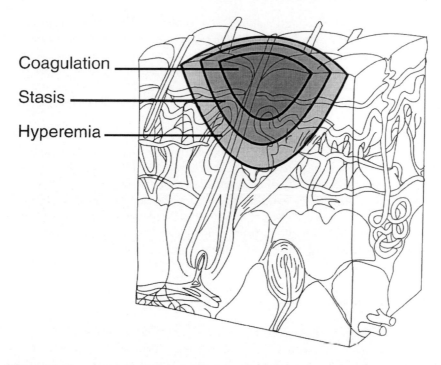

Coagulation

Stasis

Hyperemia

Figure 3.3 Concentric zones of thermal injury. The zone of coagulation is the area in most direct contact with the heat source and sustains irreparable damage. Extending outward is the zone of stasis, which, although injured, retains some ability for cellular repair. Finally, the zone of hyperemia is the least injured area and has the greatest likelihood of repair and healing. Adapted from Robson and Heggers (1988).

A superficial burn, analogous to a first-degree burn, is the least severe. A common example is sunburn. The burned area involves only the uppermost layers of the epidermis and presents as reddened, painful skin without blister. Within a few days, the superficial layers of injured skin slough and heal as healthy cells are produced from the underlying skin cells. No scarring is expected from a superficial or first-degree burn.

A partial thickness burn, analogous to the second-degree burn, causes blistering of the skin and is painful because nerve endings are exposed. Partial thickness burns are deeper than the simple superficial burn and extend past the epidermis into the dermis. Because of blood vessel disruption, these burns have a beefy red appearance. Depending on the depth of dermis involved, the partial thickness burn may be categorized further as either a superficial partial thickness or deep partial thickness burn. The superficial partial thickness burn extends just past the epidermis and minimally involves the dermis. The deep partial thickness burn is more extensive and goes deeper into the dermis. Healing in partial thickness burns progresses as healthy cells deep in the dermis replenish injured cells. Superficial partial thickness burns usually heal completely in approximately 2 weeks if infection does not occur. The deep partial thickness burn may heal in 3 to 4 weeks. Healing of partial thickness burns may result in scarring and hypertrophic changes, especially with deeper injury. Deep partial thickness burns may compromise the dermis's basal layer of cells and progress to a full thickness burn injury if not treated properly. Thus, observation over several days is necessary prior to final classification of burn depth.

A full thickness burn (analogous to third and/or fourth degree depending on depth of involvement) is the most severe and extends through the entire skin surface, past epidermis and dermis to underlying tissues such as subcutaneous tissue (third degree) or muscle and bone (fourth degree). The entirety of the overlying skin has been destroyed, including the basal layer of the dermis. Full thickness burns present as white and anesthetic because of complete destruction of blood vessels and nerve endings. Such a profoundly injured area cannot regenerate its own skin cells. Healing occurs through inward growth of skin from tissues surrounding the wound or surgically by way of skin grafting from nonburned areas of the body. Significant scarring and disfigurement occur as the full thickness burn heals.

Burns and Abuse

Inflicted burns have been recognized since the early years of professional inquiry into child maltreatment (Gillespie, 1965). Although estimates vary depending on the population studied, approximately 10% of children hospitalized for burns are believed to have sustained inflicted injury (Feldman, 1987; Meagher, 1990; Purdue et al., 1988). These children tend to be young and have a higher mortality than do comparable children who were accidentally burned. Although few burn mechanisms are pathognomonic for abuse, certain patterns have a higher association with abuse than do others. For example, tap water scalds are more commonly seen in abusive burns than in accidental burns.

Investigators have studied specific historical and physical patterns associated with inflicted burns (Ayoub & Pfeiffer, 1979; Hammond, Perez-Stable, & Ward, 1991; Hight, Bakalar, & Lloyd, 1979; Keen, Lendrum, & Wolman, 1975; Lenoski & Hunter, 1977; Stone, Rinaldo, Humphrey, & Brown, 1970; Kos & Shwayder, 2006) and have developed criteria that raise the suspicion of abusive burns. These criteria include

1. Implausible history to account for burn based on child's development, age of burn, and/or pattern of burn identified on examination
2. No history for burn provided by caregivers because child was "found" with the burn (magical injury)
3. Caregiver responsible for child at time of burn not present with child during medical evaluation
4. Burn attributed to sibling or playmate
5. Patterns of burns that imply restraint during burn injury
6. Burns on areas of the body that are "targets" for abuse, including the dorsum of the hands, feet, legs, perineum, and buttocks (see Photo 3.7)

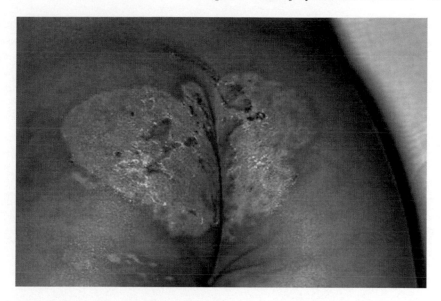

Photo 3.7 Child with healing burns to buttocks.

7. Unexplained delay in seeking treatment
8. Other suspicious injuries, such as bruises and scars of varying age and at different stages of healing
9. Evidence of neglect, such as poor hygiene or malnutrition
10. History of prior injury

Scalds

Scalding is the most common mechanism of burn injury for abused children who are admitted to the hospital (Showers & Garrison, 1988). Scalding occurs when a hot liquid comes in contact with the child's skin. Some hot liquids responsible for scalds are (a) boiling water; (b) tap water; (c) water-like liquids, such as tea or coffee; and (d) thicker liquids, such as soups or grease. Scald burns are classified as (a) splash/spill (hot liquid falls, is poured on, or is thrown at child); (b) immersion (child falls into or is submerged in hot liquid); and (c) forced immersion (pattern of burn suggests that restraint was used to plunge and hold child in the hot liquid).

Splash/spill burns may occur either in an accidental or in an inflicted manner. Overlap exists in the physical findings for both mechanisms of injury. Accidental scalds often occur in kitchen accidents as a child explores his or her environment and reaches unknowingly for containers of hot liquid that have been left within reach. Pots of boiling water and cups of hot beverages are likely culprits in such accidents. An accidental mechanism of injury is expected to give rise to a typical burn pattern. For example, if the child is looking up and reaching for a container, the hot liquid will fall first upon the child's cheek, neck, shoulder, upper arm, and upper chest. This area will be most severely burned, and as the spilled liquid runs down the body, it cools and leaves a less severe injury going outward from the points of initial contact (see Figure 3.4). Clothing holds the hot liquid in close contact to the skin, which makes the burn more severe. As the liquid falls on the child, splash marks may also appear as droplets of the hot liquid fall upon the child in other areas separate from the point of maximal contact.

Splash/spill burns also may occur in an abusive manner. Hot liquids may be poured or thrown at the child. Depending on the circumstances, the injury pattern of the burn may help differentiate an inflicted burn from an accidental spill/splash

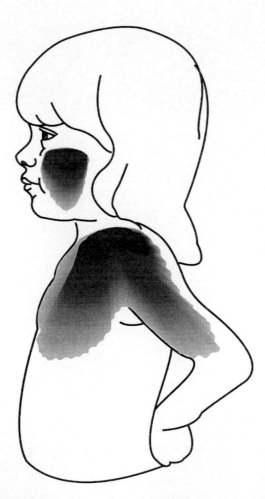

Figure 3.4 Typical spill burn pattern. The typical pattern for a spill burn where a child reaches up and pulls a container of hot liquid on top of him- or herself. The hot fluid usually falls onto the child's face and shoulder first, causing the most severe burn at the point of initial contact (expressed by the *darkest shading*). As the liquid runs down the body and cools, the burn becomes narrower and less severe at the perimeter (expressed by *lighter shading*).

burn. For example, if a child is running from a perpetrator, the liquid may be thrown at his or her back and give rise to a burn pattern that is inconsistent with a history of the child looking up and pulling a pot of boiling water on top of him- or herself. However, if the perpetrator pours the hot liquid on top of the child, the injury pattern may be similar to that described for the accidental burn and may not be useful in identifying the abusive origin of the injury. Other aspects of the medical evaluation will be necessary to diagnose abuse in such a case where burn patterns overlap.

Immersion burns occur when parts of the child's body become submerged in a hot liquid, and the burns may be accidental or inflicted. Such burns are commonly seen in abusive burning. Abusive immersion burns may occur at any age but are more common in infants and toddlers. For example, a typical immersion burn occurs when the child is held vertically by the arms or upper torso and then immersed in the hot water. In this scenario, the toes and feet come in contact with the hot water first. The child reflexively withdraws his or her lower limbs by flexing the knees and hips and assuming a cannonball-like position. The caregiver then immerses the genitals and buttocks. Depending on the size of the child and the depth of the water in the container, the child's feet and lower legs are burned, and the buttocks and genital area are also burned. Distinct lines of demarcation will separate the burned from nonburned areas, and splash marks may be limited. Such inflicted immersion burns are often related to toileting accidents or other activities that dirty a child and require that the caregiver clean the child. The pattern of burn injury described above would be inconsistent with an accidental injury, such as would occur if the child wandered over to and fell into a tub of water, or if the child was playing in an empty tub and turned on the hot water faucet (see Photo 3.8).

A forced immersion burn has a pattern of injury that is consistent with the child being restrained by the perpetrator while submerged in the hot liquid. Forced immersion burns are among the most severe and extensive burns seen in abused children. A forced immersion pattern of injury occurs when the caregiver holds the child in such a way that certain areas of the skin are forced against the relatively cooler surface of the container or tub and are protected from the more extensive burn sustained by the skin that is in full contact with the hot liquid (see Figures 3.5, 3.6, 3.7, 3.8, and 3.9). For example, this pattern results when a child is plunged into scalding hot water and is held in such a way that his or her buttocks are forcibly held against the relatively cooler tub bottom. In this scenario, the scalding water surrounds the submerged skin while the buttocks skin in contact with the bottom of the tub is somewhat spared. Therefore, the resulting burn that is less severe on the buttocks manifests as the so-called hole in doughnut sparing pattern. In addition, as the child is forcibly held in the water, areas of skin that are held tightly opposed, such as in the femoral areas and the backs of the flexed knees, may be spared as well because the hot water is unable to seep into this space to burn the skin. The resulting burn shows thermal injury where the water was in contact with the skin and relative sparing where the hot water was unable to come in contact with the skin.

Stocking and glove burns are circumferential burns of lower and upper limbs that are another pattern of immersion burns pathognomonic of abuse. An extremity

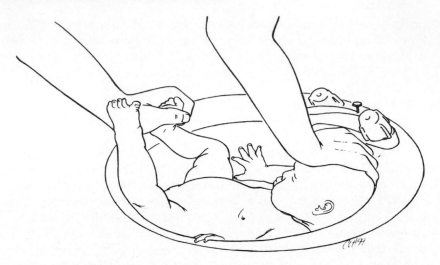

Figure 3.5 Forced immersion burn as child is forced into hot liquid. Used with permission. Daria, S., Sugar, N., Feltman K., Boos, S., Benton, S., Ornstein, A. "Into Hot Water Head First" Pediatric Emergency Care. 20;5:304.

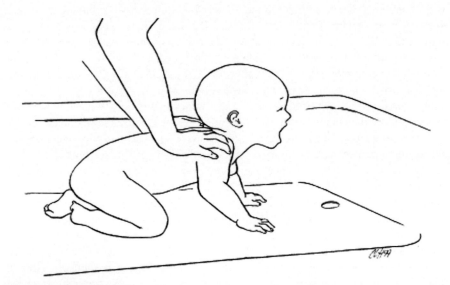

Figure 3.6 Forced immersion burn as child is forced into hot liquid. Used with permission. Daria, S., Sugar, N., Feltman K., Boos, S., Benton, S., Ornstein, A. "Into Hot Water Head First" Pediatric Emergency Care. 20;5:304.

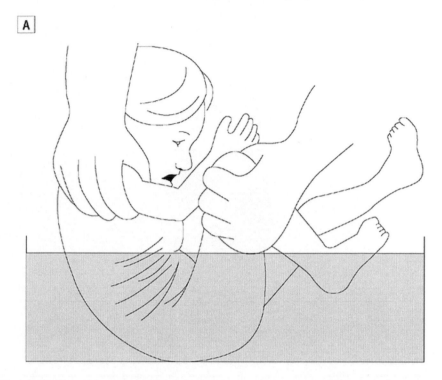

Figure 3.7 Forced immersion burn as child is forced into hot liquid. Stratman & Melski (2002), used with permission. Archives of Dermatology. March, 138;319. Copyright © 2002.

submerged in hot liquid causes a burn of the distal aspect of the extremity that has a clear line of demarcation separating the uniformly burned area from the nonburned area. The palms and soles may appear to be spared because the thicker skin there burns more slowly. Symmetric stocking and glove burns are highly suspicious for inflicted burn injury because few plausible histories could explain why a child would submerge both extremities equally into a hot liquid.

Tap Water: A Special Case

Tap water burns are associated with accidental, neglectful, and inflicted injuries. Injury prevention literature discusses the danger to children as well as to debilitated adults that is posed by hot tap water, depending on the temperature of the water and the duration of exposure (Baptiste & Feck, 1980). Early research done in the 1940s outlined the temperatures and duration of exposure at which adult skin suffers burns (Moritz & Henriques, 1947). The adult's thicker skin and the child's thinner skin are at significant risk for scalding injuries from a variety of common household sources. Home water heaters are set at temperatures that deliver water to the faucet that is between 120°F (49°C) and 150°F (65°C) (Erdman, Feldman, Rivara, Heimbach, & Wall, 1991). Comfortable water temperature for bathing occurs at approxi-

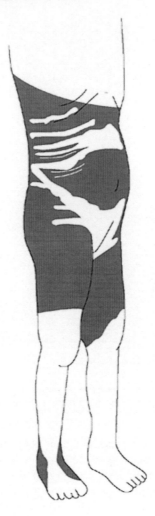

Figure 3.8 Forced immersion burn as child is forced into hot liquid. Stratman & Melski (2002), used with permission. Archives of Dermatology. March, 138;319. Copyright © 2002.

mately 101°F, and hot tubs are typically set at 106 to 108°F (Feldman, 1987). Water becomes painfully hot at 109 to 118°F. Adult skin can tolerate being in water at a temperature of 113°F for approximately 6 hr prior to sustaining a partial thickness burn (Feldman, 1983). Higher temperatures produce burns in shorter time periods. Adult skin placed in water that is at 127°F would suffer a full thickness burn in approximately 1 min. At three degrees higher, 130°F, only 30 s of exposure causes a full thickness burn, and a full thickness burn occurs in only 2 s at 150°F (Feldman, 1987; Moritz & Henriques, 1947) (see Table 3.2 and Figure 3.10). Feldman (1987) notes that a child's thinner skin suffers similar burns in a shorter period of time. It

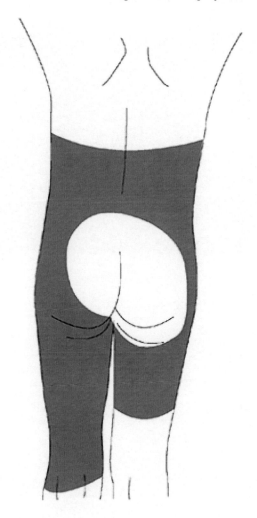

Figure 3.9 Forced immersion burn as child is forced into hot liquid. Stratman & Melski (2002), used with permission. Archives of Dermatology. March, 138;319. Copyright © 2002.

is recommended that home water heaters be set at 120°F to reduce the frequency, morbidity, and mortality of tap water burns in children (Erdman et al., 1991).

Contact Burns

Contact (or dry) burns are another type of burn seen in physical abuse cases (Feldman, 1987). A dry burn occurs when the child's skin is placed in contact with a hot object, such as an iron, heating grate, or the mouth of a hand-held hair dryer (Feldman, 1987; Lenoski & Hunter, 1977; Darok & Reischle, 2001).

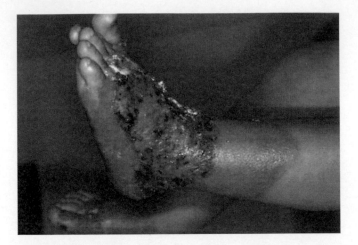

Photo 3.8 Healing burn to foot with stocking distribution; notice line of demarcation on lower leg.

Table 3.2 Effects of water temperature.

Water temperature	Effect
101°F	Comfortable for bathing
106° to 108°F	Typical hot tub temperature
109° to 118°F	Pain threshold for adult
113°F	Partial thickness burn in 6 hr
127°F	Full thickness burn in 1 min
130°F	Full thickness burn in 30 s
150°F	Full thickness burn in 2 s

Source: Adapted from Moritz and Henriques (1947) and Feldman (1987).

The resulting burn frequently forms in the shape of the hot object being touched (see Figures 3.11 and 3.12). Whereas inflicted contact burns are often geometric, accidental burns tend to be less geometric in shape because of the more glancing, brief contact between the exposed body part and the hot object (Feldman, 1987). For example, cigarette burns have different characteristics depending on whether or not they are accidental or inflicted. Accidental cigarette burns occur when the child brushes up against a lit cigarette. This causes a glancing contact, with the child quickly retracting from the cigarette as his or her skin senses the heat, and it results in an irregularly shaped, superficial burn. Inflicted cigarette burns occur as the lit cigarette is forcibly held in contact with the child's skin. This gives rise to a uniform depth and a diameter of approximately 8–10 mm. Inflicted burns are more likely than accidental ones to appear on areas of the body usually protected by clothing, such as the back, chest, and buttocks, or on "target" areas of abuse, including

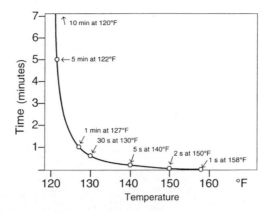

Figure 3.10 Relationship between water temperature and full thickness skin burns. Graphic representation demonstrating the relationship between water temperature and the amount of skin contact time needed to result in a full thickness burn (adapted from Moritz & Henriques, 1947; Katcher, 1981; Richardson, 1994).

the palms, soles, and genitals (Faller-Marquardt, Pollak, & Schmidt, 2008). There are two types of microwave-associated burns: scald-type burns from food or liquid heated in a microwave, which may involve the lips, oral cavity or throat, or present as a spill-type scald; and a second sort, much less common and involving very young infants (1–2 months old) who are placed in microwaves, which are then turned on. This second type of injury may or may not be lethal, and produces a characteristic burn pattern on histologic or pathologic examination, involving burning of skin and muscle (tissues containing large amounts of water), with relative sparing of the sub-cutaneous fat layer between them (fat contains much less water) (Surrell, Alexander, Cohle, Lovell, & Wehrenberg, 1987; Alexander, Surrell & Cohle, 1987). Electri-cal, flame, and chemical burns also may be inflicted upon a child. Although these are less common modes of injury, any child sustaining such injury requires careful evaluation.

Evaluation for Abuse

The history and physical examination are important in determining if abuse or neglect is the cause of the child's burn. The child's developmental ability, plausibility of the explanation, rapidity of seeking treatment, and extent and charac-teristics of the burn are important aspects of the evaluation of the child.

History

In all possible abuse cases, the history elicited from the caregiver, and from the child if verbal, is vital to the evaluation for maltreatment. The responses of the

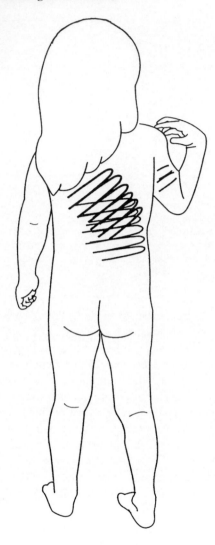

Figure 3.11 Contact burn. The child is held against a hot object such as a heating grate, which leaves a characteristic pattern.

caregiver(s) to the health care provider's questions are noted and considered in the diagnostic process. Table 3.3 lists questions that are asked when a child has been burned.

Physical Examination

The physical examination may offer clues in addition to the presenting burn to suggest the possibility of abuse. Table 3.4 lists the areas assessed in the physical exam-

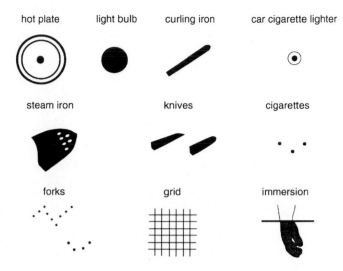

hot plate　　　light bulb　　　curling iron　　　car cigarette lighter

steam iron　　　　　　　knives　　　　　　cigarettes

forks　　　　　　　　grid　　　　　　immersion

Figure 3.12 Hot objects that may leave identifiable shapes and patterns. Johnson (1990) used with permission. Pediatrics Clinics of North america. 37:791–817, Copyright © Elsevier 1990.

ination. Interestingly, in a 2007 study of six children with inflicted burns, all six (100%) were burned on either the left upper or left lower extremity, or both; this is presumably because a right-handed abuser seized the parallel limb of a child facing him/her (Ojo, Palmer, Garvey, Atweh, & Fidler, 2007).

Indicated Laboratory Assessment

The diagnosis of a burn is essentially a clinical diagnosis. No specific laboratory or diagnostic study is indicated to diagnose a burn. Specific laboratory or diagnostic tests may be indicated depending on the severity of the burn or other diagnostic possibilities suggested by the history or physical examination. Children 2 years of age and younger with suspected nonaccidental burns should undergo skeletal surveys to look for occult fractures (Hicks & Stolfi, 2007).

Differential Diagnosis of Burns

The differential diagnosis of a burned child includes accidental injury, inflicted injury, a variety of dermatologic and infectious disorders, and folk-healing practices (Bays, 1994; Davis & Carrasco, 1992; Ellerstein, 1979; Johnson, 1990; Kornberg, 1992; Richardson, 1994; Wissow, 1990a) (see Table 3.5).

The history, physical examination, and, to a lesser extent, laboratory assessment guide the assessment and workup and are crucial to the inclusion and exclusion of possible diagnoses. Comprehensive reviews of the medical literature exist on conditions reportedly mimicking burning (Bays, 1994; Saulsbury & Hayden, 1985). Bacterial infections are common mimickers of burn injuries in children. One of the most

Table 3.3 Evaluation of history of burned child.

A. History of injury
    1. How did the burn occur?
        a. How did child come in contact with burning agent? Who noted the burn?
        b. For how long was child in contact with burning agent? Was skin covered or uncovered?
        c. Was the burn "magical"? (Child was discovered burned and no one saw the actual situation.)
        d. What was the child's reaction to being burned? (cried, etc.)
    2. What is the temperature of tap water in the house? Was the water standing or running?
B. Caregivers' response to injury
    1. Was the child taken for medical care immediately? What is the reason given for any delays in seeking treatment?
    2. Was the child taken for care by an adult other than the one supervising the child at the time of the burn? Why?
    3. Was the burn attributed to the actions of a sibling, playmate, or the child his- or herself?
    4. Is explanation of the burn implausible because of the age or developmental ability of the child, the age of the burn, or the pattern of the burn?
    5. Do the explanations change over time, or do different caregivers render differing accounts?
    6. What is the caregiver's reaction to the situation? (Is there a lack of appropriate concern over the seriousness of the injury?)
C. Medical history and examination
    1. Does the child have a medical condition that mimics burning? What is the location and configuration of the burn? How deep is the burn?
    2. Are there other signs of abuse?
D. History of prior maltreatment
    1. Is there a prior history of maltreatment or frequent visits for injury?
    2. Is the family known to social services for previous concerns of maltreatment?

common is bullous impetigo, a common bacterial skin infection which may be mistaken for cigarette burns. In contrast to inflicted burns, which are usually deep and uniform in size and depth, impetiginous lesions involve only the superficial skin layers, are frequently of different sizes, are associated with crusting (classically honey-colored), and, if necessary, can be cultured for bacteria. They heal with antibiotics, without scarring. Other causes of burn-mimicking skin lesions include: staphylococcal scalded skin syndrome, a toxin-mediated condition resulting in desquamation of the epidermis (Nields, Kessler, Boisot, & Evans, 1998); streptococcal toxic shock syndrome with ecthymatous lesions overlying necrotizing fasciitis (Heider, Priolo, Hultman, Peck, & Cairns, 2002); and eczema (Porzionato & Aprile, 2007).

Phytophotodermatitis presents with skin erythema and bulla formation and is caused by exposure to the sun of skin that has contacted psoralens in the juices of particular plants, such as limes, lemons, parsley, celery, carrots, or figs

Table 3.4 Physical examination for burns.

A. Description of each burn
   1. Type of burn(s): superficial, partial (either superficial or deep), full thickness
   2. Amount of body surface area (BSA) involved (Use Figure 3.9 for
      this estimation in the pediatric patient)
B. Burn characteristics and pattern
   1. Do burns appear older than disclosed in history?
   2. Is the distribution of the burn consistent with the history provided?
      a. Burn incompatible with the events as described (e.g., cigarette burn in
         normally clothed area, burn on area different from what would be expected
         to burn, isolated perineal and genital burns)
   3. Note signs of restraint
      a. During immersion in hot fluid (stocking and glove demarcation on
         extremities, sparing of flexure areas)
      b. Implausible splash marks or lack of them
      c. "Hole-in-doughnut" pattern
C. Identification of other signs of inflicted injury
   1. Presence of injuries such as bruises, fractures, or other burns of differing ages
   2. Evidence of maltreatment such as scars or malnourishment
   3. Injuries related to restraint such as multiple bruises mimicking fingers and
      hands on upper extremities (Ayoub & Pfeiffer, 1979)

(Coffman et al., 1985; Hill, Pickford, & Parkhouse, 1997; Mill et al., 2008). The lesions present in patterns such as drip marks (from dripping juice) or handprints (occurring when a child is handled by an adult with the juice on his/her hands). The history should specifically target contact with plants and plant juices, as well as exposure to sunlight.

Senna, a common ingredient in laxatives, may cause an irritant contact dermatitis (consisting of erythema and desquamation) following ingestion of large doses by young children, when diarrheal stool containing the laxative contacts the buttocks during passage or is contained in contact with the buttocks by a diaper. This burn may be mistaken for an immersion burn, but is characteristically diamond-shaped and follows the edges of the diaper; the gluteal cleft and perianal tissue are typically spared, and no burns to the lower extremities occur. Lesions are less severe in toilet-trained children than in those wearing diapers, presumably because diapers extend the time of contact with the irritant (Leventhal et al., 2001; Spiller et al., 2003; Durani, Agarwal & Wilson, 2006).

Cupping and moxibustion are two forms of folk medicine that can cause superficial burns to the skin and be diagnosed as abuse; the difference is that they are intended to be therapeutic to the patient, not to harm him or her. Cupping consists of a heated glass placed on the skin; a vacuum forms as the air inside cools, producing circular burns, possibly accompanied by bruising or petechiae. Moxibustion involves burning of small pieces of the moxa herb (mugwort) on the skin, producing small circular burns (Look & Look, 1997; Reinhardt & Ruhs, 1985).

Table 3.5 Differential diagnosis of burns.

Condition	Comments
Accidental burns	—May be difficult to differentiate from abusive burns —In one report, children were accidentally placed in contact with hot automobile upholstery, which subsequently burned their skin (Schmitt, Gray, & Britton, 1978). History and physical examination should support the caregiver's explanation of what took place prior to and at the time of the burn.

Dermatologic
    Epidermolysis
        bullosa (EB)
	—Group of blistering skin conditions that vary in terms of inheritance pattern, presentation, histopathology, and biochemical markers and may mimic burns (Cohen, 1993)
	—Characteristic feature is the development of blisters and erosions in response to mechanical trauma
	—Congenital presentation for some of the milder forms may be later in onset, and discovery of some may not be until later childhood or even in adulthood (Tunnessen, 1990)

Dermatitis herpetiformis	—Chronic, recurrent papular skin condition that is generally symmetric in distribution —May be mistaken for cigarette burns if the lesions are excoriated and become hemorrhagic (Fitzpatrick, Polano, & Suurmond, 1983) —Lesions tend to be small, clustered in groups, and intensely pruritic, and they are frequently found symmetrically distributed on the extensor surfaces of the extremities, buttocks, back, and abdomen —Confirmed by biopsy and response to dapsone (Cohen, 1993)
Miscellaneous	—Dermatitis, such as seen with a severe diaper rash mimicking the denuded skin seen in scald burns —Chemical burns from contact of the skin with irritating chemicals, such as analgesic creams —Drug eruptions may have the appearance of a burn —Phytophotodermatitis, in addition to the red, bruise-like lesions discussed above, may also give rise to a blistered appearance
Infections Impetigo	—Superficial bacterial infection of the skin typically caused by *staphylococcus aureus* or group A beta-hemolytic streptococcus —Lesions tend to begin as pustules and then form crusts —Lesions are of different sizes —Local adenopathy is common, lesions tend to spread locally and are pruritic, and other family members may be affected —Lesions respond to oral or topical antibiotics and heal without scarring —Differentiate cigarette burns from streptococcal impetigo; cigarette burns cause scarring (Richardson, 1994)

Folk-healing
    practices
        Coining
	—The skin may be eroded, causing linear lesions resembling burns

Table 3.5 (continued)

Condition	Comments
Cupping	—The cup may be overheated, causing circular burns to the child's skin
Moxibustion	—A variant of acupuncture in which sticks of incense or other material are burned near or on the skin at specific therapeutic points
	—The skin may become reddened, or if the heat is too intense, actual burning may result (Feldman, 1984)
	Parental education is necessary in these cases to help engage parents in less injurious health care practices.

It must be borne in mind that children with disorders that may be confused with burns are not immune to maltreatment (Bays, 1994; Johnson & Coury, 1988). Careful consideration of the possibility of conditions that mimic abuse serves the child's interests and avoids the misdiagnosis of abuse (see Table 3.5).

Treatment: Overview

The treatment and management of children who have burn injuries is complex. The reader is referred to medical texts that offer comprehensive discussion of such burn-related care (Fleisher & Ludwig, 1993; Purdue & Hunt, 1988).

When presented with any child who has a burn, whether or not in the context of maltreatment, the health care provider initially determines if the burn injury is (a) minor, (b) major, or (c) critical (Ahlgren,1990). Initial treatment strategy depends on the extent and severity of the burn as well as the stability of the patient. The extent of the burn is based on an accurate assessment of the amount of the child's body surface area (BSA) that has been burned. Figure 3.13 offers one approach to calculating the BSA in children. Superficial burns (first degree) are not included in the BSA calculation.

Critical Burn

A critical burn is the most severe and, in general, involves more than 30% of the child's BSA and/or has an associated inhalation injury. The ABCs of cardiopulmonary life support may be required. This is a life-threatening situation, and the skills of a trained burn specialist/trauma surgeon are required. Referral to a regional burn center is recommended.

Major Burn

A major burn involves more than 10% of BSA or is at least 2% full thickness. Children with major burns require hospitalization after initial treatment. Initial manage-

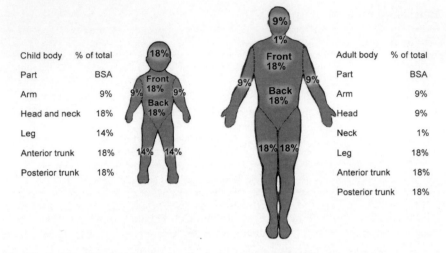

Child body	% of total
Part	BSA
Arm	9%
Head and neck	18%
Leg	14%
Anterior trunk	18%
Posterior trunk	18%

Adult body	% of total
Part	BSA
Arm	9%
Head	9%
Neck	1%
Leg	18%
Anterior trunk	18%
Posterior trunk	18%

Figure 3.13 Rule of nines. Besner and Otabor (2009) used with permission. http://emedicine. medscape.com/article/934173-media

ment includes (a) attention to ABCs, (b) fluid management, (c) analgesia, (d) wound debridement and dressing, and (e) tetanus prophylaxis. Antibiotics are used to treat infection; prophylactic antibiotics are generally discouraged.

Hospitalization may be indicated in children with less than major burns if they are under 2 years of age and/or have burns involving face, hands, perineum, or feet (Meagher, 1990). Of particular concern are circumferential burns of the extremities and chest, which may require emergency escharotomies.

Minor Burns

Finally, minor burns are those that involve less than 10% of the BSA and are less than 2% full thickness. After evaluation and initial management, minor burns may be treated in the outpatient setting with exceptions for the following situations: (a) children under 2 years; (b) burns on the face, hands, feet, and/or perineum; and (c) if abuse is the cause. Initial management includes (a) cooling the burn with water or ice; (b) careful cleansing of the wound with sterile saline, leaving blisters intact; (c) wound dressing with either an occlusive dressing or an antibiotic ointment with activity against methicillin-resistant *Staphylococcus aureus* (Singer, Brebbia, & Soroff, 2007); (d) tetanus prophylaxis; (e) pain control; (f) no routine antibiotics; and (g) close follow-up with scheduled revisit in 24 to 48 hr. At the revisit, dressing supplies may be prescribed if the burn appears to be healing and no signs of infection are present. Periodic reassessment by the clinician is suggested to adequately monitor compliance.

In Brief

- Examination of the child's skin is among the most important components of the suspected physical abuse and neglect evaluation.
- The history, physical examination, and laboratory assessment guide the assessment and workup of bruises and burns.
- The most common soft tissue injuries associated with physical abuse and neglect are bruises and burns.
- The differential diagnosis of a bruised child includes accidental trauma; inflicted trauma (physical abuse); a variety of dermatologic, hematologic, vasculitic, and infectious conditions; and congenital defects in collagen synthesis.
- Injuries to relatively protected areas such as the genitals, buttocks, proximal extremities (thighs, upper arms), neck, and back are suspicious of abuse.
- A bruise may take on the shape of the object used to injure and then heal with a scar that preserves the shape of the object.
- The history of a child who presents with bruising is an important part of the clinician's attempt to differentiate accidental from nonaccidental trauma.
- Attention to the pattern of injury helps the health care professional differentiate bruises caused by abuse from those that occurred accidentally.
- The differential diagnosis of a burned child includes accidental or inflicted injury, dermatologic and infectious conditions, and folk-healing practices.
- Scalds are the most common mechanism of burn injury found in children hospitalized for maltreatment.
- Approximately 4–10% of children hospitalized for burns are believed to have sustained abusive injury.

References

Ahlgren, L. S. (1990). Burns. In S. S. Gellis & B. M. Kagan (Eds.), *Current pediatric therapy* (13th ed., pp. 682–683). Philadelphia, PA: W. B. Saunders.

Alexander, R. C., Surrell, J. A., & Cohle, S. D. (1987, February). Microwave oven burns to children: an unusual manifestation of child abuse. *Pediatrics, 79*(2), 255–260.

American Academy of Pediatrics Committee on Child Abuse and Neglect. (2002, September). When inflicted skin injuries constitute child abuse. *Pediatrics, 110*(3), 644–645.

American Board of Forensic Odontology. (2000, December). Guidelines and standards: bitemark guidelines and standards. Colorado Springs (CO): The Board; 2000. Referenced in: Bell K. Sexual assault: clinical issues: identification and documentation of bite marks. *Journal of Emergency Nursing, 26*(6), 628–630.

Ayoub, C, & Pfeiffer, D. (1979). Burns as a manifestation of child abuse and neglect. *American Journal of Diseases of Children, 133*, 910–914.

Baptiste, M. S., & Feck, G. (1980). Preventing tap water burns. *American Journal of Public Health, 70*, 727–729.

Bays, J. (1994). Conditions mistaken for child abuse. In R. M. Reece (Ed.), *Child abuse: Medical diagnosis and management* (pp. 358–385). Philadelphia, PA: Lea & Febiger.

Besner, G. E. & Otabor, I. A. (2009). Burns: Surgical perspective. eMedicine. March 10, 2009. http://emedicine.medscape.com/article/934173-media.

Carpenter, R. F. (1999, April). The prevalence and distribution of bruising in babies. *Archives of Disease in Childhood, 80*(4), 363–366.

Casella, J. F. (1990). Disorders of coagulation. In F. A. Oski, C. D. DeAngelis, R. D. Feigin, & J. B. Warshaw (Eds.), *Principles and practice of pediatrics* (pp. 1550–1563). Philadelphia, PA: J. B. Lippincott.

Coffman, K., Boyce, W. T., & Hansen, R. C. (1985). Phytodermatitis simulating child abuse. *American Journal of Diseases of Children, 139*, 239–240.

Cotran, R. S., Kumar, V., & Robbins, S. (Eds.) (1989). *Cellular injury and adaptation.* In *Robbins' pathologic basis of disease* (4th ed., pp. 25–26). Philadelphia, PA: W. B. Saunders.

Darok, M., & Reischle, S. (2001, January 1). Burn injuries caused by a hair-dryer—An unusual case of child abuse. *Forensic Science International, 115*(1–2), 143–146.

Daria, S., Sugar, N., Feltman, K., et al. (2004). Into Hot Water Head First: Distribution of Intentional and Unintentional Burns. *Pediatric Emergency Care, 20*, 302–310.

Davis, H. W., & Carrasco, M. (1992). Child abuse and neglect. In B. J. Zitelli & H. W. Davis (Eds.), *Atlas of pediatric physical diagnosis* (2nd ed., pp. 6.1–6.30). London: Wolfe.

Durani, P., Agarwal, R., & Wilson, D. I. (2006). Laxative-induced burns in a child. *Journal of Plastic, Reconstructive and Aesthetic Surgery, 59*(10), 1129.

Ellerstein, N. S. (1979). Cutaneous manifestations of child abuse and neglect. American *Journal of Diseases of Children, 133*, 906–909.

Ellerstein, N. S. (1981). Dermatologic manifestations of child abuse and neglect. In N. S. Ellerstein (Ed.), *Child abuse and neglect: A medical reference.* New York: Wiley.

Erdman, T. C., Feldman, K. W., Rivara, F. P., Heimbach, D. M., & Wall, H. A. (1991). Tap water burn prevention: The effect of legislation. *Pediatrics, 88*, 572–577.

Faller-Marquardt, M., Pollak, S., & Schmidt, U. (2008, April 7). Cigarette burns in forensic medicine. *Forensic Science International, 176*(2–3), 200–208.

Feldman, K. W. (1983). Help needed on hot water burns. *Pediatrics, 71*, 145–146.

Feldman, K. W. (1987). Child abuse by burning. In R. E. Helfer & R. S. Kempe (Eds.), *The battered child* (4th ed., pp. 197–213). Chicago: University of Chicago Press.

Fleisher, G. R., & Ludwig, S. (1993). *Textbook of pediatric emergency medicine* (3rd ed.). Baltimore: Williams & Wilkins

Gedalia, A. (2004, June). Henoch-Schönlein purpura. *Current Rheumatology Reports, 6*(3), 195–202.

Gillespie, R. W. (1965). The battered child syndrome: Thermal and caustic manifestations. *Journal of Trauma, 5*, 523–533.

Hammond, J., Perez-Stable, A., & Ward, G. (1991). Predictive value of historical and physical characteristics for the diagnosis of child abuse. *Southern Medical Journal, 84*, 166–168.

Hathaway, W. E., Hay, W. W., Groothuis, J. R., & Paisley, J. W. (1993). *Current p pediatric diagnosis and treatment.* Norwalk, Ct. Appleton & Lange.

Heider, T. R., Priolo, D., Hultman, C. S., Peck, M. D., & Cairns, B. A. (2002, September–October). Eczema mimicking child abuse: a case of mistaken identity. *Journal of Burn Care and Rehabilitation, 23*(5):357–359.

Hicks, R. A., & Stolfi, A. (2007, May). Skeletal surveys in children with burns caused by child abuse. *Pediatric Emergency Care, 23*(5), 308–313.

Hight, D. W., Bakalar, H. R., & Lloyd, J. R. (1979). Inflicted burn in children: Recognition and treatment. *Journal of the American Medical Association, 242*, 517–520.

Hill, P. F., Pickford, M., & Parkhouse, N. (1997, October). Phytophotodermatitis mimicking child abuse. *Journal of the Royal Society of Medicine, 90*(10), 560–561.

Jackson, D. M. (1953). The diagnosis of the depth of burning. *British Journal of Surgery, 40,* 588.

Johnson, C. F. (1990). Inflicted injury versus accidental injury. *Pediatric Clinics of North America, 37,* 791–814.

Johnson, C. F., & Coury, D. L. (1988). Bruising and hemophilia: Accident or child abuse? *Child Abuse & Neglect, 12,* 409–415.

Johnson, C. F., & Showers, J. (1985). Injury variables in child abuse. *Child Abuse & Neglect, 9,* 207–215.

Keen, J. H., Lendrulm, J., & Wolman, B. (1975). Inflicted burns and scalds in children. *British Medical Journal, 4,* 268–269.

Kemp, A., Maguire, S. A., Sibert, J., Frost, R., Adams, C., & Mann, M. (2006, November). Can we identify abusive bites in children? *Archives of Disease in Childhood, 91*(11), 951.

Kessler, D. B., & Hyden, P. (1991). Physical, sexual, and emotional abuse of children. *CIBA Foundation Symposium, 43*(2), 1–32.

Kornberg, A. E. (1992). Skin and soft tissue injuries. In S. Ludwig & A. E. Kornberg (Eds.), *Child abuse: A medical reference* (2nd ed., pp. 91–104). New York: Churchill Livingstone.

Kos, L., & Shwayder, T. (2006, July–August). Cutaneous manifestations of child abuse. *Pediatric Dermatology, 23*(4), 311–320.

Langlois, N. E. I., & Gresham, G. A. (1991). The aging of bruises: A review and study of the color changes with time. *Forensic Science International, 50,* 227–238.

Lenoski, E. F., & Hunter, K. A. (1977). Specific patterns of inflicted burn injuries. *Journal of Trauma, 17,* 842–846.

Leventhal, J. M., Griffin, D., Duncan, K. O., Starling, S., Christian, C. W., & Kutz, T. (2001, January). Laxative-induced dermatitis of the buttocks incorrectly suspected to be abusive burns. *Pediatrics, 107*(1), 178–179.

Look, K. M., & Look, R. M. (1997, January). Skin scraping, cupping, and moxibustion that may mimic child abuse. *Journal of Forensic Sciences, 42*(1), 103–105.

Maguire, S., Mann, M. K., Sibert, J., & Kemp, A. (2005, February). Are there patterns of bruising in childhood which are diagnostic or suggestive of abuse? A systematic review. *Archives of Disease in Childhood, 90*(2), 182–186.

Meagher, D. P. (1990). Burns. In J. G. Raffensperger (Ed.), *Swenson's pediatric surgery* (5th ed., pp. 317–337). Norwalk, CT: Appleton & Lange.

Mill, J., Wallis, B., Cuttle, L., Mott, J., Oakley, A., & Kimble, R. (2008, August). Phytophotodermatitis: case reports of children presenting with blistering after preparing lime juice. *Burns, 34*(5), 731–733.

Moritz, A. R., & Henriques, F. C. (1947). Studies of thermal injury: The relative importance of time and surface temperature in the causation of cutaneous burns. *American Journal of Pathology, 23,* 695–720.

Nields, H., Kessler, S. C., Boisot, S., & Evans, R. (1998, March). Streptococcal toxic shock syndrome presenting as suspected child abuse. *American Journal of Forensic Medicine and Pathology, 19*(1), 93–97.

Nielsen, A., Knoblauch, N. T., Dobos, G. J., Michalsen, A., & Kaptchuk, T. J. (2007, September–October). The effect of Gua Sha treatment on the microcirculation of surface tissue: A pilot study in healthy subjects. *Explore (NY), 3*(5), 456–466.

Ojo, P., Palmer, J., Garvey, R., Atweh, N., & Fidler, P. (2007, March). Pattern of burns in child abuse. *American Surgery, 73*(3), 253–255.

O'Neill, J., Meacham, W., Griffin, P. P., & Sawyers, J. L. (1973). Patterns of injury in the battered child syndrome. *Journal of Trauma, 13*, 332–339.

O'Neill, J. A. (1979). Burns in children. In C. P. Artz, J. A. Moncrief, & B. A. Pruitt (Eds.), *Burns: A team approach* (pp. 341–350). Philadelphia, PA: W. B. Saunders.

Pascoe, J. M., Hildebrandt, H. M., Tarrier, A., & Murphy, M. (1979). Patterns of skin injury in nonaccidental and accidental injury. *Pediatrics, 64*, 245–247.

Peck, M. D., & Priolo-Kapel, D. (2002, November). Child abuse by burning: A review of the literature and an algorithm for medical investigations. *Journal of Trauma, 53*(5), 1013–1022.

Porzionato, A., & Aprile, A. (2007). Staphylococcal scalded skin syndrome mimicking child abuse by burning. *Forensic Science International, 168*(1), e1–e4.

Purdue, G. F., Hunt, J. L., & Prescott, P. R. (1988). Child abuse by burning—An index of suspicion. *Journal of Trauma, 28*, 221–224.

Rapaport, S. I. (1983). Preoperative hemostatic evaluation: Which tests, if any? *Blood, 61*, 229–231.

Reece, R. M., & Ludwig, S. (2001, January). *Child abuse: Medical diagnosis and management* (2nd ed.). Philadelphia, PA: Lippincott Williams and Wilkins.

Reinhardt, M. A., & Ruhs, H. 1985). Moxibustion. Another traumatic folk remedy. *Clinical Pediatrics (Phila), 24*(1), 58–59.

Richardson, A. C. (1994). Cutaneous manifestations of abuse. In R. M. Reece (Ed.), *Child abuse: Medical diagnosis and management* (pp. 167–184). Philadelphia, PA: Lea & Febiger.

Robson, M. C., & Heggers, J. P. (1988). Pathophysiology of the burn wound. In H. F. Carvajal & D. H. Parks (Eds.), *Burns in children: Pediatric burn management* (pp. 27–32). Chicago: Year Book.

Saulsbury, F. T., & Hayden, G. F. (1985). Skin conditions simulating child abuse. *Pediatric Emergency Care, 1*, 147–150.

Schwartz, A. J., & Ricci, L. R. (1996). How accurately can bruises be aged in abused children? Literature review and synthesis. *Pediatrics, 97*, 254–256.

Showers, J., & Garrison, K. M. (1988). Burn abuse: A four-year study. *Journal of Trauma, 28*, 1581–1583.

Singer, A. J., Brebbia, J., Soroff, H. H. (2007, July). Management of local burn wounds in the ED. *American Journal of Emergency Medicine, 25*(6), 666–671.

Spiller, H. A., Winter, M. L., Weber, J. A., Krenzelok, E. P., Anderson, D. L., & Ryan, M. L. (2003, May). Skin breakdown and blisters from senna-containing laxatives in young children. *Annual Pharmacology, 37*(5), 636–639.

Stone, N. H., Rinaldo, L., Humphrey, C. R., & Brown, R. H. (1970). *Surgical Clinics of North America, 50*, 1419–1424.

Stratman, E., & Melski, J. (2002). Scald Abuse. *JAMA, 138*(3), 318–320.

Surrell, J. A., Alexander, R. C., Cohle, S. D., Lovell, F. R. Jr., & Wehrenberg, R. A. (1987, August). Effects of microwave radiation on living tissues. *Journal of Trauma, 27*(8), 935–939.

Sussman, S. H. (1968). Skin manifestations of the Battered Child Syndrome. *Journal of Pediatrics, 72*, 99–101.

Sweet, D., Lorente, M., Lorente, J. A., Valenzuela, A., & Villanueva, E. (1997, March). An improved method to recover saliva from human skin: The double swab technique. *Journal of Forensic Science, 42*(2), 320–322.

Vogeley, E., Pierce, M. C., & Bertocci, G. (2002, March). Experience with wood lamp illumination and digital photography in the documentation of bruises on human skin. *Archives of Pediatrics & Adolescent Medicine, 156*(3), 265–268.

Wilson, E. F. (1977). Estimation of the age of cutaneous contusions in child abuse. *Pediatrics*, *60*, 750–752.

Wissow, L. S.(1990a). *Child advocacy for the clinician: An approach to child abuse and neglect*. Baltimore: Williams & Wilkins.

Appendix

Series 1: Bruising of buttocks and upper high.

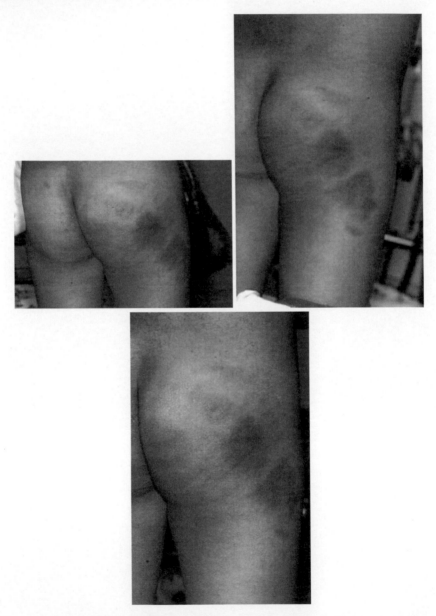

Photo 1a, b and c Photos taken at different distances showing bruises on left thigh and buttock.

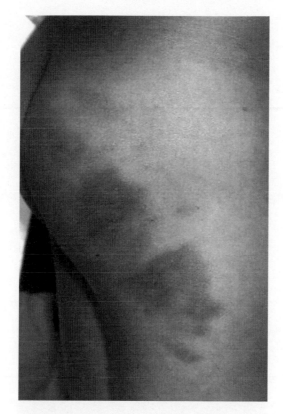

Photo 1d   Photo of bruises on thigh taken from a different angle.

Series 2: Child with bruising of ears.

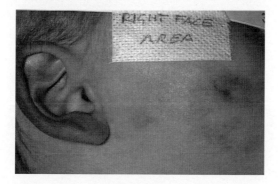

Photo 2a   Photo of patient's right ear from a distance.

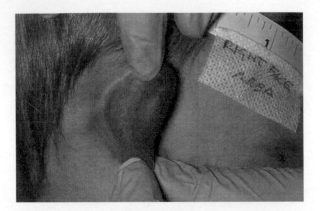

Photo 2b Photo of right ear exposed from behind.

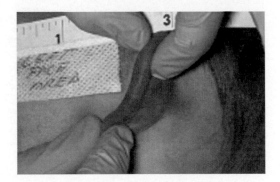

Photo 2c Photo of left ear exposed from behind.

Series 3: Lacerations/abrasions to abdomen.

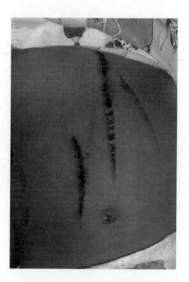

Photo 3a Photo taken at a distance showing the lacerations/abrasions on the patient's abdomen.

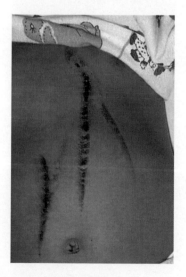

Photo 3b Photo of patient in 3a at a closer distance.

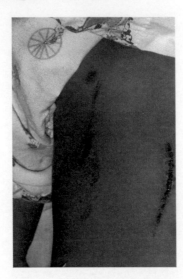

Photo 3c Photo of 3a taken at a different angle to capture a side view of the laceration/abrasion.

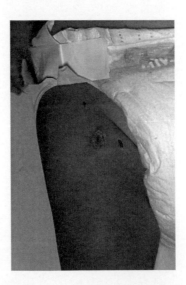

Photo 3d Photo of patient 3a with injury to right upper thigh.

Series 4: Burns of right hand with denuded skin and lower torso. Please take note of the various angles of the photos.

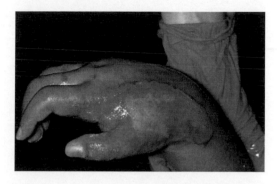

Photo 4a   Photo taken from the side angle of right hand with denuded skin.

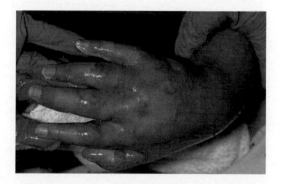

Photo 4b   Photo of the dorsum of the burned right hand.

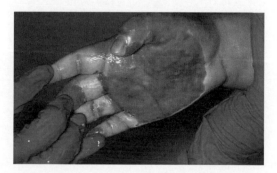

Photo 4c   Photo of the burned right palm with denuded skin.

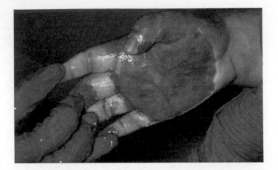

Photo 4d Photo of patient in 4c at closer view.

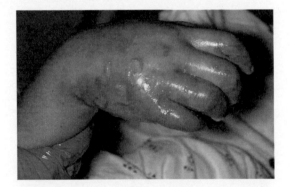

Photo 4e Photo taken from the side angle of burned right hand.

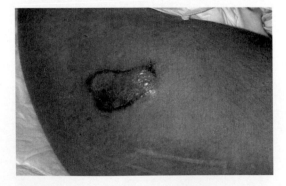

Photo 4f Photo of patient in 4e showing burned right thigh.

Series 5: Child with burns on the surfaces of both feet and the left hand.

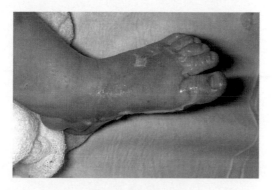

Photo 5a Photo of burns on the dorsum of the burned left foot.

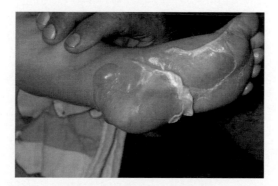

Photo 5b Photo of left foot with burns on the plantar surface.

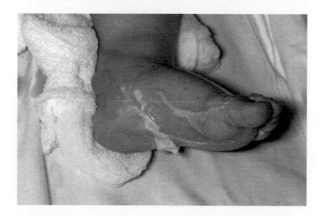

Photo 5c Photo taken at a different angle of the burns on left foot.

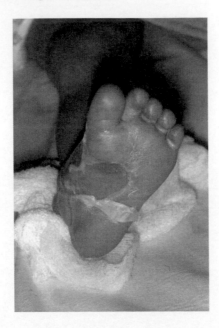

Photo 5d Photo taken at a different angle of the left foot showing the burns on plantar surface.

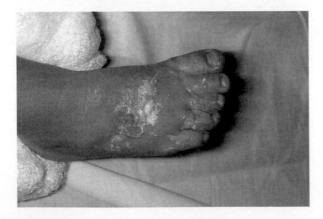

Photo 5e Photo of burns on dorsal surface of the right foot.

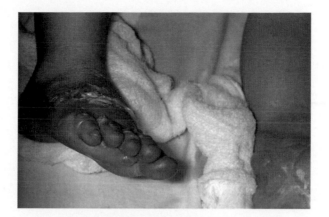

Photo 5f Photo taken at a different angle of the burns on dorsal surface of the right foot.

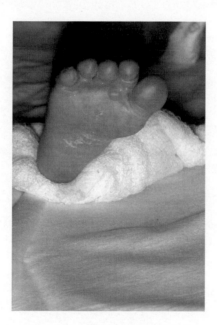

Photo 5g Photo of the burns on plantar surface of right foot.

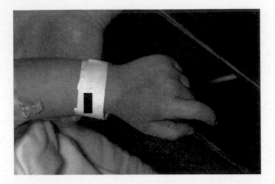

Photo 5h Photo of the same patient in 5a with a burned left hand.

Series 6: Circumscribed burns which may be confused with infections such as impetigo.

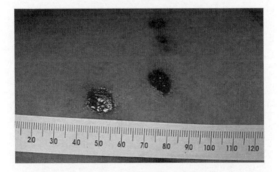

Photo 6a Circumscribed burns which may be confused with infections such as impetigo.

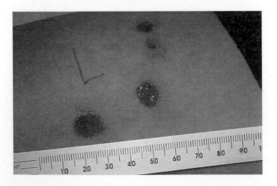

Photo 6b Photo from a distance of circumscribed burns.

Series 7: Child with burns to the body including face, shoulders and chest.

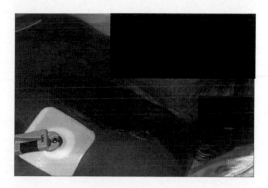

Photo 7a Photo of burns on left shoulder.

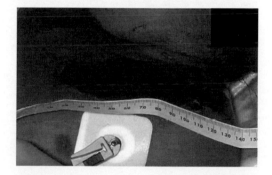

Photo 7b Photo taken from a closer distance of burns on left shoulder.

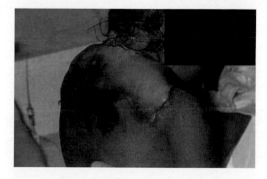

Photo 7c Photo of burns on child's right upper back.

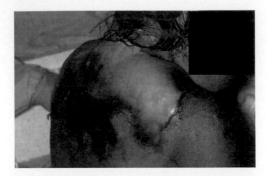

Photo 7d Photo of burns on child's right upper back taken at a closer distance.

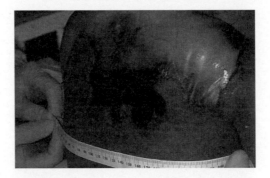

Photo 7e Photo taken at a different angle and distance of burns on child's right upper back.

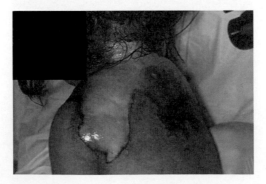

Photo 7f Photo of burns on child's left upper back and neck.

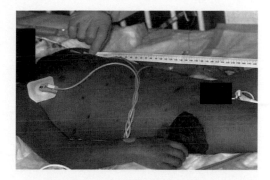

Photo 7g Photo of patient with burns to the body including face, shoulders, chest and right hip area.

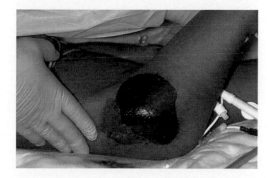

Photo 7h Photo of the burn on the right hip taken at a closer angle.

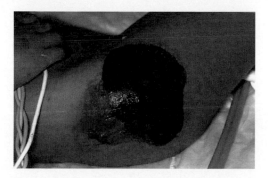

Photo 7i Photo taken from a different view of burn of right hip.

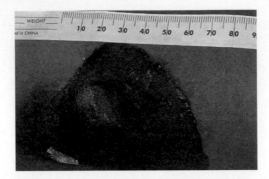

Photo 7j Photo taken at a closer distance of injury in 7i.

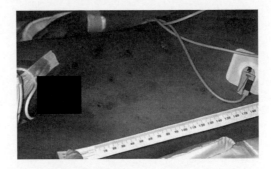

Photo 7k Photo of burns of lower abdomen

Chapter 4

Fractures and Skeletal Injuries

Nancy S. Harper and Arne H. Graff

General Principles

The identification of a skeletal injury may be the first indication of abuse. Estimates of the frequency of fractures in abused children vary from approximately 10% to 50% depending on the population studied, the type of diagnostic imaging used to detect fractures, and the age of the patients seen (Ebbin, Gollub, Stein, & Wilson, 1969; Herndon, 1983; Leventhal, Thomas, Rosenfield, & Markowitz, 1993). Recently, large population-based studies have been used to estimate the incidence of inflicted skeletal trauma. While the majority of fractures are still attributed to falls, child abuse accounts for 12% of fractures in children less than 36 months of age (Leventhal, et al., 2008). Infants and young children sustain significantly more abusive skeletal injuries than do older children, with the majority of inflicted fractures occurring in children under 12 months of age (Leventhal, 2008; Loder & Feinberg, 2007; Sibert, et al., 2002). Fractures of the ribs, arm, and leg account for over half of the inflicted skeletal injuries in young children (Leventhal, Martin, & Asnes, 2008; Starling, Sirotnak, Heisler, & Barnes-Eley, 2007). These injuries are often occult and detected only with detailed skeletal imaging.

The presence of a fracture does not prove abuse. The combination of clinical examination and history of the injury with the application of biomechanics (force, stress, bone tolerance, etc.) will help to differentiate accidental from non-accidental injuries. A detailed review of biomechanics is not included in this chapter (Pierce, Bertocci, Vogeley, & Moreland, 2004).

Bone Anatomy and Fracture Description

The anatomic and physiologic characteristics of the immature skeleton affect the frequency, type, location, and healing of pediatric fractures. Bones such as the femur are comprised of two types of bone: compact (cortical) bone and trabecular (spongy, cancellous) bone. Cortical bone has multiple concentric rings of lamellae housing the haversian canals. Mineralization and thickness of the cortical bone contribute

141

A.P. Giardino et al. (eds.), *A Practical Guide to the Evaluation of Child Physical Abuse and Neglect*, DOI 10.1007/978-1-4419-0702-8_4, © Springer Science+Business Media, LLC 1997, 2010

to its strength and stiffness. Developing and cancellous bone is more porous than cortical bone, affecting both the stiffness and flexibility of the bone, as well as the extent and type of fractures seen in children. Less dense, porous bone may help stop the propagation of a fracture line, but this quality also makes the bone more vulnerable to compression. This is well-demonstrated in the metaphyseal region where the thinner porous cortex surrounding the trabecular bone makes compression injury and buckle fracture more likely. This region where the metaphysis transitions to cortical bone has been referred to by Pierce et al. (2004) as the internal "stress riser" (Pierce et al., 2004) (Photos 4.10 and 4.11). The strength of the bone is related to its mineralization. The bones of children are less mineralized, less stiff than adult bone, but are more elastic.

The periosteum is the fibrous membrane that covers the surface of a bone. It is quite vascular supplying nutrients to the bone. It is loosely adherent to the diaphysis and tightly adherent to the metaphysis and epiphyseal region contributing to the formation of the bone collar (Pierce et al., 2004). The periosteum of the child is more osteogenic, or bone forming. The diaphyses of a child are formed through intramembranous bone formation. The periosteum retains this ability and can form bone without a cartilage scaffold (Shopfner, 1966). Bone healing is much more rapid in children than in adults, and more rapid in infants than in older children. For example, the healing of a midshaft femur fracture may take only 3 weeks in an infant, but 20 weeks in a teenager (Ogden, 1990). This difference is mostly due to the contribution of the periosteum in the healing of young bones.

The morphological features of the fracture include the bone involved, the location of the fracture within the bone, the type of fracture sustained, and the relationship of the fracture segments (Pierce et al., 2004). The mechanism of the injury as reported by the caretaker is also noted in the fracture assessment. Table 4.1 describes

Table 4.1 Anatomy of the long bone.

Bone	Characteristics
Condyle	The rounded articular (joint) surface at the end of a bone
Diaphysis	The shaft of a long bone
Epiphysis	The part of the long bone developed from a center of ossification —Separate from the shaft and separated from it by a layer of cartilage (the epiphyseal plate) —In infants and young children, not often visualized by X-ray because it is not ossified
Metaphysis	Growth zone between epiphysis and diaphysis; radiographically identified by the flaring portion of the long bone
Periosteum	Thick, fibrous membrane covering surface of a bone and consisting of two layers: inner osteogenic (bone forming) and outer connective tissue layer containing blood vessels and nerves that supply the bone

Table 4.2 Types of fracture.

Type of fracture	Characteristics
Comminuted	Bone broken into multiple pieces
Compound	Open fracture (i.e., through the skin)
Depressed	Skull fractures in which a part of the skull is inwardly displaced (toward the brain)
Diastatic	Fracture with significant separation of bone fragments; often used in relation to skull fractures
Distal	Fracture located away from center of body (near the feet or hands when describing fractures of the extremities)
Greenstick	An incomplete fracture—the compressed side of the bone is bowed, but not completely fractured. Young bones are more malleable, porous, and less brittle than an adult's, and may bend and only partially break when injured.
Hairline	Fracture without separation of the fragments (similar to a thin crack of a vase)
Impacted	A compression fracture
Linear	Resembling a line; often used to describe skull fractures
Oblique	Fracture line angled across long axis of bone (from approximately 30–45 degrees)
Occult	—Condition in which there is clinical, but not radiographic, evidence of a fracture. X-rays repeated in a few weeks show evidence of fracture healing.
	—May also indicate a fracture seen radiographically but without clinical manifestations (e.g., rib fractures and metaphyseal fractures)
Pathologic	Fracture that occurs in area of bone weakened by an underlying disease
Proximal	Fractures located toward trunk of body (for fractures of the extremities, near the hips or shoulders)
Spiral	Fracture line oblique and encircles a portion of the bone (resembles twist of a candy cane)
Stellate	Fracture lines of break radiate from central point; seen in some skull fractures
Supracondylar	Fracture to area above condyle, typically of the humerus
Torus	Impacted injury specific to children; bone buckles, rather than fracturing completely, and usually involves the metaphysis of the bone
Transverse	Fracture line perpendicular to the long axis of the bone

the anatomy of the bone, and Table 4.2 describes different types of fractures (see Figures 4.1 and 4.2).

The history of the injury is important in identifying abusive fractures because historical information should be compatible with the morphological features of the fracture and the mechanics required to cause the fracture (Photos 4.1, 4.2, 4.3, and 4.4). Torsional loading, as seen with twisting or rotation of the extremity, often results in spiral fractures (O'Connor-Read, Teh, & Willett, 2007; Pierce, 2004) (Photo 4.7). A bending load (both tensile and compressive forces occur)

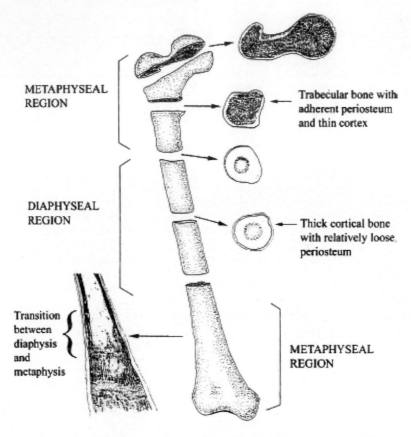

METAPHYSEAL REGION

Trabecular bone with adherent periosteum and thin cortex

DIAPHYSEAL REGION

Thick cortical bone with relatively loose periosteum

Transition between diaphysis and metaphysis

METAPHYSEAL REGION

Figure 4.1 Illustration of bone architecture. Pierce et al. (2004) used with permission.

applied to the extremity can result in a transverse fracture, perpendicular to the bone (Photo 4.1). Direct trauma also produces transverse fractures with the degree of fragmentation or comminution (Photos 4.12 and 4.13) associated with the force of the impact. Oblique fractures are likely the result of combination loading (torsional, tensile, and compressive) (Photo 4.5). The buckle fracture, as noted previously, is the result of a failure under compressive forces and typically occurs from axial loading. Immature bone fails in compression first, with the fracture line at the weakest point of the bone. Distal femur buckle fractures occur as the result of the compression of hard, cortical bone into the softer, trabecular bone of the metaphysis (Pierce et al., 2004) (Photos 4.10 and 4.11). The field of biomechanics has advanced the understanding of the association between loading forces, history and corresponding injuries. Pierce et al. (2005) found that the linear momentum associated with transverse fractures was almost 10 times greater than that seen with spiral or buckle fractures (Pierce et al., 2005) (Photos 4.1, 4.5 and 4.10).

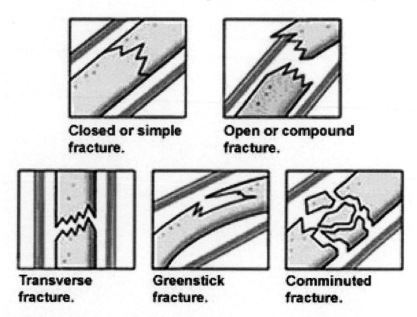

Closed or simple fracture.

Open or compound fracture.

Transverse fracture.

Greenstick fracture.

Comminuted fracture.

Figure 4.2 Illustration of fracture types. Reproduced with permission from Moseley (2009).

Fractures resulting from abuse are varied in their presentation. Clinically, the preverbal child may present with signs and symptoms indicative of pain such as irritability, crying with movement of the affected area, and decreased use of a broken limb. The majority of children with accidental injury do not have associated bruising (Worlock, Stower, & Barbor, 1986). Bruising has been documented in association with fracture in only 8–9% of children, including children with inflicted fractures (Mathew, Ramamohan, & Bennet, 1998; Peters, Starling, Barnes-Eley, & Heisler, 2008). Single skeletal injuries are most common. However, the identification of multiple fractures and/or fractures in different stages of healing should raise the suspicion of child abuse.

The identification by a health care professional of an inflicted fracture is dependent on multiple factors. They include the ability to obtain a complete and detailed history of the trauma causing the fracture, knowledge regarding fracture mechanisms in childhood, an understanding of pediatric development, and a complete and thorough evaluation of children who may have skeletal injuries that are the result of abuse. There are certain pediatric fractures that, in isolation, are so highly suspicious for child abuse that they raise concern of abuse in the absence of clinical history. These include metaphyseal and rib fractures in infants. Although diaphyseal fractures are the most common fractures that result from abuse, they are not specific for abusive injuries (Photos 4.1, 4.5, 4.7, 4.31 and 4.32).

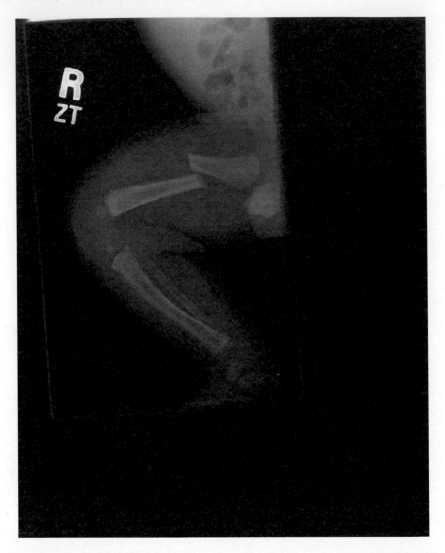

Photo 4.1 6-week-old male presents with leg swelling. Father reports falling on baby. Skeletal survey notable for right proximal transverse femur fracture with classic metaphyseal lesions of proximal and distal tibia.

Imaging Techniques

Skeletal Survey

The diagnosis of skeletal injuries is made by history and physical examination, and confirmed by radiographic imaging. Some skeletal injuries may not be apparent by clinical examination. A radiographic skeletal survey is part of the workup in infants and young children suspected of abuse (Photos 4.31 and 4.32).

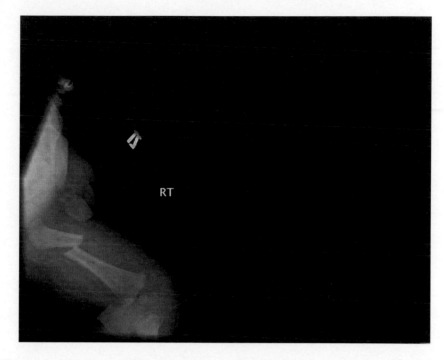

Photo 4.2 Additional angled lateral view of 6 week old male's leg shows a "bucket-handle" classic metaphyseal lesion of the proximal right tibia.

A skeletal survey is a series of X-rays taken of the child's skeleton to look for indications of new or old injury. The skeletal survey is mandatory in cases of suspected physical abuse for all infants and children under 2 years of age. It is not generally used in patients over 5 years of age. Clinical judgment is used to determine whether a screening survey is indicated for children between the ages of 2 and 5. The X-rays must include restricted views of the areas radiographed in order to obtain proper quality and resolution of the bones (Diagnostic Imaging of Child Abuse., 2009). The skeletal survey includes additional radiographs, such as lateral and/or oblique views when clinically or radiographically indicated. Many institutions now include oblique views of the chest in their imaging protocol (Photos 4.25 and 4.26). A "babygram" (i.e. a single full body image) is not acceptable. The following films are included as part of the skeletal survey (American College of Radiology, 2006):

1. Anteroposterior view of the arms, forearms, hands, femurs, lower legs, and feet on separate exposures
2. Lateral and anterior views of the axial skeleton to evaluate for vertebral, sternal, rib, and pelvic fractures
3. Anteroposterior and lateral views of the skull to evaluate for skull fractures

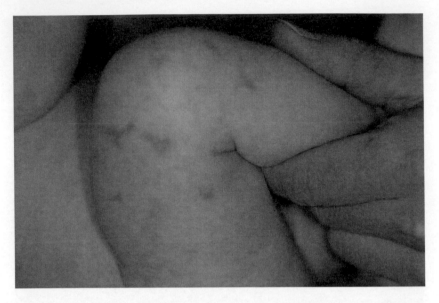

Photo 4.3 Bruising noted on the right leg of the 6 week old male appears consistent with grip marks.

Even when the skeletal survey is performed correctly, it may fail to reveal acute rib fractures and classic metaphyseal lesions. It is recommended that the initial skeletal survey be repeated in approximately 2 weeks in cases of suspected physical abuse in children less than 1 year of age. The repeat or follow-up skeletal survey has been shown to yield additional information in 46–61% of cases, often changing the outcome of the case (ruling abuse in or out) (Photos 4.20 and 4.21). The additional injuries detected are often rib fractures and metaphyseal lesions (Kleinman, Marks, Nimkin, Rayder, & Kessler, 1996; Zimmerman, Makoroff, Care, Thomas, & Shapiro, 2005) (Photos 4.22, 4.23, 4.25, 4.26, 4.28, 4.29, and 4.30).

Skeletal surveys are also recommended postmortem in cases of suspected physical abuse in children under 2 years of age. At a minimum, postmortem radiography should include well-collimated views of the long bones (appendicular skeleton) with additional views as necessary as the axial skeleton is visualized during the autopsy (The Society for Pediatric Radiology, 2004).

Radionuclide Bone Scan

The radionuclide bone scan is a sensitive test for detecting new (less than 7–10 days old) rib fractures, subtle diaphyseal fractures, and early periosteal elevation. It is sometimes used as an adjunct to plain films. Most fractures can be identified by bone scan within the first 48 h after an injury. Bone scan is not sensitive for the detection of skull fractures and does not allow for the dating of injuries.

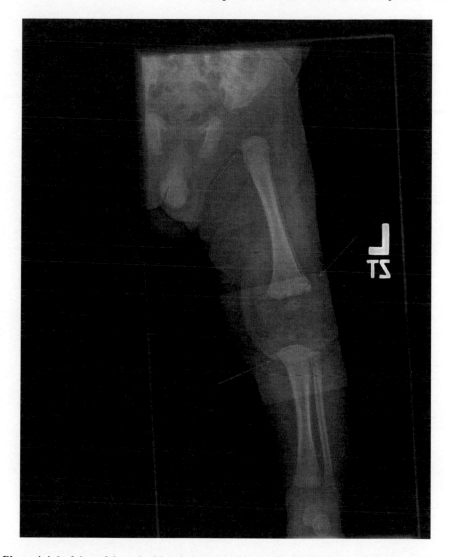

Photo 4.4 Left leg of 6 week old male is notable for multiple fractures including a proximal femur and proximal tibia classic metaphyseal lesions. Extensive traumatic periosteal reaction is seen along the lateral femur extending into the metaphysis. The distal femur has a classic metaphyseal lesion versus physeal fracture.

It is most often used in cases of suspected abuse of infants and young children in which the skeletal survey is negative and a more sensitive (but less specific) test is needed (see Chapter 2). A bone scan is used occasionally as a method of initial screening.

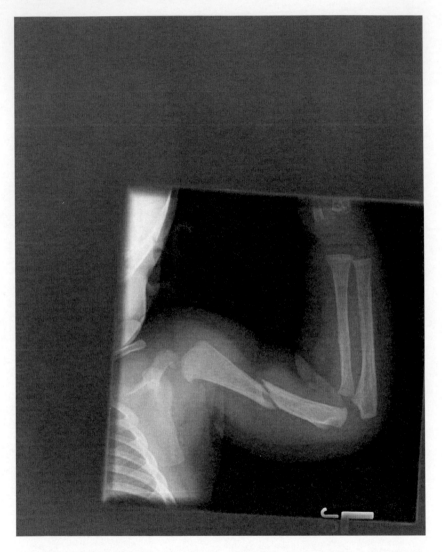

Photo 4.5 4 month old male found crying in crib lying on chest. Skeletal survey notable for oblique fracture of left humerus.

Computed Tomography

Computed tomography has been traditionally utilized in imaging the head, chest, abdomen, and pelvis for traumatic injuries. With the arrival of multidetector CT scanning (with 16, 32 and 64 slice technology), coronal and sagital as well as 3D reconstructions can be performed in addition to standard axial imaging. CT recon-struction technology has been useful in the delineation and identification of meta-physeal fractures, rib fractures (Kleinman & Schlesinger, 1997; Wootton-Gorges

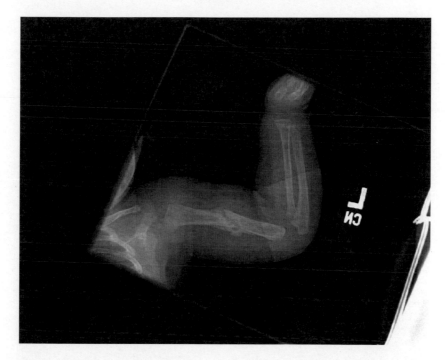

Photo 4.6 Abdundant callus formation is seen of the 4 month old's humerus on imaging performed 3 weeks after injury.

et al., 2008), complex skull fractures, and skull variants in cases of head injury (Photos 4.17, 4.18, 4.19 and 4.27).

Stages of Fracture Healing

The radiographic appearance of bone healing has been divided into stages. These stages are not discrete and exist on more of a continuum as they vary between individuals depending on age, disease, repeated trauma, immobilization, and surgical fixation. A number of fractures, such as metaphyseal and skull fractures, do not follow these stages and are difficult to date. The presence of soft tissue swelling on the scalp may help differentiate recent from older fractures.

Stage 1: Induction

The radiologic appearance of fractured long bones corresponds to the anatomic and histologic changes that occur with bone healing. Radiographically, soft tissue swelling around the injured bone represents the initial change and may be the only indication of the fracture. An injury to a bone and the soft tissues around the bone results in immediate hemorrhage and subsequent inflammation. This is

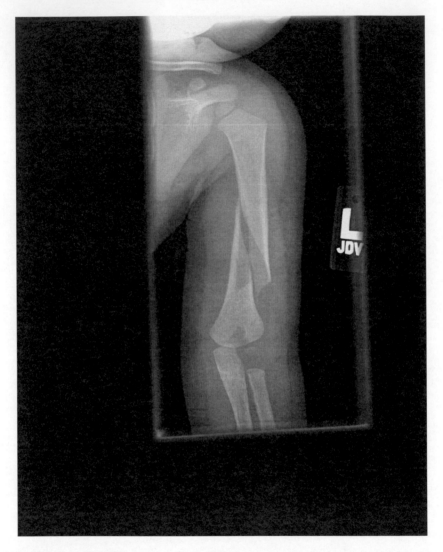

Photo 4.7 16 mo female who presented to the ER with arm swelling and pain with a reported fall. Child had multiple bruises, traumatic alopecia, and failure to thrive. Skeletal survey notable for a left humerus spiral fracture as well as a skull fracture.

clinically represented by swelling and tenderness. The majority of broken bones are not accompanied by associated external bruising or injury (Worlock et al., 1986; Mathew et al., 1998; Peters et al., 2008). Radiographically evident soft tissue swelling with obliteration of normal fat and fascial planes may persist for a few days or may last longer if the injury is severe (Merten, Cooperman, & Thompson, 1994). In general, soft tissue swelling resolves as formation of the callus develops (Kleinman, 1998). An initial widening of the gap and softening of the fracture

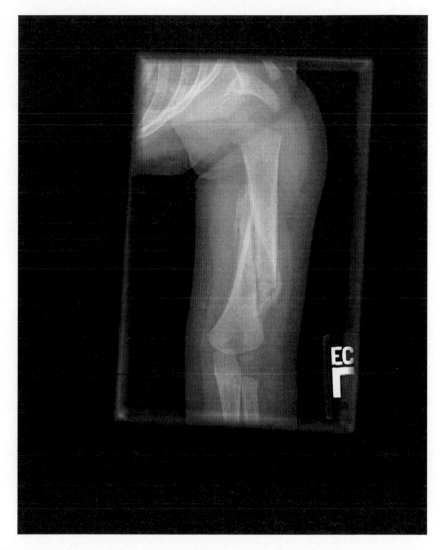

Photo 4.8 Left humerus spiral fracture at 20 days with callus formation.

margins occurs as the osteoclasts respond to the necrotic ends of the bone with bone resorption (Photo 4.24). This becomes apparent radiographically around 2–3 weeks after injury (Chapman, 1992; Islam et al., 2000).

Stage 2: Soft Callus

Callus formation begins with the laying down of periosteal new bone. Hemorrhage and inflammation occurring at the site of injury are osteo-inductive as the periosteum is rich in precursors cells and osteoblasts. Periosteal new bone is not specific

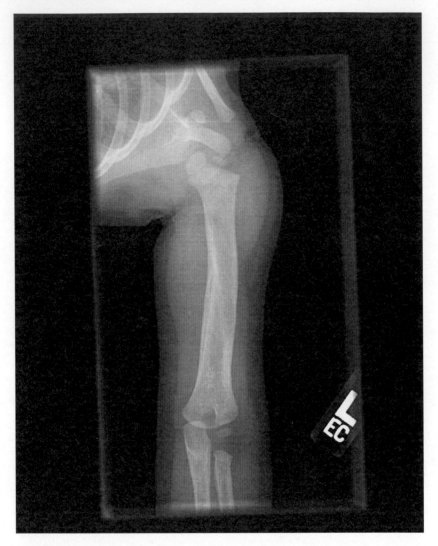

Photo 4.9 Left humerus spiral fracture at 4 months with remodeling.

for fractures and is laid down in response to a number of different injuries, including burns, frostbite, and infection (Kleinman, 1998), Periosteal new bone formation occurs approximately 1–4 weeks after an injury and may be earlier in young infants (Islam et al., 2000; Prosser et al., 2005). The initial callus consists of new blood vessels, fibrous tissue, cartilage, and new bone. Calcium deposition begins within a few days of healing, but does not peak for several weeks. The radiographic appearance of callus formation is the result of both the laying of periosteal new bone and the calcification of new cartilage (Kleinman, 1998). The stage of soft callus may last anywhere from 2 to 6 weeks (Islam et al., 2000; Kleinman, 1998) (Photos 4.6

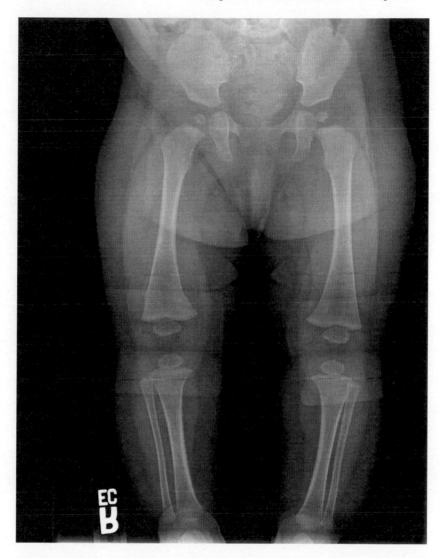

Photo 4.10 9 month old female fell from the arms of her caregiver striking knee on floor. X-rays notable for a buckle fracture of the distal right femur on anteroposterior views of the lower extremities.

and 4.8). There is also now an increase in the density of the fracture margins which occurs during this stage and has been noted in 90% of forearm fractures by 6 weeks (Islam et al., 2000).

There is considerable variability in the timing, appearance, and quantity of new bone and callus formation as a result of repetitive injury and/or the degree of immobilization of the injured bone (Kleinman, 1998). Femoral fractures in patients with

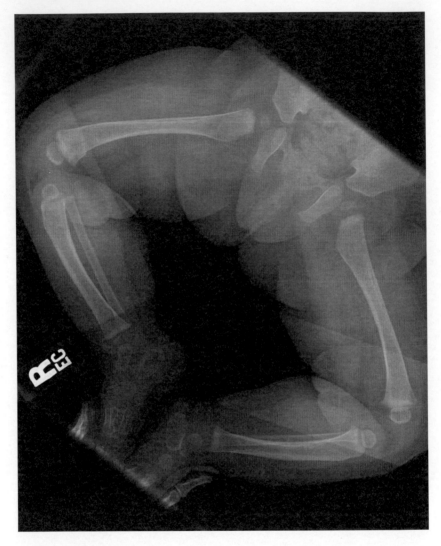

Photo 4.11 The lateral view of the buckle fracture demonstrates the posterior cortical disruption. This fracture is the result of axial loading of the femur as the knee struck the floor.

head injuries have an average healing time that is shorter than control subjects (Perkins & Skirving, 1987). The studies on the dating process of periosteal new bone and callus formation largely involve subjects with immobilized fractures. There is limited published data on the healing process of young infants and children with fractures. In addition, many non-accidental fractures are occult with late presentations for care and continued repetitive injury (Prosser et al., 2005).

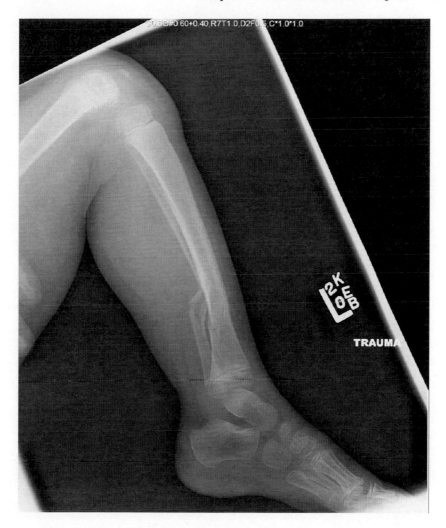

Photo 4.12 4 year old male fell from window landing on his feet. The lateral view of the tibia and fibula demonstrate comminuted fractures.

Stage 3: Hard Callus

The stage of soft callus ends with the bridging of bony fragments. The hard callus stage is characterized by lamellar bone formation with bridging of the fracture line. Clinical union occurs when the fracture is stable and without pain (Kleinman, 1998). Radiographically, the fracture line resolves and periosteal new bone becomes incorporated into the adjacent cortex. In a study of forearm fractures, the incorporation of periosteal new bone was not seen before 6 weeks after injury. The density of the callus was similar to the cortex at 10 weeks in 90% of the forearm fractures (Islam et al., 2000).

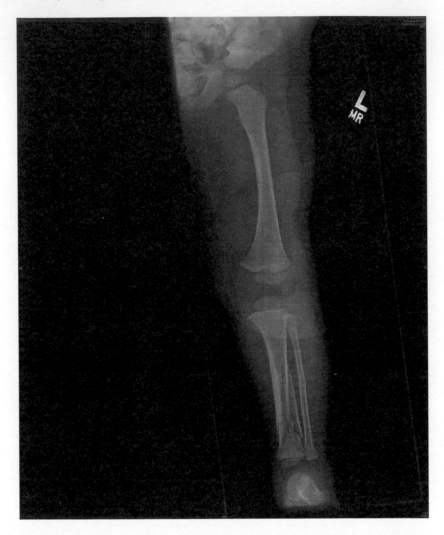

Photo 4.13 This 18 month old also has a comminuted fracture of his distal right tibia and fibula and buckling of the fibula in the middle of the diaphysis without a known history of trauma. Both picture 12 and 13 are the results of axial loads to the tibia and fibula.

Stage 4: Remodeling

During remodeling (Photo 4.9), the original configuration of the bone is restored as the callus is smoothed circumferentially. The ability of a child's bone to remodel is great, and remodeling may occur over a number of years. This process begins at 3 months and may peak at 1–2 years (Chapman, 1992). Some pediatric fractures are unrecognizable by X-ray within months after they occur.

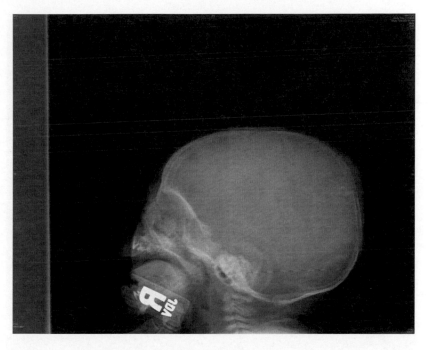

Photo 4.14 1 month old female with linear parietal skull fracture after fall from parent's arms.

The ability to detect an old fracture depends on multiple factors, including the bone injured, the type and extent of the injury, and the care the child received (Photo 4.32).

Dating of Skeletal Injuries

The dating of fractures estimates the age of injury and can identify multiple episodes of trauma. It is based on the constellation of radiologic findings including the presence or absence of soft tissue swelling as well as the appearance of periosteum, widening of fracture margins, callus formation, periosteal new bone incorporation and remodeling. There is little published evidence on the dating of fractures in children. Recent fractures can be clearly delineated from older fractures. Estimates of the age of older fractures can often be made in weeks rather than days. A recent systematic review of the literature on the healing of fractures found only three studies that clearly delineated the healing of fractures in children less than 17 years of age. There was variability in the bones studied and the appearance of the stages of healing. Periosteal reaction was seen as early as 4 days and present in at least 50% of the cases by 2 weeks after injury. Remodeling peaked around 8 weeks after injury (Prosser et al., 2005). Although largely anecdotal, general rules of thumb for

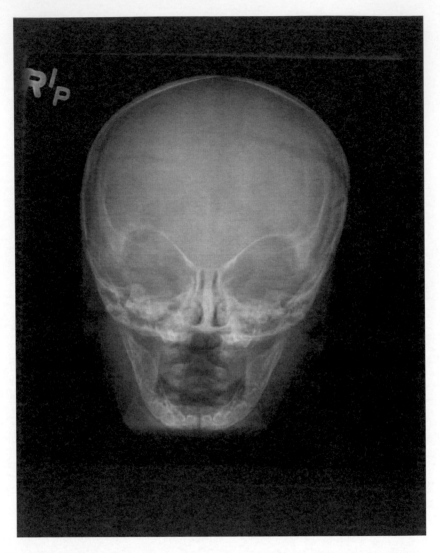

Photo 4.15 3 month old female presents with poor feeding and lethargy and no history of trauma. Skeletal survey notable for bilateral skull fractures with diastasis on the left. The infant had multiple other injuries include subdural hemorrhages, bruises, and rib fractures.

healing (average): soft tissue injury (swelling) resolution 4–10 days; SPNBF 10–14 days; fracture line indistinct 14–21 days; soft callus 14–21 days; hard callus 21–42 days; remodeling (up to one year) (Kleinman, 1998; Prosser et al., 2005).

Other factors that affect the healing process need to be considered when dating fractures including the severity of injury, degree of fracture displacement, degree of immobilization of the injured body part, metabolic bone diseases that influence the healing process, and repetitive trauma. Repetitive trauma to the fracture site cannot

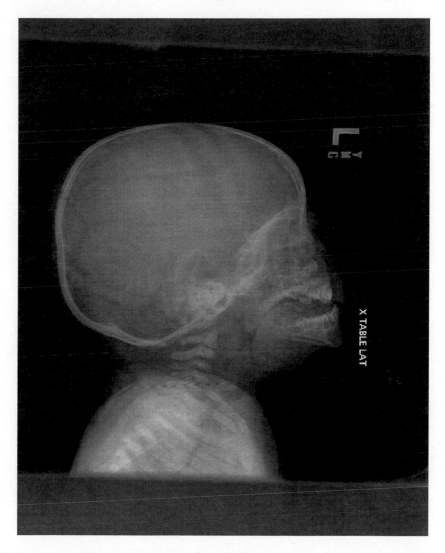

Photo 4.16 5 month old female with multiple extremity fractures is found to have a complex, comminuted skull fracture on skeletal survey. Caregiver reports only a single fall from a bouncer chair.

be ruled out in fractures that have not had medical care. Certain fracture sites, such as skull fractures or classic metaphyseal lesions, are difficult to date due to their healing patterns. The follow-up skeletal survey performed approximately 2 weeks after the initial survey is quite useful as it assists in dating and in the identification of occult injury, skeletal dysplasias, and metabolic disease.

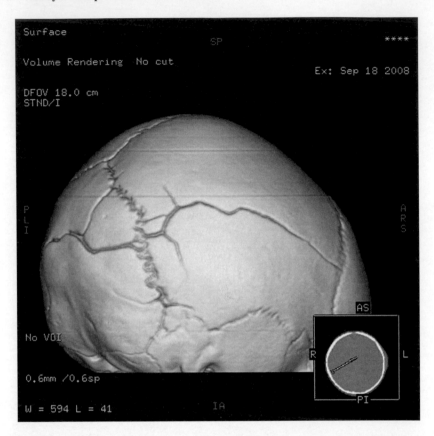

Photo 4.17 10 month old male has a scalp swelling noted at bath time. Only history of trauma is a single fall from a bed. The skeletal imaging and 3D reconstruction of the CT scan is notable for multiple fractures. Picture 17 demonstrates a right parietal-occipital complex skull fracture.

Long Bone Fractures

Fractures of the bones of the arms and legs are common childhood injuries (Rivara, Parish, & Mueller, 1986). Accidental trauma accounts for the majority of long bone fractures, and abuse accounts for only a minority. The likelihood that a long bone fracture is due to abuse is greatest in infants. The type of fracture sustained depends on the mechanical forces applied to the bone during the trauma (Table 4.3).

Due to the decreased amount of mineral content in a child's bones (as compared to an adult's bones), there is greater elasticity. The child's bone will tolerate more stress before a fracture occurs (Pierce et al., 2005). Correlating the history with the fracture type is often useful in identifying cases of non-accidental injury. However, it is important to realize that accidental fractures may be unwitnessed and therefore the exact mechanism of trauma may not be recounted. Each case requires careful evaluation to determine if an injury is suspicious for abuse. For example, spiral

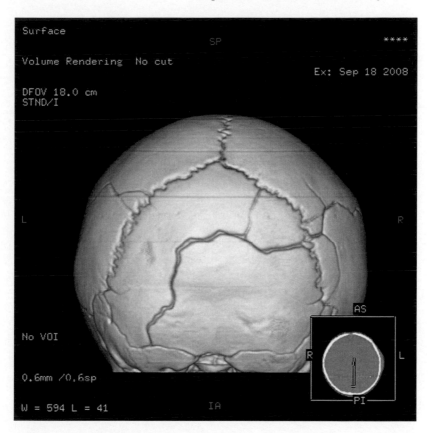

Photo 4.18 Same child with skull fracture crossing into the occipital bone.

fractures of the femur or tibia are more suspicious for abuse in the nonambulatory infant than in the ambulating toddler. Careful evaluation is needed to uncover indicators of abuse for each case (Photos 4.1 and 4.31).

Diaphyseal Fractures

Diaphyseal fractures are injuries to the midshaft of the long bones. They are generally described by the bone injured (femur, humerus, ulna, radius, tibia, fibula), the location of the fracture within the bone (distal, proximal, midshaft), and the type of fracture as defined by radiography (transverse, spiral, torus, etc.) (Photos 4.1, 4.5 and 4.7). In young infants, a diaphyseal fracture of the femur (while often due to abuse) should raise the question of birth-related injury (both in vaginal and cesarean deliveries) (Morris, Cassidy, Stephens, McCormack, & McManus, 2002). In birth-related fractures, metabolic bone disease with osteopenia should also be considered as a contributing cause. Toddler fractures (oblique or spiral tibial fractures) have been described and attributed to the mechanics of toddlers balance and walking skills (John, Moorthy, & Swischuk, 1997; Mellick, Milker, & Egsieker, 1999).

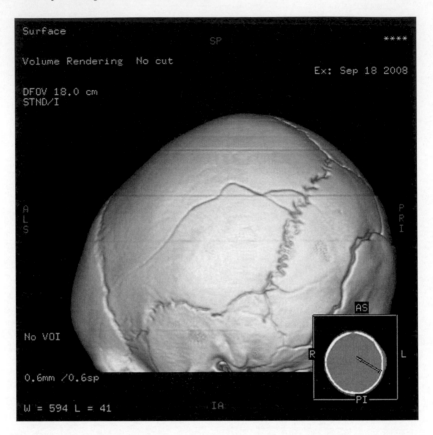

Photo 4.19 Same child with left linear parietal skull fracture as well. Extensive history of violence in the home.

Table 4.3 Common types of diaphyseal fractures seen in childhood.

Type	Characteristics	Causes
Transverse	Fracture line perpendicular to long axis of the bone Force applied to bone is perpendicular to length of the bone	Direct trauma Associated with accidental and inflicted injury
Spiral	An oblique fracture where fracture line encircles a portion of the bone	Indirect torsional forces to the bone Often associated with abusive injuries Seen with accidental injury (in ambulatory children) and child abuse (primarily in infants and young toddlers)

Table 4.3 (continued)

Type	Characteristics	Causes
Oblique	Fracture line angled across long axis of the bone (from approximately 30–45 degrees)	Often the result of combination loading (torsional, tensile, and compressive) Seen in accidental and abusive injury
Toddler's Fracture	A nondisplaced spiral fracture of the tibia Manifested by limp. There may be a delay in seeking medical care because the injury does not initially appear to be significant. May be occult: nondisplaced, little swelling, initial radiographs may fail to identify the fracture Diagnosed by bone scan at time of presentation or plain films repeated in approximately 2 weeks if clinical scenario indicates toddler's fracture but there is no fracture identified on initial radiographs	Common accidental injury in children between the ages of 1 and 3 Often occurs with routine play activities May result from running and slipping, jumping and falling, and even sliding with a difficult landing Uncommonly results from abuse History of trauma given may seem incomplete or insignificant (Mellick & Reesor, 1990)
Greenstick fracture	An incomplete fracture Compressed side of bone is bowed, but not completely fractured.	Occurs secondary to plasticity of a child's bone Commonly accidental and not commonly reported in the abused child
Torus (buckle) fracture	Localized buckling of the cortex of the bone Injuries located toward metaphysis of the bone Due to anatomy of the developing bone	Results from forces applied parallel to long axis of the bone
Impacted fracture	Involves entire bone	Both commonly accidental and not common in child abuse

Note: No type of diaphyseal fracture is diagnostic of abuse.

It requires substantial force to break the femur (although precise forces needed have not been elucidated), and healthy, nonambulatory infants do not take part in activities that generate the forces needed to sustain these fractures (Photo 4.1). Thomas et al. (1991) reported the frequency of abuse found in infants with femur fractures and found that abuse was the cause of 60% of femur fractures in children less than 1 year of age. The study also found that 30% of femur fractures were thought to be accidental (10% were of uncertain mechanism). The accidental femur fractures occurred when infants were dropped (Thomas,

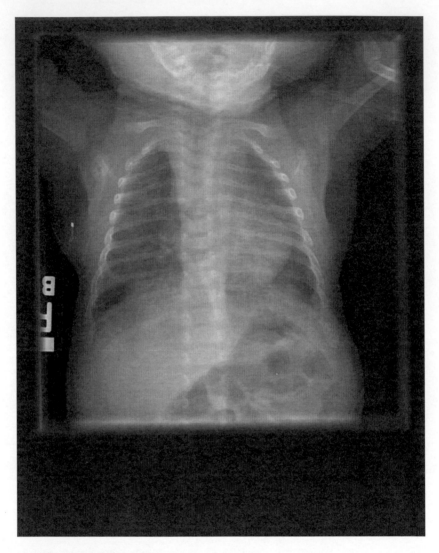

Photo 4.20 5 week old infant with multiple skull fractures and cutaneous trauma. Initial chest X-ray appeared reassuring.

Rosenfield, Leventhal, & Markowitz, 1991). These findings underlie the need for an objective, thorough evaluation of femur fractures in infants. Risk factors for abuse suggested for infants include: age less than 1 year, nonambulatory activity (not walking), inconsistency of the history with the injury and/or the developmental ability of the infant, delay in seeking care, and the presence of any other suspicious injuries. Whether a fracture is spiral or transverse is not discriminatory for abuse. In studies of femur fractures, 48–71% of non-accidental femur fractures were found to be transverse (Hui et al., 2008).

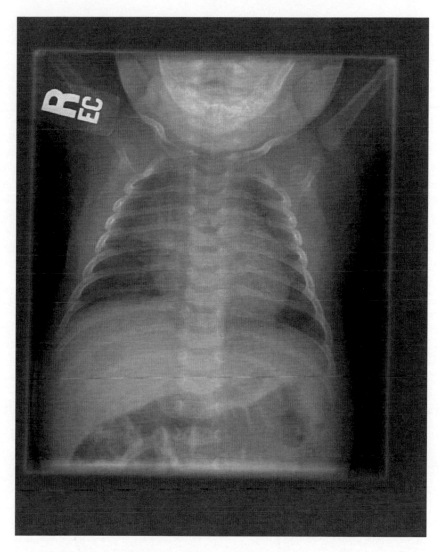

Photo 4.21 The infant had a repeat skeletal skeletal survey now demonstrating healed left posterior rib fractures of ribs 7 and 8.

Stair falls are often attributed as the cause of fractures. In general, serious injuries with stair falls are uncommon (Pierce et al., 2005). In a study of stair falls, spiral fractures of the femur were more commonly seen in children over 12 months and buckle fractures were seen in the group under the age of 12 months. The likelihood of more serious injury was increased if the fall occurred with an adult. Buckle fractures of the femur appear to be associated with compressive injury occurring with the striking of the knee onto a surface (Photos 4.10 and 4.11). A torsional injury can occur with a leg being twisted under the child during a fall. Pierce (2005) found that the linear momentum associated with transverse femur fractures was almost 10 times greater than that seen with spiral or buckle fractures (Pierce et al., 2005).

There are few published studies comparing the prevalence of humeral fractures in abused and nonabused children with estimates of abuse ranging from 20 to 88% (Kemp et al., 2008; Strait, Siegel, & Shapiro, 1995; Thomas et al., 1991;Worlock et al., 1986). Some authors estimate that as many as 88% of humerus fractures are due to abuse. This fracture can be associated with birth injury. The majority of humeral fractures are accidental and occur in older children (Caviglia, Garrido, Palazzi, & Meana, 2005). Fracture patterns described include transverse or oblique occurring with force to the shoulder or outstretched arm; and spiral or oblique fractures due to rotational (torsional) movement of the body onto an outstretched (weighted) arm (Photos 4.5 and 4.7). Supracondylar fractures of the humerus occur when children fall on the elbow or outstretched hand (with the elbow in full extension). As seen with femur fractures, the type of fracture (transverse, spiral, etc.) does not necessarily predict whether an injury is due to abuse or accident. However, spiral and oblique fractures of the humerus are the most common fracture type from abuse (Kemp et al., 2008).

Forearm diaphyseal fractures often occur secondary to sports activities or falls. These fractures are common in the pediatric population representing 42% of all pediatric fractures (Rodriguez-Merchan, 2005). The peak incidence is in children over the age of 5 years. The injury often occurs with a fall onto an outstretched hand.

Treatment of diaphyseal fractures depends on patient age, fracture age when identified, and the type and location of the fracture. In general, diaphyseal fractures impede the normal functioning of the involved bone. Treatment requires immobilization and limitation of weight bearing for lower extremity fractures.

Metaphyseal Fractures

Metaphyseal fractures of the long bones are strongly predictive of abuse and are highly specific for inflicted injuries in children under 1 year of age (Kleinman, 1998) (Photos 4.28, 4.29 and 4.30). In children over the age of 1 year, similar lesions should be viewed with caution as there are non-specific Salter-Harris II fractures and developmental variants (Kleinman, 2008). Until recently, metaphyseal fractures were thought to represent "chip fractures" of the metaphyses (Caffey, 1957). Caffey (1957) postulated that these lesions were due to small avulsions of the metaphyseal cartilage and bone at the point of insertion of the periosteum. Recent findings in which histologic correlations to radiographic findings were performed document that metaphyseal fractures represent fracture through the most immature portion of the metaphysis creating a planar type injury (Kleinman, Marks, & Blackbourne, 1986). Depending on the radiologic projection, metaphyseal fractures may appear as linear lucencies or densities across the metaphysis, "bucket-handle" fractures, or corner fractures (Photo 4.33). All of these lesions are subtle and may be recognized on a skeletal survey or incidental X-ray.

Metaphyseal fractures are injuries generally found in infants and young toddlers. The mechanism of injury is related to either acceleration–deceleration forces associated with the abusive head trauma or torsional and tractional forces applied to the bone when an infant is twisted, jerked, or pulled by an extremity (Kleinman et al., 1986) (Photos 4.2, 4.3 and 4.4). Metaphyseal fractures are often multiple and bilateral. Common sites for metaphyseal fractures include the proximal humerus, distal femur, proximal tibia, and distal tibia and fibula (Kleinman & Marks, 1996a, 1996b, 1996c; Kleinman & Marks, 1998). The number of bones involved varies from case to case, and fractures isolated to one or only a few bones are not uncommon. Metaphyseal fractures do not typically result in significant soft tissue swelling or external bruising. Injuries are not usually identified clinically by either a parent or the physician during the physical examination. In addition, most of these fractures heal without specific treatment or the need for immobilization.

The differential diagnosis should include metabolic bone disease (particularly in a premature infant), a history of rickets with excessive range of motion exercise (Helfer, Scheurer, Alexander, Reed, & Slovis, 1984; Kleinman, 1998), bone dysplasias (Langer et al., 1990), treatment for club foot (forced eversion and inversion) (Grayev, Boal, Wallach, & Segal, 2001), iatrogenic injury associated with neuromuscular disorders, osteogenesis imperfecta (Astley, 1979; Kleinman, 1998) birth-related injuries (both vaginal and cesarean deliveries) (O'Connell & Donoghue, 2007), external cephalic version (Lysack & Soboleski, 2003), osteomyelitis (Ogden, 1979), and normal variants such as step-offs, beaks, and collars (Kleinman, Belanger, Karellas & Spevak, 1991). In infants and toddlers with significant genu varum, CML-like lesions may be seen. With time these lesions do not show evidence of healing (Photos 4.22, 4.23, and 4.24).

The metaphysis is an area of rapid bone turnover due to normal growth of the infant skeleton. Because metaphyseal fractures are subtle and usually clinically silent, the skeletal survey remains the identification method of choice. A pediatrician or radiologist familiar with the skeletal manifestations of child abuse is often required to identify metaphyseal fractures. A bone scan, which identifies areas of rapid bone turnover, may not be helpful in identifying metaphyseal fractures because the metaphysis is normally an area of bone growth and turnover.

Metaphyseal fractures are difficult to detect or date radiographically due to an absence of periosteal elevation and hemorrhage. As a result, the fracture may not show signs of periosteal reaction, or the reaction may be only modest. Metaphyseal lesions may or may not heal with subperiosteal new bone formation. The clinician needs to differentiate this from physiologic new bone formation. However, physiologic new bone formation is largely diaphyseal in location. There may be sclerotic lines or loss of fracture line during the healing process. Another change, that may assist in identifying a healing fracture, is to look for local extension of the physeal lucency into the metaphysis (caused by cartilaginous hypertrophy). Most classic metaphyseal lesions will be healed by 4 weeks (Kleinman, 2008). Massive periosteal reaction usually indicates a displaced fracture or a shearing injury to the periosteum itself (Photo 4.4) (Kleinman, 1998). Metaphyseal fractures also may be dated by evaluating the sharpness of the fracture margins. As

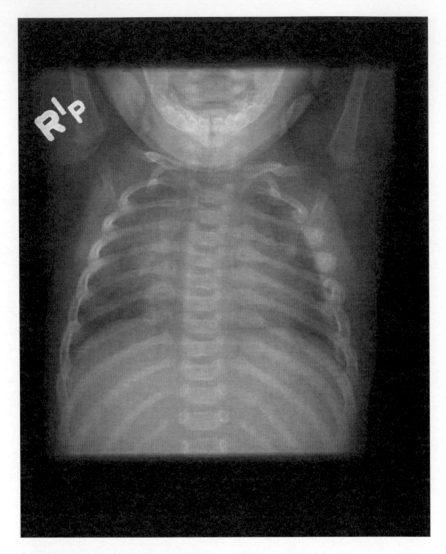

Photo 4.22 The 3 month old infant in Photo 4.15 had multiple rib fractures in addition to her skull fractures and subdural hemorrhages. The stepfather reported squeezing her around the rib cage until she would "pass out". Healing rib fractures are seen in multiple locations including the right posterior 4th–9th, left posterior 3rd–10th, and left lateral 3rd–7th.

the injury heals, the margin becomes more poorly defined. Unfortunately, this is a subjective measure and one that has not been studied systematically. It is thought that future studies using magnetic resonance imaging (MRI) may help to date meta-physeal injuries more precisely.

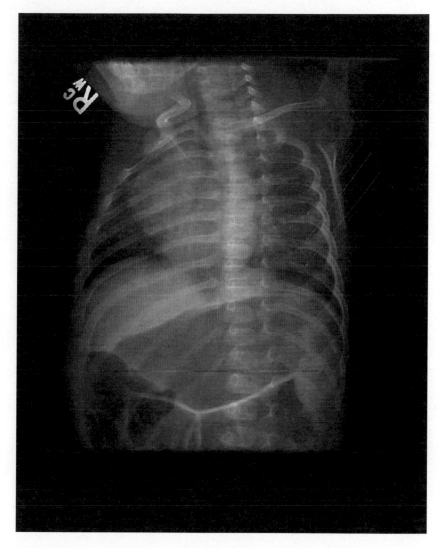

Photo 4.23 This 3 month old infant had crepitus on examination and posterior arc fractures seen only on the oblique view of the skeletal survey at the left 6th–8th ribs.

Growth Arrest Lines

Growth arrest lines are radiopaque transverse lines across the metaphyses seen occasionally in abused or neglected children. They are not specific for maltreatment and may occur in children with illness, injury, starvation, or other stresses that affect growth. Growth arrest lines represent periods of slowed growth and are most evident in bones that normally grow rapidly. They form because the usual orientation of the trabeculae of fast-growing bones is longitudinal (parallel to the long axis of the bone), as opposed to transverse (seen in the trabeculae of normally slow-growing

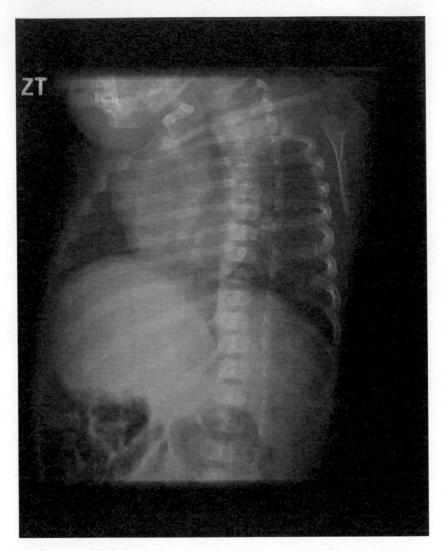

Photo 4.24 At 3 weeks the 3 month old has three clearly healing rib fractures with callus and fracture line definition.

bones) (Ogden, 1990). During periods of slow growth, the trabeculae become oriented transversely, causing a thicker appearance to the affected bone. When the stress is removed and the bone begins to grow at a normal rate, the normal longitudinal orientation of the bone resumes, and the thickened area appears as a discrete transverse line. Many children have evidence of multiple growth arrest lines in a single bone, representing prolonged periods of physiological stress. With time, the transverse orientation of the bone resolves, and growth arrest lines break down so that they are no longer visible.

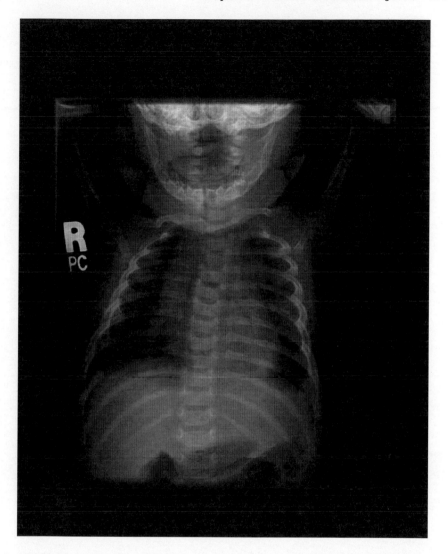

Photo 4.25 This 2 month old female presented with chest wall crepitus and was found to have multiple acute rib fractures. The AP chest is notable for a displaced rib fracture posteriorly on the left 7th rib.

Skull Fractures

Skull Anatomy

The skull consists of cranial and facial bones. The eight intramembranous cranial bones—frontal, occipital, sphenoid, ethmoid, and left and right parietal and temporal bones—develop directly within a membrane and not from cartilage, as with

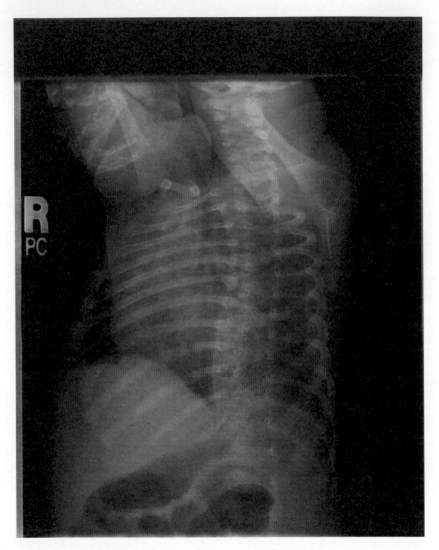

Photo 4.26 The oblique view for the infant more clearly demonstrates acute displaced fractures of left posterior 5th–8th ribs.

the long bones. The cranium is composed of a number of separate bones joined by strips of connective tissue called sutures. The main sutures include the sagital, coronal, and lambdoid. Lesser known sutures include the squamosal, metopic, and mendosal. The mendosal sutures extend medially from the lambdoid sutures into the occipital bone. In the sutures are larger areas of connective tissue known as the fontanelles. In addition to the anterior, posterior and anterolateral fontanelles, there can also be small accessory fontanelles within the sutures, especially the sagital suture. Islands of bone (ossification) found within the posterior sagital and lambdoid

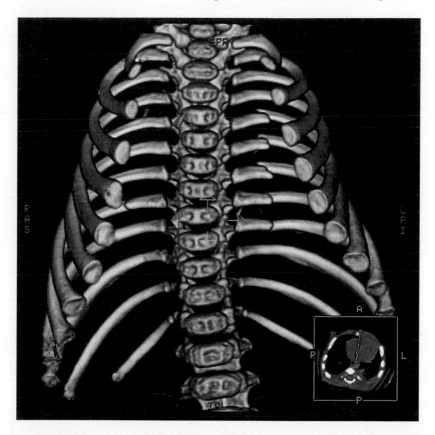

Photo 4.27 The 3D CT reconstruction of the infant shows acute fractures of left posterior 5th–9th ribs as well as the right 8th posterior. Additional fractures were identified on repeat skeletal image at 2 weeks. The child's father reported squeezing the child around the rib cage until the child stopped crying on 3 occasions.

sutures, if large enough, are referred to as "wormian bones". There is another variant of the occipital bone referred to as the interparietal (Inca) bone at the vertex of the lambdoid sutures. The Inca bone can be bipartite divided by a superior median fissure (Stokes & Cremin, 1974).

Both accessory sutures and fissures are common in the parietal bone. These fissures can be mistaken for skull fractures (Fenton, Sirotnak, & Handler, 2000; Weir, Suttner, Flynn, & McAuley, 2006). The parietal bone may be partially or completely bisected by a fissure running parallel to the sagital suture (Stokes & Cremin, 1974). The presence of these fissures is largely the result of multiple ossification centers within the developing bones of the skull. The skull of the newborn is quite thin and does not achieve the adult "three-layer" diploe configuration for 3–4 years (Holck, 2005). The parietal bone is quite thin, monolayer, and particularly susceptible to fracture. In studies of infant cadavers

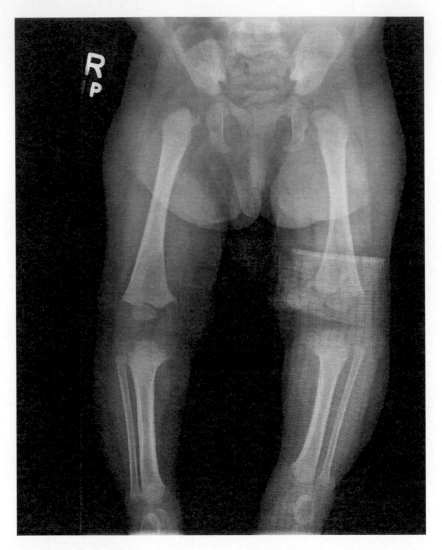

Photo 4.28 The 5 month old female presented with swelling and pain with movement of her right lower leg. There was no known trauma reported other than the child caught her leg during a feeding. Multiple classic metaphyseal lesions were found including bilateral distal femurs, bilateral proximal and distal tibias.

with falls (head-first with parieto-occipital impact) onto differing surfaces from 0.82 m, fractures occurred almost exclusively in the parietal bone (Weber, 1984, 1985, 1987). The growth and repair of the skull bones are distinct from that of the long bones, making dating of skull fractures more difficult. Additionally, bone scans do not identify skull fractures with any sensitivity. Plain skull films are more sensitive than standard CT scans as the axial bony windows can miss a fracture that

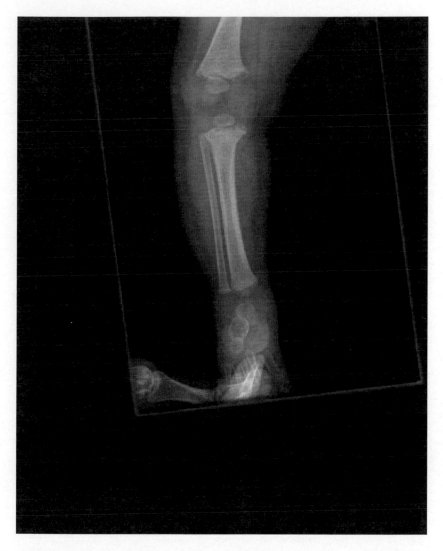

Photo 4.29 Additional views of the 5 month old female's left lower extremity and classic metaphyseal lesions.

parallels or is between slices. 3D CT reconstruction does enable a detailed view of the skull, sutures, fissures, and fractures (Photos 4.17, 4.18 and 4.19). Plain films are still the method of choice for identifying skull fractures (Photo 4.32).

Skull Fractures and Abuse

Skull fractures are due to a direct impact of the head with a solid object. A description of the fracture includes the location identifying the skull bone involved and the

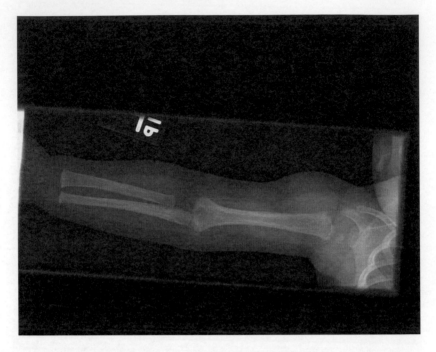

Photo 4.30 This demonstrates the 5 month old female's right proximal humeral classic metaphyseal lesion. The left upper extremity has no fractures and normal metaphyses.

type of fracture. Skull fractures related to child abuse generally refer to the cranial bones, although facial fractures occur (see Chapter 8). Table 4.4 describes common types of skull fractures.

Skull fractures are the perhaps the most common fracture in hospitalized children. However, only 17% of these were attributable to abuse in children under 12 months of age (Leventhal et al., 2008). Skull fractures are more commonly reported after accidental head injuries (Kemp et al., 2008). Simple linear parietal skull fractures are just as commonly found in accidental as in abusive head injuries (Billmire & Myers, 1985; Meservy, Towbin, McLaurin, Myers, & Ball, 1987; Leventhal et al., 1993) (Photo 4.14). In young children, accidental linear fractures may occur from falls of less than 4 ft (such as off a bed, couch, or changing table), falls of greater distances (down stairs), or walker injuries (Coats & Marguiles, 2008; Duhaime et al., 1992). Likewise, linear fractures may result from abuse and are indicative of a direct impact to the head (Photo 4.15). Some report complex skull fractures, depressed fractures, and diastatic fractures as characteristic of inflicted injury (Hobbs, 1984). Other studies report no real difference in the incidence of complex skull fractures (Leventhal et al., 1993 Meservy et al., 1987), but strong associations with multiple fractures, bilateral fractures, and fractures crossing sutures (Meservy et al., 1987) (Photo 4.15, 4.16, 4.17, 4.18 and 4.19). Bilateral skull fractures may result from crushing injuries (Hiss & Kahana, 1995), but can also occur a single midline cranial

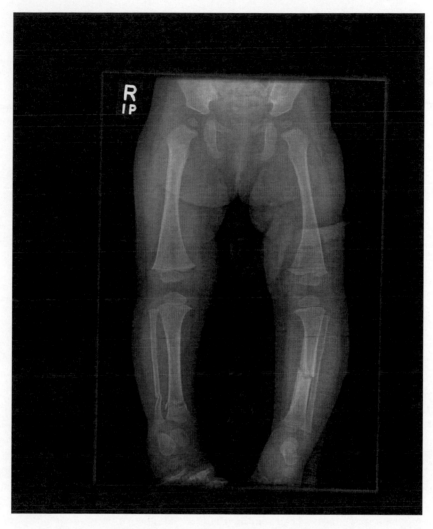

Photo 4.31 This 9 month old female presented with swelling of her left lower extremity and multiple bruises after being left in the care of the mother's boyfriend. The mother's boyfriend reports tripping on the baby. Multiple extremity fractures were found including the transverse fracture of the left tibia and comminuted fractures of the right tibia and fibula.

impact (Arnholz, Hymel, Hay, & Jenny, 1998) Young infants may sustain linear, depressed, and ping-pong fractures from simple falls because of the relative ease with which the skull can be deformed at this young age and its thin, monolayer construction (Weber, 1985). Although no fracture type is pathognomonic for abuse, abuse is suspected when no history of trauma is provided, the history is inconsistent or changes, or a history of minor injury results in complex or multiple fractures.

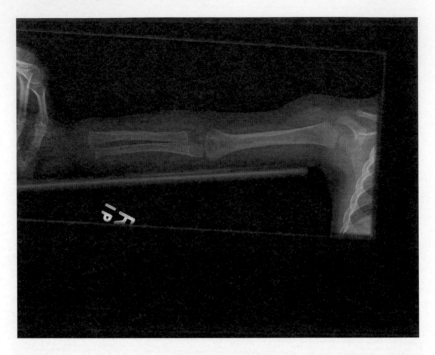

Photo 4.32 The 9 month old also had a healing transverse fracture of the distal right radius.

The presence or absence of cutaneous injury and/or skull fracture does not predict intracranial injury. In one study of the association between bruising and fractures, 43% of patients had bruising or subgaleal hematoma at the site of skull fracture. Of those patients with skull fractures, almost half had evidence of intracranial injury. Skull fractures were present in 75% of those with abusive head trauma (Peters et al., 2008). In the Duhaime et al. (1992) of head injury in young children, 37% of children with abusive head trauma had skull fractures (Duhaime et al., 1992). Much of the variability lies in study design. Controversy regarding the exact mechanism and biomechanics of abusive head trauma relates to whether impact is required to produce intracranial injury. Multiple and diastatic skull fractures, from direct impacts such as from falls from significant height or blows, do occur without life-threatening intracranial injury. Yet many children without skull fracture have intracranial injury so severe as to result in death. Infants whose injuries are credited to acceleration–deceleration injury may have a skull fracture documented by skull films. As indicated by the fracture, these children have sustained direct impact to the head in addition to acceleration–deceleration injury (see Chapter 6).

Dating Skull Fractures

Skull fractures are more difficult to date than long bone fractures, both clinically and radiographically. Soft tissue swelling may not be apparent clinically in the acute period and may become noticeable only after the associated scalp hematoma begins to degrade and liquefy. This can lead to a delay in seeking medical care by the

Table 4.4 Common types of skull fractures.

Type	Characteristics
Basilar	Fracture of base of skull Difficult to identify radiologically CT scan is a more sensitive test than plain films Usually diagnosed by clinical criteria: CSF otorrhea, rhinorrhea, raccoon eyes (periorbital blood), or Battle's sign (ecchymoses over the mastoid area)
Comminuted	Complex fracture results in separate piece(s) of bone
Complex	Comprised of more than one line May be branched or stellate, or consist of more than one distinct fracture
Depressed	Occurs when bony fragment is displaced inward toward the brain Often a comminuted fracture and may be associated with neurologic deficits, usually due to underlying brain involvement
Diastatic	Fracture margins significantly separated Injuries to the sutures can result in diastasis, either in association with a fracture or as an isolated injury Diastasis of multiple sutures may occur with increased intracranial pressure or occasionally with rapid brain growth
Linear	A single, unbranched line that can be straight, curved, or angled
Ping-pong	Bone indented, but without a distinct fracture
Stellate	A type of complex fracture Fracture lines radiate from central point

child's caregiver as well. Soft tissue swelling in the first 24 h after a skull fracture should be evident by computed tomography (CT) scan. Kleinman and Spevak (1992) evaluated soft tissue swelling associated with acute (less than 24 h old) accidental skull fractures in children. All fractures were associated with soft tissue swelling overlying the fracture of at least 4 mm, as seen by CT scan (Kleinman & Spevak, 1992). Skull fractures do not heal with exuberant callus formation. Recognition of older injuries rests on the subjective determination of fracture line definition, and is therefore imprecise. Like those in other types of fractures, infant skull fractures heal relatively rapidly compared with older children and adults. In most cases, isolated skull fractures require no specific therapy. "Growing fracture" or "leptomeningeal cyst" is a known but rare complication of diastatic skull fractures in approximately 1–2% of children under 3 years of age. Clinical examination is recommended in 6–8 weeks after injury with consideration for follow-up radiography (Ersahin, Gulmen, & Palali, 2000).

Rib Fractures

Rib fractures are unusual pediatric injuries that commonly result from major trauma (such as motor vehicle crashes [MVC] or child abuse). An evaluation for child abuse is performed when an infant or young child presents with unexplained rib fractures. Rib fractures are the most common fracture found in

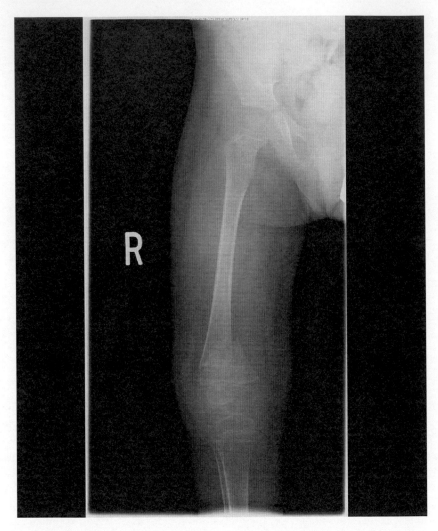

Photo 4.33 The 2 year old male presented with leg swelling and fussiness. He had a history of spastic quadriplegia after being struck by a car. His X-rays demonstrate disuse osteopenia with thin cortices. He has a distal transverse femur fracture with swelling noted after physical therapy.

association with other non-accidental injuries (Day, Clegg, McPhillips, & Mok, 2006; Kleinman, Marks, Richmond, & Blackbourne, 1995; Worlock et al., 1986). Multiple studies have confirmed the association between child abuse and rib fractures (Barsness et al., 2003; Bulloch et al., 2000); Cadzow & Armstrong, 2000; Garcia, Gotschall, Eichelberger, & Bowman, 1990; Schweich & Fleisher, 1985). A large retrospective study of trauma patients with rib fractures calculated a 95% positive predictive value for non-accidental trauma in children less than 3 years of age

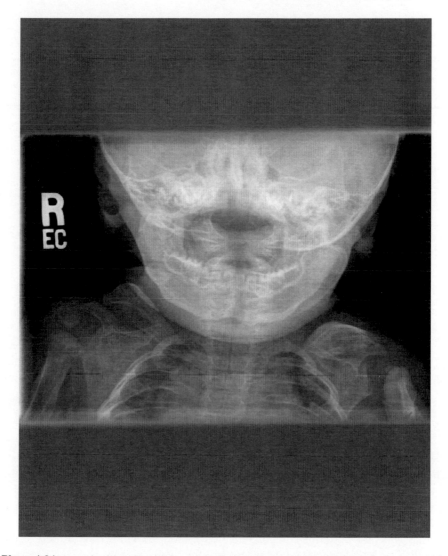

Photo 4.34 1-week-old male with bony angulations noted at birth. Multiple lesions noted in the mandible, clavicles, humeri and ribs. The child has Caffey Disease or infantile cortical hyperostosis.

with rib fractures (Barsness et al., 2003). A systematic review of the literature found rib fractures to have the highest probability for abuse at 0.71 (as compared to other skeletal injuries) (Kemp et al., 2008). Rib fractures from abuse are found in multiple locations including posterior (most common), posterolateral (mid-posterior), lateral, and anterior (Barsness et al., 2003; Bulloch et al., 2000; Kleinman et al., 1996) (Photos 4.28 and 4.29). Barsness et al. (2003) found a statistically significant association between the posterior location and non-accidental trauma.

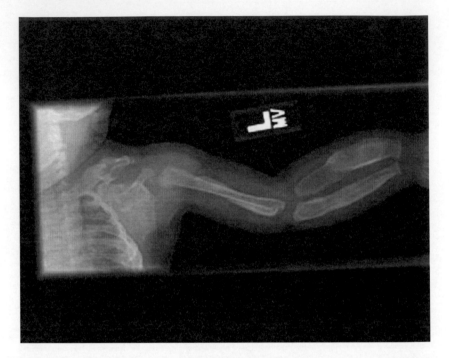

Photo 4.35 The left upper extremity of the 1 week old with Caffey Disease demonstrates the periostitis and subsequent lamellar bone formation.

Direct blows to the chest can result in rib fractures and probably represent the mechanism of injury in older children. Kleinman et al. (1992) studied postmortem changes of fractured ribs in infants who died of abuse. The location (near the costotransverse process articulation) and the healing patterns (on the ventral or internal surface of the rib) of the fractures suggested that rib fractures occur as the rib is levered over the transverse process of the adjacent vertebral body during violent manual anterior–posterior compression of the chest (Kleinman et al., 1992). CT was utilized by Kleinman and Schlesinger (1997) to assess physical factors associated with manual compression and rib fractures in rabbits. With digital chest compression on a firm surface simulating CPR, no rib fractures occurred. With manual compression with hands around the chest (until palpable/audible popping heard), levering of the ribs was seen as the vertebral body migrated dorsally. A total of 13 fractures occurred in three rabbits (Kleinman & Schlesinger, 1997). Rib fractures in non-accidental trauma usually involve multiple ribs Barsness et al. 2003) and are often bilateral. Children with accidental rib fractures from trauma often have blunt impact and/or thoracic compression. These children are struck or run over by motor vehicles, or become unrestrained projectiles striking firm surfaces with anterior–posterior compression of the chest (Bulloch et al. 2000; Kleinman & Schlesinger, 1997).

Cardiopulmonary Resuscitation and Rib Fractures

In adults, rib fractures frequently occur in association with cardiopulmonary resuscitation (CPR) (Krischer, Fine, Davis, & Nagel, 1987). In infants and young children, rib fractures do not appear to be a clinically significant complication of CPR as the thorax is less rigid and has more elasticity. In a systematic review of the literature on the relationship between cardiopulmonary resuscitation and rib fractures, a total of three children had rib fractures as a consequence of CPR out of a documented 923 cases. Two children were less than 6 months of age and one child was 5 years of age. All rib fractures were multiple and anterior. Two of the cases had mid-clavicular fractures and one case had bilateral fractures at the sterno–chondral junction. No cases were identified with posterior rib fractures. Five of the six studies meeting inclusion criteria were postmortem (Maguire et al. 2006).

Radiographic Findings of Rib Fractures

Rib fractures due to abuse are almost always occult and not recognized either by an unsuspecting caregiver or during routine physical examination. Occasionally, healing fractures with exuberant callus can be palpated, but this usually occurs only after the fractures have been diagnosed radiographically. Acute (new) rib fractures are difficult to identify by plain X-ray. Posterior rib fractures have little displacement or angulation, or disruption of the periosteum (Kleinman, Marks, Adams, & Blackbourne, 1988). Fractures are generally recognized only after callus formation and periosteal reaction are evident. The addition of oblique views to the skeletal survey has been helpful in identifying fractures (Hansen, Prince, & Nixon, 2008) (Photo 4.20 and 4.21).

Bone scan is more sensitive for the identification of acute rib fractures (less than 7–10 days old) than plain films (Mandelstam, Cook, Fitzgerald, & Ditchfield, 2003). However, the majority of studies comparing bone scan to skeletal survey did not utilize oblique views of the chest (Kemp et al., 2006). Likewise, a study comparing CT with chest X-ray found CT more sensitive in identifying rib fractures at all locations except lateral (Photos 4.25, 4.26 and 4.27). However, the study did not utilize oblique views of the chest and CT requires higher doses of radiation (Wootton-Gorges et al., 2008). Chest CT does have the additional benefit in children with multisystem trauma in identifying additional injuries including hemothorax and pulmonary contusion. In suspected abuse with an initial negative skeletal survey, a bone scan may identify acute fractures, including those of the ribs. An infant who presents without a history of trauma but with intracranial injury should have a skeletal survey with oblique views of the chest performed as part of the initial evaluation. Repeat skeletal survey in 2 weeks, as outlined in the imaging section, is crucial in the identification of occult rib fractures (Photos 4.20 and 4.21).

In the majority of cases, rib fractures are not associated with clinical pulmonary or liver injuries and do not interfere with normal respiration. These fractures typically heal rapidly and without specific therapy. However, in studies of children with thoracic trauma, the likelihood of intrathoracic injury and multisystem trauma increased in children with multiple rib fractures or posterior rib fractures (Garcia et al., 1990). Children with thoracic injury from child abuse were found to have a 50% mortality rate (Kleinman, 1990). However, the majority of children with rib fractures and thoracic injury from child abuse often have concomitant head injury (Photo 4.22).

Other Fractures Associated with Child Abuse

Child abuse can result in injury to virtually any bone in the body, although the most common injuries are fractures of the extremities, ribs, and skull. Many fractures are clinically unrecognized, which emphasizes the need for careful radiologic assessment of all bones. The following sections review injuries occasionally seen in the abused child, although none is pathognomonic for maltreatment.

Vertebral Fractures

Spinal fractures in infants and toddlers are relatively rare injuries from child abuse, but probably occur more frequently than they are recognized (Kleinman, 1990). The injury to the vertebral bodies and spinous processes are subtle and require lateral views of the spine. Most vertebral injuries are occult, although a few children present with spinal cord compression. Lateral views of the spine may reveal vertebral body compression fractures or anterior vertebral end plate injury. MRI may be used to further assess significant vertebral and spinal cord injuries. These skeletal manifestations of abuse often result from severe hyperflexion of the torso and axial spinal loading (Kleinman & Marks, 1992; Tran, Silvera, Newton, & Kleinman, 2007). Vertebral compression fractures in isolation do require further evaluation for osteogenesis imperfecta. Vertebral injuries, if stable, do not require specific therapy. Children with cord compression, however, require surgical intervention and often have permanent neurologic disability.

Pelvic Fractures

Fractures of the pelvic bones are uncommon injuries in abused children (Ablin, Greenspan, & Reinhart, 1992; Starling, Heller, & Jenny, 2002). Injuries to the pelvis that occur in infants and young children are often unrecognized prior to radiologic discovery. Most of the reported injuries are unilateral and occur in conjunction with other skeletal trauma. The ischiopubic ramus is most commonly fractured. Although the precise mechanism of inflicted pelvic trauma is not described in the literature, accidental pelvic injuries in children are due to direct trauma in association with falls, motor vehicle crashes, and crush injury (Quinby, 1966). Although accidental pelvic injuries may be life threatening, inflicted pelvic fractures are generally stable injuries that do not require surgical intervention.

There are anatomic variants associated with the ossification centers in the superior pubic ramus. The ossification centers can be single or multiple, unilateral or bilateral, and can have associated sclerosis of the margins. Fractures are more likely to be oriented obliquely to the axis of the pubic ramus with displacement of fragments and callus formation. A vertical radiolucency with smooth margins, in the absence of other pelvic or skeletal trauma, should be considered an anatomic variant (Perez-Rossello et al., 2008)

Clavicle Fractures

Clavicle fractures are common accidental pediatric injuries and are occasionally associated with abuse (Ogden, 1990). This fracture is the most common birth-related fracture and is often associated with infants who are large for gestational age. The fracture may go unnoticed while the infant is in the newborn nursery. If the question is raised on birth-related versus post-hospital care, attempts to age the healing fracture should be used. If callus is not present by the time the child is 10–14 days of age, it is unlikely to be birth-related (Kleinman, 1998). Accidental injury, accounting for 75–80% of all clavicle fractures, generally occurs in the midshaft of the bone due to the thinness of the bone at this site as well as the lack of muscular and ligamentous supports (Pecci & Kreher, 2008). Accidental fractures of the clavicle are associated with birth trauma, direct injury, or falling on an outstretched arm. Midshaft fractures are common with both accidental as well as inflicted injury. Clavicular fractures involving the acromioclavicular joint are associated with violent traction of the arms (Kogutt, Swischuk, & Fagan, 1974). Inflicted clavicular fractures are typically associated with other skeletal injuries and are an uncommon isolated finding (Merten, Radkowski, & Leonidas, 1983). In teens where ossification of the growing centers is not complete, growth plate injury must be considered (Pecci & Kreher, 2008). Clavicle fractures in older children are usually treated with a clavicle strap or figure-8 sling, primarily to ease discomfort. These injuries in young children and infants often heal well without immobilization.

Fractures of the Hands and Feet

Fractures of the hands and feet, while common in older children, are suspicious injuries in infants and young toddlers. These fractures are rare, but may be the only indication of inflicted injury. Close attention should be paid to images of the hands and feet in the skeletal survey, ensuring that the fingers are not curled or obscured by intravenous equipment. Specific treatment depends on the extent and location of the fracture.

Foot fractures may occur from forces acting on the foot such as objects dropped onto the foot, falling from height, lawn mower injuries, or from using the foot to stop motion (biking, sledding, etc.). Likewise, indirect force (adduction, eversion, and inversion) may result in fractures. Due to the many small bones, growth centers, cartilaginous bones, and lack of displacement of fracture fragments, it may be difficult to identify a fracture in the foot. X-rays, if inconclusive, may be repeated in 2–3 weeks (in the otherwise stable patient). Use of bone scans or MRI studies can be used in more concerning evaluations such as concern over talus fractures and the potential risk of avascular necrosis. Some conditions may be confused with foot fractures, including osteochondroses, tumors, inflammatory conditions, and infections.

Hand fractures are relatively common in children. Two peak ages have been identified with the first occurring at age 1–2 years (distal phalangeal fractures) and next at age 12 years (with proximal phalangeal and metacarpal) (Valencia, Leyva, & Gomez-Bajo, 2005). Sports injuries are more common in older pediatric patients (teenagers). Fractures of the fingers may present with swelling, whereas fractures to the metatarsals, metacarpals, and phalanges are frequently asymptomatic and only incidentally discovered by skeletal survey (Kleinman, 1990). The fractures can be caused by direct impact, torsion, and twisting. Buckle fractures of the proximal phalanx may be the result of forced hyperextension of the fingers (Nimkin, Spevak, & Kleinman, 1997). Oblique views may be useful in the evaluation of buckle fractures (Nimkin et al., 1997). With Salter Type I injuries, the initial X-rays may appear normal. Scaphoid fractures are unique since they may be difficult to identify acutely without the use of MRI or scaphoid views. If not identified and treated early, these fractures can result in avascular necrosis.

The Differential Diagnosis of Inflicted Fractures

Metabolic and physiological processes may lead to pathological fractures (Photo 4.33), or they may simulate fractures. Although some of these conditions are readily apparent and easily diagnosed, others can be confused with and misdiagnosed as abuse. The presence of a metabolic bone disease does not preclude abuse. The following sections describe some of the more common conditions included in the differential diagnosis of inflicted fractures.

Birth Trauma

Difficult or emergency deliveries, large infants, or breech presentations may cause diaphyseal or epiphyseal fractures of the clavicle, humerus, or femur. Multiple fractures in the newborn suggest an underlying neuromuscular or metabolic bone disease (Ogden, 1990).

Clavicle fractures are most common and may not be recognized in the days after delivery. They are often asymptomatic and may be detected initially by a parent who palpates the callus when the infant is a few weeks old.

Diaphyseal femur and humerus fractures may be noted at the time of delivery. These injuries typically cause a pseudoparalysis (the infant does not move the extremity in order to avoid pain and discomfort; to the observer, it appears "paralyzed") or asymmetry in the use of the extremities. Treatment generally requires splinting of the involved extremity for a few weeks during rapid healing.

Epiphyseal fractures most commonly involve the proximal humerus and are associated with difficult deliveries. The diagnosis may be made clinically and may be difficult to detect radiographically.

Fractures of the distal extremities or ribs are extremely rare in association with birth trauma. In a review of the literature and case series report, van Rijn, Bilo, and Robben (2008) identified 13 cases of definitive birth-related posterior rib fractures. The majority of infants had large birth weights and difficult deliveries, over 50% with shoulder dystocia. In infants with an associated clavicular fracture, the rib fractures were ipsilateral. Van Rijn et al. (2008) reported in detail three definitive and one possible case of birth-related posterior rib fractures. In all four cases, the rib fractures were mid-posterior. The authors postulate that leverage over the pubic symphysis in the macrosomic infants applies forces similar to those seen with bimanual compression, without anterior displacement of the vertebrae (van Rijn, Bilo & Robbin, 2008). Fractures due to the birth process heal rapidly. By 2 weeks of age, they should all show radiographic signs of healing. In most cases, birth trauma is easily distinguished from abuse, although the possibility that an injury was the result of birth trauma occasionally arises. Fractures that do not show the callus by 2 weeks of age are not consistent with birth trauma, and the injuries should be accounted for by another mechanism.

Caffey disease (infantile cortical hyperostosis) is a rare, benign condition which presents with a classic triad of fever, soft-tissue swelling, and irritability. The radiographic appearance is striking and notable for thickening or bony expansion, especially affecting the flat bones such as the mandible, clavicle, rib, scapula, skull, and ilium (Davis, 2007). The underlying cause of Caffey disease remains unclear. It has characteristics of an inflammatory process which is may be inherited, immunologic, or infectious in nature. It typically presents in early infancy, is self-limited, but it may have a protracted course over months. Owing to its dramatic presentation, it may be confused with child maltreatment (Davis, 2007) (Photo 4.34 and 4.35).

Normal Variations Mistaken for Abuse

A number of normal variants of the developing skeleton may be mistaken for fractures and may sometimes suggest abuse. The most common of these variations is the subperiosteal new bone formation of the long bones seen commonly in young infants between 1 and 4 months of age (Kwon, Spevak, Fletcher, & Kleinman, 2002). The subperiosteal new bone formation is a normal physiologic pattern of rapid bone growth in infants who still undergo intramembranous ossification. The new bone formation is smooth, involves multiple bones, and is generally symmetric (although it can be unilateral). The infant is asymptomatic, in contrast to infants with congenital syphilis or other disorders. If the new bone formation occurs in older infants or appears thick, irregular, or extends to the end of the metaphysis, other etiologies, including trauma, should be explored (Glaser, 1949; Kwon et al., 2002; Shopfner, 1966).

Variations can also be seen in the newborn and infant skull in size, shape, and ossification. Suture variants and fissures can be mistaken for fractures. Common mimickers of trauma include the median occipital fissure, intraparietal (accessory) sutures, the interparietal bone, accessory fontanelles in the sagital suture (called the third fontanelle) (Swischuk, 2003).

Congenital Syphilis

The osteochondritis, epiphysitis, and periostitis (inflammation of the periosteum) of congenital syphilis may mimic the metaphyseal fractures and periosteal new bone formation associated with child abuse (Fiser, Kaplan, & Holder, 1972), Sixty to eighty percent of infants infected during pregnancy will have clinical signs (Feigin, 2009). Bone involvement (most often involving the humerus or femur, but may affect any bone of the skeletal system) is the most common sign of syphilis. The early findings in congenital syphilis are varied and unpredictable. There are limited studies available to follow the long term effects. The presentation may be early (birth to 3 months) or late. Treatment with antibiotics for the mother (during the pregnancy) does not assure that infection will not occur in the fetus. Up to 50% of pregnant women, with negative VDRL testing early in the pregnancy, will deliver infants having congenital syphilis (Mandell, Douglas, Bennett, & Dolin, 2005).

Radiographic changes are often diagnostic and usually involve multiple symmetric bones. The lower extremities are involved more often than the upper extremities. Metaphyseal destruction and periosteal new bone formation are characteristic of the skeletal changes associated with syphilis. Epiphyseal changes are evident radiographically approximately 5 weeks after infection, whereas periosteal changes are first seen after 4–5 months of infection. Therefore, the radiographic manifestations of syphilis vary depending on the trimester in which the fetus was infected. Radiologic findings also include (1) Wegner's sign (serrated appearance of epiphyseal margin), (2) a zone of rarefaction at the metaphysis, (3) a moth eaten appearance, (4) irregular periosteal thickening, (5) Wimberger's Sign (demineralization and boney destruction in the upper medial tibial metaphysis) (6) Saber shin (anterior bowing of tibia) (7) Higoumonaki's Sign (periosteal reaction to the sternoclavicular portion of the clavicle) and (8) saddle nose deformity. Perforation of the hard palate has been suggested to be pathognomonic for congenital syphilis.

Clinical signs of skeletal involvement include pseudoparalysis of affected limbs (due to pain) and swelling and tenderness of the ends of involved bones. Affected infants may have other clinical manifestations of congenital syphilis, including hepatomegaly, splenomegaly, anemia, jaundice, rash, sniffles, and adenopathy. Often the first symptom is rhinitis. The rash is desquamative, diffuse, maculopapular and is found on the palms, soles, mouth, and anus.

Diagnosis is based on serologic testing which should be obtained in all high risk infants. A skeletal survey is recommended in the evaluation of congenital syphilis, because bony changes may be evident before the VDRL is positive (Schulz, Murphy, Patamasucon, & Meheus, 1990).

Copper Deficiency and Scurvy

Copper deficiency is a rare cause of metabolic bone disease and pathologic fractures. Causes include both nutritional deficiencies in premature infants as well as diseases associated with intestinal copper transport. Radiologic features include severe osteopenia, symmetric cupping of the metaphyses, metaphyseal spurs, subperiosteal new bone formation, and prominent zones of provisional calcification (ASBMR, 2006; Chapman, 1987; Shaw, 1988). Predisposing risk factors include prematurity, deficient nutrition, malnutrition, and malabsorption. Children with copper deficiency will have associated laboratory changes including sideroblastic anemia resistant to iron, neutropenia, low levels of copper and ceruloplasmin. Menke's Syndrome (kinky hair syndrome) is notable for psychomotor retardation, hypotonia, seizures, failure to thrive, and hypopigmentation, with hair that is kinky, coarse, and lacking in pigment.

Scurvy, a deficiency of Vitamin C (ascorbic acid) and ascorbic acid oxidase (copper dependent enzyme), has similar clinical and radiologic features to copper deficiency. It is also the consequence of malnutrition (not often seen before 6 months of age) and is extremely rare (ASBMR, 2006). The "scurvy line" is a lucent band under the zone of provisional calcification (not usually present in copper deficiency). Features include pathologic fractures occur through the metaphyses as well as subperiosteal and soft tissue hemorrhages. Diaphyseal fractures are not common (Kleinman, 1998).

Both copper deficiency and scurvy have severe osteopenia which can aid in the differentiation between these deficiencies and child abuse. Other clinical, laboratory, and radiologic features should be present if the copper deficiency is severe enough to cause fractures. Metabolic bone disease, such as copper deficiency, should affect the entire skeleton symmetrically.

Osteopenia of Prematurity

It is estimated that 50% of infants less than 1,000 g will develop osteopenia of prematurity (Moyer-Mileur, Luetkemeier, Boomer, & Chan, 1995) with fracture rates ranging from as low as 1.2% (Amir et al. 1988) to 27% (Dabezies & Warren, 1997). There is tremendous variability between studies depending on the gestational age of the infant, weight, and other risk factors. In addition, many of the studies with the highest rates of fracture were performed in the 1980s to early 1990s. There is now significant improvement in nutritional management, immobilization, and ventilator times (Rauch & Schoenau, 2002).

Decreased bone mineralization can occur as the result of insufficient matrix being deposited or as the result of insufficient mineral being incorporated into the matrix. Osteomalacia results from an accumulation of unmineralized bone matrix and can be seen clinically as "rickets". Osteopenia (scarcity of bone) is the result of decreased amounts of matrix or bone tissue whether through insufficient deposition or increased resorption. During the last trimester, 80% of calcium and phosphorous deposition occurs in fetal bone as well as 2/3 of the fetal weight gain. The full-term infant will develop "physiological osteoporosis of infancy" in the first few months of life as the marrow cavity size in the long bone increases faster than the cross-sectional area of the bone cortex. There is no bone fragility associated with "physiological osteoporosis of infancy" in the full-term infant. This also occurs in the premature infant albeit earlier than the term infant (Rauch & Schoenau, 2002).

The preterm infant (< 32 weeks gestation) has a bone mineral content (BMC) that is 40–50% less than the full-term infant at 40 weeks gestation (Congdon, Horsman, Ryan, Truscott, & Durward, 1990; Horsman et al., 1989). In multiple prospective studies of premature infant bone accretion, there is rapid mineral deposition occurring between 40 and 60 weeks postconception (Congdon et al., 1990; Horsman et al., 1989a; McDevitt, Tomlinson, White, & Ahmed, 2007 Mineral accretion rates are often 5–10 times higher in preterm infants (Congdon et al., 1990) than full-term infants suggesting the presence of a "biostat" (McDevitt et al. 2007). The deficit noted at birth between preterm and full-term infants is largely resolved by 50 weeks postconception in preterm infants (Horsman et al. 1989b). Preterm infants increase their BMC by 30–60% of the mean value seen in full-term infants whereas full-term infants increase their BMC by only 11–45% (Horsman et al., 1989b).

Risk factors for mineralization issues in premature infants include prematurity < 28 weeks gestational age, cholestatic jaundice, TPN for greater than 3 weeks, BPD with prolonged use of steroids, and prolonged diuretic therapy (greater than 2 weeks) (Amir et al., 1988; Carroll, Doria, & Paul, 2007). Premature infants who are ELBW (< 1,000 g) appear to be at greatest risk for osteopenia of prematurity at 6–12 weeks of age. Osteopenia of prematurity should be suspected when there is elevation in alkaline phosphatase and low phosphorous levels (Rauch & Schoenau, 2002). Close attention to calcium and phosphorous content in TPN, as well as the use of supplemented breast milk and premature formulas, has decreased the incidence of bone disorders in premature infants. In a large study of fractures in 973 premature infants, only 1.2% of infants surviving more than 6 months had fractures (Amir et al., 1988). Dahlenberg, Bishop, and Lucas (1989) compared the incidence of prematurity in three groups of children less than 5 years of age. Children with fracture were compared to children with accidental injury without fracture and to the entire population. There was no difference between the three groups in the incidence of prematurity. The study suggests that a substantially increased risk of fracture does not persist into childhood.

Rickets

The radiographic appearance of rickets is identical regardless of its etiology and reflects the undermineralization of growing bones. There are multiple causes of rickets, including vitamin D deficiency, renal and hepatic disease, medications (antacids, anticonvulsants, furosemide), and other rare diseases. Children at risk for rickets include small, ill, premature infants (related to nutritional compromise, high growth rates, medication use); breast-fed infants who do not receive Vitamin D supplementation and have limited UV-B light exposure; children using sunscreen or in the practice of covering most of the skin with clothing; children and adolescents with restrictive diets or poor nutritional habits; and children with kidney or liver disease (Bergstrom, 1991; Wharton & Bishop, 2003).

Radiographic findings include fraying of the costochondral junctions and metaphyses, widening of the distance from the epiphysis to the mineralized portion of the metaphysis, flaring of the metaphyses, and cortical thinning (Photo 4.36). The changes that occur in the metaphyses and ribs are not usually confused with abuse. These changes can develop rapidly, in contrast to osteomalacia. During healing, bony changes may mimic abuse because dense mineralization occurs adjacent to radiolucent bone, which may resemble metaphyseal fractures. Periosteal new bone formation may mimic trauma. In long bones, rickets will differ from abuse with the findings of Looser's Zones (symmetric transverse insufficiency fractures) (Kleinman, 1990). The most common long bone sites are the proximal tibia and fibula, and the distal end of the radius and ulna. Changes in the phalanges include subperiosteal erosions.

The diagnosis of rickets is dependent on clinical suspicion and laboratory screening for rickets. Clinically, affected children may appear apathetic and irritable and prefer to sit rather than stand and walk. The epiphyseal ends of long bones may be tender and swollen (big wrists). Other clinical findings included delayed eruption of teeth, enamel hypoplasia, rachitic rosary, frontal bossing, craniotabes, and genu varum (bowed legs) (Wharton & Bishop, 2003). Laboratory findings in rickets include hypophosphatemia, elevated alkaline phosphatase, and elevated parathyroid hormone (PTH). Calcium levels are often variable (normal to low). The diagnosis of rickets requires a detailed evaluation of clinical, laboratory and radiologic findings (Misra, Pacaud, Petryk, Collett-Solberg, & Kappy, 2008). Low levels of 25-hydroxy Vitamin D can confirm the diagnosis, but are not diagnostic in isolation.

There is a lack of agreement in the literature surrounding the definition of normal levels for 25-hydroxy Vitamin D. Most experts agree that levels of 25-hydroxy Vitamin D less than 20 ng/ml are deficient with less than 8 ng/ml indicative of severe deficiency. Levels between 21 and 30 ng/ml are considered insufficient (Gordon et al. 2008; Holick, 2009). There is increasing evidence that Vitamin D deficiency is common among infants and toddlers (Holick, 2007). In a prospective study of children ages 8–24 months, 40% had insufficient levels of Vitamin D with 12% deficient (<20 ng/ml) and approximately 2% severely deficient (<8 ng/ml). Of those children found deficient in Vitamin D, one-third appeared demineralized on plain X-ray and a few children (3 of 40) demonstrated rachitic changes (Gordon et al., 2008). Vitamin D deficiency has certainly been associated with breastfeeding without vitamin supplementation and with inadequate milk consumption.

There are other metabolic causes of osteopenia, osteomalacia, and rickets. Metabolic bone disease should affect the entire skeleton symmetrically. Low levels of 25-hydroxy Vitamin D are not diagnostic of metabolic bone disease in isolation and are a common finding in the population. A detailed evaluation including careful history taking, physical examination, laboratory and radiologic testing should exclude these conditions. Treatment of rickets is guided by the primary cause.

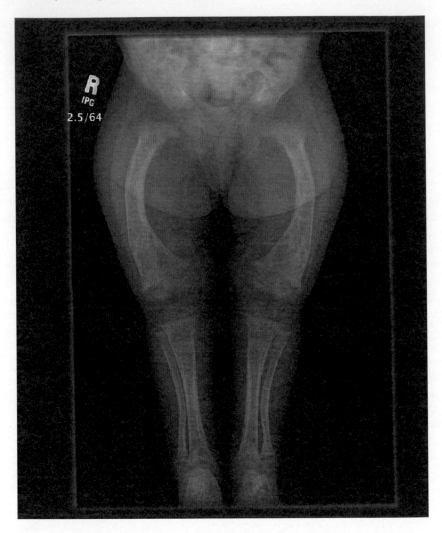

Photo 4.36 3.5-year-old female with renal rickets. Note the bowing of the long bones as well as the flaring and ragged metaphyses.

Osteogenesis Imperfecta

Osteogenesis imperfecta (OI), also referred to as Brittle Bone Disease, is a rare (1 in 10,000 births), inherited disorder of connective tissue that results from an abnormal quantity or quality of type I collagen. The clinical result is osteoporosis with increased bone fragility and decreased bone density. There are different variable expressions of the disease, which is classified into four major clinical types (and 7 subtypes) based on phenotype and radiologic features. Most forms of this disease are easily distinguished from child abuse, but only the rare case may pose difficulties. The following sections describe the major features of each type of OI. Table 4.5

Table 4.5 Common characteristics of osteogenesis imperfecta types I–IV.

Type	Major characteristics	Comments	Confused with abuse
Type I	80% of all cases Bone fragility mild to moderately severe Fractures occasionally at birth Fractures common during preschool years (Silence, 1988) Blue sclera Hearing impairment or family history of hearing impairment Easy bruising Short stature Dentinogenesis	Most common form Autosomal dominant inheritance	Rarely
Type II	Death by 1 month of age Severe skeletal deformities Blue sclerae Intrauterine growth retardation Multiple fractures at birth	Perinatal lethal form	No (not confused)
Type III	Severe bone fragility and osteopenia Fractures at birth (2/3 cases) (Silence et al., 1986) Growth retardation Skeletal deformities Sclerae: normal but may be mild blue at birth Triangular facies (85% cases) Dentinogenesis imperfecta (50%) Ligamentous laxity (50%) Easy bruisability (25%) Occasional hearing impairment	Rare and more severe form	Easily distinguishable from abuse
Type IV	Bone fragility mild to moderate Birth fractures (> 1/3 cases) Osteopenia Wormian bones Dentinogenesis imperfecta may be present Normal sclerae Hearing impairment uncommon Easy bruising uncommon	Rare Autosomal dominant Inheritance Mild form of disease Bones may appear normal at time of first fracture	Most difficult form to distinguish Most at risk for diagnosis of abuse (Ablin, Greenspan, Reinhart, & Grix, 1990)

shows common characteristics of the four types of OI. An important piece of the diagnosis of OI is the emphasis on connective tissue defects including dental, skin, bone and sclera. Due to the range of severity expressed, patients may not always fall clearly into one category (Glorieux, 2008; Byers, Krakow, Nunes, & Pepin, 2006).

Laboratory testing for bone studies are generally normal, except following a fracture when the alkaline phosphatase may be elevated. Teeth may look normal on gross examination, but may show defects on X-ray (Glorieux, 2008).

Type I

The most common (and mildest form) of OI is type I, which accounts for 80% of all cases and has autosomal dominant inheritance. Although type I is a relatively mild form of OI, the bone fragility varies from mild to moderately severe. Fractures are occasionally present at birth but characteristically begin during preschool years (Sillence, 1988). Children often have blue sclerae. Common findings include hearing impairment or a family history of hearing loss, and easy bruising due to abnormal collagen in blood vessels. Associated findings, such as joint hypermobility, growth deficiency, and dentinogenesis imperfecta may occur. Short stature is also characteristic of type I OI (Byers et al., 2006).

Type II

Type II is the perinatal lethal form of the disease and is not confused with child abuse. Affected neonates all have severe skeletal deformities, blue sclerae, intrauterine growth retardation, short bowed legs and arms, and multiple fractures at birth. Affected children generally die in early infancy, although there are reports of infants surviving to one year of life.

Type III

Type III is the most severe form surviving beyond infancy and is also called "progressive deforming type", with autosomal dominant or a new dominant mutation as the mode of inheritance. Bone fragility and osteopenia are more severe than in types I and IV, and fractures at birth are present in two-thirds of affected patients (Sillence et al., 1986). Growth retardation (height achieved is that of a prepubertal child) and skeletal deformities such as scoliosis and bowed limbs are common often resulting in patients requiring wheelchair use. Sclerae are typically normal, but may be mildly blue or grey at birth. Eighty-five percent of patients eventually manifest triangular facies because of soft craniofacial bones and temporal bossing (Sillence, 1988). This is usually not apparent in early childhood. Dentinogenesis imperfecta and ligamentous laxity occur in about half the patients, and easy bruising in 25%. Hearing impairment is found only occasionally (Photo 4.37).

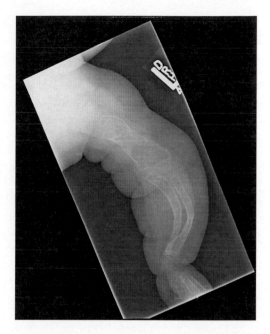

Photo 4.37 Left upper extremity of an infant with Osteogenesis Imperfecta type 3.

Type IV

Type IV is a rare form of OI with autosomal dominant inheritance. This is the most variable form of OI from moderately severe to a mild form of OI (with the first clinical signs occurring at birth or later in school years). Type IV may be the most difficult to distinguish from abuse (Ablin, Greenspan, Reinhart, & Grix, 1990). Bone fragility varies from mild to moderate, and fractures at birth are present in less than one-third of patients. The bones may be normal in radiologic appearance at the time of the first fracture. The sclerae are typically normal. Hearing impairment and easy bruising are uncommon. Dentinogenesis imperfecta may be present.

Taitz (1987) estimates the probability of encountering sporadic cases of type IV OI to be between 1 per million to 1 per 3 million births. For large cities, this translates to one case every 100–300 years (Taitz, 1987; Marlowe, et al., 2002), in comparing the incidence of OI and NAI (non-accidental injury) in the first 3 years of life, found child abuse to be 24 times more likely than OI as the cause of fractures in childhood (Marlowe, Pepin, & Byers, 2002).

There are a number of clinical findings that help to identify children with OI. Blue sclerae, hearing impairment, dental abnormalities, hypermobility of joints, easy bruising, short stature, wormian skull bones, osteopenia, bowing tendency, angulation of healed fractures, and progressive scoliosis all suggest OI.

The fractures seen in OI are generally diaphyseal, although metaphyseal fractures resembling those seen in abuse are described (Astley, 1979). Radiographic changes of generalized osteopenia, bowing and remodeling deformities can be seen. Vertebral compression fractures may also be identified.

A few children with type IV OI have a normal physical examination, no obvious radiographic evidence of OI, and a negative family history. These children are at risk for an incorrect diagnosis of abuse. Children with OI usually have a history of minor trauma that accounts for the location, but not the severity of the injury. Recurrent fractures often occur in different environments, helping to distinguish OI from abuse (Gahagan & Rimsza, 1991).

Biochemical analysis of type 1 collagen in cultured skin fibroblasts can confirm the diagnosis after careful clinical evaluation. In patients with clinical manifestations of OI, biochemical alterations of type I collagen are identified in greater than 90% (Wenstrup, Willing, Starman, & Byers, 1990). Testing may be performed from skin biopsy or blood specimens. Testing involves fibroblast collagen analysis or DNA sequencing. Costs and sensitivities depend on the laboratory site used. Approximate testing turn around time is 4–12 weeks, depending on the choice of test and laboratory site. Some mutations may be missed and some changes in gene findings may not be clearly identified as causing OI in that patient. Children with multiple and repeated fractures with features of OI, whose clinical features are not characteristic of abuse, are candidates for biochemical analysis. If there is any question about the correct diagnosis, the child should be placed in a protective environment while awaiting test results. Finally, it is important to note that osteogenesis imperfecta and child abuse can coexist.

In Brief

- Fractures are a common manifestation of abuse, particularly in infants and young children.
- Diaphyseal fractures are the most common type of fracture associated with abuse, but are not specific for inflicted injury.
- The history of injury, development abilities of the child, morphologic type of fracture, and biomechanics are considered in determining the likelihood of abuse in children with diaphyseal fractures.
- Rib fractures and metaphyseal fractures are highly specific for child abuse.
- A skeletal survey should be done in all children less than 2 years of age who have injuries suspicious for abuse.
- The yield from the skeletal survey decreases with increasing age of the child and is not a useful test in children older than 5 years.
- Standards for performing skeletal surveys exist and should be followed (American College of Radiology, 2006).
- Radionuclide bone scan may identify infants and young children with subtle injuries that are not detected by skeletal survey.
- Bone scans are excellent in detecting rib injury, but are not useful in identifying skull fractures and do not consistently identify metaphyseal fractures.

- Skeletal surveys should be repeated in 2 weeks in all infants less than 1 year of age with injuries suspicious for abuse.
- A number of disease states predispose to fractures. Careful evaluation usually distinguishes children with pathological fractures from those who are abused.
- Trauma is the leading cause of bony injury to otherwise healthy bones.
- The presence of a medical disease and child abuse can coexist and are not mutually exclusive.

Additional Recommended Reading

Coats, B., & Margulies, S. S., (2008). Potential for head injuries from low-height falls: Laboratory Investigation. *Journal of Neurosurgery Pediatrics, 2*, 321–330.

Kleinman, P. K., & Schlesinger, A. E. (1997). Mechanical factors associated with posterior rib fractures: laboratory and case studies. *Pediatrics Radiology, 27*, 87–91.

Pierce, M. C., Bertocci, G. E., Vogeley, E., & Moreland, M. S. (2004). Evaluating long bone fractures in children: a biomechanical approach with illustrative cases. *Child Abuse and Neglect, 28*, 505–524.

Pierce, M. C., Bertocci, G. E., Janosky, J. E., Aguel, F., Deemer, E., Moreland, M., et al. (2005). Femur fractures resulting from stair falls among children: An injury plausibility model. *Pediatrics, 115*, 1712–1722.

References

ASBMR. (2006). *Primer on the metabolic bone diseases and disorders of mineral metabolism*. Washington, DC: The American Society for Bone and Mineral Research.

Ablin, D. S., Greenspan, A., & Reinhart, M. A. (1992). Pelvic injuries in child abuse. *Pediatrics Radiology, 22*, 454–457.

Ablin, D. S., Greenspan, A., Reinhart, M., & Grix, A. (1990). Differentiation of child abuse from osteogenesis imperfecta. *American Journal of Roentgenology, 154*, 1035–1046.

American College of Radiology. (2006). ACR practice guideline for skeletal surveys in children. Res 47,17,35: 253–257.

Amir, J., Katz, K., Grunebaum, M., Yosipovich, Z., Wielunsky, E., & Reisner, S. H. (1988). Fractures in premature infants. *Journal of Pediatric Orthopaedics, 8*, 41–44.

Arnholz, D., Hymel, K. P., Hay, T. C., & Jenny, C. (1998). Bilateral pediatric skull fractures: accident or abuse?. *Journal of Trauma, 45*, 172–174.

Astley, R. (1979). Metaphyseal fractures in osteogenesis imperfecta. *British Journal of Radiology, 52*, 441–443.

Barsness, K. A., Cha, E. S., Bensard, D. D., Calkins, C. M., Partrick, D. A., Karrer, F. M., et al. (2003). The positive predictive value of rib fractures as an indicator of nonaccidental trauma in children. *Journal of Trauma, 54*, 1107–1110.

Bergstrom, W. H. (1991). Hypophosphatemic rickets with hypocalciuria following long-term treatment with aluminum-containing antacid. *Bone, 12*, 301.

Billmire, M. E., & Myers, P. A. (1985). Serious head injury in infants: accident or abuse?. *Pediatrics, 75*, 340–342.

Bulloch, B., Schubert, C. J., Brophy, P. D., Johnson, N., Reed, M. H., & Shapiro, R. A. (2000). Cause and clinical characteristics of rib fractures in infants. *Pediatrics, 105*, E48.

Byers, P. H., Krakow, D., Nunes, M. E., & Pepin, M. (2006). Genetic evaluation of suspected osteogenesis imperfecta (OI). *Genetics in Medicine, 8*, 383–388.

Cadzow, S. P., & Armstrong, K. L. (2000). Rib fractures in infants: red alert! The clinical features, investigations and child protection outcomes. *Journal of Paediatrics and Child Health, 36*, 322–326.

Caffey, J. (1957). Some traumatic lesions in growing bones other than fractures and dislocations: clinical and radiological features: The Mackenzie Davidson Memorial Lecture. *British Journal of Radiology, 30*, 225–238.

Carroll, D. M., Doria, A. S., & Paul, B. S. (2007). Clinical-radiological features of fractures in premature infants – a review. *Journal of Perinatal Medicine, 35*, 366–375.

Caviglia, H., Garrido, C. P., Palazzi, F. F., & Meana, N. V. (2005). Pediatric fractures of the humerus. *Clinical Orthopaedics and Related Research*, 49–56.

Chapman, S. (1987). Child abuse or copper deficiency? A radiological view. *British Medical Journal (Clinical research ed.), 294*, 1370.

Chapman, S. (1992). The radiologic dating of injuries. *Archives of Disease in Childhood, 67*, 1063–1065.

Coats, B., & Margulies, S. S. (2008). Potential for head injuries in infants from low-height falls. *Journal of Neurosurgery: Pediatrics, 2*, 321–330.

Congdon, P. J., Horsman, A., Ryan, S. W., Truscott, J. G., & Durward, H. (1990). Spontaneous resolution of bone mineral depletion in preterm infants. *Archives of Disease in Childhood, 65*, 1038–1042.

Dabezies, E. J., & Warren, P. D. (1997). Fractures in very low birth weight infants with rickets. *Clinical Orthopaedics and Related Research*, 233–239.

Dahlenberg, S. L., Bishop, N. J., & Lucas, A. (1989). Are preterm infants at risk for subsequent fractures?. *Archives of Disease in Childhood, 64*, 1384–1393.

Davis, B. C. (2007). Caffey disease. eMedicine. Accessed December 1, 2009, http://emedicine.medscape.com/article/406697-overview

Day, F., Clegg, S., McPhillips, M., & Mok, J. (2006). A retrospective case series of skeletal surveys in children with suspected non-accidental injury. *Journal of Clinical Forensic Medicine, 13*, 55–59.

Diagnostic Imaging of Child Abuse. (2009, May). *Pediatrics, 123*(5), 1430–1435.

Duhaime, A. C., Alario, A. J., Lewander, W. J., Schut, L., Sutton, L. N., Seidl, T. S., et al. (1992). Head injury in very young children: mechanisms, injury types, and ophthalmologic findings in 100 hospitalized patients younger than 2 years of age. *Pediatrics, 90*, 179–185.

Ebbin, A. J., Gollub, M. H., Stein, A. M., & Wilson, M. G. (1969). Battered child syndrome at the Los Angeles Count General Hospital. *American Journal of Diseases of Children, 118*, 660–667.

Ersahin, Y., Gulmen, V., & Palali, M. S. (2000). Growing skull fractures (craniocerebral erosion). *Neurosurgical Review, 23*, 139–144.

Feigin, R. D. (2009). *Feigin & Cherry's textbook of pediatric infectious diseases*. Philadelphia: Saunders/Elsevier.

Fenton, L. Z., Sirotnak, A. P., & Handler, M. H. (2000). Parietal pseudofracture and spontaneous intracranial hemorrhage suggesting nonaccidental trauma: report of 2 cases. *Pediatric Neurosurgery, 33*, 318–322.

Fiser, R. H., Kaplan, J., & Holder, J. C. (1972). Congenital syphilis mimicking the battered child syndrome. How does one tell them apart?. *Clinical Pediatrics (Phila)*, *11*, 305–307.

Gahagan, S., & Rimsza, M. E. (1991). Child abuse or osteogenesis imperfecta: How can we tell?. *Pediatrics*, *88*, 987–992.

Garcia, V. F., Gotschall, C. S., Eichelberger, M. R., & Bowman, L. M. (1990). Rib fractures in children: A marker of severe trauma. *Journal of Trauma*, *30*, 695–700.

Glaser, K. (1949). Double contour, cupping and spurring in roentgenograms of long bones in infants. *American Journal of Roentgenology, Radium Therapy, and Nuclear Medicine*, *61*, 482–492.

Glorieux, F. H. (2008). Osteogenesis imperfecta. *Best Practice & Research Clinical Rheumatology*, *22*, 85–100.

Gordon, C. M., Feldman, H. A., Sinclair, L., Williams, A. L., Kleinman, P. K., Perez-Rossello, J., et al. (2008). Prevalence of vitamin D deficiency among healthy infants and toddlers. *Archives of Pediatrics and Adolescent Medicine*, *162*, 505–512.

Grayev, A. M., Boal, D. K., Wallach, D. M., & Segal, L. S. (2001). Metaphyseal fractures mimicking abuse during treatment for clubfoot. *Pediatrics Radiology*, *31*, 559–563.

Hansen, K. K., Prince, J. S., & Nixon, G. W. (2008). Oblique chest views as a routine part of skeletal surveys performed for possible physical abuse – is this practice worthwhile?. *Child Abuse and Neglect*, *32*, 155–159.

Helfer, R. E., Scheurer, S. L., Alexander, R., Reed, J., & Slovis, T. L. (1984). Trauma to the bones of small infants from passive exercise: a factor in the etiology of child abuse. *Journal of Pediatrics*, *104*, 47–50.

Herndon, W. A. (1983). Child abuse in a military population. *Journal of Pediatric Orthopaedics*, *3*, 73–76.

Hiss, J., & Kahana, T. (1995). The medicolegal implications of bilateral cranial fractures in infants. *Journal of Trauma*, *38*, 32–34.

Hobbs, C. J. (1984). Skull fracture and the diagnosis of abuse. *Archives of Disease in Childhood*, *59*, 246–252.

Holck, P. (2005). What can a baby's skull withstand? Testing the skull's resistance on an anatomical preparation. *Forensic Science International*, *151*, 187–191.

Holick, M. F. (2007). Vitamin D deficiency. *The New England journal of medicine*, *357*, 266–281.

Holick, M. F. (2009). Vitamin D Status: Measurement, interpretation, and clinical application. *Annals of Epidemiology*, *19*(2), 73–78.

Horsman, A., Ryan, S. W., Congdon, P. J., Truscott, J. G., & James, J. R. (1989). Osteopenia in extremely low birthweight infants. *Archives of Disease in Childhood*, *64*, 485–488.

Horsman, A., Ryan, S. W., Congdon, P. J., Truscott, J. G., & Simpson, M. (1989a). Bone mineral accretion rate and calcium intake in preterm infants. *Archives of Disease in Childhood*, *64*, 910–918.

Horsman, A., Ryan, S. W., Congdon, P. J., Truscott, J. G., & Simpson, M. (1989b). Bone mineral content and body size 65–100 weeks' postconception in preterm and full term infants. *Archives of Disease in Childhood*, *64*, 1579–1586.

Hui, C., Joughin, E., Goldstein, S., Cooper, N., Harder, J., Kiefer, G., et al. (2008). Femoral fractures in children younger than three years: the role of nonaccidental injury. *Journal of Pediatric Orthopaedics*, *28*, 297–302.

Islam, O., Soboleski, D., Symons, S., Davidson, L. K., Ashworth, M. A., & Babyn, P. (2000). Development and duration of radiographic signs of bone healing in children. *American Journal of Roentgenology*, *175*, 75–78.

John, S. D., Moorthy, C. S., & Swischuk, L. E. (1997). Expanding the concept of the toddler's fracture. *Radiographics*, *17*, 367–376.

Kemp, A. M., Butler, A., Morris, S., Mann, M., Kemp, K. W., Rolfe, K., et al. (2006). Which radiological investigations should be performed to identify fractures in suspected child abuse?. *Clinical Radiology*, *61*, 723–736.

Kemp, A. M., Dunstan, F., Harrison, S., Morris, S., Mann, M., Rolfe, K., et al. (2008). Patterns of skeletal fractures in child abuse: systematic review. *British Medical Journal*, *337*, a1518.

Kleinman, P. K. (1990). Diagnostic imaging in infant abuse. *American Journal of Roentgenology*, *155*, 703–712.

Kleinman, P. (1998). *Diagnostic imaging of child abuse*. St. Louis, MO: Mosby.

Kleinman, P. K. (2008). Problems in the diagnosis of metaphyseal fractures. *Pediatrics Radiology*, *38*(Suppl 3), S388–S394.

Kleinman, P. K., Belanger, P. L., Karellas, A., & Spevak, M. R. (1991). Normal metaphyseal radiologic variants not to be confused with findings of infant abuse. *American Journal of Roentgenology*, *156*, 781–783.

Kleinman, P. K., & Marks, S. C., Jr. (1992). Vertebral body fractures in child abuse. Radiologic-histopathologic correlates. *Investigative Radiology*, *27*, 715–722.

Kleinman, P. K., & Marks, S. C., Jr. (1996a). A regional approach to classic metaphyseal lesions in abused infants: The distal tibia. *American Journal of Roentgenology*, *166*, 1207–1212.

Kleinman, P. K., & Marks, S. C., Jr. (1996b). A regional approach to the classic metaphyseal lesion in abused infants: The proximal humerus. *American Journal of Roentgenology*, *167*, 1399–1403.

Kleinman, P. K., & Marks, S. C., Jr. (1996c). A regional approach to the classic metaphyseal lesion in abused infants: The proximal tibia. *American Journal of Roentgenology*, *166*, 421–426.

Kleinman, P. K., & Marks, S. C., Jr. (1998). A regional approach to the classic metaphyseal lesion in abused infants: the distal femur. *American Journal of Roentgenology*, *170*, 43–47.

Kleinman, P. K., Marks, S. C., Adams, V. I., & Blackbourne, B. D. (1988). Factors affecting visualization of posterior rib fractures in abused infants. *American Journal of Roentgenology*, *150*, 635–638.

Kleinman, P. K., Marks, S. C., & Blackbourne, B. (1986). The metaphyseal lesion in abused infants: a radiologic-histopathologic study. *American Journal of Roentgenology*, *146*, 895–905.

Kleinman, P. K., Marks, S. C., Jr., Nimkin, K., Rayder, S. M., & Kessler, S. C. (1996). Rib fractures in 31 abused infants: postmortem radiologic-histopathologic study. *Radiology*, *200*, 807–810.

Kleinman, P. K., Marks, S. C., Jr., Richmond, J. M., & Blackbourne, B. D. (1995). Inflicted skeletal injury: a postmortem radiologic-histopathologic study in 31 infants. *American Journal of Roentgenology*, *165*, 647–650.

Kleinman, P. K., Marks, S. C., Spevak, M. R., & Richmond, J. M. (1992). Fractures of the rib head in abused infants. *Radiology*, *185*, 119–123.

Kleinman, P. K., Nimkin, K., Spevak, M. R., Rayder, S. M., Madansky, D. L., Shelton, Y. A., et al. (1996). Follow-up skeletal surveys in suspected child abuse. *American Journal of Roentgenology*, *167*, 893–896.

Kleinman, P. K., & Schlesinger, A. E. (1997). Mechanical factors associated with posterior rib fractures: laboratory and case studies. *Pediatrics Radiology*, *27*, 87–91.

Kleinman, P. K., & Spevak, M. R. (1992). Soft tissue swelling and acute skull fractures. *Journal of Pediatrics, 121,* 737–739.

Kogutt, M. S., Swischuk, L. E., & Fagan, C. J. (1974). Patterns of injury and significance of uncommon fractures in the battered child syndrome. *American Journal of Roentgenology, Radium Therapy, and Nuclear Medicine, 121,* 143–149.

Krischer, J. P., Fine, E. G., Davis, J. H., & Nagel, E. L. (1987). Complications of cardiac resuscitation. *Chest, 92,* 287–291.

Kwon, D. S., Spevak, M. R., Fletcher, K., & Kleinman, P. K. (2002). Physiologic sub-periosteal new bone formation: prevalence, distribution, and thickness in neonates and infants. *American Journal of Roentgenology, 179,* 985–988.

Langer, L. O., Jr., Brill, P. W., Ozonoff, M. B., Pauli, R. M., Wilson, W. G., Alford, B. A., et al. (1990). Spondylometaphyseal dysplasia, corner fracture type: a heritable condition associated with coxa vara. *Radiology, 175,* 761–766.

Leventhal, J. M., Thomas, S. A., Rosenfield, N. S., & Markowitz, R. I. (1993). Fractures in young children. Distinguishing child abuse from unintentional injuries. *American Journal of Diseases of Children, 147,* 87–92.

Leventhal, J. M., Martin, K. D., & Asnes, A. G. (2008). Incidence of fractures attributable to abuse in young hospitalized children: results from analysis of a United States database. *Pediatrics, 122,* 599–604.

Loder, R. T., & Feinberg, J. R. (2007). Orthopaedic injuries in children with Nonaccidental trauma: demographics and incidence from the 2000 kids' inpatient database. *Journal of Pediatric Orthopaedics, 27,* 421–426.

Lysack, J. T., & Soboleski, D. (2003). Classic metaphyseal lesion following external cephalic version and cesarean section. *Pediatrics Radiology, 33,* 422–424.

Maguire, S., Mann, M., John, N., Ellaway, B., Sibert, J. R., & Kemp, A. M. (2006). Does cardiopulmonary resuscitation cause rib fractures in children? A systematic review. *Child Abuse and Neglect, 30,* 739–751.

Mandell, G. L., Douglas, R. G., Bennett, J. E., & Dolin, R. (2005). Mandell, Douglas, and Bennett's Principles and Practice of Infectious Diseases. In: Editor (Ed.) Book Mandell, Douglas, and Bennett's Principles and Practice of Infectious Diseases. Elsevier/Churchill Livingstone, City, pp. 2 v. (xxxviii, 3661, cxxx p.)

Mandelstam, S. A., Cook, D., Fitzgerald, M., & Ditchfield, M. R. (2003). Complementary use of radiological skeletal survey and bone scintigraphy in detection of bony injuries in suspected child abuse. *Archives of Disease in Childhood, 88,* 387–390, discussion 387–390.

Marlowe, A., Pepin, M. G., & Byers, P. H. (2002). Testing for osteogenesis imperfecta in cases of suspected non-accidental injury. *Journal of Medical Genetics, 39,* 382–386.

Mathew, M. O., Ramamohan, N., & Bennet, G. C. (1998). Importance of bruising associated with paediatric fractures: prospective observational study. *British Medical Journal, 317,* 1117–1118.

McDevitt, H., Tomlinson, C., White, M. P., & Ahmed, S. F. (2007). Changes in quantitative ultrasound in infants born at less than 32 weeks' gestation over the first 2 years of life: influence of clinical and biochemical changes. *Calcified Tissue International, 81,* 263–269.

Mellick, L. B., Milker, L., & Egsieker, E. (1999). Childhood accidental spiral tibial (CAST) fractures. *Pediatric Emergency Care, 15,* 307–309.

Merten, D. F., Cooperman, D. R., & Thompson, G. H. (1994). Skeletal manifestation. In R. M. Reece (Ed.), *Child abuse: Medical diagnosis and management* (pp. 23–53). Malvern, PA: Lea & Febiger.

Merten, D. F., Radkowski, M. A., & Leonidas, J. C. (1983). The abused child: a radiological reappraisal. *Radiology, 146*, 377–381.

Meservy, C. J., Towbin, R., McLaurin, R. L., Myers, P. A., & Ball, W. (1987). Radiographic characteristics of skull fractures resulting from child abuse. *American Journal of Roentgenology, 149*, 173–175.

Misra, M., Pacaud, D., Petryk, A., Collett-Solberg, P. F., & Kappy, M. (2008). Vitamin D deficiency in children and its management: review of current knowledge and recommendations. *Pediatrics, 122*, 398–417.

Morris, S., Cassidy, N., Stephens, M., McCormack, D., & McManus, F. (2002). Birth-associated femoral fractures: incidence and outcome. *Journal of Pediatric Orthopaedics, 22*, 27–30.

Moseley, C. F. (Ed.) *Your orthopaedic connection*. Fractures: an overview. Rosemont, IL: American Academy of Orthapaedic Surgeons. http://orthoinfo.aaos.org/topic.cfm?topic=A00139 Accessed December 1, 2009

Moyer-Mileur, L., Luetkemeier, M., Boomer, L., & Chan, G. M. (1995). Effect of physical activity on bone mineralization in premature infants. *Journal of Pediatrics, 127*, 620–625.

Nimkin, K., Spevak, M. R., & Kleinman, P. K. (1997). Fractures of the hands and feet in child abuse: imaging and pathologic features. *Radiology, 203*, 233–236.

O'Connell, A., & Donoghue, V. B. (2007). Can classic metaphyseal lesions follow uncomplicated caesarean section?. *Pediatric Radiology, 37*, 488–491.

O'Connor-Read, L., Teh, J., & Willett, K. (2007). Radiographic evidence to help predict the mechanism of injury of pediatric spiral fractures in nonaccidental injury. *Journal of Pediatric Orthopaedics, 27*, 754–757.

Ogden, J. A. (1979). Pediatric osteomyelitis and septic arthritis: the pathology of neonatal disease. *Yale Journal of Biology & Medicine, 52*, 423–448.

Ogden, J. A. (1990). *Skeletal injury in the child*. Philadelphia, PA: Saunders.

Pecci, M., & Kreher, J. B. (2008). Clavicle fractures. *American Family Physician, 77*, 65–70.

Perez-Rossello, J. M., Connolly, S. A., Newton, A. W., Thomason, M., Jenny, C., Sugar, N. F., et al. (2008). Pubic ramus radiolucencies in infants: the good, the bad, and the indeterminate. *American Journal of Roentgenology, 190*, 1481–1486.

Perkins, R., & Skirving, A. P. (1987). Callus formation and the rate of healing of femoral fractures in patients with head injuries. *Journal of Bone and Joint Surgery, 69*, 521–524.

Peters, M. L., Starling, S. P., Barnes-Eley, M. L., & Heisler, K. W. (2008). The presence of bruising associated with fractures. *Archives of Pediatrics and Adolescent Medicine, 162*, 877–881.

Pierce, M. C., Bertocci, G. E., Janosky, J. E., Aguel, F., Deemer, E., Moreland, M., et al. (2005). Femur fractures resulting from stair falls among children: an injury plausibility model. *Pediatrics, 115*, 1712–1722.

Pierce, M. C., Bertocci, G. E., Vogeley E., & Moreland, M. S. (2004). Evaluating long bone fractures in children: A biomechanical approach with illustrative cases. *Child Abuse and Neglect, 28*, 505–524.

Prosser, I., Maguire, S., Harrison, S. K., Mann, M., Sibert, J. R., & Kemp, A. M. (2005). How old is this fracture? Radiologic dating of fractures in children: a systematic review. *American Journal of Roentgenology, 184*, 1282–1286.

Quinby, W. C., Jr. (1966). Fractures of the pelvis and associated injuries in children. *Journal of Pediatric Surgery, 1*, 353–364.

Rauch, F., & Schoenau, E. (2002). Skeletal development in premature infants: a review of bone physiology beyond nutritional aspects. *Archives of Disease in Childhood. Fetal and Neonatal Edition, 86*, F82–F85.

Rivara, F. P., Parish, R. A., & Mueller, B. A. (1986). Extremity injuries in children: predictive value of clinical findings. *Pediatrics, 78,* 803–807.

Rodriguez-Merchan, E. C. (2005). Pediatric fractures of the forearm. *Clinical Orthopaedics and Related Research,* 65–72.

Schulz, K., Murphy, F., Patamasucon, P., & Meheus, A. (1990). Congenital syphilis. In: Holmes K. K. (Ed.), *Sexually transmitted diseases* (pp. 821–842). New York: McGraw-Hill, Inc.

Schweich, P., & Fleisher, G. (1985). Rib fractures in children. *Pediatric Emergency Care, 1,* 187–189.

Section on Radiology. (2000). Diagnostic imaging of child abuse. *Pediatrics, 105,* 1345–1348.

Sibert, J. R., Payne, E. H., Kemp, A. M., Barber, M., Rolfe, K., Morgan, R. J., et al. (2002). The incidence of severe physical child abuse in Wales. *Child Abuse and Neglect, 26,* 267–276.

Shaw, J. C. (1988). Copper deficiency and non-accidental injury. *Archives of Disease in Childhood, 63,* 448–455.

Shopfner, C. E. (1966). Periosteal bone growth in normal infants. A preliminary report. *American Journal of Roentgenology, Radium Therapy, and Nuclear Medicine, 97,* 154–163.

Sillence, D. O. (1988). Osteogenesis imperfecta nosology and genetics. *Annals of the New York Academy of Sciences, 543,* 1–15.

Sillence, D. O., Barlow, K. K., Cole, W. G., Dietrich, S., Garber, A. P., & Rimoin, D. L. (1986). Osteogenesis imperfecta type III. Delineation of the phenotype with reference to genetic heterogeneity. *American Journal of Medical Genetics, 23,* 821–832.

Starling, S. P., Heller, R. M., & Jenny, C. (2002). Pelvic fractures in infants as a sign of physical abuse. *Child Abuse and Neglect, 26,* 475–480.

Starling, S. P., Sirotnak, A. P., Heisler, K. W., & Barnes-Eley, M. L. (2007). Inflicted skeletal trauma: the relationship of perpetrators to their victims. *Child Abuse and Neglect, 31,* 993–999.

Stokes, N. J., & Cremin, B. J. (1974). The skull vault in neonates and infants. *Australasian Radiology, 18,* 275–282.

Strait, R. T., Siegel, R. M., & Shapiro, R. A. (1995). Humeral fractures without obvious etiologies in children less than 3 years of age: when is it abuse?. *Pediatrics, 96,* 667–671.

Swischuk, L. E. (2003). *Imaging of the newborn, infant, and young child.* Baltimore: Williams & Wilkins.

Taitz, L. S. (1987). Child abuse and osteogenesis imperfecta. *British Medical Journal (Clinical research ed.), 295,* 1082–1083.

The Society for Pediatric Radiology – National Association of Medical Examiners (2004). Post-mortem radiography in the evaluation of unexpected death in children less than 2 years of age whose death is suspicious for fatal abuse. *Pediatrics Radiology, 34,* 675–677.

Thomas, S. A., Rosenfield, N. S., Leventhal, J. M., & Markowitz, R. I. (1991). Long-bone fractures in young children: distinguishing accidental injuries from child abuse. *Pediatrics, 88,* 471–476.

Tran, B., Silvera, M., Newton, A., & Kleinman, P. K. (2007). Inflicted T12 fracture-dislocation: CT/MRI correlation and mechanistic implications. *Pediatrics Radiology, 37,* 1171–1173.

Valencia, J., Leyva, F., & Gomez-Bajo, G. J. (2005). Pediatric hand trauma. *Clinical Orthopaedics and Related Research,* 77–86.

van Rijn, R. R., Bilo, R. A., & Robben, S. G. (2008). Birth-related mid-posterior rib fractures in neonates: a report of three cases (and a possible fourth case) and a review of the literature. *Pediatrics Radiology, 39*, 30–34.

Weber, W. (1984). [Experimental studies of skull fractures in infants]. *Z Rechtsmed, 92*, 87–94.

Weber, W. (1985). [Biomechanical fragility of the infant skull]. *Z Rechtsmed, 94*, 93–101.

Weber, W. (1987). [Predilection sites of infantile skull fractures following blunt force]. *Z Rechtsmed, 98*, 81–93.

Weir, P., Suttner, N. J., Flynn, P., & McAuley, D. (2006). Normal skull suture variant mimicking intentional injury. *British Medical Journal, 332*, 1020–1021.

Wenstrup, R. J., Willing, M. C., Starman, B. J., & Byers, P. H. (1990). Distinct biochemical phenotypes predict clinical severity in nonlethal variants of osteogenesis imperfecta. *American Journal of Human Genetics, 46*, 975–982.

Wharton, B., & Bishop, N. (2003). Rickets. *Lancet, 362*, 1389–1400.

Wootton-Gorges, S. L., Stein-Wexler, R., Walton, J. W., Rosas, A. J., Coulter, K. P., & Rogers, K. K. (2008). Comparison of computed tomography and chest radiography in the detection of rib fractures in abused infants. *Child Abuse and Neglect, 32*, 659–663.

Worlock, P., Stower, M., & Barbor, P. (1986). Patterns of fractures in accidental and non-accidental injury in children: a comparative study. *British Medical Journal (Clinical Research Edition), 293*, 100–102.

Zimmerman, S., Makoroff, K., Care, M., Thomas, A., & Shapiro, R. (2005). Utility of follow-up skeletal surveys in suspected child physical abuse evaluations. *Child Abuse and Neglect, 29*, 1075–1083.

Chapter 5

Abdominal and Thoracic Trauma

Rohit Shenoi

Of all the types of injuries resulting from child abuse, abdominal, and thoracic injuries are the most dangerous. They rank as the second most lethal type of inflicted injuries in children after head injuries. Victims of child abuse with significant abdominal and thoracic injuries often succumb to their injuries before diagnosis and treatment. They are young and defenseless and unable to brace themselves against the very violent forces that cause these types of injuries. Blunt force caused by kicking or punching is a common mechanism. Several factors such as inaccurate and incomplete history offered by the accompanying adult, the lack of external markers, and the lack of immediately evident specific signs and symptoms often lead to a delayed presentation and diagnosis. Victims presenting late with cardiovascular instability may be assumed to have a medical cause and receive standard cardio-pulmonary resuscitation instead of management based on trauma protocols. This explains the high fatality rates associated with these injuries.

This chapter describes the prevalence, nature, and extent of inflicted abdominal and thoracic injuries in children. It will guide the reader in making an early diagnosis by maintaining a high index of suspicion, in the appropriate use of diagnostic tests and in conducting a comprehensive evaluation of injuries in childhood victims of inflicted visceral trauma.

Epidemiology

Blunt abdominal injuries are uncommon in childhood victims of trauma accounting for 1.7% to 7.2% of all types of trauma in children (DiScala, Sege, Li, & Reece, 2000, Tracy, O'Connor, & Weber, 1993; Yamamoto, Wiebe, & Mathews, 1991). However, among those identified as having abdominal trauma, the frequency of inflicted trauma varies from 4 to 19%. In a study of British children,

A.P. Giardino et al. (eds.), *A Practical Guide to the Evaluation of Child Physical Abuse and Neglect*, DOI 10.1007/978-1-4419-0702-8_5, © Springer Science+Business Media, LLC 1997, 2010

Barnes et al. (2005) described the incidence of abdominal injury due to abuse as 0.9 cases per million children per year (95% CI 0.58–1.39) for children up to 14 years of age and 2.33 cases per million children per year (1.43–3.78) in those younger than 5 years. Trokel, DiScala, Terrin, and Sege (2006) studied all cases of blunt abdominal trauma, excluding those caused by motor vehicle crashes, in patients aged 0–4 years from the National Pediatric Trauma Registry (NPTR) phases 2 and 3 (October 1995–April 2001). Child abuse was the most common mechanism of injury (40.5%) among the 664 cases that were analyzed. The contribution of race in visceral injuries is complex. It is possible that different races and ethnic groups abuse their children in different ways and may lead to different patterns of injury but data are not available to prove this. Child abuse may be over diagnosed in injured minority children or under diagnosed in White non-Hispanic patients. However Trokel et al. (2006) suggest that the same risk factors are associated with a medical diagnosis of suspected child abuse in both minority and White children. Trauma to the internal thoracic structures is less common than abdominal injuries.

Abdominal Injuries—General Principles

Blunt trauma accounts for the majority of injuries to the abdomen in victims of abuse. Although penetrating injuries do occur (such as stabs or gunshot wounds), they are relatively infrequent when compared to blunt trauma (Canty, Canty, & Brown, 1999). Three basic mechanisms of blunt trauma account for the abdominal injuries commonly found in abused children:

1. *Crushing* of solid organs (liver, spleen, and pancreas) of the upper abdomen against the vertebral bodies or bony thorax as a result of a blow to the upper abdomen. Hepatic or splenic injuries may be mild, with small amounts of blood loss, or may result in severe hemorrhage and death. The patient's presentation generally reflects the degree of blood loss, ranging from asymptomatic injuries to hemorrhagic shock or cardiac arrest. Children with pancreatic injury may present with symptoms of pancreatitis.
2. *Sudden compression* of hollow abdominal viscera (intestines, stomach, colon, bladder) against the vertebral column as a result of a blow to the abdomen. Most patients with hollow visceral injuries present for medical care with signs of peritonitis or sepsis, often because of a delay in seeking treatment. Vomiting and abdominal pain also may result from hematoma formation.
3. *Shearing* of the posterior attachments or vascular supply of the abdominal viscera (mesenteric tears, disruption of small intestines at sites of ligament support) occur as a result of rapid acceleration or deceleration, such as when a child is thrown against a wall. Shearing forces may also result in intestinal perforations (Kleinman, 1987). Children generally present with hypotension, shock, or cardiac arrest, reflecting severe blood loss. Patients with intestinal perforations from shearing forces generally present with symptoms related to peritonitis or sepsis.

The spectrum of abdominal injuries include rupture or hematoma to hollow organs (stomach, small intestine, including duodenum and rectum), pancreatic injury and unexplained pancreatitis, solid organ lacerations or contusions (liver, spleen, or kidney), and injury to major blood vessels (mesenteric vessels are especially susceptible).

Although major abdominal trauma occurs infrequently, it is the second leading cause of death due to physical abuse. The relatively high mortality rate due to abdominal and thoracic injuries is likely due to a number of factors, including (a) young age of the victims with a poorly developed musculature and relatively small antero-posterior abdominal diameter placing intra-abdominal organs at increased risk, (b) failure to brace and protect themselves from trauma due to poor coordination, (c) delay in seeking appropriate medical care, (d) delay in correct diagnosis that occurs when misleading or incomplete histories are provided by the caretaker, (e) lack of external signs of trauma, (f) severity of injuries sustained to vital organs, (g) brisk hemorrhage associated with certain injuries, and (h) co-existing head injuries.

Studies have found greater mortality with abusive abdominal trauma than with accidental injury (Ledbetter, Hatch, Feldman, Ligner, & Tapper, 1988; Roaten et al., 2006). Mortality rates were reported to be as high as 45% (Cooper et al., 1988). However, the mortality rates due to visceral injuries may have decreased in part due to increased awareness of visceral injuries caused by abuse and improved treatment. Trokel, DiScala, Terrin, & Sege, (2004); in an analysis of children under 5 years of age with blunt abdominal injury from the National Pediatric Trauma Registry (NPTR) database described an overall mortality rate of 21.9% in abused children with abdominal injuries. Victims with solely abdominal injuries had the least mortality rate of 8.8%. Victims with abdominal and skeletal injuries (11.1% mortality) and abdominal injuries with Traumatic brain injury (TBI) and skeletal injury (29.6% mortality) were next. The highest mortality was seen in abused children with abdominal and TBI but without skeletal injury (57.7% mortality). It is speculated that abused victims with fractures may be more obviously injured to caretakers and thus may be brought to medical attention sooner than children without fractures. The presence of fractures may also initiate an earlier trauma evaluation by the physicians and leads to earlier definitive management.

Peritonitis and sepsis account for most other deaths. Many children with inflicted abdominal injury do not manifest symptoms immediately, and the severity of the injuries may not be readily apparent. Caregivers may incorrectly assume that their actions did not result in severe injuries and may not bring the child for medical care. The severity of the peritonitis and the rapidity with which signs and symptoms develop depend on the location and severity of the initial injury, nature of bacterial contamination of the peritoneal cavity, and the child's preexisting health. In general, signs of peritonitis develop within hours of the injury, although death may be delayed by a few days in untreated cases.

The symptoms and presentation of the child generally reflect the type and severity of the injuries sustained, the time elapsed prior to seeking medical care, and the rate of bleeding. Patients often present with nonspecific abdominal complaints and without a history of trauma. Common, nonspecific presenting symptoms of children with inflicted abdominal trauma include vomiting, which may be bilious (if an obstruction exists), fever, and abdominal pain. Physical examination may reveal fever, abdominal tenderness, abdominal distention, diminished bowel sounds, and other signs indicative of obstruction or peritonitis. Classic peritoneal signs are not always present in infants and young children. In one series, absent bowel sounds and non-localized tenderness were the only consistent physical findings in children with intestinal perforations (Cobb et al., 1986).

Affected children are best managed by personnel trained in the management of pediatric trauma. The medical prognosis for children who sustain abusive visceral injury improves if the child survives acutely and is managed aggressively.

Evaluation of Inflicted Abdominal Trauma

The approach to the evaluation is dependent on the severity of injuries. Children with severe injuries presenting in shock or cardiac arrest require full resuscitation and management based on trauma protocols. The stabilization should include a trauma response team and pediatrics specialists in emergency medicine, surgery, and critical care. For children presenting in community hospitals, early transfer to tertiary care centers by transport teams trained in the management of pediatric emergencies and trauma is necessary. Once the child is stabilized, a careful and well-documented history is the most important part of the medical evaluation. This should be followed by a thorough physical examination with meticulous documentation, indicated laboratory studies, and psychosocial assessment. Children with less severe injuries are evaluated according to their symptoms and examination findings.

History

Historical clues to child abuse are the same for abdominal trauma as with other forms of physical abuse (see Chapter 2). The history provided by the caregiver of the child may be incomplete and misleading and may not include a history of trauma. The history may be even more obscure if the child is brought by a non-offending caregiver who has not witnessed the injury. If the history provided by the perpetrator includes trauma, the trauma is often reportedly trivial. Common chief complaints may be falls down the stairs, off the bed, or off the couch. It is important to remember that stairway falls in children rarely result in life-threatening injury or significant abdominal trauma (Joffe and Ludwig, 1988, Huntimer, Muret-Wagstaff, & Leland, 2000). If the child is critically ill and has a reported minor trauma, attention may be focused incorrectly solely on central nervous system injury. Co-existing head trauma can obfuscate a clinical examination of the abdomen and further delay the detection of visceral injuries.

With inflicted abdominal injuries, the history focuses on the following:

1. Details of any injury history given
2. Details of when the child was last well and when the child became symptomatic
3. Details of who was with the child at the time of injury or when symptoms initially began

Physical Examination

The initial evaluation of a patient with suspected child abuse should follow trauma assessment protocols. After ensuring that the patient is hemodynamically stable, the examiner completes a full physical examination to identify all injuries. There may be co-existing extra-abdominal injuries such as head injuries. A careful head to toe examination, concentrating on the skull, extremities, genitalia, and skin, is required. Of note, many children with serious abdominal trauma have no soft tissue injury to the abdomen (Cooper et al., 1988). The internal organs, rather than the skin, absorb the force of the impact (see Figure 5.1). Lack of abdominal bruising never eliminates intra-abdominal trauma from diagnostic consideration in an abused or otherwise injured child. During the initial evaluation and later management, attention is paid to assessment of vital signs and mental status, observation, auscultation, and palpation of the child's abdomen. Vital signs include body temperature, heart rate, respiratory rate, and blood pressure. These are important measures of hemodynamic stability and are serially monitored in all patients with suspected abdominal trauma. Serial measurements of the vital signs and hematocrit, especially in response to fluid resuscitation, may help to predict the type and severity of the injury (Cooper et al., 1988). Below are listed important clinical situations:

- Children with intestinal or pancreatic hematomas have mild blood loss into a confined space and present with mild anemia and stable vital signs.
- Children with intestinal perforations generally are not acutely anemic but may have tachycardia and fever as the result of peritonitis.
- Children with minor solid organ injuries tend to present with low hematocrit, tachycardia, and hypotension which generally respond clinically to volume resuscitation.
- Children with major solid organ injury or vascular trauma typically present with low hematocrit and profound shock and may not respond clinically to fluid resuscitation.
- Children may maintain relatively normal blood pressure despite significant blood loss until late in the clinical course, at which time the child's condition can deteriorate rapidly.

Findings of the abdominal examination may suggest the etiology of the injury. In the comatose patient, the clinical examination of the abdomen is more limited and interpretation more difficult. The following suggests a systematic approach to the assessment.

1. *Observation of the abdomen.* Look for signs of distention. Abdominal distention may be due to gastric air. Distention that persists after the placement of a nasogastric tube may indicate solid visceral injury or peritonitis.
2. *Auscultation (precedes palpation).* Note bowel sounds. Absent bowel sounds may indicate perforation and peritonitis. Peritonitis may be accompanied by fever, absent bowel sounds, bloody or bilious nasogastric aspirate, and marked abdominal tenderness with guarding.
3. *Palpation.* Carefully palpate for liver and spleen size and for masses. Note any voluntary or involuntary guarding or rebound tenderness.

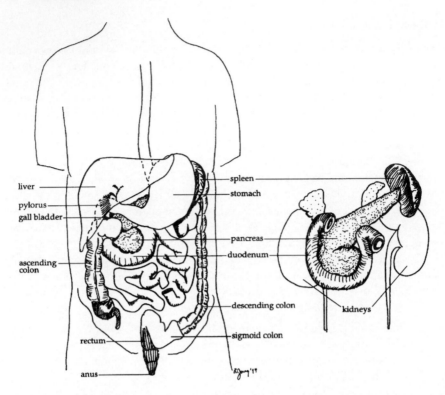

Figure 5.1 On *left*, schematic of the abdominal anatomy showing the location of the vital organs with transverse colon not drawn. On *right*, relative organ position with stomach and intestines not drawn.

Indicated Laboratory/Diagnostic Evaluation Laboratory

The laboratory evaluation is an important part of the workup of abdominal trauma and may prove helpful in evaluating children with possible inflicted abdominal trauma (see Table 5.1).

1. *Complete blood count (CBC with differential).* The CBC identifies anemia (suggests blood loss in a clinical setting of trauma) and infection (elevation of the white blood cell [WBC] count). Thrombocytopenia may indicate disseminated intravascular coagulopathy (DIC) or an underlying bleeding disorder.
2. *Prothrombin time (PT), and partial thromboplastin time (PTT).* Screen for coagulopathies or suspected DIC.
3. *Fluid and electrolyte assessment (chemistry panel).* Children with signs of intra-abdominal pathology frequently require fluid resuscitation and ongoing intravenous fluid management. A chemistry panel is often sent to the laboratory to assist in ongoing fluid management.

Table 5.1 At a glance—laboratory tests.

Laboratory study	Indications	Notes
CBC with differential, platelet count	Screen for anemia due to blood loss, nutritional deficiency Screen for infection Check platelet count	May need serial samples
Prothrombin time (PT), partial thromboplastin time (PTT) Chemistry panel (electrolytes, BUN, creatinine, glucose, etc.)	Screen for coagulopathies and DIC Screen for metabolic abnormalities Helps assess ongoing fluid management	
Serum aspartate aminotransferase (AST, SGOT) and alanine aminotransferase (ALT, SGPT)	Screen for liver injury	Not specific for trauma
Urinalysis (U/A)	Screen for renal, bladder, genital injury, myoglobinuria or hemoglobinuria, UTI	
Serum amylase and lipase	Screen for pancreatic injury	Not specific for trauma

4. *Liver Function Tests (LFTs) (hepatic transaminases).* Elevations of the serum aspartate aminotransferase (AST) > 450 IU/L and the serum alanine aminotransferase (ALT) > 250 IU/L are sensitive predictors of liver injury associated with blunt abdominal trauma (Hennes et al., 1990). Coant, Kornberg, Brody, & Edward-Holmes (1992) found that in abused children, milder elevations in these levels can identify patients with liver lacerations who are asymptomatic at presentation. Holmes et al. (2002) mentioned that AST greater than 200 units per liter (U/L) or ALT greater than 125 U/L and urinalysis with greater than 5 red blood cells (RBCs) per high power field and hematocrit less than 30% were helpful in detecting intra-abdominal injuries in children with blunt accidental trauma. Besides traumatic injuries, liver enzyme elevation may occur after a period of ischemia. This is a more diffuse injury that will not be visualized on radiographic studies (Garland, Werlin, & Rice, 1988).

It is important to measure hepatic transaminases in all children with suspected abdominal trauma and in young victims of physical abuse as a screen for occult hepatic injury. Serial measurements may be used to support the dating of an injury because enzyme levels return to normal rapidly after blunt trauma. Hepatic transaminases rise rapidly after uncomplicated blunt liver injury and then fall predictably. Persistently stable or increasing concentrations may indicate complications (Baxter, Lindberg, Burke, Shults, & Holmes, 2008). Elevations of hepatic transaminases are not specific for trauma and, depending on the clinical situation, may necessitate evaluation for other etiologies, including hepatitis.

5. *Amylase/lipase*. Elevations of the serum amylase and lipase are markers of pancreatic injury and are measured in all children with suspected abdominal trauma. However, the level of the enzyme increase does not appear to correlate with the extent of injury.
6. *Urinalysis (U/A)*. Renal injury is usually indicated by the presence of gross blood in the urine, a positive urine dipstick for blood, or a microscopic urinalysis with greater than 20 RBCs per high power field. Occasionally, the urine is positive for blood by dipstick, but microscopy reveals no RBCs. Myoglobinuria, or occasionally hemoglobinuria, may be the cause. In the acute situation, elevation of the serum creatine phosphokinase (CPK) supports the diagnosis of myoglobinuria. Elevated CPK in this setting indicates deep contusions and muscle injury.

Radiological Evaluation

Children with abdominal injuries who are hemodynamically stable are approached differently from those with life-threatening injuries. The following are commonly used methods for imaging the abdomen in children (see Table 5.2).

Table 5.2 At a glance—radiologic evaluation.

Study	Detects	Limitations
Plain abdominal radiographs	Intestinal obstruction, ascites, intra-abdominal foreign bodies, free air in abdomen, bone injuries surrounding abdomen	Difficult to detect solid organ injuries
Upper gastrointestinal (UGI) series, barium enema (BE)	Injuries to esophagus, stomach, duodenum, intestines, and colon	Requires contrast Patient must be stable
Ultrasonography (US)	Pancreatic, renal, liver, spleen, and pelvic injuries; free fluid within the abdominal cavity; intestinal hematomas; retroperitoneal injuries	Requires direct contact with abdominal wall
Abdominal CT scan	Solid organ injuries	Requires contrast
	May detect hollow visceral injury, occasionally detects rib fractures	Patient needs to be hemodynamically stable
Radionuclide scans	Anatomy and function of specific organs	Length of time
Intravenous pyelography (IVP)	Abnormalities of urinary system	Requires contrast
	Used as adjunct to other tests described	
Skeletal survey	New and healing fractures Other abnormalities of skeleton	Difficult to detect solid organ injuries

1. *Plain abdominal radiographs*. Plain films are used for initial evaluation in all stable children with suspected intra-abdominal injury. Films are taken with the patient in the frontal view with the patient supine and erect. A cross-table lateral or left lateral decubitus film is used instead of an erect film for infants or children who cannot assume an erect posture. Hollow visceral perforations are sometimes, but not always, associated with pneumoperitoneum (free air in the abdominal cavity). Perforations of the stomach are most commonly associated with free peritoneal air. If a significant amount of free intraperitoneal air is present, it may be visible on supine views as it outlines the falciform ligament of the liver or if the serosal aspect of the gut opposes it (Kleinman, 1998). Free intraperitoneal fluid appears as diffusely increased density or a central location of the bowel on supine abdominal views. Retroperitoneal perforations (such as to the duodenum) are very difficult to detect on plain radiograph. Plain films can be used to detect intestinal obstruction, ascitis, intra-abdominal foreign bodies, and occasional injuries to the bony structures surrounding the abdomen.

2. *Upper Gastrointestinal (UGI) Series*. The use of contrast is debatable. Oral contrast in the stomach or small intestine can better delineate the lesser sac of the peritoneum, pancreas, duodenum, or jejunum. However, oral contrast may place a patient at greater risk of aspiration especially if the patient is obtunded, sedated, or immobilized (Sane et al., 2000). Contrast examinations of the GI tract define the location and extent of intestinal tract injuries. UGI is frequently used to evaluate esophageal, gastric, duodenal, and jejunal injuries, especially a duodenal hematoma. Small bowel follow-through is used in conjunction with the UGI to evaluate the small intestine. Contrast enemas visualize colonic abnormalities. Contrast examinations can localize the site of intestinal perforation and can be used for evaluating ulcers and hematomas. Water-soluble contrast media are recommended for patients with possible intestinal perforation.

3. *Ultrasonography (US)*. Ultrasound of the abdomen is useful as a screening examination of the abdomen. US identifies free fluid within the abdominal cavity, assesses pancreatic injuries (rupture, pancreatitis, pseudocyst), and evaluates renal anatomy. It can identify solid organ and intestinal hematomas and evaluates the retroperitoneum and pelvis. Focused abdominal sonography (FAST) can rapidly diagnose intra-abdominal injury, especially in patients who are hemodynamically unstable. However, the bony thorax and the presence of air can limit the usefulness of this test. Therefore, ultrasonography has a complementary role of improving the selection of patients for further imaging without compromising diagnostic accuracy. CT is still the preferred imaging modality for seriously injured children and for victims of child abuse.

4. *CT scan*. Abdominal CT scan is the radiographic method of choice for evaluating abdominal trauma. The chest should be included if serious chest trauma is expected. Helical or dynamic axial scanning techniques with proper timing of intravenous contrast bolus are important for accurate diagnosis. The following list describes conditions and situations where abdominal CT scan is recommended:

1. Solid organ injuries (if hemodynamically stable)
2. Intra-abdominal bleeding (if hemodynamically stable)
3. Physical examination findings uninterpretable because of obtundation
4. Child undergoing head CT scan because of neurologic signs of trauma

CT scan with IV contrast with or without gastrointestinal contrast is the method of choice for detecting injuries to solid viscera such as the liver, spleen, or kidney and may detect hollow visceral injury. The reliability of CT scans to detect intestinal injury, such as perforation, intramural hematomas, and mesenteric injury is less clear. CT scan is contraindicated in children who have a history of anaphylaxis to contrast agents, severe shock, and renal failure (Sane et al., 2000). It is not recommended for patients who are hemodynamically unstable despite resuscitative efforts; these patients require emergency laparotomy in the operating room.

5. *Radionuclide scans (liver-spleen scan, radionuclide renal scan).* Radionuclide scans are inadequate for evaluating suspected visceral injury from child abuse. They have been used to evaluate specific organs for both anatomy and function.
6. *Skeletal survey.* Approximately two-thirds of children with inflicted abdominal injuries have other manifestations of abuse by physical examination or skeletal survey (Ledbetter et al., 1988). Therefore, it is extremely important to obtain a skeletal survey in children with inflicted abdominal trauma. Most victims of abusive abdominal injury are young, and approximately one-third of patients with inflicted abdominal trauma will specifically have skeletal injuries (Cooper et al., 1988; Ledbetter et al., 1988). The skeletal survey is best performed when the patient is stable, but it should be done prior to discharge from the hospital (see Chapter 2 and Chapter 4).

Specific Organ Injuries

Solid Organ Injuries Liver

The relative size and location of the liver predispose it to injury from blunt trauma. Liver injuries, such as lacerations and subcapsular hematomas, are among the most common abdominal injuries due to abuse. They are most often due to blows to the upper abdomen, although penetrating injuries can result in liver laceration. The severity of liver injuries varies from asymptomatic to life threatening. (See Table 5.3 for an overview of organ injuries.) Clinical manifestations and management depend on the size of the laceration and its location.

Elevations of hepatic enzymes (ALT, AST) have a reported sensitivity of 100% and a specificity of 92% for predicting hepatic injury in children (Hennes et al., 1990; Karaduman, Sarioglu-Buke, Kilic, & Gurses, 2003), and contribute significantly to the identification of children with intra-abdominal injuries after blunt trauma (Holmes et al., 2002). The high rate of occult liver injuries in children with suspected physical abuse has lead to the recommendation for broader screening of these children for abdominal injury (Jenny, 2006). It is measured in all patients with

Table 5.3 At a glance—organ injuries.

Solid organ injuries		
Liver	Commonly injured in abuse-related abdominal trauma	Lacerations Subcapsular hematomas
Spleen	Infrequently reported as abuse-related Protection from underlying ribs	
Pancreas	Commonly injured in abuse-related trauma	Crush injury Pancreatitis
Renal system	Infrequently reported as abuse-related Protection from surrounding tissues	
Hollow visceral injuries		
Oropharynx/ Esophagus		Aspiration, traumatic perforations, burns resulting from caustic ingestion
Stomach	Infrequently reported as abuse related	
Duodenum	Commonly injured in abuse-related abdominal trauma Vulnerable because of fixed position near vertebral column	Hematomas Perforations
Jejunum/Ileum	Infrequently reported as abuse related	
Colon	Infrequently reported as abuse related	Penetrating rectal trauma of special concern, i.e., rule out sexual abuse

suspected abdominal trauma and in infants and young children with other signs of physical abuse. CT scan is the method of choice for imaging the liver in cases of abdominal trauma and is done unless the child requires immediate surgical intervention. Small lacerations and many subcapsular hematomas are treated nonoperatively, although more extensive injuries require surgical repair.

Liver laceration is a reported complication of CPR in adults, usually in association with rib fractures. Liver lacerations also have been reported in association with CPR in young children (Krischer, Fine, Davis, & Nagel, 1987). The first reports date back to the early 1960s prior to widespread acknowledgment of physical abuse. Abuse may not have been recognized in these early case reports. Although children who died with liver lacerations were not identified as abused, the cause of death remained undetermined. In one case, the child had previously suffered "traumatic brain injury" (Thaler & Krause, 1962). Liver lacerations resulting from CPR are extremely rare in children and should not be assumed to be the result of CPR, especially if the child dies and cause of death is undetermined.

Spleen

Splenic injury is often caused by accidental trauma but is infrequently reported as the result of abuse (Caniano, Beaver, & Boles, 1986; Ledbetter et al., 1988). This may relate to its position underlying the ribs (Cooper, 1992). Splenic injury should be suspected in any child with left-sided chest wall pain. Contusions of the spleen and subcapsular hematomas are more common than splenic lacerations in nonaccidental trauma. A splenic rupture in a preambulatory child is strongly suggestive of abuse. Like liver injuries, the severity of splenic injuries ranges from minor to life threatening. Evaluation for splenic injuries is done by CT scan or liver and spleen scan. Management is dependent on the extent of the injury, and surgical repair may be required. Attempts at salvaging the spleen are a mainstay in the therapeutic approach to this form of injury.

Pancreas

Pancreatic injury resulting from blunt trauma to the upper abdomen occurs with some frequency. The body of the pancreas overlies the spine and can be crushed with significant blows to the epigastrium. Injury to the pancreas typically results in pancreatitis because of the release and activation of pancreatic enzymes. Causes of pancreatitis in childhood include biliary tract disease, congenital anomalies, cystic fibrosis, infection, and medications (Ziegler, Long, Philippart, & Klein, 1988). Trauma is a leading cause of pancreatitis in children (Cooney & Grosfeld, 1975). Abuse is a leading cause of traumatic pancreatitis in children less than 4 years of age and is often associated with other manifestations of abuse (Ziegler et al., 1988). Other trauma-related causes include those caused by bicycle handle bars, motor vehicle crashes and falls. Pancreatic pseudocysts, which may develop after abuse (Pena & Medovy, 1973), form as resultant fluid collections and become confined, beginning within a few days of the injury.

The development of pancreatitis after trauma may be insidious so that not all children present with it in the acute period. Most children with pancreatitis eventually develop abdominal pain, vomiting, fever, abdominal distention, or other nonspecific symptoms. Elevation of the serum amylase and/or lipase level in children with abdominal symptoms indicates pancreatic involvement. CT scan and ultrasound are most useful in identifying pancreatic injuries.

The management of pancreatitis is usually conservative and consists of bowel and bed rest, nasogastric decompression, and pain and nutritional therapy. Surgery is reserved for children with severe pancreatic injury and those who require drainage of pseudocysts.

Kidney, Bladder, Urinary Tract

Abuse may result in injuries to the kidneys, ureters, and bladder. Severe blows to the flank most commonly cause renal contusions or lacerations. Because the kidneys are well protected by their location and surrounding anatomy, trauma severe enough to cause renal injury is often associated with injuries to other abdominal organs. Although children may present with flank pain and tenderness, these symptoms are not universally present. Hematuria (gross hematuria or greater than 20 RBCs per high power field) generally indicates renal involvement in children with abdominal trauma. The severity of the renal injury is not reflected by the degree of hematuria, so that all children with hematuria require renal imaging by CT scan or other methods. Both myoglobinuria (secondary to rhabdomyolysis and muscle injury) and hemoglobinuria may result from abuse and can be mistaken for hematuria (Mukerji & Siegel, 1987; Rimer & Roy, 1977). Unlike hematuria, neither will show microscopic evidence of urinary RBCs. Myoglobinuria and hemoglobinuria may result in renal failure. Most renal injuries are managed conservatively and do not require surgery. Myoglobinuria and hemoglobinuria require aggressive medical treatment and careful hydration.

Bladder injuries from abuse are unusual but have been reported (Halsted & Shapiro, 1979). Traumatic rupture of superior surface of the bladder can occur as a consequence of inflicted blows to the abdomen and present with pseudorenal failure (Yang, Kuppermann, & Rosas, 2002). With rupture of the bladder, urine and blood extravasate into the peritoneal cavity. Peritoneal resorption of urine produces electrolyte imbalance, acidosis, and uremia. Victims who present early do not have significantly increased BUN or creatinine concentrations. However a delay in presentation and diagnosis of bladder rupture results in significant resorption of urea and creatinine through peritoneal dialysis. The recognition of a possible relationship between an elevated BUN and intraperitoneal rupture of the bladder may be the only indication of this diagnosis in clinically unsuspected cases. The diagnostic test of choice is a retrograde cystogram radiograph. The outcome of surgical treatment of traumatic bladder rupture is generally good, but delayed diagnosis may lead to abscess and urinary fistula formation.

Stomach and Bowel Perforation Injuries

Injuries to the hollow viscera of the abdominal cavity may occur from abuse and are often difficult to diagnose. Hollow viscera are more commonly injured in abused children as compared to children who sustain accidental abdominal trauma (Ledbetter et al., 1988), (Trokel et al., 2006). Hollow visceral injury is generally due to either direct blows to the abdomen or shearing forces associated with rapid deceleration. Bowel perforations may occur anywhere along the course of the intestine, but most tend to be located in the duodenum (Tracy et al., 1993, Nijs, Vanclooster, de Gheldere, & Garmijn, 1997) because of its fixed position in the retroperitoneum and at the duodeno-jejunal junction. Children (particularly infants and toddlers) with perforations or hematomas to the intestinal tract, without a history of significant accidental trauma, require a full evaluation for child abuse. Findings on CT suggestive of small bowel or mesenteric injury include free intraperitoneal fluid, thickened bowel wall, and extraluminal air (Frick, Pasquale, & Cipolle, 1999).

Oropharynx/Esophagus

Injuries to the pharynx and esophagus due to child abuse are reported occasionally. Reported injuries include foreign body aspirations (Nolte, 1993), traumatic perforations, and burns resulting from caustic ingestion (Friedman, 1987; McDowell & Fielding, 1984). Children with esophageal foreign bodies typically present with respiratory symptoms either from direct compression of the membranous tracheal wall by the object or infection that develops in surrounding tissues. Patients with significant injury to the posterior oropharynx, hypopharynx, esophagus, or trachea often present with fever, subcutaneous emphysema, erythematous swelling of the neck, hemoptysis, hematemesis, or pneumomediastinum. Caustic ingestions manifest by drooling, respiratory distress, oral burns, and/or stridor.

Stomach

Gastric perforation is reported in the child abuse literature, although it is not a frequent injury (McCort & Vaudagna, 1964; Schechner & Ehrlich, 1974). Gastric perforation is more common if the child has a full stomach at the time of the trauma. Children with gastric perforation have rapid manifestations of the injury because of pain associated with gastric spasms and the noxious effects of gastric acid in the peritoneum. Gastric perforation is usually indicated by a distended, tense abdomen, and pneumoperitoneum on plain radiograph. Gastric perforations require timely operative repair. Gastric perforation is reported as a complication of CPR, albeit rare (Krischer et al., 1987). Gastric distention can accompany duodenal hematomas secondary to the obstructive effect of the hematoma.

Duodenum

Duodenal hematomas and perforations are among the more frequent abdominal injuries that result from abuse (Ledbetter et al., 1988; McCort & Vaudagna, 1964; Woolley, Mahour, & Sloan, 1978; Gaines, Schultz, Morrison, & Ford, 2004). The duodenum is at risk for injury due to its relatively fixed position in the upper mid-abdomen, its proximity to the vertebral column, and its rich blood supply from the pancreaticoduodenal arteries. A crushing injury that forces the duodenum against the vertebral column typically results in rupture of the duodenal blood vessels. This results in a hematoma that develops between the mucosa and serosa. As the hematoma expands, the duodenal lumen narrows, leading to partial (or occasionally complete) obstruction. Duodenal hematoma can result from both accidental and inflicted trauma. Children with duodenal hematoma often have some delay in presentation because the signs of obstruction develop with time. Children typically present with vomiting and abdominal pain and have abdominal tenderness on examination. Associated injuries to the pancreas may be found.

Plain films may be normal but may show gastric dilatation and decreased bowel gas. The diagnosis of a duodenal hematoma can be made by UGI, CT, and ultrasound. Affected children may have significant anemia (Woolley et al., 1978).

Children who present with unexplained duodenal hematoma should be screened for coagulopathies, and young victims should have a skeletal survey.

Injuries to the duodenum result in prolonged hospitalization. Treatment of duodenal hematoma is conservative, with bowel rest and nasogastric suctioning. Surgery to evacuate the hematoma is occasionally required. Transections, avulsions, and lacerations of the duodenum may also result from abuse (Tracy et al., 1993; Woolley et al., 1978). Children with perforations of the duodenum present with vomiting, abdominal pain, and signs of sepsis. Classic signs of peritonitis may be absent because of the duodenum's location in the retroperitoneum. Plain films are often normal if the perforation is in the retroperitoneum. Radiographic diagnosis is best made by UGI with water-soluble contrast media. Treatment requires surgical repair.

Jejunum/Ileum

Perforations and hematomas of the small intestine may occur in abused children with abdominal trauma. They are infrequent in accidentally injured children (Ledbetter et al., 1988). A majority of intestinal perforations are located in the jejunum, near the ligament of Treitz, and is the result of either direct compression associated with blows to the abdomen or shearing forces. A delay in presentation is common. Peritoneal signs typically develop within 6–12 h after perforation, but children are sometimes brought for medical treatment only after days have passed. Children may present with signs of peritonitis and sepsis, although classic peritoneal findings may not be present (Cobb, Vinocur, Wagner, & Weintraub, 1986). Plain radiographs may reveal free air. UGI may locate the perforation, although in many patients the need for laparotomy precludes the usefulness of extensive radiographic evaluation. Surgical resection or repair constitutes definitive treatment.

Colon

Abused children sustain injuries to the colon infrequently. There are occasional reports of colonic injury from blunt abdominal trauma (Caniano et al., 1986). Injuries to the colon are also associated with penetrating rectal trauma that may be the result of physical or sexual abuse (Press, Grant, Thompson, & Milles, 1991). Signs related to peritonitis are often present. Rectal blood is usually present in children who present with injuries to the colon and/or rectum. Colonic perforations require surgical repair.

Retroperitoneal Vascular Injuries

Severe deceleration injuries that result in shearing of the mesentery and retroperitoneal vascular supply to the abdomen are occasionally encountered (Cooper et al., 1988; Dworkind, McGowan, & Hyams, 1990). Shearing injuries result in retroperitoneal hemorrhage, which can be life threatening. Injuries to larger retroperitoneal vessels may result in hemorrhagic shock; emergency laparotomy is required to save the child's life. CT scan sometimes identifies smaller retroperitoneal hematomas. Children with less severe injuries may be managed conservatively, without operative repair.

Differential Diagnosis

In additional to common conditions such as infective gastrointestinal and respiratory conditions, the following conditions are important to consider in the differential diagnosis of inflicted visceral trauma.

(1) Seat Belt syndrome. Child passengers between 4 and 8 years of age may be inappropriately restrained in lap belts, alone or in combination with shoulder restraints, instead of belt positioning booster seats. In these children there is a tendency for the lap belt to ride over the abdomen rather than over the hips. The sudden deceleration forces generated in automobile crashes can cause significant blunt force injuries to the abdomen and spine. The findings in the seat belt syndrome include abdominal wall ecchymosis, small bowel injury, and lumbar spine injury or Chance fractures.
(2) Bicycle Handle Bar Injuries. A child who is accidently struck in the abdomen by a bicycle handle bar can present with injuries to the bowel, pancreas, or liver.
(3) Falls. Though falls can result in intra-abdominal injuries, it is important to obtain a history of blunt or penetrating force trauma in a child who presents with injuries sustained after a fall. Stairway falls in children rarely result in life-threatening injury or significant abdominal trauma (Joffe and Ludwig, 1988, Huntimer et al., 2000).

Most children who sustain significant inflicted abdominal trauma are young, generally between 6 months and 3 years of age (Cobb, Vinocur, Wagner, & Weintraub, 1986; Cooper et al., 1988), and tend to be younger than those with accidental abdominal trauma (Ledbetter, Hatch, Feldman, Ligner, & Tapper, 1988). When compared to children who die of inflicted head trauma, those with fatal abdominal injuries tend to be slightly older (Cooper et al., 1988). Ledbetter et al. (1988) compared accidental and abusive injuries in 156 cases of abdominal trauma. Eleven percent were due to abuse. The abused group tended to be younger (mean age, $2\frac{1}{2}$ years), have a history inconsistent with their physical findings, and have a higher incidence of hollow viscus injuries. Wood, Rubin, Nance, and Christian (2005) described that young abused children were more likely to have hollow viscus injuries alone or in combination with solid organ injuries and a delay in seeking care than young children with accidental abdominal trauma. However the delay in seeking care was not specific for inflicted injury and occurred in some children with low-velocity accidental abdominal trauma. Trokel et al. (2006) evaluated the associations between patient and injury characteristics and the medical diagnosis of suspected child abuse. They concluded that young children with severe pancreatic or hollow viscus injuries or severe abdominal injuries in the context of either brain injury or undernourishment should be evaluated for the possibility that these injuries resulted from abuse. Small bowel injuries due to abuse are 2.3 times more likely than those due to motor vehicle crashes and 5.7 times more likely than those due to falls. Therefore, injuries to the small bowel in young children need special consideration, particularly if a minor fall is the explanation (Barnes et al., 2005).

(4) Other conditions. Acute appendicitis with bowel perforation and hematuria in patients with glomerulonephritis or resulting from minor trauma in patients with hydronephrosis and Wilm's tumor can also mimic child abuse.

Thoracic Injuries

While not as common as inflicted head injuries, thoracic injuries are an important source of morbidity and mortality in children. They are an independent predictor of mortality in pediatric trauma patients (Peclet et al., 1990). Roaten et al. (2006) reported that thoracic injuries including pulmonary contusions, rib and clavicle fractures were three times more common in child abuse victims (17%) than those with accidental trauma (6%) in a regional pediatric trauma center. DiScala et al. (2000) compared hospitalized children under age five years who were victims of child abuse with victims of unintentional injuries using data from the National Pediatric Trauma Registry between 1988 and 1997. Thoracic injuries were more common following child abuse (12.5%) than after accidental trauma (4.5%).

Children have important anatomic and physiologic differences when compared to adults. Unlike adults, children undergo constant growth and change. The greater flexibility of the thoracic cage in young children permits the anterior ribs to be compressed to meet the posterior ribs. As a result, pulmonary contusions are more common, whereas rib fractures occur less frequently in children than adults (Nakayama, Ramenofsky, & Rowe, 1989). As the bony rib cage ossifies, fractures and flail segments begin to occur. Similarly, bony thoracic spine injuries are uncommon in infancy through preadolescence. Because the bones are incompletely ossified, the ligamentous attachments are more flexible, and the supportive musculature is not fully developed, younger patients are more likely to experience injuries without plain film abnormalities.

The internal thoracic organs in children are not only smaller than in adults but exhibit different physiologic characteristics. Early in life, the trachea is narrow, short, more compressible, and narrowest at the level of the cricoid cartilage. Therefore, small changes in airway diameter or seemingly inconsequential wounds in the thoracic cage may lead to rapid respiratory embarrassment. In addition, children have a diminished functional residual capacity coupled with higher oxygen consumption per unit body mass and are therefore more prone to the rapid evolution of hypoxemia.

Direct lung injury usually manifests as non-anatomic areas of consolidation often in the absence of rib fractures, chest wall bruising, or other external anatomic correlates of lung trauma. At a parenchymal level, findings include alveolar hemorrhage, consolidation, and edema. The physiologic consequences include ventilation/perfusion mismatch, decreased compliance, hypoxemia, and hypoventilation.

Cardiac function in children is able to compensate for a remarkable degree of hypovolemia. Cardiac output is largely determined by heart rate and preload, whereas contractility is largely fixed. Whereas adults may manifest hypotension after a 15–20% blood volume loss, children may remain compensated with up to a 40% blood loss. Myocardial dysfunction, although rare, may follow cardiac contusion. In this setting, posttraumatic dysrhythmias may also precipitate rapid physiologic deterioration. Furthermore, the less prominent fixation of the mediastinum in children allows for more visceral shift, compromise of preload and profound hypotension (Bliss & Silen, 2002).

Pulmonary Injuries

These injuries include pulmonary contusions, hemothorax, pneumomediastinum, and pneumothorax. Contusions and lacerations of the lower lungs are occasionally identified by abdominal CT (Sivit, Taylor, & Eichelberger, 1989). Although rib fractures in abused infants are common (see Chapter 4), symptomatic pulmonary injury is unusual. In isolation, rib fractures are a rare source of morbidity or mortality but indicate significant energy transfer. In the age group 0–3 years, child abuse is a paramount concern after ruling out conditions of bony fragility such as osteogenesis imperfecta and rickets. As with significant abdominal trauma, external signs of trauma such as bruising over the chest wall may be absent despite serious intrathoracic injury. Chest radiographs followed by CT scan of the chest with intravenous contrast are performed if the patient is stable and internal chest injury is suspected.

Pulmonary contusions are among the most common thoracic injuries in traumatized children. Patients with significant pulmonary contusions present with tachypnea and hypoxia. The initial chest radiograph can detect pulmonary contusions in most patients. They resemble infiltrates on radiographs shortly after injury. However, radiographic findings in pulmonary contusions are observed much earlier than those caused by aspiration which is typically delayed. Management of most pulmonary injuries is supportive, and operative repair is not usually required for blunt force injuries. Pneumothoraces can be present in older children with rib fractures, but infants may present with them without rib fractures due to a compliant chest wall. Prompt drainage of intra-thoracic collections of air or fluid that may limit pulmonary expansion facilitates a rapid return to normal physiology.

Non-cardiogenic pulmonary edema can occur after intentional suffocation or inflicted head injury. This usually has a rapid onset. At presentation, these children have diffuse inspiratory rales, pink frothy pulmonary secretions, and chest radiographs with infiltrates. The appearance of these secretions, coupled with the rapid clinical and radiographic improvement in the course of illness, help exclude the diagnosis of infiltrates because of aspiration, infection, or ingestion of toxic drugs or chemicals. Victims of intentional suffocation have characteristic family and medical histories that should alert the physician to consider the diagnosis during evaluation of unexplained acute life-threatening events in infants especially those with a recent history of wellness (Rubin, McMillan, Helfaer, & Christian, 2001).

Occasionally, chylothorax from injury to the thoracic duct may be attributed to child abuse (Anderst, 2007, Guleserian, Gilchrist, Luks, Wesselhoeft, & DeLuca, 1996, Geismar, Tilelli, Campbell, & Chiaro, 1997). The anatomy of the thoracic duct predisposes it to traumatic rupture with compressive and/or acceleration–deceleration forces. It enters the posterior mediastinum from the abdominal cavity by passing through the aortic hiatus of the diaphragm on the anterior surface of the vertebral column. Continuing extrapleurally in the posterior mediastinum up the right side of the vertebrae, the duct then crosses to the left side of the vertebral column, typically between the fourth and sixth vertebrae, before traveling cephalad and exiting the thoracic inlet. Disruption of the duct in the thorax leads to an accumulation of extrapleural chyle, which may eventually rupture the mediastinal pleura and form a chylothorax. Abusive chylothorax occurs when the thoracic duct is subjected to shearing forces against compressed ribs and/or vertebrae in association with spinal hyperextension during shaking.

Though blunt trauma to the chest is more common, penetrating injuries to the chest occasionally occur from child abuse. These injuries are best managed by pediatric surgeons trained in trauma.

Cardiac Injuries

Direct cardiac injuries are rarely seen following child abuse. Cardiac injuries as the result of abuse have been reported (Cumberland, Riddick, & McConnell, 1991; Marino & Langston, 1982; Rees, Symons, Joseph, & Lincoln, 1975). Rees et al. (1975) reported a traumatic ventriculoseptal defect (VSD) that resulted from a kick to the chest of a 5-year-old girl and Karpas, Yen, Sell, and Frommelt (2002) reported a 5-month-old infant who sustained a traumatic VSD and left ventricular aneurysm after inflicted blunt trauma to the chest. She presented in cardiac failure and was treated medically with eventual surgical repair. This injury was felt to have occurred from the heart being distorted and crushed against the vertebrae. Cumberland et al. (1991) report intimal tears of the right atrium found at autopsy of six children, three of whom were teenagers who died in motor vehicle accidents (MVAs) and three of whom were young victims of abuse. All six children had associated liver lacerations and other signs of abdominal trauma. The authors postulate that the cardiac injuries were the result of transmitted hydrostatic forces from the abdomen, through the inferior vena cava, and to the fixed right atrium.

Commotio cordis is a condition where a disorganized cardiac rhythm and collapse rapidly ensue following blunt trauma to the chest. Denton and Kalelkar (2000) described two children aged 14 months and 3 years who collapsed immediately after being struck on the chest by a closed fist and died. No external chest trauma was visible in one child. Commotio cordis was also reported by Boglioli, Taff, and Harleman (1998) in a 28-month-old boy and by Baker, Craig, and Lonergan (2003) in a 7-week-old infant due to child abuse.

Blunt cardiac injuries can result in electrical conduction abnormalities. Children with suspected cardiac injuries require continuous ECG monitoring, chest radiography, electrocardiogram (ECG), echocardiography, and serial cardiac enzymes. Elevated cardiac enzymes (troponin I and CPK MB fractions) are helpful to diagnose cardiac muscle damage. Close monitoring and serial physical examinations are essential to identify the development of life-threatening complications of blunt cardiac injuries which include dysrhythmias, traumatic VSD, and ventricular wall aneurysms (Karpas et al., 2002). In general, significant myocardial contusion can be ruled out when 12-lead ECG and echocardiography findings are normal (Wesson, 1998).

In Brief

- Visceral injuries are rare in children, but when they occur they are more likely to be nonaccidental in etiology.
- Most victims of serious inflicted visceral injury are infants and toddlers.
- The vast majority of injuries are due to blunt trauma, not penetrating injury.
- Nonaccidental trauma should be suspected in children with visceral injuries, with an unclear history, or accompanying head trauma or malnourishment.
- The mechanism of injury is related to *crushing* of solid organs, *compression* of hollow viscera against the vertebrae or bony thorax, or *shearing* forces that result from sudden deceleration.
- Morbidity and mortality associated with abusive abdominal injury are related to delays in diagnosis and treatment which stem from delayed presentation of the victim.
- Rib fractures commonly result from inflicted thoracic trauma. Inflicted cardiac and pulmonary injuries are less common.
- Infant and child victims of physical abuse should be screened for abdominal injuries by history, physical examination, and appropriate screening tests, including AST, ALT, and amylase.
- Solid organ injuries are the most common visceral injuries resulting from abuse, but are also seen with accidental trauma. Hollow visceral injury is more common with inflicted trauma than with accidental injury.
- Vital signs, serial hematocrit, and the response to fluids generally indicate the severity and probable type of abdominal injury present.
- CT scan is the imaging modality of choice to detect visceral injury, although plain abdominal radiography, ultrasound, GI contrast studies, and radionuclide studies all contribute to the noninvasive evaluation of visceral trauma.
- Most solid organ injuries are treated conservatively without the need for surgery. Laparotomy is required for repair of intestinal perforation, significant mesenteric and vascular injuries.
- Children who survive the acute assault generally have good medical outcome.

References

Anderst, J. D. (2007). Chylothorax and child abuse. *Pediatric Critical Care Medicine, 8,* 394–396.

Baker, A. M., Craig, B. R., & Lonergan, G. J. (2003). Homicidal commotio cordis: The final blow in a battered infant. *Child Abuse and Neglect, 27,* 125–130.

Barnes, P. M., Norton, C. M., Dunstan, F. D., Kemp, A. M., Yates, D. W., & Sibert, J. R. (2005). Abdominal injury due to child abuse. *Lancet, 366,* 234–235.

Baxter, A. L., Lindberg, D. M., Burke, B. L., Shults, J., & Holmes, J. F. (2008). Hepatic enzyme decline after pediatric blunt trauma: A tool for timing child abuse?. *Child Abuse and Neglect, 32,* 838–845.

Bliss, D., & Silen, M. (2002). Pediatric thoracic trauma. *Critical Care Medicine, 30*(Supplement), S409–S415.

Boglioli, L. R., Taff, M. L., & Harleman, G. (1998). Child homicide caused by commotio cordis. *Pediatric Cardiology, 19,* 436–438.

Caniano, D. A., Beaver, B. L., & Boles, E. T. (1986). Child abuse: An update on surgical management in 256 cases. *Annals of Surgery, 203,* 219–224.

Canty, T. G., Sr., Canty, T. G., Jr., & Brown, C. (1999). Injuries of the gastrointestinal tract from blunt trauma in children: A 12-year experience at a designated pediatric trauma center. *Journal of Trauma, 46,* 234–240.

Coant, P. N., Kornberg, A. E., Brody, A. S., & Edward-Holmes, K. (1992). Markers for occult liver injury in cases of physical abuse in children. *Pediatrics, 89,* 274–278.

Cobb, L. M., Vinocur, C. D., Wagner, C. W., & Weintraub, W. H. (1986). Intestinal perforation due to blunt trauma in children in an era of increased nonoperative treatment. *Journal of Trauma, 26,* 461–463.

Cooney, D. R., & Grosfeld, J. L. (1975). Operative management of pancreatic pseudocysts in infants and children: A review of 75 cases. *Annals of Surgery, 182,* 590–596.

Cooper, A. (1992). Thoracoabdominal trauma. In S. Ludwig & A. E. Kornberg (Eds.), *Child abuse: A medical reference* (2nd ed., pp. 131–150). New York: Churchill Livingstone.

Cooper, A., Floyd, T., Barlow, B., Niemirska, M., Ludwig, S., Seidl, T., et al. (1988). Major blunt trauma due to child abuse. *Journal of Trauma, 28,* 1483–1487.

Cumberland, G. D., Riddick, L., & McConnell, C. F. (1991). Intimal tears of the right atrium of the heart due to blunt force injuries to the abdomen. *American Journal of Forensic Medicine and Pathology, 12,* 102–104.

Denton, J. S., & Kalelkar, M. B. (2000). Homicidal commotio cordis in two children. *Journal of Forensic Science, 45,* 734–735.

DiScala, C., Sege, R., Li, G., & Reece, R. M. (2000). Child abuse and unintentional injuries- a 10 year retrospective. *Archives of Pediatrics and Adolescent Medicine, 154,* 16–22.

Dworkind, M., McGowan, G., & Hyams, J. (1990). Abdominal trauma—Child abuse. *Pediatrics, 85,* 892.

Friedman, E. M. (1987). Caustic ingestions and foreign body aspirations: An overlooked form of child abuse. *Annals of Otology, Rhinology and Laryngology, 96,* 709–712.

Frick, E. J., Jr., Pasquale, M. D., & Cipolle, M. D. (1999, May). Small-bowel and mesentery injuries in blunt trauma. *Journal of Trauma, 46* (5), 920–926.

Gaines, B. A., Shultz, B. S., Morrison, K., & Ford, H. R. (2004). Duodenal injuries in children: Beware of child abuse. *Journal of Pediatric Surgery, 39,* 600–602.

Garland, J. S., Werlin, S. L., & Rice, T. B. (1988). Ischemic hepatitis in children: diagnosis and clinical course. *Critical Care Medicine, 16*, 1209–1212.

Geismar, S. L., Tilelli, J. A., Campbell, J. B., & Chiaro, J. J. (1997). Chylothorax as a manifestation of child abuse. *Pediatric Emergency Care, 13*, 386–389.

Guleserian, K. J., Gilchrist, B. F., Luks, F. I., Wesselhoeft, C. W., & DeLuca, F. G. (1996). Child abuse as a cause of traumatic chylothorax. *Journal of Pediatric Surgery, 31*, 1696–1697.

Halsted, C. C., & Shapiro, S. R. (1979). Child abuse: Acute renal failure from ruptured bladder. *American Journal of Diseases of Children, 133*, 861–862.

Hennes, H. M., Smith, D. S., Schneider, K., Hegenbarth, M. A., Duma, M. A., & Jona, J. Z. (1990). Elevated liver transaminase levels in children with blunt abdominal trauma: A predictor of liver injury. *Pediatrics, 86*, 87–90.

Holmes, J. F., Sokolove, P. E., Brant, W. E., Palchak, M. J., Vance, C. W., Owings, J. T., et al. (2002). Identification of children with intra-abdominal injuries after blunt trauma. *Annals of Emergency Medicine, 39*, 500–550.

Huntimer, C. M., Muret-Wagstaff, S., & Leland, N. L. (2000). Can falls on stairs result in small intestine perforations?. *Pediatrics, 106*, 301–305.

Jenny, C. (2006). Evaluating infants and young children with multiple fractures. *Pediatrics, 118*(3), 1299–1303.

Joffe, M., & Ludwig, S. (1988). Stairway injuries in children. *Pediatrics, 82*, 457–461.

Karpas, A., Yen, K., Sell, L. L., & Frommelt, P. C. (2002). Severe blunt cardiac injury in an infant: a case of child abuse. *Journal of Trauma, 52*, 759–764.

Karaduman, D., Sarioglu-Buke, A., Kilic, I., & Gurses, E. (2003). The role of elevated liver transaminase levels in children with blunt abdominal trauma. *Injury, 34*, 249–252.

Kleinman, P. K. (1987). Visceral trauma. In P. K. Kleinman (Ed.), *Diagnostic imaging of child abuse* (pp. 115–158). Baltimore: Williams and Wilkins.

Kleinman, P. K. (1998). Visceral trauma. In Kleinman, P. K. ed., *Diagnostic imaging of child abuse* (2nd ed., 248–284). St. Louis, MO: Mosby.

Krischer, J. P., Fine, E. G., Davis, J. H., & Nagel, E. L. (1987). Complications of cardiac resuscitation. *Chest, 92*, 287–291.

Ledbetter, D. J., Hatch, E. I., Jr., Feldman, K. W., Ligner, C. L., & Tapper, D. (1988). Diagnostic and surgical implications of child abuse. *Archives of Surgery, 123*, 1101–1105.

Marino, T. A., & Langston, C. (1982). Cardiac trauma and the conduction system. *Archives of Pathology and Laboratory Medicine, 106*, 173–174.

McCort, J., & Vaudagna, J. (1964). Visceral injuries in battered children. *Radiology, 82*, 424–428.

McDowell, H. P., & Fielding, D. W. (1984). Traumatic perforation of the hypopharynx: An unusual form of abuse. *Archives of Disease in Childhood, 59*, 888–889.

Mukerji, S. K., & Siegel, M. J. (1987). Rhabdomyolysis and renal failure in child abuse. *American Journal of Roentgenology, 148*, 1203–1204.

Nakayama, D. K., Ramenofsky, M. L., & Rowe, M. I. (1989). Chest injuries in children. *Annals of Surgery, 210*, 770–775.

Nijs, S., Vanclooster, P., de Gheldere, C., & Garmijn, K. (1997). Duodenal transection in a battered child: a case report. *Acta Chirurgica Belgica, 97*, 192–193.

Nolte, K. B. (1993). Esophageal foreign bodies as child abuse. Potential fatal mechanisms. *American Journal of Forensic Medicine and Pathology, 14*, 323–326.

Peclet, M. H., Newman, K. D., Eichelberger, M. R., Gotschall, C. S., Garcia, V. F., & Bowman, L.M. (1990). Thoracic trauma in children: an indicator of increased mortality. *Journal of Pediatric Surgery, 25*, 961–965.

Pena, S. D. J., & Medovy, H. (1973). Child abuse and traumatic pseudocyst of the pancreas. *Journal of Pediatrics, 83*, 1026–1028.

Press, S., Grant, P., Thompson, V. T., & Milles, K. L. (1991). Small bowel evisceration: Unusual manifestation of child abuse. *Pediatrics, 88*, 807–809.

Rees, A., Symons, J., Joseph, M., & Lincoln, C. (1975). Ventricular septal defect in a battered child. *British Medical Journal, 1*, 20–21.

Rimer, R. L., & Roy, S. (1977). Child abuse and hemoglobinuria. *JAMA, 238*, 2034–2035.

Roaten, J. B., Partrick, D. A., Nydam, T. L., Bensard, D. D., Hendrickson, R. J., Sirotnak, A. P., et al. (2006). Nonaccidental trauma is a major cause of morbidity and mortality among patients at a regional level 1 pediatric trauma center. *Journal of Pediatric Surgery, 41*, 2103–2015.

Rubin, D. M., McMillan, C. O., Helfaer, M. A., & Christian, C. W. (2001). Pulmonary edema associated with child abuse: Case reports and review of the literature. *Pediatrics, 108*, 769–775.

Sane, S. M., Kleinman, P. K., Cohen, R. A., Di Pietro, M. A., Seibert, J. J., Wood, B. P., et al. (2000). American Academy of Pediatrics. Diagnostic imaging of child abuse. Section on Radiology. *Pediatrics, 105*, 1345–1348.

Schechner, S. A., & Ehrlich, F. E. (1974). Gastric perforation and child abuse. *Journal of Trauma, 14*, 723–725.

Sivit, C. J., Taylor, G. A., & Eichelberger, M. R. (1989). Visceral injury in battered children: A changing perspective. *Radiology, 173*, 659–661.

Thaler, M. M., & Krause, V. W. (1962). Serious trauma in children after external cardiac massage. *The New England Journal of Medicine, 267*, 500–501.

Tracy, T., O'Connor, T. P., & Weber, T. R. (1993). Battered children with duodenal avulsion and transection. *American Journal of Surgery, 59*, 342–345.

Trokel, M., DiScala, C., Terrin, N. C., & Sege, R. D. (2004). Blunt abdominal injury in the young pediatric patient: child abuse and patient outcomes. *Child Maltreatment, 9*, 111–117.

Trokel, M., DiScala, C., Terrin, N. C., & Sege, R. D. (2006). patient and Injury Characteristics in Abusive abdominal injuries. *Pediatric Emergency Care, 22*, 700–704.

Wesson, D. E. (1998). Thoracic injuries. In O'Neill J. A., Rowe M. I., Grosfeld J. L., Fonkalsrud E. W., Coran A. G. (Eds.), Pediatric surgery (5th ed., 248–258). St. Louis, MO: Mosby.

Wood, J., Rubin, D. M., Nance, M. L., & Christian, C. W. (2005). Distinguishing inflicted versus accidental abdominal injuries in young children. *Journal of Trauma, 59*, 1203–1208.

Woolley, M. M., Mahour, G. H., & Sloan, T. (1978). Duodenal hematoma in infancy and childhood: Changing etiology and changing treatment. *American journal of surgery, 136*, 8–14.

Yamamoto, L. G., Wiebe, R. A., & Mathews, W. J. (1991). A one-year prospective ED cohort of pediatric trauma. *Pediatric Emergency Care, 7*, 267–274.

Yang, J. W., Kuppermann, N., & Rosas, A. (2002). Child abuse presenting as pseudorenal failure with a history of a bicycle fall. *Pediatric Emergency Care, 18*, 91–2.

Ziegler, D. W., Long, J. A., Philippart, A. I., & Klein, M. D. (1988). Pancreatitis in childhood: Experience with 49 patients. *Annals of Surgery, 207*, 257–261.

Chapter 6

Abusive Head Trauma

Erin E. Endom and Donna Mendez

Introduction

Abusive head trauma (AHT) is the leading cause of trauma deaths in infants (Gerber and Coffman, 2007). AHT is most common in the first year of life; as many as 95% of severe head injuries in the first year of life are due to inflicted injury (Duhaime et al., 1987; Ettaro, Berger, & Songer, 2004; Hadley, Sonntag, Rekate, & Murphy, 1989; Jaspan, Griffiths, McConachie, & Punt, 2003; Keenan, Runyan, & Nocera, 2006; King, MacKay, & Sirnick, 2003; Ludwig & Warman, 1984). Head injury is the most common cause of death from physical abuse; one study found that 36 of 42 abuse deaths were due to AHT. It is estimated that up to 28/100,000 infants sustain AHT in the first year of life, with a mortality rate of 21.4%. This results in nearly 500 deaths/year from AHT in the United States. This number, however, is almost certainly an underestimate due to incomplete reporting (Graupman & Winston, 2006; Kesler et al., 2008; Parmar, Sinha, Hayhurst, May & O'Brien, 2007).

Perpetrators are primarily male; fathers and mothers' boyfriends make up the majority of abusers (37 and 20.5% respectively in one study), followed by female sitters (17.3%) and mothers (12.6%) (Duhaime, 2008; Graupman & Winston, 2006; Starling et al., 2004). Factors increasing victim risk of AHT include male gender; prematurity, low birth weight, or disability; young age (12 months and younger); more than two siblings; a mother who smoked during pregnancy; and parents who are young, unmarried, and/or have low levels of education. All these factors, except gender, are associated with lower socio-economic status; however, the absence of these factors cannot be used to exclude

231

A.P. Giardino et al. (eds.), *A Practical Guide to the Evaluation of Child Physical Abuse and Neglect*, DOI 10.1007/978-1-4419-0702-8_6, © Springer Science+Business Media, LLC 1997, 2010

AHT as a possibility (Gerber and Coffman, 2007; Graupman & Winston, 2006; Kesler et al., 2008; Wu et al., 2004).

Anatomy and General Principles

Children are more vulnerable than adults to intracranial injury because of their anatomy (Figure 6.1). The head of an infant is larger than an adult's in proportion to the body (the brain of an average 2 year-old child is approximately 75% the weight of an average adult brain) and also heavy and unstable. The large head and weak neck musculature permit greater movement when the head is subjected to acceleration–deceleration forces. In addition, the weak cervical muscles cannot adequately stop the head's motion once acceleration starts (Gean, 1994; Williams, 1994).

The base of the infant skull is relatively flat, permitting the brain to move more readily in response to acceleration–deceleration forces. With increasing age, the brain does not move as much due to the development of prominent bony ridges and concavities. The infant skull is thinner and more pliable, transferring impact force more effectively across the subarachnoid space to the brain. The subarachnoid space is larger and more shallow than that in adults, contributing to this increased transfer of forces (Gean, 1994; Kriel, Krach, & Sheehan, 1988; Pounder, 1997).

Infants and young children have relatively soft brains with high water content and a jelly-like texture. There are several reasons why the young child's brain is

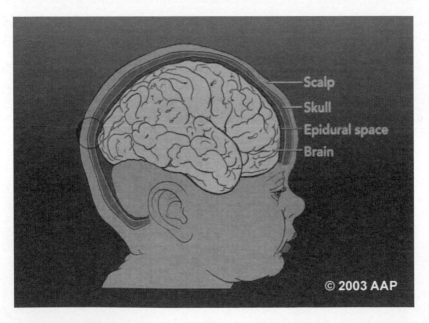

Figure 6.1 Anatomy of infant head. American Academy of Pediatrics. Visual Diagnosis of Child Abuse on CD-ROM. 2nd Edition. Elk Grove Village, Ill. 2003. Reprinted with permission.

softer than an adult's: the central nervous system is not completely myelinated, the axons are smaller than that of adults, and the brain is primarily composed of neurons without dendritic connections (Gean, 1994; Williams, 1994).

Because of the unique characteristics of the developing skull and brain, children under the age of 5 years are particularly vulnerable to brain injury. Impact to the immature brain is more likely to produce shearing injury rather than the typical brain contusions that might occur in older children and adults (Gean, 1994).

Forces

AHT may be caused by blunt force, shaking, or a combination of forces. Rotational (angular) forces are prominent in AHT.

Biomechanical forces generated during inflicted and noninflicted head injuries are different. Most non-abusive head injuries (non-AHT) are due to contact and translational forces. Contact forces, which occur when the head is struck or strikes an object, produce focal injuries to the scalp, skull, and brain, including skull fractures, intracranial cerebral lacerations, contusions, and epidural or subdural hemorrhages (Bandak, 1995; Duhaime et al., 1987; Duhaime et al., 1992; Gennarelli, 1993; Hanigan, Peterson, & Njus, 1987; McIntosh et al., 1996; Margulies & Thibault, 1989; Ommaya, 1995). Noninflicted brain injuries are typically caused by translational forces that produce linear movement of the brain in addition to the effects of contact force. Short falls are an example of this type of trauma (Gennarelli et al., 1982; Ommaya, Faas, & Yarnell, 1968). Although such falls may occasionally result in a skull fracture, these incidents are generally benign and do not result in loss of consciousness, neurologic deficit, or death (Duhaime et al., 1992; Ommaya et al., 1968; Stahlthammer, 1986; Wilkins and Rengachary, 1985).

Rotational and acceleration–deceleration forces are generated by either impact or nonimpact inertial mechanisms, such as whiplash shaking, which produce sudden acceleration or deceleration of the head. Rotational forces applied to the head cause the brain to turn abruptly on its central axis or its attachment at the brainstem cerebral junction, while acceleration–deceleration produce forward and backward movements of the brain against the inner table of the skull. Evidence from biomechanical models is controversial since no realistic model is available. Extensive clinical and experimental data, however, have suggested that such movements of the brain result in diffuse injury of two types: subdural hematoma (SDH) and diffuse axonal injury (DAI) (Ommaya & Gennarelli, 1974; Stahlthammer, 1986; Wilkins & Rengachary, 1985). Biomechanical forces have been shown to be greater with shaking and impact than with shaking alone (Alexander, Sato, Smith, & Bennett, 1990; Duhaime et al., 1987; Gennarelli & Meaney, 1996; Gilliland & Folberg, 1996; Hymel, Bandak, Partington, & Winston, 1998), but confessions, eyewitness accounts, and the absence of contusions confirm that shaking alone can cause fatal cerebrocranial trauma secondary to SDH and DAI (Duhaime et al., 1987) (Table 6.1).

Table 6.1 Injury types produced by abusive (AHT) and non-abusive (non-AHT) head trauma.

Type of TBI	Type of force	Type of ICI injury seen	Morbidity/Mortality
AHT	Contact	DAI	Poor
	Rotational	SDH	
Non-AHT	Rotational	EDH	Fair
		SDH	
		Contusion	
		Laceration	

Shaken Infant/Shaken Impact Syndrome (SIS)

Shaken infant/shaken impact syndrome (SIS) is a subgroup of AHT, caused specifically by either shaking of the child alone, or shaking in combination with blunt impact to the head. Clinical features of SIS include subdural and/or subarachnoid hemorrhage, occult fractures (especially involving the skull, ribs and long bones), and retinal hemorrhages. Only one-third of patients exhibit all three clinical features.

The question of the ability of shaking alone versus shaking/impact of shaking to cause the injuries seen in AHT remains controversial because there is not yet a satisfactory model of the infant head and brain. Another mechanism of injury that has been suggested is damage to the lower brainstem and upper cervical spine. This has only been demonstrated on autopsy and not in living children who have sustained AHT. Hadley et al. described a "whiplash-shake syndrome" showing significant cervical spine injury associated with subdural and/or epidural hematomas and contusions of the spinal cord at the cervicomedullary junction (Hadley et al., 1989). Damage to the cervicomedullary junction, particularly the respiratory centers, may be an important mechanism contributing to morbidity and mortality in SIS (Geddes, Hackshaw, Vowles, Nickols, & Whitwell, 2001; Hadley et al., 1989; Shannon et al., 1998).

In SIS, shearing forces on the bridging veins and retina are thought to be the cause of subdural and retinal hemorrhages (Caffey, 1972; Case, Graham, Handy, Jentzen, & Monteleone, 2001; Gennarelli and Meaney, 1996; Hymel et al., 1998, Hymel, Jenny, & Block, 2002). It is not known, however, how long and how often a child must be shaken to cause serious injury, or why retinal hemorrhages almost invariably result from shaking but rarely from falls (Billmire & Myers, 1985). It has been calculated that a child with a body mass of 3.8–4.5 kg must be shaken 40–50 times over 20 s in order to suffer serious brain injury (Levitt, Sutton, Goldman, Mikhail, & Christopher, 1994).

Retinal Hemorrhages (RH)

Retinal hemorrhages are frequently noted in children with AHT (60–85% in retrospective series) (Bechtel et al., 2004; Keenan et al., 2003; King et al., 2003;

Morad et al., 2002). They are rarely seen with accidental TBI (Bechtel et al., 2004; Christian, Taylor, Hertle, & Duhaime, 1999; Vinchon, Defoort-Dhellemmes, Desurmont, & Dhellemmes, 2005). RH associated with AHT are characteristically numerous, involve multiple layers of the retina, and extend beyond the posterior pole to the peripheral retina (Adams et al., 2004; Wygnanski-Jaffe et al., 2006).

Skeletal Fractures

Approximately 20 to 50% of victims of AHT have extracranial skeletal fractures (Alexander et al., 1990; Bechtel et al., 2004; Bonnier, Nassogne, & Errard, 1995; Haviland & Russell, 1997; Merten, Osborne, Radkowski, & Leonidas, 1984). In one retrospective study of 71 children younger than 3 years of age with AHT, 32% of victims had extracranial fractures; 87% of these had multiple bony injuries (Lazoritz, Baldwin, & Kini, 1997). In a prospective study comparing young children with serious inflicted versus noninflicted head injury, the abused patients were more likely to have rib, long bone, and metaphyseal fractures than those who had sustained accidental trauma (Bechtel et al., 2004). Classic metaphyseal avulsion lesions of the long bones were one of the early injuries described in AHT. They are thought to be the result of either torsion and traction when an extremity is twisted or pulled, or from shearing forces applied across the metaphysis when a child is shaken and the limbs begin to flail (Caffey, 1974).

Rib fractures in infants with normal bones, especially fractures of the posterior ribs, are highly specific for child abuse. In a retrospective review of infants with rib fractures, 82% were attributed to child abuse; the remaining cases were associated with accidental trauma involving major forces (8%), bone fragility (8%), or birth trauma (2%) (Bulloch et al., 2000). Another review of rib fractures in young children found a 95% positive predictive value for this bony injury as an indicator of abuse (Barsness et al., 2003).

Studies of the radiologic and histopathologic characteristics of rib fractures and perpetrator admissions as to how they shook an infant have revealed how posterior and anterior rib fractures are caused by the perpetrator's hands wrapping around the child's thorax, with the vertebrae acting as a fulcrum.

Head Injuries: Extracranial

Almost half of children with AHT present without evidence of external trauma, such as bruising to the head or face (Alexander et al., 1990; Morris, Smith, Cressman, & Ancheta, 2000; Haviland & Russell, 1997). In one retrospective series describing children with inflicted head injury, 54% had no bruising noted at initial presentation (King et al., 2003). Even those without scalp swelling may have evidence on autopsy of intracranial or subgaleal hematoma.

Scalp

Children with AHT may have scalp swelling (Duhaime et al., 1987; Jenny, Hymel, Ritzen, Reinert, & Hay, 1999; Starling et al., 2004). In a recent study, abused children less than 3 years of age admitted to a hospital were evaluated to find the prevalence of occult head injury with a normal neurological exam. Occult head injuries included scalp injury (74%), skull fracture (74%), and intracranial injury (53%) noted by CT or MRI but not on physical examination (Rubin, Christian, Bilaniuk, Zazyczny, & Durbin, 2003).

Subgaleal Hematoma

Subgaleal hematoma is bleeding into the potential space between the fibrous layers of the scalp and the skull. Subgaleal hematomas are associated with blunt injury to the head but have also been reported from hair-pulling during an abusive event. Forceful hair-pulling results in the scalp being lifted off the calvarium (Hamlin, 1968; Seifert & Puschel, 2006). Children without scalp swelling may have evidence on autopsy of a subgaleal hematoma. A subgaleal hematoma may be associated with an underlying skull fracture.

Skull Fractures

Skull fractures are caused by direct force to the head and are seen in both inflicted and noninflicted head injury (Photo 6.1). The reported incidence of a skull fracture

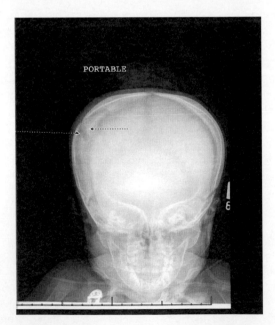

Photo 6.1 Skull fracture. Displaced fracture within the fronto-occiptal bone. There are also diastasis of all visual sutures

in AHT is 9–31%. The parietal bone is the skull bone most commonly fractured in both AHT and non-AHT (Bonnier et al., 1995; Child Abuse Prevention Center, 1998; Harwood-Nash, Hendrick, & Hudson, 1971; Leventhal, Thomas, Rosenfield, & Markowitz, 1993; Meservy, Towbin, McLaurin, Myers, & Ball, 1987; Zimmerman et al., 1979).

The specificity of certain types of skull fractures as an indicator of AHT is not entirely clear. Complex fractures (multiple, bilateral, diastatic, or depressed) have historically been associated with AHT (Brown and Minns, 1993; Ewing-Cobbs et al., 1998; Hobbs, 1984). More recent studies, however, have called these assumptions into question (Arnhotz, Hymel, Hay, & Jenny, 1998; Leventhal et al., 1993).

Accidental falls at home are rarely associated with injury more serious than a linear skull fracture. Looking at more serious falls from greater heights, Barlow investigated 61 children who had fallen from heights of at least one story (Barlow, Niemirska, Gandhi, & Leblanc, 1983). Seventeen of these (28%) had skull fractures, but only one had an SDH (1.8%). Williams reported 106 patients younger than 3 years old with a history of a free fall witnessed by two or more people or by a noncaretaker (Williams, 1991). Of the 106 patients, 77 sustained only mild bruises, abrasions, or simple skull fractures. Of these 77 patients, 43 had fallen more than 10 ft. Intracranial injuries, depressed skull fractures, or compound fractures occurred in 14 patients who fell between 5 and 40 ft. However, in the three patients who fell less than 10 ft, no life-threatening injury occurred. An interesting aspect of this study is that in 53 patients with unwitnessed falls (or falls witnessed by only one caretaker), there were 18 severe injuries, including intracranial injuries, in patients who fell less than 5 ft. This finding suggests that these patients were, in fact, victims of non-AHT. A similar phenomenon has been noted in other studies (Chadwick, Chin, Salerno, Landsverk, & Kitchen, 1991; Reiber, 1993). In a study by Hobbs, eight children in the AHT group who had skull fractures had associated SDHs; no SDHs were seen in the non-AHT skull fracture group (Hobbs, 1984).

Head Injuries: Intracranial

Intracranial bleeding is a nonspecific term to describe bleeding inside the skull.

Subdural Hemorrhage (SDH)

A subdural hemorrhage occurs in the space between the dura and the arachnoid membranes, usually as a result of tearing of the bridging veins that join the surface of the brain to the dura. Subdural hemorrhages seen in victims of non-AHT are caused typically by severe force such as an MVA, ejection from a motor vehicle, or a fall from a significant height. The trivial home accidents that children so frequently sustain are associated with primarily translational forces and not with the rotational forces necessary to develop tearing of bridging veins, which would produce subdural hemorrhage (Duhaime et al., 1992; Haviland & Russell, 1997; Helfer, Slovis, & Black, 1977; Kravitz, Driessen, Gomberg, & Korach, 1969; Lyons & Oates, 1993;

Nimityonskul & Anderson, 1987; Tzioumi & Oates, 1998; Williams, 1991). Even in children that have fallen down the stairs, the incidence of intracranial injury is rare. Joffe and Ludwig found no evidence of intracranial hemorrhage in 363 patients, 1 month to 18.7 years old, with a history of having fallen down stairs (Johnson, Fischer, Chapman, & Wilson, 2005).

Noninflicted SDHs are usually limited to the cerebral convexities and can produce signs and symptoms of intracranial mass effect (Ewing-Cobbs et al., 2000). They usually occur at a single site (the site of impact) and are often associated with an overlying fracture. Subdural blood seen away from the point of impact is unusual in accidental trauma, unless severe (Warrington & Wright, 2001).

SDHs following accidental trauma are relatively rare in contrast to AHT in which SDHs are the most common type of intracranial bleeding with a reported incidence of 82–92% (Brown & Minns, 1993; Case, 2008; Dashti, Decker, Razzaq, & Cohen, 1999; Hoskote, Richards, Anslow, & McShane, 2002; Reece & Sege, 2000; Duhaime et al., 1992; Zimmerman et al., 1979). Hymel reported SDHs in 16/39 (41%) of an inflicted group compared with 4/39 (10%) of a noninflicted group (Hymel, Rumack, Hay, Strain, & Jenny, 1997). Jayawant found the incidence of SDH in AHT to be 27 of 33 (82%), which reflects their study population of children less than 2 years of age in whom it is known that there is a high risk of AHT (Jayawant et al., 1998).

As in noninflicted trauma, the commonest site for SDHs in AHT is over the cerebral convexities. SDHs typically associated with AHT are those in more than one location or bilateral; chronic; of mixed density (implying repeated episodes of bleeding); or in the posterior fossa (Duhaime et al., 1996; Ewing-Cobbs et al., 2000; Feldman et al., 2001; Hoskote et al., 2002; McHugh, 2005; Tung, Kumar, Richardson, Jenny, & Brown, 2006; Wells, Vetter, & Laud, 2002). Interhemispheric subdural hemorrhages in AHT are usually posterior (Wells et al., 2002). While SDHs in AHT may be extensive, they are usually shallow and most do not cause significant mass effect.

A recent study by Tung noted that mixed-density SDHs were significantly more common in AHT (67%) than in accidental trauma (18%). Homogenous hyperdense SDHs were more common in accidental injury (Tung et al., 2006).

The possibility of AHT needs to be seriously considered in any child with subdural hemorrhage and no history of significant trauma, particularly in the presence of other unexplained injuries. There may be little or no evidence of external cranial trauma in those with AHT (Chabrol, Decarie, & Fortin, 1999; Morris et al., 2000).

Chronic Subdural Hematoma

Most inflicted SDHs are reabsorbed over a period of days to weeks, but in some cases it evolves into a chronic subdural hematoma (Dias, Backstrom, Falk, & Li, 1998; Duhaime et al., 1996; Ewing-Cobbs et al., 2000; Hymel, Rumack, Hay, Strain, & Jenny, 1997). There is an association between chronic SDHs and AHT with chronic subdural collections suggesting prior episodes of abuse (Alexander, Crabbe, Sato, Smith, & Bennett, 1990; Dias et al., 1998; Ewing-Cobbs et al., 1998;

Wells, Vetter, & Laud, 2002). The development of the classic multilayered chronic SDH results from venous bleeding under low pressure and requires that the subdural space be able to enlarge without a significant increase in pressure. The factors that permit this exist only in specific categories of people, such as those with brain atrophy, those with hydrocephalus and ventricular shunts, or those with traumatic encephalomalacia (Lee, Bae, Doh, Bae, & Yun, 1998). A chronic SDH very rarely follows severe head injury in a previously normal person, in whom an acute SDH transforms by aging to become a chronic subdural membrane. Instead, the blood of the acute subdural hemorrhage in these head injuries is readily resolved or rapidly organized (Duhaime et al., 1996; Lee et al., 1998; Parent, 1992). A young child whose SDH subsequently organizes into a membrane composed of large vascular channels at risk for rebleeding would have most likely been symptomatic before the time of rebleeding, because there would have been a preexisting brain abnormality. The time required for an acute subdural to evolve to a chronic SDH varies from days to weeks (Dias et al., 1998). It is not possible to presume that chronic SDHs are caused by AHT in the absence of other supporting evidence such as unexplained bone fractures.

Rebleeds are believed to occur frequently in resolving SDHs, but the amount of bleeding around the existing hematoma is seldom large. Rebleeding after trivial injury or spontaneous rebleeding from a preexisting chronic SDH should not be offered as an explanation for the presence of acute subdural blood if the old subdural membrane is not demonstrated on autopsy (Chadwick et al., 1998). There is no evidence that rebleeding can cause serious brain injury (Showers, 1998). The hypothesis is sometimes advanced that the existence of an old, small, chronic SDH or effusion can predispose to the development of massive and life-threatening acute SDH as the result of very minor trauma or normal handling. One mechanism that has been suggested for this putative phenomenon is that excess extracerebral fluid allows the brain more freedom to move about within the cranium, thereby rendering the bridging veins more prone to tearing. If this mechanism did indeed apply, one would expect to see SDH in association with other causes of excess extracerebral cerebrospinal fluid, such as post-meningitis subdural effusion, communicating hydrocephalus or cerebral atrophy, but with rare exceptions infants with these conditions have not developed subdural hematoma. MRI is a radiological modality (Photo 6.2) which can differentiate between acute and chronic subdural collections and is essential for a second investigation. It is best performed 5–10 days after the insult, when it can reliably differentiate between acute and chronic subdural collections (Barlow et al., 1983; Child Abuse Prevention Center, 1998).

Epidural Hematoma (EDH)

An epidural hematoma is due to bleeding into the space between the inner skull surface and the dura. Arterial EDHs are due to a tear of the middle meningeal artery or one of its major branches. EDHs may also result from venous bleeding. EDHs are typically associated with accidental trauma but have been described in abused children (Dashti et al., 1999; Duhaime et al., 1992; Reiber, 1993).

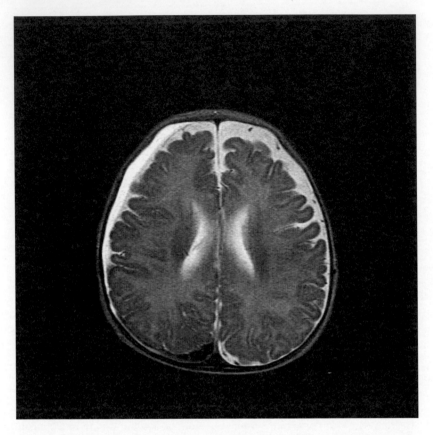

Photo 6.2 MRI with new and old SDH. View of the new subdurals on the right cerebral convexities and the old subdurals on the left cerebral convexities.

Subarachnoid Hemorrhage (SAH)

A subarachnoid hemorrhage is bleeding into the area between the arachnoid membrane and the pia mater surrounding the brain. This may occur spontaneously or as a result of arteriovenous malformations, cerebral aneurysms, coagulopathies, infection, and accidental trauma (Broderick, Talbot, Prenger, Leach, & Brott, 1993). SAH in accidental TBI is associated with a major accident. SAH is not typically associated with AHT; when present, it usually occurs at the site of a focal impact and in association with depressed skull fractures or cortical contusions.

SAH is also seen frequently in association with subdural hemorrhages as bridging veins rupture and bleed into both spaces. Inflicted SAH may be produced by a shaking-only event or shaking/impact event (Ewing-Cobbs et al., 2000). SAH in the posterior interhemispheric fissure may be difficult to differentiate from SDH or the normal falx.

Intraventricular Hemorrhage (IVH)

Intraventricular hemorrhage is bleeding into the brain's ventricular system. The most common etiology is the rupture of subependymal veins, usually due to rotational forces. Injury to the corpus callosum is common; in its absence, IVH is usually caused by extension of an intraparenchymal bleed. Bleeding occurs most commonly into the lateral ventricles (McHugh, 2005). IVH in the infant outside the newborn period is usually from vascular malformation, coagulopathy or trauma, or as a surgical complication. IVH has been described as a consequence of AHT but is rare (Cohen, Kaufman, Myers, & Towbin, 1986).

Contusion

A cerebral contusion is a bruise of the brain tissue. Contusions are often indicative of direct impact. In AHT, contusions are often seen in association with other cerebral injuries such as DAI and subarachnoid hemorrhages (Hardman & Manoukian, 2002). MRI and CT are equally sensitive in detecting hemorrhagic contusions. Contusions are likely to heal on their own without medical intervention.

Numerous small contusions from broken capillaries that occur in gray matter under the cortex are called multiple petechial hemorrhages or multifocal hemorrhagic contusions and are caused by shearing forces at the time of impact. These hemorrhages are a type of diffuse brain injury, which are better visualized on MRI than on CT (Barlow et al., 1983; Kleinman, 1987; Zimmerman et al., 1979).

Diffuse Axonal Injury (DAI)

Diffuse axonal injury is diffuse microscopic tearing of axons in the white matter of the brain, caused by movement of the brain within the skull (Gennarelli et al., 1982). Extreme forces of angular deceleration are required to produce DAI. This injury is responsible for prolonged coma in many patients after severe head injury, and may coexist with SDH. DAI is detected with MRI or upon autopsy and is at best poorly visualized on CT (Barlow et al., 1983; Downie, 2001; Zimmerman et al., 1979). DAI is best demonstrated with diffusion-weighted MRI, which shows diffusion restriction in the area of injury (Ewing-Cobbs et al., 1998).

Hypoxic-Ischemic Injury

Hypoxic-ischemic injury is another important consequence of AHT. Injury may be multifocal and widespread and does not necessarily respect vascular territories. Cerebral edema may accompany cerebral hypoxia-ischemia (Ewing-Cobbs et al., 1998). MRI, particularly diffusion-weighted imaging, detects hypoxic-ischemic change earlier and more frequently than CT alone (Sato et al., 1989).

Hygromas

Hygromas are enlarged subdural or subarachnoid spaces filled with cerebrospinal fluid (CSF). Children with AHT are more likely to show hygromas than those with non-AHT. Subarachnoid hygromas can represent either brain atrophy or communicating hydrocephalus, reflecting previous head injuries (Ewing-Cobbs et al., 1998, 2000; Hymel et al., 1998). Subdural hygromas are believed to be derived mainly from chronic subdural hematomas but can also develop following neurosurgical procedures (Biousse et al., 2002). After trauma, subdural fluid collections (hygromas) can develop from a tear in the arachnoid and subsequent accumulation of CSF (Hymel et al., 1998). It is not uncommon for chronic SDHs to be misinterpreted on CT as subdural hygromas, and vice versa. MRI can differentiate a chronic SDH from a subdural hygroma and brain atrophy, when clinically warranted (Biousse et al., 2002).

Most hygromas are small and clinically insignificant. Larger hygromas may cause secondary localized mass effects on the adjacent brain parenchyma, enough to cause neurologic symptoms. Acute hygromas can be a potential neurosurgical emergency requiring decompression.

Intracerebral Hemorrhage (ICH)

Intracerebral hemorrhage is bleeding from a ruptured intracerebral blood vessel. It frequently follows trauma involving a rapid jerking motion of the neck. Vertebrobasilar dissections have been known to occur at fixation points, i.e., where the vertebral artery enters the dura. It seems that the tethering of the arteries at these points increases the shearing forces at these locations during trauma, producing small tears of the intima progressing to traumatic arterial dissection. Late manifestations include thrombus formation, vascular occlusion, and stroke (Taveras & Joseph, 2002). These types of arterial injuries are commonly suspected following trauma involving adults, but less commonly considered in children. Since children have risk factors that theoretically increase the rate of arterial injury during trauma, it is unclear why this is not more frequently reported in the pediatric population. Nguyen reported a case in which a 3 month-old male victim of AHT developed intracranial vertebral artery dissection in association with SAH, but without an associated stroke (Agner & Weig, 2005). Three cases of arterial dissection with ensuing stroke caused by abuse have been reported (Nguyen, Burrowes, Ali, Bowman, & Shaiban, 2007).

Clinical Presentation

The history given by parents or caretakers is of critical importance in determining whether any trauma is accidental or inflicted. In AHT the history is often one of nonspecific symptoms with no mention of trauma, or a history of minor impact (a short distance fall from standing, falling off a couch or bed). Symptoms may include vomiting, sleepiness, or change in behavior. Intracranial injuries, particularly in infants, often present with nonspecific symptoms such as irritability, lethargy, poor feeding and/or vomiting, without specific or focal neurologic symptoms.

Head injury in the absence of any history of trauma has been shown to be strongly associated with abuse (Ettaro et al., 2004; Lam, Montes, Farmer, O'Gorman, & Meagher-Villemure, 1996; Hettler & Greenes, 2003; Reece & Sege, 2000). A common presenting complaint is of a mysterious swelling on the head, often noted by the mother while bathing the child or combing his/her hair, and associated with an underlying skull fracture. In contrast, accidental head injuries usually present with a specific history of trauma (Michaud, Rivara, Grady, & Reay, 1992). Children with AHT are also significantly more likely to present with seizure activity or altered mental status compared to children with accidental head injury, who are more likely to present with scalp hematomas (seizures 53% vs. 6%; altered mental status 53% vs. 1%) (Bechtel et al., 2004).

An acute life-threatening event (ALTE) is defined as an event of any of the following: apnea, breath-holding, choking, cyanosis, change in muscle tone, and/or seizure activity. ALTE may be associated with intracranial trauma, especially in infants, and even in the absence of external signs of trauma. Parents rarely give a history of trauma or of shaking the infant (Gupta & Kumar, 2007). A study conducted in Denver involving children who died of AHT found that the most common presenting complaint was apnea; only 1 of 36 had a presenting complaint of trauma (Graupman & Winston, 2006). In Vellody's study of infants with a history of ALTE (Duhaime et al., 1992), 4 of 108 infants were eventually found to have sustained AHT (Waseem & Pinkert, 2006). All four had other findings suspicious for abuse including skin contusions, fractures, retinal hemorrhages, or a history given by a parent that the infant had been shaken.

Children with AHT often present with a history of minor head trauma inconsistent with the severity/type of injury. Epidural hemorrhage (EDH) has been shown to occur with low-impact trauma due to tearing of the vulnerable middle meningeal artery (Vellody, Freeto, Gage, Collins, & Gershan, 2008). In contrast, subdural hemorrhage (SDH), especially in conjunction with retinal hemorrhage, occurs much more common in and is highly suspicious for abuse (Gilliland & Folberg, 1996; Vellody et al., 2008). SDH results from tearing of the bridging veins, indicative of shear injury rather than a single blunt impact. Short-distance falls from a couch or bed may result in scalp contusions or lacerations, soft tissue hematomas, and linear skull fracture; multiple or depressed fractures, subarachnoid or subdural bleeds associated with this history are highly suspicious. Tarantino et al. studied 167 infants presenting for evaluation after short vertical falls or drops of 4 ft or less; only two sustained intracranial hemorrhages and both were later found to have been abused (Myhre, Grøgaard, Dyb, Sandvik, & Nordhov, 2007), When major/nonaccidental trauma is admitted, the caretaker may allege that someone else did it (older sibling, babysitter). A common story is that the father, stepfather, or mother's boyfriend was alone with the child when the injuries were sustained.

Suspicious historical factors may include

1. A history that changes among caregivers or during evaluation or that is confusing or inconsistent with the child's injuries.
2. Delay in seeking care.
3. Fresh blood in nose or mouth following an alleged ALTE, which has been associated with smothering.
4. Recurrent ALTE or SIDS in a family (Waseem & Pinkert, 2006).

A heightened index of suspicion on the part of the examining physician, combined with a careful review of the history of the incident, signs and symptoms, and other physical findings, is critical to detection of abuse.

Differentiating Between Accidental and Nonaccidental Head Trauma

Wilkins reviewed multiple studies of falls in children and found that falls of 1.2 m (50 in., or just over 4 ft) were never fatal (Tarantino, Dowd, & Murdock, 1999). Short household falls can produce linear parietal skull fractures; higher force is required to produce depressed fractures, diastatic fractures (wider than 3 mm), multiple or stellate fractures, or fractures that cross suture lines or involve the occipital area or the base of the skull (Tarantino et al., 1999; Wilkins, 1997) (see Table 6.2). Diastasis of a single skull suture results from direct trauma to the suture; generalized diastasis is more likely to result from increased intracranial pressure.

Table 6.2 Range of injuries produced by common mechanisms of trauma. Adapted from Gerber and Coffman (2007).

Minor household falls (< 4 ft):
Soft tissue injuries
Linear skull fractures
Epidural hematomas
Falls > 4 ft:
All of above +
Depressed and basilar skull fractures
Subarachnoid hemorrhages
Cerebral contusions
Severe trauma (motor vehicle accident, nonaccidental trauma):
Diffuse subdural hematomas
Diffuse axonal injuries

As noted above, epidural hemorrhage may occur with relatively minor trauma to the parietal skull if the vulnerable middle meningeal artery is torn. Subdural and subarachnoid hemorrhages are much more strongly associated with abuse; however, they cannot be considered pathognomonic as they have been documented in accidental head trauma. Mixed-density SDH on computed tomography (CT)

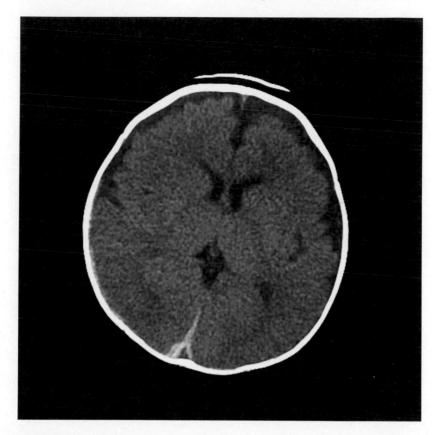

Photo 6.3 CT with new and old SDH. This is a 3 month old who was diagnosed with inflicted TBI at our institution. On her CT see new subdural hemorrhages and old subdurals in extraaxial spaces.

(Photo 6.3), which may indicate fresh bleeding into an older hematoma, is significantly more frequent in AHT, while homogeneous hyperdense SDH is more frequent in accidental trauma (Tung et al., 2006); again, however, mixed-density bleeding cannot be considered pathognomonic for abuse. Interhemispheric bleeds have been thought to be strongly associated with AHT; however, recent studies document its presence in non-AHT (Kellogg, 2007)

Parents and caregivers often seek medical attention for accidental injuries before any symptoms develop; care for inflicted injuries is frequently sought for either symptoms or unexplained signs of injury (Fujiwara, Okuyama, & Miyasaka, 2008).

Associated Findings

Retinal hemorrhages (RH) are strongly associated with AHT (60% vs. 10% in one 2004 study (Bechtel et al., 2004)) (Photo 6.4). Location, depth, and extent of RH may help distinguish abusive from accidental trauma:

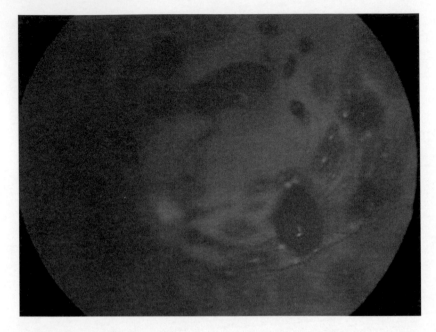

Photo 6.4 Retina hemorrhage. Courtesy of Paul G. Steinkuller, MD, Baylor College of Medicine and Texas Children's Hospital.

Bilateral: 40% vs. 1.5%
Pre-retinal (vitreous) bleeds: 30% vs. 0%
Premacular: 20% vs. 0%
Extending to periphery of retina: 27% vs. 0% (Bechtel et al., 2004; Wilkins, 1997)

A dilated examination by a pediatric ophthalmologist experienced in the assessment of retinal hemorrhage should be performed whenever AHT is suspected.

Tears to the frenulum of the tongue or upper lip are common following accidental trauma, such as falls in children beginning to walk or children struck in the face by deploying airbags during a motor vehicle accident. They may also occur during attempts at intubation. However, in the absence of such a history, a frenulum tear in an infant too young to walk may be a manifestation of abuse, either from "bottle jamming" (forcing a nipple or pacifier into the child's mouth) or from blunt trauma to the mouth, and may be associated with significant head injury (Barnes & Krasnokutsky, 2007.

Skin findings may include bruises, burns, and/or patterned injuries. Areas of injury particularly associated with AHT are the ears, especially the posterior pinnae and postauricular areas, the neck and angle of the jaw, and the scalp (hematomas may not be readily visible, but can be detected by palpation) (Wilkins, 1997). Fractures of long bones and ribs are associated with shaking; these may not be evident on physical examination but require radiographs to detect.

Laboratory abnormalities may also be associated with AHT. A significant intracranial bleed can produce an acute drop in hemoglobin and hematocrit, especially in a young infant with small total blood volume and little reserve. Bloody cerebrospinal fluid obtained via atraumatic lumbar puncture can be a marker of intracranial bleeding. Developmental delay or abnormal head growth may result from chronic, repeated head trauma.

Differential Diagnosis

It has been suggested that a widened subarachnoid space in infants may predispose to SDH with minor or no trauma (Kellogg, 2007). This theory is controversial, since other researchers have felt there is no increased vulnerability of bridging veins in the child with widened extracerebral spaces (Thackeray, 2007). This condition is otherwise known as benign extracerebral collection, benign extracerebral subarachnoid space, or benign external hydrocephalus. It consists of an asymptomatic increase in the subarachnoid space without ventricular dilatation and has been defined as a distance of 5 mm or greater between the brain surface and the inner table of the skull. It occurs in young children undergoing rapid head growth and usually normalizes by 2 years of age; macrocephaly has been described but is not universally present (McNeely, Atkinson, Saigal, O'Gorman, & Farmer, 2006; Reece & Nicholson, 2003). It is thought that stretching of the bridging veins may predispose to SAH or SDH without trauma or after only minor trauma. The clinical course of SAH/SDH in this setting is generally benign, in contrast to the high morbidity and mortality seen with inflicted trauma (Gerber & Coffman, 2007; Reece & Nicholson, 2003).

Other medical conditions that may present with SDH, RH, or both

1. Osteogenesis imperfecta (OI), not only because of bone fragility but vascular fragility as well; 10 to 30% of OI patients also have bleeding diatheses (Parmar et al., 2007).
2. Glutaric aciduria type I, a rare neurometabolic disorder with macrocephaly and subdural hematomas mimicking AHT (Ravid & Maytal, 2003).
3. Menkes (kinky hair) disease, a disorder of copper absorption (Bishop, Liu, McCall, & Brockmeyer, 2007).
4. Coagulopathies. Hemorrhagic disease (vitamin K deficiency) of the newborn occurs in both early-onset (first 72 hr of life) and late-onset forms (after the first week, rarely as late as 6 months of age). The late-onset form is associated with up to 100% incidence of IC hemorrhage. Prothrombin time (PT) and activated partial thromboplastin time (PTT) are markedly elevated, while thrombin time and fibrinogen level remain normal; the K-dependent clotting factors II, VII, and X are decreased as well. Early-onset disease usually occurs in neonates who did not receive vitamin K at birth; prematurity, low birth weight, and some maternal drugs can cause it as well. The late-onset form can be caused by malabsorption, liver disease, or gastroenteritis (Nassogne et al., 2002). Meningitis

and encephalitis are also associated with intracranial bleeding, especially in the presence of disseminated intravascular coagulation; labs reveal marked increase in PT and PTT, thrombocytopenia, decreased fibrinogen, elevated D-dimer and fibrin degradation products (Rutty, Smith, & Malia, 1999).

Clinical Evaluation and Management

The initial steps in the medical evaluation of AHT depend on the child's condition. As always, the ABCs (airway, breathing, circulation) take precedence. While a detailed discussion of the medical management of head trauma is beyond the scope of this chapter, the clinically unstable patient is approached and managed as any seriously head-injured child would be: stabilization of ABCs; management of increased intracranial pressure with head-of-bed elevation and drugs; emergent head CT as stability allows; and neurosurgical consultation and intervention as clinically indicated. A detailed history and physical examination (as detailed below) may be performed when the child's condition permits (Table 6.3).

For the medically stable patient, the first step in evaluation is a detailed history, including the factors detailed in Table 6.3.

Table 6.3 Historical factors in evaluation of AHT

Circumstances of injury	What precisely happened; when; how; who witnessed it (question direct witnesses; document direct quotes from caregivers whenever possible)
Symptoms	Loss of consciousness/duration; emesis; altered behavior or mental status; seizure-like activity
Time to seeking medical care	Red flag: delay in seeking care
Other injuries	Red flag: multiple injuries/types of injuries without corresponding history
Past medical history	Underlying medical conditions, trauma, hospitalizations, surgeries
Perinatal history	Premature, adopted, planned/unplanned, pregnancy or birth complications, maternal depression
Developmental history	Red flag: developmental stage inconsistent with alleged events
Family history	Bleeding, bone, other genetic/metabolic disorders
Social history	Stressors: family, job, social, financial, child's temperament, substance abuse, or violence in home

Physical examination should, of course, include a detailed examination of the head. Palpation of the entire scalp may reveal soft tissue hematomas or skull deformities not readily visible under the hair. Bruises around the eyes, ears (including behind the pinnae), mastoid prominences, and on the neck should be sought. Bleeding from the ears, nose, or mouth, septal hematomas, and frenulum tears are markers for trauma. Complete neurological assessment should be performed. In addition, a careful examination of the entire body (with clothes removed, but with attention to the patient's modesty) should be conducted for signs of other injuries.

Imaging of intracranial structures (see Table 6.4) serves three purposes in the evaluation and management of nonaccidental trauma: (1) diagnosis and clinical monitoring of intracranial injury; (2) establishment of necessity for therapeutic intervention; and (3) documentation of injury for social/legal investigation (Jaspan, Griffiths, McConachie, & Punt, 2003).

Table 6.4 Proposed protocol for sequential imaging of significant AHT. Adapted from Jaspan et al. 2003.

1. Head CT as soon as patient stable	Reliably detects acute problems requiring emergent medical or surgical intervention
2. Skull films (full 4-view series)	Detects linear skull fractures in line with plane of CT cuts which may be missed on CT
3. MRI or repeat CT on day 3–4	MRI more sensitive at detecting subacute hemorrhage, ischemic changes, and cervical spine injuries (esp. diffusion-weighted imaging)
4. Repeat CT on day 10	Assess for secondary damage
5. Repeat MRI at 2–3 months	Assess for end-stage damage, late sequelae (chronic SDH, hydrocephalus, leptomeningeal cyst)

Computed tomography (CT) is generally available on an emergent basis; is excellent at detecting bleeding, mass effect, and other conditions requiring emergent intervention; and, especially in conjunction with plain skull radiographs, is superior to MRI in detecting skull fractures. A repeat CT 24–48 h after the initial study may be indicated to monitor for worsening hemorrhage or edema. Subtle findings of hypoxia, edema, and loss of gray–white differentiation on initial CT may evolve within 48 h into what is colloquially known as the "big black brain"—massive, uniform edema, and hypodensity of one or both hemispheres, possibly due to local increase in ICP, release from damaged brain tissue of vasoactive factors, or both (Fenton, Sirotnak, & Handler, 2000; Graupman & Winston, 2006).

Magnetic resonance imaging (MRI) is difficult to obtain on an emergent basis but is superior to CT for evaluation of edema, dating IC injuries, detection of subtle injuries in patients with normal CT but abnormal neurologic examinations, and detection of cervical spine injury (Wilkins, 1997). Diffuse axonal injury (DAI) is shown as petechial hemorrhages in the gray–white junction and in the corpus callosum; it is poorly visualized on CT, and MRI is more sensitive at detecting the signs of this injury pattern (Fenton et al., 2000; Graupman & Winston, 2006).

Evaluation for other injuries should include, at least:

Skeletal survey in children < 2 y/o or nonverbal (repeat in 2 weeks or consider bone scan for high-risk patients).
CBCdp, PT/PTT, liver functions, urinalysis.
DIC panel if intracranial injury, as intraparenchymal damage can alter coagulation (Wilkins, 1997).
Further evaluation as clinically indicated (cardiac enzymes if suspicion of cardiac injury, abdominal CT to rule out abdominal trauma).

Imaging alone cannot reliably detect AHT; the entire constellation of findings including historical, physical, laboratory, social and law enforcement evaluations all affect the differentiation between accidental and inflicted head injury. It is incumbent upon the examining physician to evaluate not just a single injury but the whole patient.

Outcomes

Outcomes for children with AHT are poor, with mortality rates ranging from 13 to 38% (Keenan et al., 2003; Ludwig & Warman, 1984). A six-fold increase in mortality rate (13% vs. 2%) has been seen in children with TBI with AHT versus non-AHT (Reece & Sege, 2000). Among survivors, the rate of persisting disability is higher in those with AHT versus non-AHT. Thirty to fifty percent of survivors suffer cognitive or other neurological deficits, and only 30% recover fully (Case et al., 2001). Multiple factors are associated with worse mortality and morbidity, including age of the child at injury, severity of the injury, the type and extent of primary and secondary brain injuries, and the nature and severity of associated extracranial injuries (Rustamzadeh, Truwit, & Lam, 2002).

Age

The effect of age at time of brain injury (TBI) on neurologic and functional outcome is complex, with the results among studies being inconsistent (Michaud et al., 1992). Most studies show worse outcomes for children injured at younger ages (Berger, Pitts, Lovely, Edwards, & Bartkowski, 1985; Ewing-Cobbs, Duhaime, & Fletcher, 1995; Lazar & Menaldino, 1995; Mahoney et al., 1983). It was once believed that the plasticity of the infant brain would allow very young children to compensate for their TBI but the opposite is now thought to be true (Ewing-Cobbs & Fletcher, 1987; Ewing-Cobbs et al., 1997; Raimondi & Hirschauer, 1984).

Severity of Injury

Higher severity of injury has been associated with worse outcome in children with AHT. Ewing-Cobbs found that more severe injury, as measured by lower Glasgow Coma Scale (GCS) scores and longer periods of unconsciousness, has been associated with worse cognitive, motor, and behavioral outcomes (Taylor & Alden, 1997). Even in children with comparable GCS scores, AHT has been shown to result in larger cognitive deficits and less favorable Glasgow Outcome Scale (GOS) scores at short-term follow-up (average 1.3 months), in comparison with children with non-AHT (Ewing-Cobbs et al., 1998).

Goldstein et al. found more severe injury, as indicated by the admission GCS, in 14 of 40 children whose brain injuries were abusive. Outcomes in that study, as indicated by GOS at hospital discharge, were worse in the group with AHT. Children with AHT were also significantly younger (mean age 1.6 years) than those with non-AHT (mean 7.3 years) (Ewing-Cobbs, Prasad, Kramer, & Landry, 1999).

Type of TBI

SDH and DAI, which are among the characteristic lesions of AHT in young children, are associated with worse outcomes than other types of intracranial injury (Berger et al., 1985; Goldstein, Kelly, Bruton, & Cox, 1993; Rustamzadeh et al., 2002).

Secondary brain injury is also associated with worse outcome. Secondary brain injury may occur from hypoxia, hypotension, edema, infarction, delayed hemorrhage, or pressure necrosis from displacement and herniation of the brain (Duhaime, Christian, Rorke, & Zimmerman, 1998). Children with widespread infarction and atrophy have worse physical and cognitive deficits. In a study by Gilles and Nelson, poorer outcome was seen in those with AHT and signs of ischemia who eventually developed cerebral infarction (Gilles & Nelson, 2008).

Long-Term Neurocognitive Functioning

Survivors of AHT show poorer long-term neurocognitive functioning compared to those with non-AHT. This may be related to the fact that children who survive AHT tend to be younger than those who are injured accidentally. They have attained fewer neurocognitive skills prior to the injury. Skills that are in a rapid stage of development may be more vulnerable to disruption by trauma than skills that have already been acquired (Raimondi & Hirschauer, 1984). In a study by Bonnier et al. of 13 patients with AHT, six initially appeared to recover fully. By the end of the study, however, 11 of 12 survivors had been diagnosed with abnormalities including psychomotor delay, mental retardation, learning disabilities, blindness, seizures, tetraplegia, and hemiparesis (Bonnier et al., 1995). In another study, 25 children with AHT were followed for a mean of 59 months, with 68% having abnormalities at follow-up. Identified abnormalities included motor (60%), visual (48%) speech and language impairment (64%), and epilepsy (20%). Behavioral disturbances were noted in 52% of children. The behavioral abnormalities included self-injurious and self-stimulatory behaviors, hyperactivity, impulsivity, temper tantrums, and rage reactions. Many of the behavioral problems developed in the second and third year of life (Barlow et al., 1983). Ewing-Cobbs reported outcomes of 40 children with TBI (20 with AHT and 20 with non-AHT); only 20% of the AHT children were doing well neurocognitively, compared with 55% of children with non-AHT (Brown & Minns, 1993). In a recent study, children evaluated a year after severe TBI had worse cognitive and behavioral outcomes when the TBI was inflicted than when it was accidental (Keenan et al., 2006).

In Brief

- Head trauma is the leading cause of morbidity and mortality related to child physical abuse.
- Acute subdural hemorrhage in an infant or toddler should raise the suspicion of shaking impact syndrome unless a clear history of sufficient trauma is elicited.
- The etiology of chronic extra-axial fluid collections is not always clear. All infants and children with unexplained extra-axial collections should have an evaluation for possible abuse along with a skeletal survey and social work evaluation.
- Infants and toddlers with abusive head trauma present for medical care with nonspecific symptoms, such as irritability, lethargy, vomiting, apnea, and seizures. The possibility of trauma is often not initially considered.
- CT scan is the preferred initial imaging study for children with acute injuries. MRI is more sensitive in identifying or clarifying many of the injuries seen in abused children.
- Skeletal survey and ophthalmologic examination are mandatory for the evaluation of the abused infant and toddler with head injuries.

References

Adams, G., Ainsworth, J., Butler, L., Bonshek, R., Clarke, M., Doran, R., et al. (2004). Update from the ophthalmology child abuse working party: Royal College ophthalmologists. *Eye*, *18*(8), 795–798.

Agner, C., & Weig, S. G. (2005). Arterial dissection and stroke following child abuse: case report and review of the literature. *Child's Nervous System*, *21*(5), 416–420.

Alexander, R., Crabbe, L., Sato, Y., Smith, W., & Bennett, T. (1990). Serial abuse in children who are shaken. *American Journal of Diseases of Children*, *144*(1), 58–60.

Alexander, R., Sato, Y., Smith, W., & Bennett, T. (1990). Incidence of impact trauma with cranial injuries ascribed to shaking. *American Journal of Diseases of Children*, *144*(6), 724–726.

Arnhotz, D., Hymel, K. P., Hay, T. C., & Jenny, C. (1998). Bilateral pediatric skull fractures: Accident or abuse?. *Journal of Trauma*, *45*, 172.

Barlow, B., Niemirska, M., Gandhi, R. P., & Leblanc, W. (1983). Ten years of experience with falls from a height in children. *Journal of Pediatric Surgery*, *18*(4), 509–511.

Barnes, P. D., & Krasnokutsky, M. (2007). Imaging of the central nervous system in suspected or alleged nonaccidental injury including the mimics. *Topics in Magnetic Resonance Imaging*, *18*(1), 53–54.

Bandak, F. A. (1995). On the mechanics of impact neurotrauma: a review and critical synthesis. *Journal of Neurotrauma, 12*(4), 635–649.

Barsness, K. A., Cha, E. S., Bensard, D. D., Calkins, C. M., Partrick, D. A., Karrer F. M., & Strain, J. D. (2003). The positive predictive value of rib fractures as an indicator of nonaccidental trauma in children. *Journal of Trauma, 54*(6), 1107–1110.

Bechtel, K., Stoessel, K., Leventhal, J. M., Ogle, E., Teague, B., Lavietes, S., et al. (2004). Characteristics that distinguish accidental from abusive injury in hospitalized young children with head trauma. *Pediatrics, 114*(1), 165–168.

Berger, M. S., Pitts, L. H., Lovely, M., Edwards, M. S., & Bartkowski, H. M., (1985). Outcome from severe head injury in children and adolescents. *Journal of Neurosurgery, 62*(2), 194–199.

Billmire, M. E., & Myers, P. A. (1985). Serious head injury in infants: accident or abuse?. *Pediatrics, 75*(2), 340–342.

Biousse, V., Suh, D. Y., Newman, N. J., Davis, P. C., Mapston, T., & Lambert, S. R. (2002). Diffusion-weighted magnetic resonance imaging in shaken baby syndrome. *American Journal of Ophthalmology, 133*(2), 249–255.

Bishop, F. S., Liu, J. K., McCall, T. D., & Brockmeyer, D. L. (2007). Glutaric aciduria type 1 presenting as bilateral subdural hematomas mimicking nonaccidental trauma. Case report and review of the literature. *Journal of Neurosurgery, 106*(3 Suppl), 222–226.

Bonnier, C., Nassogne, M., & Errard, P. (1995). Outcome and prognosis of whiplash shaken infant syndrome; late consequences after a symptom-free interval. *Developmental Medicine & Child Neurology, 37*(11), 943–956.

Broderick, J., Talbot, G. T., Prenger, E., Leach, A., & Brott, T. (1993). Stroke in children within a major metropolitan area: the surprising importance of intracerebral hemorrhage. *Journal of Child Neurology, 8*(3), 250–255.

Brown, J., & Minns, R. (1993). Non-accidental head injury, with particular reference to whiplash shaking injury and medico-legal aspects. *Developmental Medicine & Child Neurology, 35*(10), 849–869.

Bulloch, B., Schubert, C. J., Brophy, P. D., Johnson, N., Reed, M. H., & Shapiro, R. A. (2000). Cause and clinical characteristics of rib fractures in infants. *Pediatrics, 105*(4), E48.

Caffey, J. (1972). On the theory and practice of shaking infants. Its potential residual effects of permanent damage and mental retardation. *American Journal of Diseases of Children, 124*(2), 161–169.

Caffey, J. (1974). The whiplash shaken infant syndrome: manual shaking by the extremities with whiplash-induced intracranial and intraocular bleedings, linked with residual permanent brain damage and mental retardation. *Pediatrics, 54*(4), 396–403.

Case, M. E. (2008). Forensic pathology of child brain trauma. *Brain Pathology, 18*(4), 562–564.

Case, M. E., Graham, M. A., Handy, T. C., Jentzen, J. M., & Monteleone, J. A. (2001, June). Position paper on fatal abusive head injuries in infants and young children. *American Journal Forensic Medicine in Pathology, 22*(2), 112–122.

Chabrol, B., Decarie, J. C., & Fortin, G. (1999). The role of cranial MRI in identifying patients suffering from child abuse and presenting with unexplained neurological findings. *Child Abuse and Neglect, 23*(3), 217–228.

Chadwick, D. L., Chin, S., Salerno, C., Landsverk, J., & Kitchen, L. (1991, October). Deaths from falls in children: how far is fatal?. *Journal of Trauma, 31*(10), 1353–1355.

Chadwick, D. L., Kirschner, R. H., Reece, R. M., Ricci, L. R., Alexander, R., Amaya, M., et al. (1998). Shaken baby syndrome—a forensic pediatric response. *Pediatrics, 101*(2), 321–323.

Child Abuse Prevention Center. (1998) Research project on the incidence and risk factors of shaken baby syndrome in the state of Utah.

Christian, C. W., Taylor, A. A., Hertle, R. W., & Duhaime, A. C. (1999). Retinal hemorrhages caused by accidental household trauma. *Journal of Pediatrics, 135*(1), 125–127.

Cohen, R. A., Kaufman, R. A., Myers, P. A., & Towbin, R. B. (1986). Cranial computed tomography in the abused child with head injury. *American Journal of Roentgenology, 146*(1), 97–102.

Dashti, S. R., Decker, D. D., Razzaq, A., & Cohen, A. R. (1999). Current patterns of inflicted head injury in children. *Pediatrics Neurosurgery, 31*(6), 302–306.

Dias, M. S., Backstrom, J., Falk, M., & Li, V. (1998). Serial radiography in the infant shaken impact syndrome. *Pediatrics Neurosurgery, 29*(2), 77–85.

Downie, A. (2001). www.radiology.co.uk/sr-x/tutors/cttrauma/tutor.htm

Duhaime, A. C. (2008, May) Demographics of abusive head trauma. *Journal of Neurosurgery Pediatrics, 1*(5), 349–350.

Duhaime, A. C., Alario, A. J., Lewander, W. J., Schut, L., Sutton, L. N., Seidl, T. S., et al. (1992). Head injury in very young children: mechanisms, injury types, and ophthalmologic findings in 100 hospitalized children younger than 2 years of age. *Pediatrics, 90*(2 Pt 1), 179–185.

Duhaime, A. C., Christian, C. W., Armonda, R., Hunter, J., & Hertle, R. (1996). Disappearing subdural hematomas in children. *Pediatrics Neurosurgery, 25*(3), 116–122.

Duhaime, A. C., Christian, C. W., Rorke, L. B., & Zimmerman, R. A. (1998). Nonacciden-tal head injury in infants—the "shaken baby syndrome". *The New England Journal of Medicine, 338*(25), 1822–1829.

Duhaime, A. C., Gennarelli, T. A., Thibault, L. E., Bruce, D. A., Margulies, S. S., & Wiser, R. (1987, March). The shaken baby syndrome: a clinical, pathological, and biomechanical study. *Journal of Neurosurgery, 66*(3), 409–415.

Ettaro, L., Berger, R. P., & Songer, T. (2004). Abusive head trauma in young children: char-acteristics and medical charges in a hospitalized population. *Child Abuse and Neglect, 28*(10), 1099–1111.

Ewing-Cobbs, L., Duhaime, A. C., & Fletcher, J. (1995). Inflicted and noninflicted traumatic brain injury in infants and preschoolers. *Journal of Head Trauma Rehabilitation, 10*(5), 13–24.

Ewing-Cobbs, L., Kramer, L., Prasad, M., Canales, D. N., Lovis, P. T., Fletcher, J. M., et al. (1998). Neuroimaging, physical and developmental findings after inflicted and noninflicted traumatic brain injury in young children. *Pediatrics, 102*(2 Pt 1), 300–307.

Ewing-Cobbs, L., & Fletcher, J. M. (1987). Neuropsychological assessment of head injury in children. *Journal of Learning Disabilities, 20*(9), 526–535.

Ewing-Cobbs, L., Fletcher, J. M., Levin, H. S., Francis, D. J., Davidson, K., & Miner, M. E. (1997). Longitudinal neuropsychological outcome in infants and preschoolers with trau-matic brain injury. *Journal of the International Neuropsychological Society, 3*(6), 581–591.

Ewing-Cobbs, L., Prasad, M., Kramer, L., & Landry, S. (1999). Inflicted traumatic brain injury: relationship of developmental outcome to severity of injury. *Pediatrics Neuro-surgery, 31*(5), 251–258.

Ewing-Cobbs, L., Prasad, M., Kramer, L., Lovis, P. T., Baumgartner, J., Fletcher, J. M., & Alpert, B. (2000). Acute neuroradiologic findings in young children with inflicted or non-inflicted traumatic brain injury. *Child's Nervous System, 16*(1), 25–34.

Feldman, K. W., Bethel, R., Shugerman, R. P., Grossman, D. C., Grady, M. S., & Ellenbogen, R. G. (2001). The cause of infant and toddler subdural hemorrhage: a prospective study. *Pediatrics, 108*(3), 636–646.

Fenton, L. Z., Sirotnak, A. P., & Handler, M. H. (2000). Parietal pseudofracture and spontaneous intracranial hemorrhage suggesting nonaccidental trauma: report of 2 cases. *Pediatrics Neurosurgery*, *33*(6), 318–322.

Fujiwara, T., Okuyama, M., & Miyasaka, M. (2008, October). Characteristics that distinguish abusive from nonabusive head trauma among young children who underwent head computed tomography in Japan. *Pediatrics*, *122*(4), 841–847, Epub 2008 Sep 1.

Gean, A. D. (1994). Imaging of Head Trauma. New York: Raven Press.

Williams, P. (1994). Gray's Anatomy (38th ed., pp. 607–609). New York: Churchill Livingstone.

Geddes, J. F., Hackshaw, A. K., Vowles, G. H., Nickols, C. D., & Whitwell, H. L. (2001). Neuropathology of inflicted head injury in children. 1. Patterns of brain damage. *Brain*, *124*(Pt 7), 1290–1298.

Gennarelli, T. A. (1993). Mechanisms of brain injury. *Journal of Emergency Medicine*, *11*(suppl 1), 5–11.

Gennarelli, T. A., Thibault, L. E., Adams, J. H., Graham, D. I., Thompson, C. J., & Marcincin, R. P. (1982). Diffuse axonal injury and traumatic coma in the primate. *Annals of Neurology*, *12*(6), 564–574.

Gennarelli, T. A., & Meaney, D. F. (1996). Mechanisms of primary head injury. In Wilkins R. H., Rengachary S. S. (Eds.), *Neurosurgery* (2nd ed., pp. 2607–2637). New York: McGraw-Hill.

Gerber, P., & Coffman, K. (2007). Nonaccidental head trauma in infants. *Child's Nervous System*, *23*(5), 499–507.

Gilles, E. E., & Nelson, M. D. (1998, August) Cerebral complications of nonaccidental head injury in childhood. *Pediatrics Neurology*, *19*(2), 119–128.

Gilliland, M. G. F., & Folberg, R. (1996). Shaken babies—some have no impact injuries. *Journal of Forensic Sciences*, *41*(1), 114–116.

Goldstein, B., Kelly, M. M., Bruton, D., & Cox, C. (1993). Inflicted versus accidental head injury in critically injured children. *Critical Care Medicine*, *21*(9), 1328–1332.

Graupman, P., & Winston, K. R. (2006). Nonaccidental head trauma as a cause of childhood death. *Journal of Neurosurgery*, *104*(4 Suppl), 245–250.

Gupta, S., & Kumar, A. (2007). Child abuse: inflicted traumatic brain injury. *Indian Pediatrics*, *44*(10), 783–784.

Hadley, M. D., Sonntag, V. K., Rekate, H. L., & Murphy, A. (1989). The infant whiplash-shake injury syndrome: a clinical and pathological study. *Neurosurgery*, *24*(4), 536–540.

Hamlin, H. (1968). Subgaleal hematoma caused by hair-pull. *JAMA*, *204*(4);22, 339.

Hanigan, W. C., Peterson, R. A., & Njus, G. (1987). Tin ear syndrome: rotational acceleration in pediatric head injuries. *Pediatrics*, *80*(5), 618–622.

Hardman, J. M., & Manoukian, A. (2002, May) Pathology of head trauma. *Neuroimaging Clinics of North America*, *12*(2), 175–187.

Haviland, J., & Russell, R. I. (1997). Outcome after severe non-accidental head injury. *Archives of Disease in Childhood*, *77*(6), 504–507.

Harwood-Nash, D. C., Hendrick, E. B., & Hudson, A. R. (1971). The significance of skull fracture in children. A study of 1,187 patients. *Radiology*, *101*(1), 151–156.

Helfer, R. E., Slovis, T. L., & Black, M. (1977). Injuries resulting when small children fall out of bed. *Pediatrics*, *60*(4), 533–535.

Hettler, L., & Greenes, D. S. (2003). Can the initial history predict whether a child with a head injury has been abused?. *Pediatrics*, *111*(3), 602–607.

Hobbs, C. J. (1984). Skull fracture and the diagnosis of abuse. *Archives of Disease in Childhood*, *59*(3), 246–252.

Hoskote, A., Richards, P., Anslow, P., & McShane, T. (2002). Subdural haematoma and non-accidental head injury in children. *Child's Nervous System, 18*(6–7), 311–317.

Hymel, K. P., Bandak, F. A., Partington, M. D., & Winston, K. R. (1998). Abusive head trauma? A biomechanical approach. *Child Maltreatment, 3*, 116–128.

Hymel, K. P., Jenny, C., & Block, R. W. (2002). Intracranial hemorrhage and rebleeding in suspected victims of abusive head trauma: Addressing the forensic controversies. *Child Maltreatment, 7*(4), 329–348.

Hymel, K. P., Rumack, C. M., Hay, T. C., Strain, J. D., Jenny, C. (1997). Comparison of intracranial computed tomographic (CT) findings in pediatric abusive and accidental head trauma. *Pediatrics Radiology, 27*(9), 743–747.

Jaspan, T., Griffiths, P. D., McConachie, N. S., & Punt, J. A. G. (2003). Neuroimaging for non-accidental head injury in childhood: a proposed protocol. *Clinical Radiology, 58*(1), 44–53.

Jayawant, S., Rawlinson, A., Gibbon, F., Price, J., Schulte, J., Sharples, M., et al. (1998). Subdural haemorrhages in infants: population based study. *British Medical Journal, 317*(7172);5, 1558–1561.

Jenny, C., Hymel, K. P., Ritzen, A., Reinert, S., & Hay, T. C. (1999). Analysis of missed cases of abusive head trauma. *JAMA, 281*(7);17, 621–626.

Johnson, K., Fischer, T., Chapman, S., & Wilson, B. (2005, April) Accidental head injuries in children under 5 years of age. *Clinical Radiology, 60*(4), 464–468.

Keenan, H. T., Runyan, D. K., Marshall, S. W., Nocera, M. A., Merten, D. F., & Sinal, S. H. (2003). A population-based study of inflicted traumatic brain injury in young children. *JAMA, 290*(5);6, 621–626.

Keenan, H. T., Runyan, D. K., & Nocera, M. (2006). Child outcomes and family characteristics 1 year after severe inflicted or noninflicted traumatic brain injury. *Pediatrics, 117*(2), 317–324.

Kellogg, N. D. (2007). American Academy of Pediatrics Committee on Child Abuse and Neglect. Evaluation of suspected child abuse. *Pediatrics, 119*(6), 1232–1241.

Kesler, H., Dias, M. S., Shaffer, M., Rottmund, C., Cappos, K., & Thomas, N. J. (2008). Demographics of abusive head trauma in the Commonwealth of Pennsylvania. *Journal of Neurosurgery Pediatrics, 1*(5), 351–356.

King, W. J., MacKay, M., & Sirnick, A. (2003). Canada Shaken Baby Study Group. Shaken baby syndrome in Canada: clinical characteristics and outcomes of hospital cases. *Canadian Medical Association Journal, 21168*(2), 155–159.

Kleinman, D. K. (1987). Pathology of head trauma. *Neuroimaging Clinics of North America, 12*, 175–187.

Kravitz, H., Driessen, F., Gomberg, R., & Korach, A. (1969). Accidental falls from elevated surfaces in infants from birth to one year of age. *Pediatrics, 44*(Suppl 5), 869–876.

Kriel, R. L., Krach, L. E., & Sheehan, M. (1988). Pediatric closed head injury: outcome following prolonged unconsciousness. *Archives of Physical Medicine and Rehabilitation, 69*(9), 678–681.

Lam, C. H., Montes, J., Farmer, J. P., O'Gorman, A. M., & Meagher-Villemure, K. (1996). Traumatic aneurysm from shaken baby syndrome: case report. *Neurosurgery, 39*(6), 1252–1255.

Lazar, M. F., & Menaldino, S. (1995). Cognitive outcome and behavioral adjustment in children following traumatic brain injury: a developmental perspective. *Journal of Head Trauma Rehabilitation, 10*, 55–63.

Lazoritz, S., Baldwin, S., & Kini, N. (1997). The whiplash shaken infant syndrome: has Caffey's syndrome changed or have we changed his syndrome?. *Child Abuse and Neglect, 21*(10), 1009–1014.

Lee, K. S., Bae, W. K., Doh, J. W., Bae, H. G., & Yun, I. G. (1998). Origin of chronic subdural haematoma and relation to traumatic subdural lesions. *Brain Injury, 12*(11), 901–910.

Leventhal, J. M., Thomas, S. A., Rosenfield, N. S., & Markowitz, R. I. (1993). Fractures in young children. Distinguishing child abuse from unintentional injuries. *American Journal of Diseases of Children, 147*(1), 87–92.

Levitt, M. A., Sutton, M., Goldman, J., Mikhail, M., & Christopher, T. (1994). Cognitive dysfunction in patients suffering minor head trauma. *American Journal of Emergency Medicine, 12*(2), 172–175.

Ludwig, S., & Warman, M. (1984). Shaken baby syndrome: a review of 20 cases. *Annals of Emergency Medicine, 13*(2), 104–107.

Lyons, J. L., & Oates, R. K. (1993). Falling out of bed: a relatively benign occurrence. *Pediatrics, 92*(1), 125–127.

McHugh, K. (2005). Neuroimaging in non-accidental head injury: if, when, why and how. *Clinical Radiology, 60*(7), 826–827.

McIntosh, T. K., Smith, D. H., Meaney, D. F., Kotapka, M. J., Gennarelli, T. A., & Graham, D. I. (1996). Neuropathological sequelae of traumatic brain injury: relationship to neurochemical and biomechanical mechanisms. *Laboratory Investigation, 74*(2), 315–342.

McNeely, P. D., Atkinson, J. D., Saigal, G., O'Gorman, A. M., & Farmer, J. P. (2006). Subdural hematomas in infants with benign enlargement of the subarachnoid spaces are not pathognomonic for child abuse. *American Journal of Neuroradiology, 27*(8), 1725–1728.

Mahoney, W. J., D'Souza, B. J., Haller, J. A., Rogers, M. C., Epstein, M. H., & Freeman, J. M. (1983). Long-term outcome of children with severe head trauma and prolonged coma. *Pediatrics, 71*(5), 756–762.

Margulies, S. S., & Thibault, L. E. (1989). An analytical model of traumatic diffuse brain injury. *Journal of Biomechanical Engineering, 111*(3), 241–249.

Meservy, C. J., Towbin, R., McLaurin, R. L., Myers, P. A., & Ball, W. (1987). Radiographic characteristics of skull fractures resulting from child abuse. *American Journal of Roentgenology, 149*(1), 173–175.

Merten, D. F., Osborne, D. R., Radkowski, M. A., Leonidas, J. C. (1984). Craniocerebral trauma in the child abuse syndrome: radiological observations. *Pediatrics Radiology, 14*(5), 272–277.

Michaud, L. J., Rivara, F. P., Grady, M. S., Reay, D. T. (1992). Predictors of survival and severity of disability after severe brain injury in children. *Neurosurgery, 31*(2), 254–264.

Morad, Y., Kim, Y. M., Armstrong, D. C., Huyer, D., Mian, M., & Levin, A. V. (2002). Correlation between retinal abnormalities and intracranial abnormalities in the shaken baby syndrome. *American Journal of Ophthalmology, 134*(3), 354–359.

Morris, M. W., Smith, S., Cressman, J., & Ancheta, J. (2000). Evaluation of infants with subdural hematoma who lack external evidence of abuse. *Pediatrics, 105*(3 Pt 1), 549–553.

Myhre, M. C., Grøgaard, J. B., Dyb, G. A., Sandvik, L., & Nordhov, M. (2007). Traumatic head injury in infants and toddlers. *Acta Pædiatrica, 96*(8), 1159–1163.

Nassogne, M. C., Sharrard, M., Hertz-Pannier, L., Armengaud, D., Touati, G., Delonlay-Debeney, P., et al. (2002). Massive subdural haematomas in Menkes disease mimicking shaken baby syndrome. *Child's Nervous System, 8*(12), 729–731.

Nguyen, P. H., Burrowes, D. M., Ali, S., Bowman, R. M., & Shaiban, A. (2007). Intracranial vertebral artery dissection with subarachnoid hemorrhage following child abuse. *Pediatrics Radiology, 7*(6), 600–602.

Nimityonskul, P., & Anderson, L. D. (1987). The likelihood of injuries when children fall out of bed. *Journal of Pediatric Orthopaedics, 7*(2), 184–186.

Ommaya, A. K. (1995). Head injury mechanisms and the concept of preventive management: a review and critical synthesis. *Journal of Neurotrauma, 2*(4), 527–546.

Ommaya, A. K., Faas, F., & Yarnell, P. (1968). Whiplash injury and brain damage. *JAMA*, *204*(4);22, 285–289.

Ommaya, A. K., & Gennarelli, T. A. (1974). Cerebral concussion and traumatic unconsciousness. Correlation of experimental and clinical observations of blunt head injuries. *Brain*, *97*(4), 633–654.

Parmar, C. D., Sinha, A. K., Hayhurst, C., May, P. L., & O'Brien, D. F. (2007). Epidural hematoma formation following trivial head trauma in a child with osteogenesis imperfecta. *Journal of Neurosurgery*, *106*(1 Suppl Pediatrics), 57–60.

Parent, A. D. (1992). Pediatric chronic subdural hematoma: a retrospective comparative analysis. *Pediatrics Neurosurgery*, *18*(5–6), 266–271.

Pounder, D. (1997). Shaken adult syndrome. *American Journal Forensic Medicine in Pathology*, *18*(4), 321–324.

Raimondi, A. J., & Hirschauer, J. (1984). Head injury in the infant and toddler. Coma scoring and outcome scale. *Childs Brain*, *11*(1), 12–35.

Ravid, S., & Maytal, J. (2003). External hydrocephalus: a probable cause for subdural hematoma in infancy. *Pediatrics Neurology*, *28*(2), 139–141.

Reece, R. M., & Sege, R. (2000). Childhood head injuries: accidental or inflicted?. *Archives of Pediatrics & Adolescent Medicine*, *154*(1), 11–15.

Reece R. M., & Nicholson C. E. (Eds.) (2003). Inflicted childhood neurotrauma: proceedings of a conference sponsored by HHS, NIH, NICHD, ORD, NCMRR. American Academy of Pediatrics, Elk Grove Village, IL

Reiber, G. D. (1993). Fatal falls in childhood. How far must children fall to sustain fatal head injury? Report of cases and review of the literature. *American Journal Forensic Medicine in Pathology*, *14*(3), 201–207.

Rubin, D. M., Christian, C. W., Bilaniuk, L. T., Zazyczny, K. A., & Durbin, D. R. (2003). Occult head injury in high-risk abused children. *Pediatrics*, *111*(6 Pt 1), 1382–1386.

Rustamzadeh, E., Truwit, C. L., & Lam, C. H. (2002). Radiology of nonaccidental trauma. *Neurosurgery Clinics of North America*, *13*(2), 183–199.

Rutty, G. N., Smith, C. M., & Malia, R. G. (1999). Late-form hemorrhagic disease of the newborn: a fatal case report with illustration of investigations that may assist in avoiding the mistaken diagnosis of child abuse. *American Journal Forensic Medicine*, *20*(1), 48–51.

Sato, Y., Yuh, W. T. C., Smith, W. L., Alexander, R. C., Kao, S. C., & Ellerbroek, C. J. (1989). Head injury in child abuse: evaluation with MR imaging. *Radiology*, *173*(3), 653–657.

Seifert, D., & Puschel, K. (2006). Subgaleal hematoma in child abuse. *Forensic Science International*, *157*(2–3);10, 131–133.

Shannon, P., Smith, C. R., Deck, J., Ang, L. C., Ho, M., & Becker, L. (1998). Axonal injury and the neuropathology of shaken baby syndrome. *Acta Neuropathology*, *95*(6), 625–631.

Showers, J. (1998). Never never never shake a baby. The challenge of the shaken baby syndrome. Proceedings of the Second National Conference on Shaken Baby Syndrome, September 1998, Salt Lake City, Utah. Alexandria, Virginia: National Association of Children's Hospitals and Related Institutions, 1999

Stahlthammer, D. (1986). Experimental models of head injury. *Acta Neurochirurgica Suppl (Wien)*, *36*, 33–46.

Starling, S. P., Patel, S., Burke, B. L., Sirotnak, A. P., Stronks, S., & Rosquist, P. (2004). Analysis of perpetrator admissions to inflicted traumatic brain injury in children. *Archives of Pediatrics & Adolescent Medicine*, *158*(5), 454–458.

Tarantino, C. A., Dowd, D., & Murdock, T. C. (1999). Short vertical falls in infants. *Pediatric Emergency Care*, *15*(1), 5–8.

Taveras, J. M., & Joseph, T. (Eds.) (2002). *Radiology on CD-ROM: Diagnosis, imaging, intervention*. Philadelphia: Lippincott Williams & Wilkins.

Taylor, H. G., & Alden, J. (1997). Age-related differences in outcomes following childhood brain insults: an introduction and overview. *Journal of the International Neuropsychological Society, 3*(6), 555–567.

Thackeray, J. D. (2007, October). Frena tears and abusive head injury: a cautionary tale. *Pediatric Emergency Care, 23*(10), 735–737.

Tung, G. A., Kumar, M., Richardson, R. C., Jenny, C., & Brown, W. D. (2006). Comparison of accidental and nonaccidental traumatic head injury in children on noncontrast computed tomography. *Pediatrics, 118*(2), 626–633.

Tzioumi, D., & Oates, R. K. (1998). Subdural hematomas in children under 2 years. Accidental or inflicted? A 10-year experience. *Child Abuse and Neglect, 22*(11), 1105–1112.

Vellody, K., Freeto, J. P., Gage, S. L., Collins, N., & Gershan, W. M. (2008). Clues that aid in the diagnosis of nonaccidental trauma presenting as an apparent life-threatening event. *Clinical Pediatrics, 47*(9), 912–918.

Vinchon, M., Defoort-Dhellemmes, S., Desurmont, M., & Dhellemmes, P. (2005). Accidental and nonaccidental head injuries in infants: a prospective study. *Journal of Neurosurgery, 102*(4 Suppl), 380–384.

Warrington, S. A., & Wright, C. M. (2001). Accidents and resulting injuries in premobile infants: data from the ALSPAC study. *Archives of Disease in Childhood, 85*(2), 104–107.

Waseem, M., & Pinkert, H. (2006). Apparent life-threatening event or child abuse?. *Pediatric Emergency Care, 22*(4), 245–246.

Wells, R. B., Vetter, C., & Laud, P. M. (2002, March). Intracranial hemorrhage in children younger than 3 years: prediction of intent. *Archives of Pediatrics & Adolescent Medicine, 156*(3), 252–257.

Wilkins, B. (1997). Head injury—abuse or accident?. *Archives of Disease in Childhood, 76*, 393–397.

Wilkins R. H., & Rengachary S. S. (Eds.) (1985). *Neurosurgery* (pp. 1531–1535). New York: McGraw-Hill.

Williams, R. A. (1991). Injuries in infants and small children resulting from witnessed and corroborated free falls. *Journal of Trauma, 31*(10), 1350–1352.

Wu, S. S., Ma, C. X., Carter, R. L., Ariet, M., Feaver, E. A., Resnick, M. B., & Roth, J. (2004). Risk factors for infant maltreatment: a population-based study. *Child Abuse and Neglect, 28*(12), 1253–1264.

Wygnanski-Jaffe, T., Levin, A. V., Shafiq, A., Smith, C., Enzenauer, R. W., Elder, J. E., et al. (2006). Postmortem orbital findings in shaken baby syndrome. *American Journal of Ophthalmology, 142*(2), 233–240.

Zimmerman, R. A., Bilaniuk, L. T., Bruce, D., Schut, L., Uzzell, B., & Goldberg, H. I. (1979). Computed tomography of craniocerebral injury in the abused child. *Radiology, 130*(3), 687–690.

Chapter 7

Neglect and Failure to Thrive

Tal Ben-Galim, Penelope T. Louis, and Angelo P. Giardino

Neglect is the most common form of child maltreatment, representing approximately 64% of the 905,000 substantiated cases of maltreatment in the United States in 2006 (U.S. Department of Health & Human Services, 2008). It represents a situation in which there is a risk of harm to a child because the child's basic physical, supervisional, medical, emotional, and/or educational needs are not being met (DePanfilis, 2006) (see Table 7.1 for categorization of different forms of neglect). State laws define child neglect in various ways but conceptually neglect may be defined as

a condition in which a [child's caregiver], either deliberately or by extraordinary inattentiveness, permits the child to experience avoidable suffering and/or fails to provide one or more of the [components] generally deemed essential for developing [the child's] physical, intellectual, and emotional capacities. (Polansky cited in Gaudin (1993, p. 4))

Neglect of the child's physical needs, such as food, clothing, hygiene, and medical care, accounts for more than half of the neglect cases identified each year (U.S. Department of Health & Human Services, 2008). Despite its high incidence, neglect at times has received less professional attention than physical or sexual abuse, prompting Wolock and Horowitz (1984) to decry the "neglect of neglect." The most commonly cited reason for lack of attention to this significant problem is ambivalence and discomfort among health care professionals in passing judgment on parental choices regarding child-rearing style (Dubowitz, Black, Starr, & Zuravin, 1993; Ludwig, 1992). Of note, neglect is also the most fatal form of child maltreatment accounting for at least 42% of the 1,553 deaths known to have occurred in 2006 from child maltreatment (U.S. Department of Health & Human Services, 2008).

A.P. Giardino et al. (eds.), *A Practical Guide to the Evaluation of Child Physical Abuse and Neglect*, DOI 10.1007/978-1-4419-0702-8_7, © Springer Science+Business Media, LLC 1997, 2010

Table 7.1 Types of neglect.

Physical neglect
  Neglect of basic
    physical needs
	Failure to provide clothing, food, shelter, and hygiene

Medical neglect	Failure to provide or a delay in providing needed care by a professional for a physical injury, illness, medical condition, or impairment

Supervisional neglect
  Abandonment/
    expulsion
	Desertion of a child without arranging for reasonable care and supervision, including cases where (a) children are not claimed within 2 days, (b) children are left with no or false information given regarding caregiver's whereabouts, and (c) indefinite refusal of custody without adequate arrangement for care of child by others

Custody inattention	Apparent unwillingness to maintain custody by (a) repeated shuttling of child from household to household or (b) repeatedly leaving a child with others for days or weeks at a time
Safety	Inattention to the hazards in the child's physical environment and developmental capacity that place him or her at risk for injury

Emotional neglect
  Inattention to basic
    emotional needs/
    nurturance/
    affection
	Inattention to the child's needs for affection, emotional support, attention, and competence, including (a) markedly overprotective restrictions that foster immaturity or emotional overdependence; (b) chronically applying expectations clearly inappropriate in relation to the child's age or level of development; (c) domestic violence in the child's presence; (d) encouragement of or permitting drug or alcohol use by the child; (e) encouragement of or permitting other maladaptive behavior (e.g., severe assaultiveness, chronic delinquency)

Mental health care neglect	Failure to provide, or a delay in providing, needed care for a child's emotional or behavioral impairment or problem in accord with competent professional recommendation
Educational neglect Truancy	Permitted school absences averaging at least 5 days per month
Failure to enroll	Failure to enroll a school-age child, causing the child to miss at least one month of school, or a pattern of keeping a school-age child home for nonlegitimate reasons (e.g., to work, to care for siblings, etc.) an average of at least 3 days a month

Inattention to
    special
    education
    needs
	Inattention to recommended remedial education services for child's diagnosed learning disorder or other special education need

Source: Adapted from NIS-2 (NCAAN, 1988).

This chapter presents an overview of neglect with a focus on failure to thrive (FTT) which depending on circumstances may be associated with neglect (Block, Krebe, & The Committee on Child Abuse and Neglect, and the Committee on Nutrition, 2005).

Conceptual Approaches

Health care providers have long been aware that caregiving which fails to meet a child's basic needs is likely to be deleterious to the child's growth, development, and well-being (Chapin, 1908; Fontana & Besharov, 1979; Kempe, Silverman, Steele, Droegmueller, & Silver, 1962; Spitz, 1945, 1949). Dubowitz et al. (1993) have called for a perspective of shared responsibility in describing neglect. Rather then focusing on a specific caregiver's failure, they focus their attention instead on the child's unmet needs, looking at the shared failures of the caregivers, family, community, and society to meet the child's basic needs. This human ecological approach encourages health care providers to pay more attention to the strengths and weaknesses of the child's caregiving environment (Dubowitz, Giardino, & Gustavson, 2000). This perspective also enables health care providers to formulate comprehensive treatment plans that are likely to incorporate all the resources available in the child's environment. An example is a child who fails to grow because of a lack of formula. An approach that does not solely blame the child's parents but which instead identifies the parents' lack of resources as part of the problem may be more beneficial to the child and caregiver. The problem can be solved, for example, by helping the child's mother apply for the Supplemental Food Program for Women, Infants and Children (WIC) benefits and assisting her to obtain necessary resources to provide for her child.

There is debate as to what constitutes good parenting and what represents neglectful caregiving. Most professionals would be expected to reach similar conclusions when caregiver behaviors and choices fall far from expected norms. For example, starving a child represents a failure to meet basic food needs, and not changing a diaper for 24 hr represents failure to meet a child's basic hygienic needs. However, does leaving a child home alone at age 11 constitute neglect of the child's need for supervision? The answer to this question may entail a complicated response in part depending on broad considerations, such as (a) the child's maturity, (b) the proximity and availability of a responsible adult, and (c) the duration of the caregiver's absence. In such "gray" cases, the health care provider is forced to rely on subjective, personal judgments. From a cultural sensitivity perspective, it is crucial that the health care provider not impose his or her personal child-rearing style and beliefs on other families. Instead, the approach is to focus on the specific circumstances in a given case and evaluate the child's unmet needs and ensure that the child's growth and developmental well-being are not being imperiled.

Effects of Neglect

A range of physical, emotional, and cognitive effects on the developing child occur when basic needs are unmet. Each child's response to neglect is different and depends in part on the type of neglect (i.e., which basic needs have not been met adequately), the developmental stage at which the neglect occurs, the severity of the unmet need, how long the need was unmet, and the effectiveness of the intervention by caring adults to halt the neglect (DePanfilis, 2006). The child's response to neglect depends on a complex interaction of risk to which the child is exposed and the protective factors present inherently in the child and operating within the child's environment. Some children appear to be resilient in that despite being neglected they appear to be able to overcome this adversity and mature and develop beyond what might be expected (DePanfilis, 2006). It may be possible to promote resilience in neglected children by supporting and building upon the child's and family's strengths especially around ordinary human adaptation processes such as motivation for change, family rituals and traditions, and basic parenting skills. When medical needs are not met, direct effects on the child's physical health and well-being may be observed. Typically reported effects of neglect on children are (a) withdrawn affect; (b) decreased social interactions; (c) disorganized, aggressive interactions with peers; and (d) fewer positive play behaviors such as offering, sharing, accepting, and following (Peterson & Urquiza, 1993). Behavioral effects can be conceptualized as occurring along a continuum ranging from internalizing and externalizing behaviors (DePanfilis, 2006; Pears, Kim, & Fisher, 2008). Table 7.2 lists the commonly seen behaviors along this internalizing/externalizing continuum. In addition, children who have experienced

Table 7.2 Continuum of internalized and externalized behavioral problems.

Internalized	Externalized
Agitation	Difficulty in paying attention
Nightmares	Not listening when spoken to
Avoidance of certain activities or people	Difficulty in organizing tasks and activities
Difficulty in falling asleep or staying asleep	Being easily distracted
	Being forgetful
Sleeping too much	Bedwetting
Difficulty in concentrating	Excessive talking
	Difficulty in awaiting their turn
Hypervigilance	Bullying or threatening others
Irritability	Being physically cruel to people or animals
Becoming easily fatigued	Playing with or starting fires
	Stealing
Poor appetite or overeating	Destroying property
Low self-esteem	
Feelings of hopelessness	

DePanfilis (2006).

impaired or delayed growth on the basis of neglect may experience delayed language development and social, maturational, and behavioral difficulties (El-Baba, Bassali, & Benjamin, 2009).

Health Care Evaluation

The general approach to the health care evaluation of neglect mirrors the evaluation suggested for other forms of maltreatment. It is ideally based on a multidisciplinary approach that includes (a) a comprehensive medical history; (b) a thorough physical examination; (c) specific, directed laboratory and diagnostic testing; (d) a formal psychosocial assessment of the family, including observation of the child–caregiver interactions, and (e) meticulous documentation of the evaluation's findings. For over three decades clinicians have recognized that laboratory tests should only be obtained in the health care evaluation for suspected neglect when their need is suggested by the child's history or a finding uncovered on physical examination (Sills, 1978).

Neglect and Growth: Failure to Thrive (FTT)

FTT is a working diagnosis generally applied to children who are similar only in an observable deviation from an expected growth trajectory (AAP, 2003; Block et al., 2005; El-Baba et al., 2009; Olson, 2006; Zenel, 1997). There is not a single etiology that accounts for all cases of FTT, and some suggest replacing FTT with other terms thought to be more accurate, such as growth failure, growth retardation, and growth deficiency (Goldbloom, 1987; Kempe & Goldbloom, 1987). Although these arguments have merit, FTT is a term firmly rooted in clinical practice and remains the working diagnosis for children not growing as expected (Ludwig, 1992) (See Photo 7.1).

FTT usually presents in infancy and early childhood when there are rapid periods of growth. With malnutrition, weight is the first growth parameter affected, followed by height and then head circumference (Barbero & Shaheen, 1967). In evaluating a child with FTT as the working diagnosis, the clinician carefully considers the age of presentation, the presence or absence of risk factors for growth failure (such as underlying medical condition), and psychosocial factors that might affect feeding and growth. The diagnosis is made when the evaluation is completed and information from each component of the evaluation carefully considered. Once a definite etiology for the problem is uncovered, the term FTT may be linked with the appropriate diagnosis.

For many years, FTT was thought to be either organic (physically based) or nonorganic (socially based). Health care professionals thought that the growth retardation seen in children labeled as FTT originated either from a medical condition or illness or from a psychosocial aberration in the child's caregiving environment. This dichotomous view has since been modified as clinicians realized that a third category, "mixed" FTT, accounts for a large number of cases in which a combination of both organic and psychosocial factors contributes to growth failure (Homer &

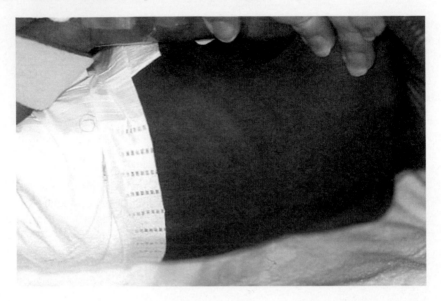

Photo 7.1 The back of an infant with FTT who has visible ribs secondary to paucity of subcutaneous fat.

Ludwig, 1981; El-Baba et al., 2009). (Table 7.3 for questions asked in the evaluation of FTT.)

Consequently, the differential diagnosis of FTT includes a wide range of possible etiologies for growth failure that may be as broad as the index of a pediatric textbook (Tunnessen & Roberts, 1999; Zenel, 1997). Table 7.4 contains a differential diagnosis for FTT. Psychosocial FTT is used when the growth failure is primarily attributed to characteristics in the child's caregiving environment, namely social, environmental, psychological, or behavioral factors that affect the amount of nutrition that the child functionally receives. (See Table 7.5 for an overview of the evaluation of FTT.)

Stephens, Gentry, & Michener (2008) summarize the basic nutritional issues that underlie the growth problems seen in all types of FTT: (a) not enough calories going into the child, (b) too many calories excreted by the child, or (c) too many calories expended internally. Organic causes may be seen in children with gastrointestinal anatomic abnormalities such as short-gut, malabsorption, or a hypermetabolic state related to chronic inflammation. However, these organic conditions may coexist with social, environmental, psychological, and/or behavioral issues that contribute to or exacerbate the nutritional problem, thus giving rise to "mixed" FTT. For example, feeding a child with a cleft lip and palate may so challenge the caregivers that efforts to feed the child become dysfunctional and ineffective. Thus, an initial organic problem may become mixed over time as the psychosocial component becomes established (See Photos 7.2 and 7.3).

Table 7.3 Guide to the observation of caregiver–child interactions.

I. General

A. Caregiver

Is there caregiver–child physical contact? What kind?

Is there cuddling?

Does caregiver smile at child? Do they look at each other?

Does caregiver appear aware of child? Child's needs? Child's comfort?

Is there playful behavior? Does caregiver engage the child with toys?

Is there verbal communication? Pleasant? Angry? Commanding?

B. Child

Is the baby/child verbal? Speech delayed?

Is the child alert? Withdrawn? Apathetic? Sad? Apprehensive?

Are there unusual body postures? Tone floppy? Rigid?

Does child respond to separation from caregiver?

II. Feeding observation (Chatoor & Egan, 1983)

Observations of feeding occur in a comfortable place that is quiet and relatively free from distractions and interruptions.

A. Homeostasis/Attachment

Does the caregiver

Begin the feeding touching the nipple to the infant's cheek?

Stimulate the infant's lips and allow the child to open his or her mouth prior to introducing the nipple into his or her mouth?

Seem aware of the amount flowing in the nipple?

Hold the bottle at a comfortable angle for the infant and avoid jostling the child or bottle?

Notice when the infant is hungry and initiate feed promptly?

Avoid excessive burping and wiping?

Permit the infant to set the pace of the feed?

Allow the child to rest, interact, and return to the feed?

Balance the infant's need for attention with the need to avoid overstimulation that could be distracting?

Notice when the infant appears satisfied and halt the feed when the infant displays behaviors indicating satiety, such as turning away and closing his or her mouth?

B. Separation and individuation

Does the caregiver

Comfortably position the child for feeding/eating?

Position him- or herself in an easily seen location and place the eating utensils in the child's view? Talk in a soothing, reassuring manner that does not overstimulate and distract the child? Demonstrate patience and permit time for the child to acclimate to meal time?

Allow the child to handle the food and, when ready, permit self-feeding?

Demonstrate patience for the child's pace?

Respect the child's likes and dislikes?

Source: Adapted from Kempe and Goldbloom (1987), Ludwig (1992), and Satler (1990).

Table 7.4 Summary of organic causes of failure to thrive.

Prenatal causes	Prematurity with complications Maternal malnutrition Toxic exposure in utero Alcohol, smoking, medications, infections IUGR Chromosomal abnormalities

Postnatal causes	Inadequate intake
	  • Lack of appetite (e.g., iron deficiency anemia, CNS pathology, chronic infection)
	  • Inability to suck or swallow: CNS or muscular
	  • Vomiting (e.g., CNS, metabolic, obstruction, renal)
	  • Gastroesophageal reflux and esophagitis
	
	Poor absorption and/or use of nutrients
	  • GI disorder (e.g., CF, celiac disease, Shwachman-Diamond syndrome, chronic diarrhea)
	  • Renal—Renal failure, renal tubular acidosis
	  • Endocrine—Hypothyroidism, diabetes mellitus, growth hormone deficiency
	  • Inborn error of metabolism
	  • Chronic infection (e.g., HIV, tuberculosis, parasites)
	
	Increased metabolic demand
	  • Hyperthyroidism
	  • Chronic disease (e.g., heart failure, BPD)
	  • Chronic inflammatory conditions (e.g., inflammatory bowel disease, systemic lupus erythematosus)
	  • Renal failure
	  • Malignancy

Used with permission, El-Baba et al. (2009). Used with permission

FTT Evaluation

The following is included in the medical evaluation of a child whose growth is below expectation:

1. Comprehensive medical history with prenatal, feeding, and dietary history.
2. Complete physical examination, including measurement of growth parameters (weight, height/length, and head circumference), body mass index (BMI), and review of prior measurements.
3. Laboratory workup, specifically indicated by history and physical examination.
4. Psychosocial assessment with observation of caregiver–child interactions, especially around feeding.
5. Careful documentation of all findings. (See Table 7.5 for an overview of the evaluation for FTT.)

Table 7.5 Overview of evaluation of FTT.

History	—Birth history (premature, IUGR, twin, birth weight)
	—Familial history (short stature)
	—Growth history (growth charts)
	—Diet history
	—Past medical history
	—Past surgical history
	—Psychosocial history (family dynamics and stressors)
Physical assessment	—Growth
	—Nutrition (e.g., signs of nutritional deficiencies)
	—Congenital anomalies
	—Evidence of neglect/abuse
Indicated laboratory studies	—CBC
	—Electrolytes
	—Urinalysis
	—Urine culture
	—Sedimentation rate
Clinical observation	—Child's interactions with caregiver
	—Weight gain under supervision/hospitalization
	—Feeding behaviors
Documentation	—Frequent visits with accurate recordings on growth chart

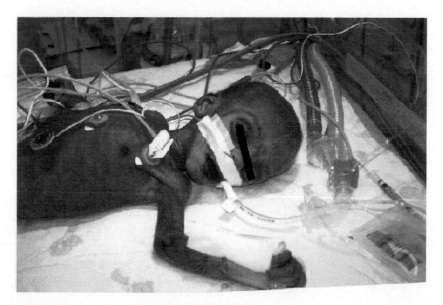

Photo 7.2 Seven month old with life-threatening malnutrition and dehydration. The baby weighed less than his birth weight at the time of hospital admission (7 months old). Note the sunken eyes, muscle wasting, and scaphoid appearance of the abdomen.

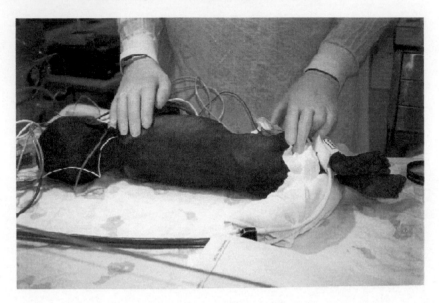

Photo 7.3 Posterior view of previous baby. Note the severe wasting. Marks on the lower back represent Mongolian spots. The baby had no evidence of physical injuries

History

The evaluation of FTT includes the medical history (see Chapter 2) and specific information about nutritional status, diet, and feeding behaviors. The following are areas to highlight in the FTT history:

1. Any history of medical conditions that may affect the amount of calories ingested, excreted, or internally expended.
2. Adequacy of caloric intake. The Committee on Dietary Allowances (1980) of the National Research Council estimates that healthy infants on average require approximately 115 kcal/kg during their first 6 months of life and that this can vary from 95 to 145 kcal/kg (10th–90th percentile, respectively). From 6 months to 1 year of age, the caloric requirement, on average, decreases to approximately 105 kcal/kg, ranging from 80 to 135 kcal/kg (10th–90th percentile, respectively). Approximate targets exist for the amount of formula an infant should receive based on the standard caloric content of commercial formulas (20 kcal/oz).
3. History of weight gain. On average, healthy infants who receive adequate caloric intake are expected to gain weight at standard rates, although a range of normal growth exists (Gahagan, 2006). The weight targets are approximately as follows:

   0–3 months of age → 27 g/day
   ≥3–6 months of age → 20 g/day

$\geq$6–12 months of age → 12 g/day
$\geq$12–18 months of age → 8 g/day

4. Family growth history, including information on the size, growth patterns, and timing of puberty of the biological parents as well as those of other family members (El-Baba et al., 2009). Methods exist to correct for genetic height expectations based on analysis of parental size (Himes, Roche, Thissen, & Moore, 1985; Tanner, Goldstein, & Whitehouse, 1970).

Physical Examination

A thorough physical examination focuses on findings suggestive of underlying disorders, growth parameters, and objective developmental assessment. The following are areas to highlight in the FTT physical examination.

1. *Findings indicative of underlying disease and/or physical signs of maltreatment.*

Signs of wasting as evidenced by loss of subcutaneous tissue in the buttocks, thighs, temporal and paraspinal areas, and around the rib cage (disease or maltreatment).

Nutritional deficiencies may reveal themselves through changes in the skin (e.g., dry, cracked), hair (e.g., sparse, fragile), teeth (e.g., caries, delayed eruption), and nails (e.g., dystrophic) (disease or maltreatment).

Physiological aberrations as evidenced by decreases in pulse, core body temperature, and body fat (disease or maltreatment).

Congenital syndromes with characteristic findings in the hands, feet, face, head, extremities, and body habitus (disease).

Signs of neglectful caretaking, such as dirty, poorly maintained clothing; excessive diaper rash; bald patch on the back of the head; poor grooming; and a general lack of proper hygiene (Hobbs et al., 1993).

2. *Growth measurements.* Standard growth parameters are plotted for weight, height/length, weight for height, and head circumference on NCHS growth charts. Many suggest expressing the child's weight as a "weight age." This is done by plotting the child's current weight and determining at what age this weight would represent the 50th percentile (Goldbloom, 1987). For example, a 2-year-old child at 9 kilos has a "weight age" of 10 months based on the NCHS charts.

Plotting and reviewing previous growth points is an important part of the growth assessment and assists in visualizing the growth pattern over time.

Head circumference is measured for at least the first 2 years, and recumbent length is measured until age 2 and then followed by a standing height.

Correction for prematurity is necessary when plotting growth parameters. This is done by subtracting the number of weeks that the baby is premature (based on a 40-week gestation) from the baby's chronological age and then plotting the measured growth parameter against the corrected age. Head circumference measurements are plotted against corrected age until a chronological age of 18 months.

Weight is corrected in this fashion until 24 months of age, and height measurements are corrected up to 40 months (Brandt, 1979).

Despite age correction, extremely premature infants and infants with severe intrauterine growth retardation (IUGR) may remain short throughout life. To evaluate the growth of IUGR infants, determine whether the IUGR was asymmetric or symmetric. Asymmetric IUGR exists when weight is lower than anticipated for gestational age but head circumference and length are spared. Symmetric IUGR exists when head circumference, length, and weight are all equally reduced for gestational age. Infants with symmetric IUGR have a relatively poor developmental prognosis and often fail to grow properly.

FTT is suspected with the following findings:

Growth parameters

a. weight and/or height/length measurements are less than the 3rd percentile (Stephens et al., 2008)
b. weight for height is less than 3rd percentile
c. weight-for-length < 80% of ideal weight (Block et al., 2005)

Growth pattern

a. measurements that follow a curve less than the 3rd percentile (keeping in mind that from a statistical perspective, 3% of healthy children will follow this pattern)
b. measurements that drop across at least two formal growth curves, namely 95th, 90th, 75th, 50th, 25th, 10th, 5th percentile curves
c. measurements that give rise to a fluctuating, "saw-toothed" pattern suggesting normal or near-normal growth punctuated by periods of poor growth

In addition to standard growth measurements, anthropometric growth assessments, such as mid-upper arm circumference and triceps skinfold thickness assessment may be assessed. This provides an objective assessment of fat and muscle mass and these measurements are typically performed by nutritionists and dieticians (Ayatollahi & Mostajabi, 2008).

3. *Assessment of developmental abilities.* Objective assessment of developmental abilities is also possible during the physical examination because components of standardized developmental screening tests are easily accomplished.

Specific, Directed Laboratory Evaluation

Laboratory tests and diagnostic procedures may be needed to evaluate FTT (Berwick, Levy, & Kleinerman, 1982; Homer & Ludwig, 1981; Sills, 1978). Laboratory tests confirm a diagnosis suggested by the clinical evaluation, but not all children evaluated for FTT need a laboratory evaluation. Specific laboratory tests are done during the workup. Random panels of tests rarely uncover etiologies not initially expected based on the history or physical.

Studies indicate that the usefulness of laboratory and radiologic tests alone in the diagnosis of neglect is low (Berwick et al., 1982; Sills, 1978). Berwick et al. (1982) retrospectively studied 122 children (between 1 and 25 months) admitted to a tertiary care center for FTT evaluation. An average of 40 laboratory and radiological procedures were performed per child, and only 0.8% were deemed helpful in making a diagnosis. Sills's (1978) retrospective study of 185 children hospitalized for FTT found similar results. Only 1.4% of all tests ordered were of positive diagnostic value, and no test was useful without a specific indication from the clinical evaluation.

The health care provider presented with a child who is failing to grow considers a wide range of possible etiologies. Basic laboratory screens that may be helpful are (a) CBC (e.g., anemia, infection); (b) erythrocyte sedimentation rate (e.g., infection, inflammation); (c) urinalysis (e.g., renal disease, infection); (d) urine culture (e.g., infection); (e) lead screen (e.g., anemia); and (f) electrolytes, including blood urea nitrogen (BUN) and serum creatinine (e.g., metabolic disorder, renal disease, renal tubular acidosis) (Zenel, 1997). A bone age may be useful as well as thyroid function tests if history and/or physical suggest a chromosomal or endocrinological disorder. The bone age is determined through a radiograph of the child's hand. The child's X-ray is then compared to "standards" by the radiologist, and a bone age is assigned (Zenel, 1997). This bone age is then compared to the child's chronological age looking for variation. After review of other evaluation components, further laboratory or radiological tests may be indicated based on clinician judgment.

Psychosocial Assessment and Feeding Observations

The evaluation of FTT includes a thorough psychosocial assessment that begins at the initial assessment and continues throughout the entire evaluation. Growth failure may be one of many indicators of psychosocial disorganization and may be associated with major life events. The health care provider explores the caregiving environment and asks questions about marital or relationship problems, lack of prenatal and postpartum care for the mother, and lack of immunizations and other health maintenance for the child (Ludwig, 1992). In addition, observation of interactions surrounding the child's feeding remains a critical component of this assessment. Areas that require specific attention include the following:

1. The caregiver's comfort with the child and his or her appreciation of the child's developmental accomplishments. Goldbloom (1987) suggests that the health care provider ask the caregivers a simple question: "Are you having fun with the baby?" Responses that include an instant smile or a cheerful affirmation are encouraging. Delayed, equivocal, or silent responses are concerning.
2. The child's feeding/dietary history along with observations of the caregiver/child interaction during feeding reveal whether mealtime is a healthy, pleasurable experience for the pair or if it is completed in anger or with force by a rejecting caregiver (Schmitt & Mauro, 1989). For example, a disturbed mother may feed

her infant with disinterest or with an obvious lack of awareness of the infant's minute-to-minute needs. The observer may uncover oral-motor difficulties with sucking, gagging, or swallowing, as well as ongoing struggles with feeding and food refusal.

Treatment

The design of the treatment plan for the child with FTT depends upon the results of the evaluation. If psychosocial concerns are prominent, a multidisciplinary treatment plan is ideal because it draws on the expertise of physician, nurse, social worker, and nutritionist. The treatment plan consists of standard therapy for the condition in the relatively uncommon situation in which FTT is caused purely by a medical condition with no psychosocial overlay. For example, if the child's FTT resulted from chronic diarrhea secondary to a bacterial infection, then the appropriate treatment is antibiotics and careful refeeding.

More commonly, medical conditions coexist with psychosocial problems. In this situation, complex management plans are necessary. Table 7.4 lists a differential diagnosis for FTT. In addition to indicated treatment for specific medical conditions, one needs to address the following: (a) nutritional requirements for catch-up growth and feeding behavior, (b) inpatient versus outpatient therapy, (c) comprehensive follow-up programs, and (d) whether a child protective services (CPS) report should be filed. Each component is discussed below.

1. *Nutrition and feeding.* Children with FTT require significantly more calories than the standard, recommended amount. To achieve "catch-up" growth, Krugman and Dubowitz (2003) recommend that a child will need on average 50% above the recommended requirement. Thus, an infant with an average need for 105 kcal/kg/day would require approximately 160 kcal/kg/day to achieve catch-up growth. If a baby weighs 6 kg and drinks a standard 20 kcal/oz formula, then he or she needs 32 oz (640 kcal) for routine growth and an additional 16 oz (total of 48 oz, 980 kcal) to ensure catch-up growth.

The requirement for catch-up growth frequently proves to be too large a volume for the child drinking a standard 20 kcal/oz formula. The caregiver can reconstitute concentrated or powdered formula using less water and achieve a higher caloric content. If the child is no longer on formula but on whole milk, the milk can be fortified with nonfat dry milk or instant breakfast preparations to increase its caloric content. In addition, several high caloric beverages are commercially available that may be used for supplementation.

In older children, caloric intake is more difficult to measure because of solid foods in the diet that are more variable in nutritional content. Baby food jars of fruits and vegetables contain approximately 15 kcal/oz and those of meats and desserts are 25–30 kcal/oz (Schmitt & Mauro, 1989). In addition, the caloric value of the child's foods can be enhanced by adding high-calorie food fortifiers such as (a) butter (40 kcal/tsp), (b) cheese (100 kcal/oz), (c) peanut butter (100 kcal/tsp), and (d) sour cream (30 kcal/tsp) (Tougas, cited in Bithoney, Dubowitz, & Egan, 1992).

Adequate management by a primary care provider of mild to moderate malnutrition is possible if he or she has experience with such cases. Nutritional consultation is recommended for more severe malnutrition in order to provide appropriate nutrients and calories and to guard against refeeding syndrome.

If feeding behaviors are poorly developed or dysfunctional, the caregiver requires (re)training that addresses general parenting skills, feeding routines, mealtime behaviors, and modeling of positive caregiver–child interactions. Videotaping of the caregiver–child interaction around feeding may provide the caregivers with insight into what some of these problems are.

2. *Inpatient versus outpatient therapy.* In the past, virtually all children who presented with FTT were admitted to the hospital for long lengths of stay to observe feeding and weight gain patterns. The changing health care environment discourages hospitalizations for children with FTT and, increasingly, shifts from inpatient care to outpatient care. However, clinical indications exist for both inpatient and outpatient care.

Inpatient stays offer the opportunity to provide close supervision and control over the amount and frequency of feeding. They are criticized as being artificial and potentially confusing to the caregiver if weight gain does not occur. In addition, requiring hospitalization to get a child to feed and gain weight may reinforce a sense of helplessness in the caregiver. Hospitalization of infants with FTT may be indicated if any of the following situations are present:

- Nonaccidental trauma
- Risk for nonaccidental trauma
- Sibling previously abused
- Caregiver appears angry, violent, or volatile
- Severe malnutrition, marasmus, kwashiorkor, or emaciation
- Weight less than birth weight at 2 months of age or older or no weight gain in more than 2 months
- Severe hygiene neglect, such as filthy, unwashed skin, or severe diaper rash
- Severely disturbed caregiver
- Negative caregiver–child interaction
- Outpatient treatment failure: no weight gain with 1-month trial of increased caloric feedings
- Caregiver refuses assistance with child's problem

Each case must be handled individually viewing the above criteria as clinical practice guidelines.

Outpatient trials have the advantage of being more natural and replicating what is possible at home. However, there is less control and supervision in the outpatient setting. Outpatient trials are recommended for less severe cases when there is no immediate danger to the child's health. Outpatient management for children with FTT is typically appropriate in the following circumstances:

- Child over 12 months of age
- State of malnutrition is in the mild to moderate range
- The caregiver–child interaction has some positive aspects

- The caregivers are accepting of help
- Absent risk factors for nonaccidental injuries

3. *Follow-up.* Active, ongoing, and continuous involvement by the health care provider with the child and caregiver (and CPS worker, if involved) is essential to ensure that the treatment plan is working. Medical appointments, in-home services, and psychological services for the caregiver(s) are frequently necessary over a period of months to years, depending on the family and how successful the original regimen was in fostering growth. (See Chapter 14 for further discussion of CPS and maltreatment follow-up.)

4. *Whether a CPS report should be filed.* Whether to report a case of FTT to CPS remains a primary management decision in the treatment of FTT. Laws guiding the reporting of neglect and FTT are intentionally vague to allow for clinical judgment. Cases where clear-cut parental misinstruction is the cause of the problem are best handled through education and close follow-up. For example, a case in which the caregiver misunderstood formula preparation instructions and mixed one part of formula with two parts of water (instead of the correct one part of water) may best be solved with caregiver education and careful follow-up in the health care provider's office.

CPS reporting is typically done in clinical situation with the following characteristics:

1. Physical abuse is present
2. Pervasive patterns of neglect or cruelty are uncovered
3. The caregivers appear incapable of adequately caring for the child (e.g., caregivers who are seriously mentally ill, substance abusers, severely cognitively impaired, homeless, or resistant to accepting assistance with their child's problem)

CPS may recommend foster placement as being in the child's best interest. In general, foster placement is considered in FTT cases if the caregiver

1. Rarely visits the child if hospitalized
2. Demonstrates a negative, punitive, or indifferent attitude toward the child
3. Remains uncooperative in the treatment protocol
4. Is an active substance abuser
5. Suffers from severe psychiatric illness
6. Is found to be severely cognitively impaired
7. Holds to dietary beliefs that are dangerous to the child's well-being (e.g., believes that child should feed only on fruits)

Medical Neglect

Caregivers may be deemed neglectful by refusing or delaying to meet the health care needs of their child (Jenny, C. & Committee on Child Abuse and Neglect, 2007) (See Photo 7.4). Such health care needs include

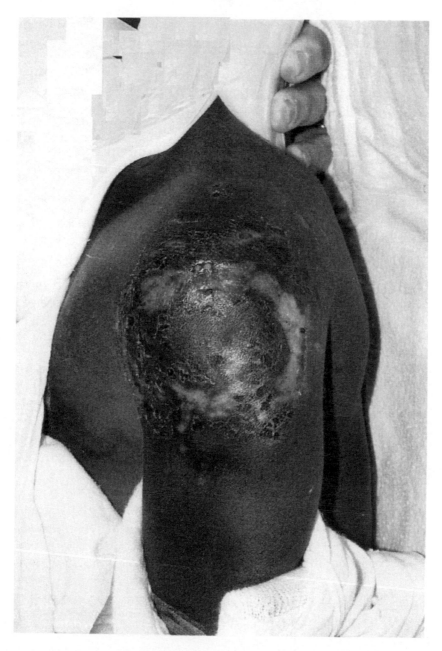

Photo 7.4 Three-year-old battered child with injuries of different ages to the shoulder. The exact mechanism of these injuries is not known. Repeated delays in seeking treatment led to poor probability for full healing.

- Routine preventive medical and dental care
- Timely access to acute care for illness or injury
- Meeting the ongoing care demands of a given condition (e.g., the chronically ill child) (DePanfilis, 2006)

Medical neglect may present to the health care provider in a number of ways. Typical presentations include

- Delay in seeking care for an injury or illness
- Failure to administer prescribed medications
- Administration of recommended medications in a manner or schedule that impairs appropriate care
- Noncompliance with routine preventive care needs (such as immunization schedules, lead and anemia screening, dental checkups)
- Noncompliance with the treatment needs for both acute and chronic conditions (such as failure to suction a tracheostomy according to the neonatologist's instructions)

Variability in the range of presentations exists. For example, reported cases of medical neglect in asthmatic patients include parents who fail to administer medicines properly as well as those who refuse to remove or separate the child from household pets that are known triggers of the child's asthma exacerbations (Boxer, Carson, & Miller, 1988; Franklin & Klein, 1987).

A distinction exists between noncompliance and medical neglect (Ludwig, 2005). Noncompliance occurs when the caregiver fails to carry through on the recommendations of the treating health care provider. This may or may not have negative consequences for the child. Medical neglect, on the other hand, occurs when the noncompliance or delay in seeking care results in further illness or worsening injury (See Photo 7.5). The distinction rests on the presence or absence of identifiable harm.

The treatment of medical neglect is tailored to each case depending on the child and caregiver. The evaluated level of risk or injury to the child will determine whether reporting medical neglect cases to CPS may be indicated. Hospitalization and/or removal from the home and placement in foster care may also be necessary if the child is at risk for injury or illness. Appropriate follow-up plans are essential to ensure compliance and assess adequacy of ongoing care.

Other Forms of Neglect

The health care provider faces children with other forms of neglect that include the following:

- *Supervisional*. Children who are abandoned may be brought to an emergency department for evaluation after a neighbor or relative alerts authorities to the possibility of supervisory neglect. Children may also sustain injuries due to inadequate supervision and require medical intervention. Abandonment is supported by a physical examination that reveals (a) poor hygiene, (b) hoarse cry,

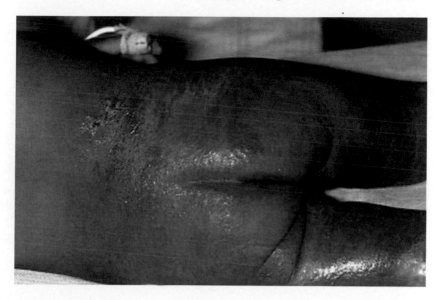

Photo 7.5 Child whose body cast was left in place beyond the recommended removal date. Note areas of erythema and skin breakdown.

(c) excessive hunger, or (d) dehydration. Appropriate management requires reporting the case to CPS and placing the child in a safe, properly supervised environment with either a family member or a foster parent. Another area that relates to supervisional neglect are children who sustain accidental injuries due to inadequate supervision.

- *Emotional.* Emotional (psychological) neglect is a form of maltreatment that involves caregiving that fails to provide a nurturing, development-promoting environment for the child's psychological and emotional well-being. The impact on the child is impaired psychological and emotional functioning. Many consider emotional neglect and emotional abuse synonymous because the damage inflicted upon the child's mental health by either is similar and often pervasive. Believed to be the most common form of maltreatment, emotional neglect is the least well-defined, the least diagnosed, and the least understood. The caregiving to which the child is exposed creates an environment in which he or she is at

1. A disadvantage in accomplishing developmental, peer, school, and community tasks.
2. Risk for experiencing chronic and severe anxiety, agitation, depression, social withdrawal, or unreasonable fears about his or her life.
3. Risk for failing to receive proper therapy for psychological or emotional problems (Ludwig, 2005).

The caregiving that the child receives is characterized by repetitive episodes that include belittling, neglect, humiliation, and verbal attacks on the child's value and worth. The child's self-image is destroyed and a myriad of dysfunctional behaviors, attitudes, and perspectives ensue (see Table 7.1). Diagnosis of this form of maltreatment requires careful observation and documentation of the caregiver's interactions with the child, both verbal and nonverbal. Management and treatment for the emotionally maltreated child will require the skills of mental health professionals, and close follow-up is essential (DePanfilis, 2006)

- Educational. Educational neglect is a manifestation of a caregiving environment that fails to provide adequately for a child's school attendance and performance. This situation may be due to a wide variety of reasons, ranging from a caregiver who is overwhelmed by life circumstances to a caregiver–child dynamic where the child's absences are encouraged through excessive dependency (DePanfilis, 2006). Psychosocial assessment is essential and the root causes for the failure to comply with the needs for formal schooling need to be addressed. Management and treatment require attention to the underlying causes and an approach that supports the child and caregiver in complying with educational obligations.

In Brief

- Neglect is the most commonly reported form of child maltreatment representing 64% of the 905,000 cases of maltreatment in the United States in 2006 (CM, 2006).
- A child's response to neglect depends on the type of neglect, the developmental stage at which the neglect occurred, the severity of the unmet need, the length of time that the child's need was not adequately met, and the effectiveness of the intervention by caring adults to halt the neglect.
- FTT is a term rooted firmly in clinical practice and remains the working diagnosis for children not growing as expected.
- The evaluation of FTT includes the medical history and specific information about nutritional status, diet, and feeding behaviors.
- The physical evaluation of FTT focuses on findings suggestive of underlying disorders, growth parameters, and objective developmental assessment.
- Observation of the child's feeding interactions is a critical component of the FTT assessment.
- The design of the treatment plan for the child with FTT depends on the cause of the growth failure.
- Reporting a case of FTT to child protective services (CPS) remains a primary management decision in treatment of FTT.
- Laws guiding the reporting of neglect and FTT are intentionally vague to allow for the clinician's judgment.
- The changing health care environment discourages hospitalizations for children with FTT and increasingly shifts care from inpatient to outpatient evaluation.
- Noncompliance occurs when the caregiver fails to carry through on the recommendations of the treating health care provider.
- Medical neglect occurs when the noncompliance or delay in seeking care results in further illness or worsening injury (Ludwig, 2005).

- Emotional (psychological) neglect is caregiving that fails to provide a nurturing, development-promoting environment for the child's psychological and emotional well-being.
- Educational neglect is a manifestation of a caregiving environment that fails to adequately provide for a child's school attendance and performance.

Note

1. *Refeeding syndrome* initially described the severe metabolic complications observed when a severely malnourished person was given concentrated calories via total parenteral nutrition. The term is now used more broadly and refers to the physiological complications that occur when a severely malnourished person is reintroduced to "normal" foodstuffs in an uncontrolled manner. In addition to phosphorus depletion, shifts in humoral potassium, magnesium, and glucose may have serious, even fatal, cardiovascular and neurological consequences (Solomon & Kirby, 1990).

Case A

E.T. demonstrates that medical causes of FTT may coexist with overwhelming social causes.

E.T. is a former 6 lb. 1 oz. term infant born to a teenage mother with an uncomplicated pregnancy and delivery. The baby was noted to be gaining weight appropriately until age 6 months. Between 6 and 9 months of age, the health care provider became increasingly concerned about the child's weight gain. Mother had difficulty keeping appointments, and the infant's weight began to drop off significantly (points C on growth chart in Figure 7.1). Evaluation revealed sketchy history of intermittent constipation and physical examination notable for hypotonicity and significant developmental delay. Due to mother's noncompliance with scheduled health care, the health care provider consulted social work services and arranged for home nursing visits.

Psychosocial evaluation uncovered a chaotic household and an inadequate diet due to the mother's lack of funds to purchase the infant's food. The health care providers considered that the "constipation" might be related to the poor diet. Between 9 and 11 months (C–C on growth chart in Figure 7.1), weight gain was noted but still below the fifth percentile. (In retrospect, this appears to have been related to severe constipation/impaction.) At age 12 months, weight loss was again noted and the child was admitted to the hospital for an inpatient evaluation. E.T.'s length leveled off between 6 and 12 months as well (see Figure 7.2).

Workup revealed Hirschsprung's disease. E.T. underwent surgical repair including placement of a colostomy (Point S on growth chart). On follow-up, E.T. began to gain weight, and his development improved. Social services remained involved to assist with the psychosocial issues uncovered during the evaluation.

Weight by age percentiles for boys aged birth – 36 months

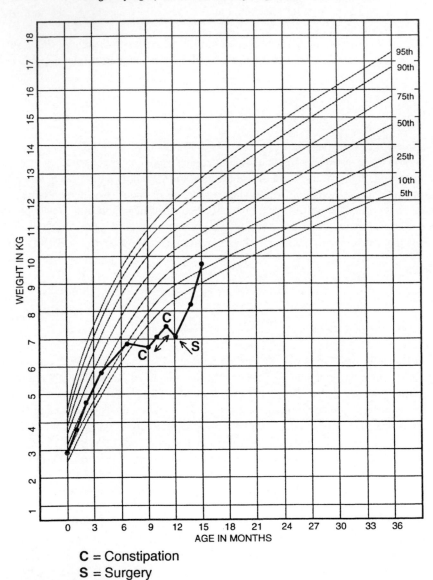

C = Constipation
S = Surgery

Figure 7.1 Case A: E.T's weight by age chart.

Length by age percentiles for boys aged birth – 36 months

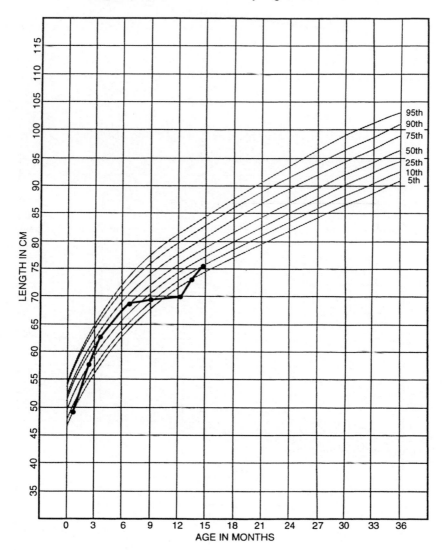

Figure 7.2 Case A: E.T.'s length by age chart.

Case B

T.H. demonstrates that observation over time provides useful information that may clarify the etiology of the growth failure.

T.H. is a term infant born to a 23-year-old mother who had an uncomplicated prenatal course with no history of smoking or drug use. Infant was first seen

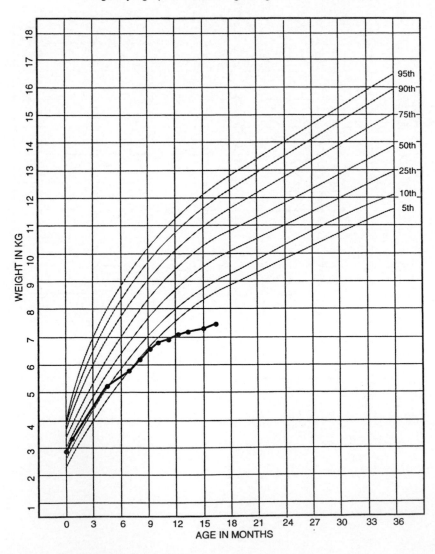

Figure 7.3 Case B: T.H.'s weight by age chart.

Length by age percentiles for girls aged birth – 36 months

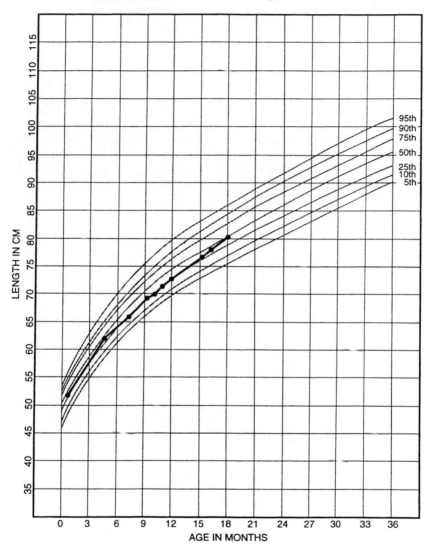

Figure 7.4 Case B: T.H.'s length by age chart.

in well-baby clinic at 2 weeks of age for routine care. She was breast-fed until 1 month of age, when mother stopped due to unsuccessful breast-feeding. Infant was initially placed on Isomil and then switched to Sin-lilac at 6 months of age. By 7 months of age, the baby's weight was noted to be dropping across percentiles (see Figures 7.3 and 7.4 for T.H.'s growth charts). This seemed to correlate with the introduction of solids. She continued to be closely followed and was referred to an early intervention feeding program.

Over the next 6 months, she was followed closely with frequent weight checks. Her weight gain continued to be poor (see Figure 7.3), and she was now below the fifth percentile. Length remained at approximately the 50th percentile (see Figure 7.4). Initial evaluation consisted of basic laboratory testing and results were unremarkable. At 13 months of age, after no sustained improvement in weight gain, T.H. was hospitalized for an inpatient workup. She was able to demonstrate weight gain during the hospital stay.

Psychosocial evaluation noted that mother appeared depressed with sullen expression and flat affect. During ongoing care, the mother was noted to be losing weight herself. When questioned about her personal eating habits, she revealed a childhood history of multiple caregivers and foster care placement. She related being force-fed to vomiting for almost 1 year and appeared terrorized when recounting experience. Mother said she was afraid of making her daughter vomit. Mother also related how she can go a day or more without eating solids. "I sometimes don't feel hungry, so I don't eat."

The mother was unreceptive to the health care provider's suggestion that the mother seek psychological counseling, although she did agree that she was depressed. The child was referred to Child Protective Services for supportive services.

Case C

S.S. demonstrates how careful assessment of the social environment and correlation to the growth pattern observed over time may uncover the cause of a child's growth failure.

S.S. is an SGA term infant born to a 17-year-old mother in 11th grade. S.S. is cared for by her mother during summer vacations (A on growth chart in Figure 7.5) and by her maternal grandmother during the school year (B on growth chart in Figure 7.5). Initially, her growth was consistent with an SGA infant whose mother was 5 ft, 2 in. tall. Her growth pattern over 18 months revealed intermittent periods of growth retardation (A on growth chart in Figure 7.5). Basic laboratory findings were unremarkable. Length seemed to follow a pattern consistent with an SGA infant (see Figure 7.6). At S.S.'s 18-month visit, the health care provider correlated the episodes of poor weight gain with the primary caregiver transition from grandmother to mother that occurred during summer vacations.

Weight by age percentiles for girls aged birth – 36 months

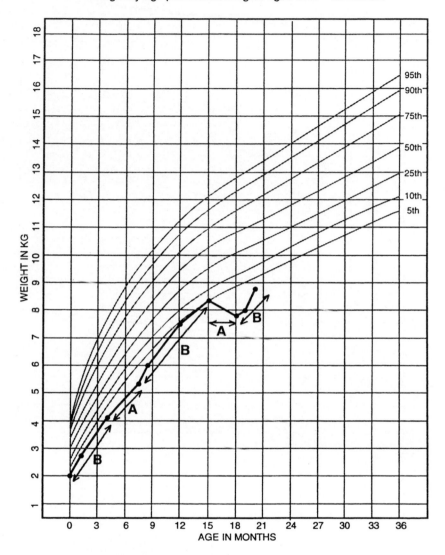

A = Summer
B = School Year

Figure 7.5 Case C: S.S.'s weight by age chart.

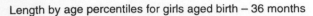

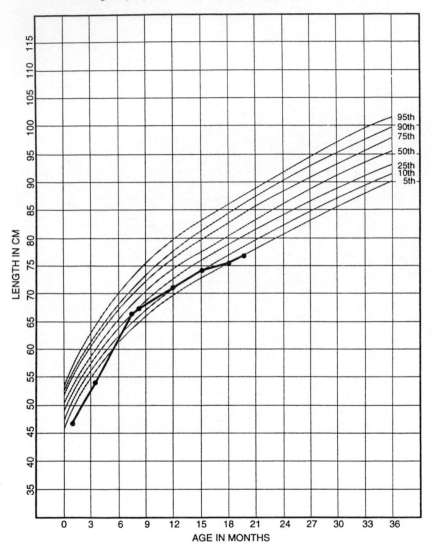

Figure 7.6 Case C: S.S.'s length by age chart.

References

American Academy of Pediatrics. (2003). Failure to thrive (pediatric undernutrition). In R. E. Kleinman (ed.), *Pediatric nutrition handbook* (5th ed., pp. 443–457). Elk Grove Village, IL: American Academy of Pediatrics.

Ayatollahi, S.-M.-T., & Mostajabi, F. (2008). Triceps skinfold thickness centile charts in primary school children in Shiraz. *Archives of Iranian Medicine, 11*(2), 210–213.

Barbero, G. J., & Shaheen, E. (1967). Environmental failure to thrive: A clinical view. *Journal of Pediatrics, 71*, 639–644.

Berwick, D. M., Levy, J. C., & Kleinerman, R. (1982). Failure to thrive: Diagnostic yield of hospitalization. *Archives of Diseases of Childhood, 57*, 347–351.

Bithoney, W. G., Dubowitz, H., & Egan, H. (1992). Failure to thrive/growth deficiency. *Pediatrics in Review, 13*, 453–459.

Block, R. W., Krebe, N. F., & The Committee on Child Abuse and Neglect, and the Committee on Nutrition. (2005). Clinical report. Guidance for the clinician in rendering care. American academy of pediatrics. *Pediatrics, 116*, 1234–1237.

Boxer, G. H., Carson, J., & Miller, B. D. (1988). Neglect contributing to tertiary hospitalization in childhood asthma. *Child Abuse & Neglect, 12*, 491–501.

Brandt, L. (1979). Growth dynamics of low birthweight infants with emphasis on the perinatal period. In F. Faulkner & J. Tanner (Eds.), *Human growth neurobiology and nutrition*. New York: Plenum.

Chapin, H. D. (1908). A plan for dealing with atrophic infants and children. *Archives of Pediatrics, 25*, 491–496.

Chatoor, J., & Egan, J. (1983). Nonorganic failure to thrive and dwarfism due to food refusal: A separation disorder. *Journal of the American Academy of Child Psychiatry, 22*, 294.

DePanfilis, D. (2006). Child neglect: A guide for prevention, assessment, and intervention. U.S. department of health and human services. Administration for children and families. Administration on children, youth and families children's bureau. Office on child abuse and neglect. http://www.childwelfare.gov/pubs/usermanuals/neglect/neglect.pdf

Dubowitz, H., Black, M., Starr, R. H., & Zuravin, S. (1993). A conceptual definition of child neglect. *Criminal Justice and Behavior, 20*, 8–26.

Dubowitz, H., Giardino, A. P., & Gustavson, E. (2000). Child neglect: Guidance for pediatricians (Review). *Pediatrics in Review, 21*(4), 111–116.

El-Baba, M. F., Bassali, R. W., & Benjamin, J. (2009, May 4). Failure to thrive. eMedicine. http://emedicine.medscape.com/article/985007-overview

Fontana, V. J., & Besharov, D. J. (1979). *The maltreated child: The maltreatment syndrome in children— a medical, legal, and social guide* (4th ed.). Springfield, IL.: Charles C Thomas.

Fontana, V. J., Donovan, D., & Wong, R. J. (1963). The maltreatment syndrome in children. *New England Journal of Medicine, 269*, 1389–1394.

Franklin, W., & Klein, R. E. (1987). Severe asthma due to household pets: A form of child abuse or neglect. *New England Regional Allergy Proceedings, 8*, 259–261.

Gahagan, S. (2006). Failure to thrive: A consequence of undernutrition. *Pediatrics in Review, 27*, e1–e11.

Gaudin, J. M. (1993). *Child neglect: A guide for intervention*. U.S. Department of Health and Human Services: Administration for Children and Families: National Center on Child Abuse and Neglect.

Goldbloom, R. B. (1987). Growth failure in infancy. *Pediatrics in Review, 9*(2), 57–61.

Himes, J. H., Roche, A. F., Thissen, D., & Moore, W. M. (1985). Parent-specific adjustments for evaluation of recumbent length and stature of children. *Pediatrics, 75*, 304–313.

Hobbs, C. J., Hanks, H. G. I., & Wynne, T. M. (1993). Failure to thrive. In *Child abuse and neglect: A clinician's handbook* (pp. 17–45). New York: Churchill Livingstone.

Homer, C., & Ludwig, S. (1981). Categorization of etiology of failure to thrive. *American Journal of Diseases of Children, 135*, 848–851.

Jenny, C. & Committee on Child Abuse and Neglect (2007). Recognizing and responding to medical neglect. *Pediatrics, 120*(6), 1385–1389.

Kempe, R. S., & Goldbloom, R. B. (1987). Malnutrition and growth retardation ("failure to thrive") in the context of child abuse and neglect. In R. E. Helfer & R. S. Kempe (Eds.), *The battered child* (4th ed., pp. 312–335). Chicago: University of Chicago Press.

Kempe, R. S., Silverman, F. N., Steele, B. F., Droegmueller, W., & Silver, H. K. (1962). The battered child syndrome. *Journal of the American Medical Association, 181,* 17–24.

Krugman, S. D., & Dubowitz, H. (2003). Failure to thrive. *American Family Physician, 68,* 879–884.

Ludwig, S. (1992). Failure to thrive/starvation. In S. Ludwig & A. E. Kornberg (Eds.), *Child abuse: a medical reference* (2nd ed.). New York: Churchill Livingstone

Ludwig, S. (2005). Psychosocial emergencies: Child abuse. In G. R. Fleisher & S. Ludwig (Eds.), *Textbook of pediatric emergency medicine* (5th ed., pp. 1761–1802). Baltimore: Williams and Wilkins.

National Center on Child Abuse and Neglect. (1988a). *Child neglect: A guide for intervention.* Washington, DC: U.S. Department of Health and Human Services.

National Center on Child Abuse and Neglect. (1988b). *Study findings: Study of national incidence and prevalence of child abuse and neglect.* Washington, DC: U.S. Department of Health and Human Services.

Olson, E. M. (2006, January/February). Failure to thrive: Still a problem of definition. *Clinical Pediatrics, 45,* 1–6.

Pears, K. C., Kim, H. K., & Fisher, P. A. (2008). Psychosocial and cognitive functioning of children with specific profiles of maltreatment. *Child Abuse & Neglect, 32*(10), 958–971.

Peterson, M. S., & Urquiza, A. J. (1993). *The role of mental health professionals in the prevention and treatment of child abuse and neglect.* Washington, DC: U.S. Department of Health and Human Services.

Satler, E. (1990). Childhood feeding problems. In *Feelings and their medical significance.* Columbus, OH: Ross Laboratories.

Schmitt, B. D., & Mauro, R. D. (1989). Nonorganic failure to thrive: An outpatient approach. *Child Abuse & Neglect, 13,* 235–248.

Sills, R. H. (1978). Failure to thrive: The role of clinical and laboratory evaluation. *American Journal of Diseases of Children, 132,* 967–969.

Spitz, R. A. (1945). Hospitalism: An inquiry into the genesis of psychiatric conditions in early childhood. *Psychoanalytic Study of the Child, 1,* 53–74.

Spitz, R. A. (1949). The role of ecological factors in emotional development in infancy. *Child Development, 20*(3), 145–155.

Stephens, M. B., Gentry, B. C., Michener, M. D. (2008). What is the clinical workup for failure to thrive? *Journal of Family Practice, 57*(4), 264–266.

Tanner, J. M., Goldstein, H., & Whitehouse, P. H. (1970). Standards for children's height at age 2–9 years allowing for height of parents. *Archives of Diseases of Childhood, 45,* 755–762.

Tunnessen, W. W., Jr., & Roberts, K. B. (1999). *Signs and symptoms in pediatrics* (3rd ed.). Philadelphia: Lippincott Williams & Wilkins.

U.S. Department of Health and Human Services Administration for Children and Families. (2008). Child Maltreatment 2006. http://www.acf.hhs.gov/programs/cb/pubs/cm06/cm06.pdf. Accessed April 15, 2009.

Wolock, I., & Horowitz, B. (1984). Child maltreatment as a social problem: The neglect of neglect. *American Journal of Orthopsychiatry, 54,* 530–543.

Zenel, J. A. (1997). Failure to thrive. *Pediatrics in Review, 18,* 371–378.

Chapter 8

Medical Child Abuse

Reena Isaac and Thomas A. Roesler

Introduction

A few years ago this chapter might have begun with an account of the Baron von Munchausen. It might have chronicled the life of an elderly German soldier turned raconteur, who lived from 1720 to 1797, who loved to frequent the salons of Europe and entertain people with his stories, and who was made famous by one of his countrymen (Meadow & Lennert, 1984). We would explain how Rudolph Raspe wrote a book of tall tales, children's stories in the same vein as Paul Bunyan that he attributed to the Baron (Raspe, 1944). This account would precede a description of Meadow's original paper "Munchausen syndrome by proxy: The hinterland of child abuse" (Meadow, 1977). It would seek to establish that the central feature of this form of child abuse was the falsehoods told by parents who tricked physicians into giving unnecessary medical care.

But today we no longer have to begin a chapter with the story of the Baron. Today we can say that for the past 30 years we have been looking at this type of child abuse through the wrong end of the telescope. Instead of focusing on the lies told by the perpetrator and on how that person fooled the doctor, we can now acknowledge the need to begin by looking at the harm to the child caused by the parent's actions.

Medical child abuse is defined as a child receiving unnecessary and harmful or potentially harmful medical care at the instigation of a caretaker (Roesler & Jenny, 2008). It results from a parent relating to a physician in a way that leads the medical care provider to expose the child to possibly harmful treatment. Any medical procedure, for example, a blood draw, or a trial of medication that is potentially harmful, could be considered abusive if there was no clear medical reason for it to happen. Over the past 30 years there have been hundreds of published reports of children receiving such care based on the actions of caretakers, primarily mothers (Rosenberg, 1987).

291

A.P. Giardino et al. (eds.), *A Practical Guide to the Evaluation of Child Physical Abuse and Neglect*, DOI 10.1007/978-1-4419-0702-8_8, © Springer Science+Business Media, LLC 1997, 2010

In order to make a diagnosis of medical child abuse, it is important to know if the child received harmful medical care based on a parent's actions. Medical child abuse has many features in common with the other forms of maltreatment as well as a number of characteristics that distinguish it from physical, sexual, or psychological abuse. It is not essential to know *why* the parent acted in a way that compelled the doctor to give mistaken treatment. The motivation of the parent comes into play later when determining whether a child can be returned safely to the home environment, much as with other forms of abuse. Furthermore, one can assume a parent would lie about their actions just as one can assume that parents often lie when confronted about maltreating their children.

The process of rethinking the Munchausen syndrome by proxy (MSBP) concept has been evolving over a number of years. Difficulty with the concept was voiced as early as 20 years ago. Many recommended that the use of MSBP gave no indication as to what happened to the child and suggested substituting what exactly occurred, for example as in poisoning or suffocation (Fisher & Mitchell, 1995; Morley, 1995).

A special taskforce of the American Professional Society on the Abuse of Children (APSAC) made a significant effort to deal with the confusion surrounding MSBP and reported in the journal *Child Maltreatment* (Ayoub et al., 2002). In an attempt to address the confusion, including the controversy regarding who should carry the diagnosis, the taskforce decided to divide the entity in two. Thus, *pediatric condition falsification* (PCF) was the name assigned to the child victim. *Factitious disorder* by proxy (FDP) was retained as a diagnosis given to the parent. The authors of the report indicate that one condition could exist without the other. However, when both elements (PCF *and* FDP) were involved, MSBP, the original designation, could be applied to the disorder (Schreier, 2002).

The attempted solution to the confusion surrounding MSBP was only partially successful. Later writers used the term *Munchausen syndrome by proxy abuse* (Meadow, 2002) to emphasize the abuse rather than the deception by the parent. And yet another attempted solution is represented by the more recent term, *fabricated or induced illness in a child by a carer* (Bools, 2007). However, none of these efforts were able to take the final step and eliminate the notion of fabrication from the definition.

The use of the term "medical child abuse" eliminates the difficulty with the terminology and implications of MSBP. The use of medical child abuse ensures that the focus is properly placed back on the child victim, that abuse has occurred, and that the abuse has taken place within a medical setting. The recent policy statement by the American Academy of Pediatrics follows this general use and places the emphasis firmly on the abuse rather than the abuser (Stirling, 2007).

Background

Medical abuse shares the same relationship with medical neglect that physical and psychological abuse have with physical neglect and psychological neglect. Medical neglect occurs when a *parent* does not provide the medical care a child needs.

Medical abuse represents a *parent* seeking out excessive medical care for the child. In neither situation is the doctor committing neglect or abuse. The doctor or medical system is a tool, a conduit through which the abuse is carried out.

In all forms of abuse, physical, sexual, psychological, or medical, there is a wide range of ways the abuse can present. Physical abuse can involve beating, burning, biting, or cutting. Psychological abuse can result from belittling, criticism, shaming, or blaming. Likewise, medical abuse has a large variety of presentations.

The various presentations of all forms of abuse can be sorted on a continuum from mild to severe. For example, a child who misses school because his mother takes him to unnecessary medical appointments would fall on the mild end of the continuum, while a child who receives unnecessary surgery is at the extreme end.

In all forms of abuse there is a threshold beyond which it is deemed necessary to protect children from the actions of their caretakers. In the above example the child who only goes to appointments and gets unnecessary physical exams would probably not warrant protection yet a child getting unnecessary major surgery would almost certainly need to be defended from the actions of his parent. There are physical and psychological consequences for the child that range from mild to severe and the consequences are not always commensurate with the severity of the abuse. For example, a child sexually molested one time might have lifelong psychological issues while a victim of long standing incest might not consider her abuse to be particularly debilitating. While long-term effects of medical abuse have not been studied as well as other forms of child maltreatment, the few existing reports of medical child abuse are consistent with other forms of abuse (Libow, 1995).

There are four treatment phases for all types of child abuse, and these phases are essentially the same across all types of child abuse. The first phase of treatment, and perhaps the biggest challenge for all abuse presentations, is to identify that abuse is taking place. Sexual abuse can continue for many years before it comes to the light of day. The same is true with medical abuse. The second step in child abuse treatment is to stop it. The third step is to provide for ongoing safety. Step four is treatment of the physical and psychological effects of the abuse. The goal is to accomplish the four steps while both protecting the integrity of the family and keeping the child safe.

Just as the forms of child maltreatment share many similarities, so do the perpetrators. Studies of perpetrators often document unhappy childhoods with histories of maltreatment. Being abused in childhood does not necessarily result in a parent who abuses her child. Nor should a parent who had no abuse history be considered incapable of committing harm to offspring. However, in general, adults tend to treat their children in the way they were treated.

Perpetrators of all forms of abuse often lie about their involvement and make excuses for their behavior. The excuses differ with the type of abuse, but the tendency to avoid responsibility is common to all presentations. Similarly, treatment of perpetrators is preconditioned on the adult entering into a sincere treatment relationship that includes some self-awareness of the consequences of his or her actions. In all forms of abuse perpetrators tend not to seek treatment until strongly encouraged by representatives of society.

The difference between medical abuse and physical, sexual, or psychological maltreatment is the type of harm. A physically molested child is damaged from a physical act. A sexually abused child has been exposed to harmful sexual behavior. A medically abused child has received unnecessary medical care.

Case Report

A 6-month-old baby boy had a history of multiple presumed diagnoses of gastroesphogeal reflux, laryngomalacia, plagiocephaly, obstructive and central sleep apnea, and other reported medical conditions. The patient was hospitalized for a month for the inability to tolerate oral feeds. After an extensive medical workup that revealed no definitive medical cause for the baby's food intolerance, a nasoduodenal tube was placed to provide the child nutrition and the patient was then discharged. The infant was readmitted after the mother reported projectile vomiting episodes and the inability to maintain feeds. During the admission process it was noted that the child had normal electrolytes, normal vital signs, and no significant weight loss or dehydration. The infant underwent a fundoplication and G-tube placement during this hospitalization.

Medical and surgical staff began raising concerns regarding the history provided by the mother as the child's symptoms were not congruent with the clinical picture. The chart documented numerous lab reports with findings that were normal or equivocal. The mother frequently reported that the child was in pain. However, during documented observations and interviews, staff usually described the child as "smiling and in no distress." The mother said the child had a helmet fitted in the neonatal unit to treat a "flattened head" (presumed diagnosis of plagiocephaly). However, the child at 8 months had a round head. The mother, nevertheless, insisted on the child wearing the helmet. She complained to the hospital intern that the baby had a "very horrible diaper rash" and needed medicated cream. The intern examined the baby and did not see a rash of any kind.

The child's mother was quite active socially on the wards, walking around the halls of the floor with the baby in his helmet, and entering other patient's rooms despite requests by the nursing staff to respect the patients' privacy and concerns for infection control. The mother inquired about the medical status of patients.

The concerns created by the behavior of the mother prompted a report to Child Protective Services. The medical staff recommended the mother be removed from the hospital to allow a realistic medical assessment of the child. During this period, the physicians were able to eliminate all of the prior presumed diagnoses, except laryngomalacia, and the child was taken off all medications. Eventually, the baby was found to eat adequately without the need of the G-tube, which was quickly removed. The child was placed in foster care, as there were concerns that the mother would likely continue to have access to the child if placed with a family member. Child Protective Services reported a month after the child's discharge that the mother insisted that the baby had a sponge accidentally left behind during a previous surgery. She insisted that the baby be reevaluated. An X-ray of the child's abdomen did not reveal a foreign object.

A 9-year-old sibling of the baby was subsequently removed from the mother when it was discovered that the sibling's medical visits and investigations increased significantly in the period after the baby's removal from the mother's care.

Identifying Medical Child Abuse

The first step in identifying that a child is possibly being harmed is to consider that maltreatment might be taking place. The inclusion of medical child abuse in the list of differential diagnoses may facilitate the thought process involved in determining whether medical child abuse is present. As with other forms of abuse, the diagnosis is made after taking a careful history, doing a thorough physical exam, and noticing inconsistencies between the history provided by the caretaker and the clinical picture. In medical child abuse, clinicians may need to consider whether specific treatments might not have been necessary. This requires that clinicians have the confidence to question previous care, the clarity to see clinical decisions based on potentially false information, and the fortitude to correct a medical plan and protect a child from further harm.

The following aspects of care are essential components that provide the blueprints of medical investigations into a diagnosis of MCA and possible management and monitoring methods (Mian, 1995; Roesler & Jenny, 2008; Stirling, 2007):

- *Clear and Open Communication*:

There is an understanding within the physician–patient relationship that the common goal is the improved health and welfare of the child. In pediatric medicine, this relationship most often extends to the parent of the child. The unspoken assumption is that the history provided by the historian (i.e. the parent) is accurate and timely. The physician and parent work together toward the common goal which is the health of the child. Physicians understand that the emotions and reactions of concerned parents may logically distort a parent's perception of symptoms of a sick child. However, the line is crossed when medical treatment is manipulated in a manner that ultimately brings harm to the child by deceptive means. Close coordination and communication with other medical care providers (i.e., subspecialists, former primary care physicians of the index case), though not a guarantee of preventing MCA, can assist in identifying and clarifying such cases. Direct communication between physicians would make unnecessary the use of the parent as the conduit of medical advice from other disciplines and may potentially prevent or identify such cases.

The primary care physician can serve as a "gatekeeper" for present and future medical care utilization. In this capacity, one physician has knowledge of all medical diagnoses and treatments of the child and siblings and can limit redundant or superfluous medical care. One approach might include "flagging" such cases by the insurance provider and thereby alerting the primary care physician or institution of extraneous medical consultations. Another manner in which the primary care physician is made aware of excessive medical utilizations is by having the parent authorize the school to communicate to the physician when there is an unexplained absence without the physician's approval. These options are very useful in tracking such cases and can be best introduced with either the help of the Child Protective Services or the parent's (more often the nonoffending parent's) authorization (Stirling, 2007).

- *Conservative Medical Investigations*:

The pursuit of an elusive medical diagnosis that defies objective medical theory and management may drive the medical team to investigate by increasingly more invasive and painful means. Sensible and balanced testing may minimize unnecessary intervention and harm to the child. The decisions for diagnostic investigations should be based on medical necessity, a consideration of risk/benefit analysis, low morbidity, and the ability to distinguish between a true organic condition and medical child abuse (Mian, 1995). Cautious consideration must be practiced when relying on parental observation. The physician may need to reevaluate a clinical decision and clinical course and ensure that reported observations of the child's medical course are not being filtered through a questionable source. When the diagnosis is elusive and diagnostic efforts become more aggressive, the physician must always weigh risks to the patient against the benefits of an accurate diagnosis.

In some cases, poisoning for example, one may need to collect samples to identify extraneous or foreign substances. It is prudent to have a system in place that allows for a "chain of custody" protocol in handling such specimens. For example, if MCA is strongly suspected in a child who has recently vomited, the vomitus may be collected and analyzed for the presence of emetine while making sure that proper handling of the specimens is in place to satisfy later forensic needs.

Other investigations may require not only the presence of a substance (qualitative) but also the measured levels (quantitative) of the material. Such information can allow us to know when substances were introduced to the patient. A discussion with a local toxicologist may assist in clarifying such situations while addressing compounding factors such as the child's symptoms, medications genuinely prescribed, and underlying medical conditions and situations.

- *Collection of Medical Information (Child's Past Medical History): Comprehensive Medical Record Review*

In complicated and potentially severe presentations, medical record review is the central feature of the evaluation (Roesler & Jenny, 2008; Sanders & Bursch, 2002). It is a long and tedious process, made more difficult by the large number of records usually involved and by the complexity of the medical issues (true medical conditions that are concurrent with suspected spurious symptoms).

The process begins with the birth records of the child and involves recording on a timeline every medical event in the child's life.

- Obtain all of the child's medical records. Various social and legal agencies can assist in obtaining information that may otherwise be difficult to retrieve. Some cases may involve several different medical institutions, different subspecialists, and/or different cities or states (Table 8.1).

Table 8.1 Chronology of events.

Date	Patient	Event	Location/ Provider	Diagnosis/ Complaint	Comment
4/19/2008	Brittany	Admitted	West Hospital	Acute gastroenteritis	No vomitus seen
4/25/2008	Brittany	Office visit	Dr. Apple	Otitis media	Antibiotics given, normal exam
4/27/08	Brittany	Phone call	Dr. Apple	Difficulty in breathing	

Table 8.1: (Chronology of Events) is an example of a timeline fashioned to detail: the child's medical history, dates and locations of treatment, the chief complaints, supporting medical information, the treatments given, and specific comments. Hospitalizations, office visits, and phone calls are reviewed.

- Search for patterns. Particular attention is paid to times when medical appointments ceased for a significant period. It is important to consider why care stopped (i.e. a sibling was hospitalized; the mother was pregnant). Or alternatively, consider when medical appointments became more frequent, and why (i.e. parents separated or divorced; a period of stress is recognized). Occasions might be noted where multiple providers are treating the same reported condition.
- Take special appraisal of the physician notes as well as documentation of nursing and ancillary staff (occupational therapist, speech therapists, and social worker's notes).

These disciplines may have more frequent interactions and might note observations that are not sometimes apparent to the physician who has been investigating a particular symptom.

- Note documented inconsistencies within the records. In a complicated case it is often necessary to request medical records for the index patient, the siblings, and the parents or caretaker suspected of abusing the child (Trent, 2008). At some point a threshold is reached and the decision must be made whether the child needs protection from ongoing unnecessary medical care.

Clear and Watchful Monitoring

There are times when objective observation of the child is required to determine what is true and what is clinically spurious. In these circumstances, it may be valuable to admit the child to a hospital setting, where it is possible to monitor his or her actual signs and symptoms (as opposed to the signs and symptoms being filtered through the report of the parent). This consideration is important if the caretaker tends to exaggerate or lie about the child's pain or disability.

Placing a child in a hospital setting is only useful if it can be ensured that the parent cannot continue to act in a way that will result in harmful care. One might need to order constant observation of the child (having a hospital aide to sit and monitor the child), or even exclude the parent from the hospital completely. Some parents have been known to directly alter their child's medical record.

Covert Video Surveillance

One diagnostic tool that has received considerable attention is covert video surveillance (CVS). This involves using a hidden video camera to observe a parent interacting with her child without being aware she is being watched. There are published reports of video evidence being used to convict perpetrators who smothered their children thereby committing physical abuse and, in addition, the medical abuse that often accompanies illness induction (Southall et al., 1987). Despite recommendation that every children's hospital have the capacity to do covert video surveillance, very few facilities are actually equipped to do so (Hall, Eubanks, Meyyazhagan, Kenney, & Johnson, 2000).

Covert video surveillance has been used to diagnose medical child abuse for more than 20 years. For almost as long there have been calls to eliminate its use on ethical or moral grounds (Evans, 1994, 1995, 1996). Southall and his colleagues have conducted a lengthy debate in the British medical literature with opponents (Southall, Plunkett, Banks, Falkov, & Samuels, 1997; Southall & Samuels, 1996). They argue that CVS is a diagnostic test, not an experimental procedure, that it does not violate privacy of adults who are taking care of their children in a semi-public environment in the hospital, and that it is sometimes necessary to save the lives of children. Hall agrees and states that one positive benefit from CVS is that it occasionally exonerates parents previously suspected of harming their children (Hall et al., 2000).

Instituting a program of CVS is not a simple task. A responsible staff person must be available 24 h a day to observe the behavior of the mother and child on a remote monitor. Without this element the child is exposed to potential and preventable harm. It is clearly unethical to establish a monitoring system, allow abuse to take place, and then view the video evidence hours or days later. Another difficulty arises when a mother who might be harming the child at home chooses not to do so in the hospital environment. A video that does not show harm could be used to prove that no harm has taken place when in fact the opposite is true.

Final Diagnosis

While many various professionals may raise the suspicion of the possibility of medical child abuse, the ultimate medical diagnosis must be determined by a physician. The evaluation for suspected MCA is essentially a sum of its parts: careful, detailed history taking, physical examination, laboratory/diagnostic analysis, and comprehensive chart review. Such medical investigations are pursued with a conservative, measured approach.

Presentation

There is no one typical way children can be victimized by receiving excessive medical care. All organ systems are potential targets. Symptom presentations are limited only by the perpetrator's medical knowledge, sophistication, and imagination. Actions taken by perpetrators that create the charade of organic conditions include the following:

- *Exaggeration*: i.e. embellishing or heightening an existing medical condition or symptom in order to obtain more medical attention and care.
- *Fabrication*: i.e. lying about non-existent symptoms.
- *Persuasion*: i.e. repeatedly demanding medical care until the physician gives in to the demand; altering perceptions of a child's condition.
- *Simulation*: i.e. contaminating specimens collected for laboratory analysis.
- *Induction*: i.e. actually directly hurting the child and then seeking unnecessary medical treatment for the induced condition (Table 8.2).

Table 8.2 Common presentations and examples of how they may produced.

Apnea: manual suffocation, poisoning, induced hypoglycemia
Seizures: lying, poisoning, suffocation
Diarrhea: laxative poisoning, salt poisoning, contamination
Vomiting: poisoning (ipecac ingestion), lying
CNS depression: drugs, suffocation
Bleeding: blood thinning meds, exogenous blood applied, paints/dye
Rash: drug, caustics
Fever: contamination w/ infected material, falsifying temps

Meadow (1977), Southall & Samuels (1996), Carter, Izsak, & Marlow (2006), Holstege & Dobmeier (2006), Aranibar & Cerda (2005), de Ridder & Hoeska (2000).

Table 8.2 displays examples of commonly reported symptoms and how they may be surreptitiously fabricated or induced.

Prevalence

Child abuse is not an illness. It is a painful event in the life of a child. It can result in both physical and psychological illness and frequently does. Child abuse is an act committed by an adult on a child that takes many forms. To determine its prevalence requires us to take into consideration many factors. First there needs to be a definition of the behavior that is considered abusive. This involves society determining at what point along the spectrum from mild to severe a child might need protection.

The definition of abuse and the threshold point shifts from culture to culture and over time. It stands to reason that mild forms might be quite common and the more severe presentations might be uncommon.

This description of child abuse in general is also true for medical child abuse. How many children have received antibiotics for a viral infection at the insistence of a parent who is adamant that her child cannot recover from the illness without what is essentially useless treatment? This "mild presentation" might have a very high prevalence. It also would not likely meet the community standard for a child needing protection.

Attempts to establish prevalence rates of MSBP have been hampered by the lack of an objective, quantifiable definition. The only serious attempts were made in Great Britain and New Zealand where two different groups sought to determine the frequency of severe events. McClure and colleagues (McClure, Davis, Meadow, & Sibert, 1996) in England searched child protection records for founded cases of MSBP, primarily involving induction of illness such as suffocation and non-accidental poisoning. Using the number of cases identified and the number of children in the geographic area covered by the records, they determined an approximate prevalence rate of 0.5 in 100,000 children. A similar attempt to establish prevalence in New Zealand involved sending questionnaires to pediatricians in the country surveying for possible cases of MSBP. The authors concluded that 2 in 100,000 children met their criteria for MSBP (Denny, Grant, & Pinnock, 2001). Of note, these prevalence rates apply only to very particular child abuse presentations in the two industrialized countries studied at the time the research took place and subsequently suggest that such events are quite rare. Perhaps when the general concept of MCA is firmly established in the fabric of pediatrics and clinicians are comfortable in its identification and scope, then it will be possible to know more accurately the prevalence of MCA. With the development of community standards and legal definitions, we can acquire a gradual understanding of how frequently children get harmful medical treatment at the insistence of their parents.

Profiles

Despite the efforts of many authors to detail a profile of a potential perpetrator of MSBP, there is no data to suggest that such a profile can accurately predict those parents who would subject the children to harmful medical care. In this regard medical child abuse once again is similar to other forms of child abuse. Characteristics, such as being employed in the medical profession, having vast knowledge about the child's illness, doting over the child during hospitalization while "blossoming" in such an environment, and having an absent husband, have all found their way onto such "profiles" (Bools, Neale, & Meadow, 1994; Hall et al., 2000; Rosenberg, 1987). Such characteristics can easily be discounted when one considers that

(1) Most people employed in the medical profession seldom abuse their children medically.

(2) Most mothers who have absent husbands do not harm their children medically.
(3) Most doting parents in the hospital just love their children and do not want to see them harmed.

This is not to say that perpetrators of medical child abuse might not be employed in the medical profession or might not have a husband away at sea for many months. These things do happen in the lives of people who medically abuse their children. The caveat to this is that these factors cannot be used to create a profile with any predictive value. The fact that many professional basketball players are of African-American ancestry does not mean that all African-Americans are good basketball players or that non-African-Americans cannot be professional basketball players.

Bools and colleagues (1994) interviewed mothers accused of harming their children in the medical environment and found that many of them were high utilizers of medical services themselves and tended to have many unexplained somatic symptoms. Even this tendency to view the world through medical glasses cannot be used as a profile characteristic as most such people do not expose their children to unnecessary medical care.

Motivation

As in other forms of child abuse the reason why the perpetrator committed the act becomes an important factor when a determination is to be made about whether the child can remain safely in the home. It is not necessary to know why a person harmed the child to determine if the child was hurt and whether it should be stopped. As with other forms of child abuse there can be many motivations for why a parent might expose her child to unnecessary medical care. As early as 15 years ago Levin and Sheridan wrote, "Motivations of the perpetrator are probably not uniform, and may include components of help seeking; a delusion that the illness is real; rage at the victim, healthcare provider(s), or significant others; and tangible secondary gain" (Levin & Sheridan, 1995). The physician's role is to diagnose harm in the child. The determination of motivation and its consequences is best left to the legal realm; however, this consideration may also have its place when determining the treatment of the perpetrator.

Once it has been determined that a child has been harmed and that the harm should stop, then it becomes necessary to listen to the perpetrator try to explain what brought her to act as she did. There may be an understandable and believable explanation. On the other hand, the perpetrator may try to explain why she put her child at risk with reasons that do not conform with the reality of the situation. These considerations all come into play when treatment decisions are being formulated. It is for these reasons that the motivation of the perpetrator of medical child abuse is just as important as the motivation of perpetrators of any other kind of child maltreatment.

The really interesting question is why motivation of perpetrators of MCA has been the object of so much speculation. Ever since the first cases described, people in the medical community have been significantly focused on why parents would abuse their children in this particular way. It has, apparently, been much easier for medical personnel to understand why a caretaker would sexually harm a child, or psychologically harm a child, then to understand why they would subject her child to unnecessary medical care.

The reason for this extended and time-consuming speculation has less to do with the perpetrator than it does the medical caregivers. The concern with motivation of perpetrators of MCA may reflect communitywide countertransference on the part of medical care providers. Doctors and nurses who have their medical care used against the interests of the child may understandably feel betrayed, angry, sad, and sometimes foolish. Their response to these feelings has been to focus an inordinate amount of attention on why a parent would put them, the medical care practitioner, in this emotionally uncomfortable position. The motivation question really has more to do with, "Why did this parent make me do this stupid and harmful thing to my patient?" than it does to the alternative question, "Why would a parent subject a child to unnecessary medical care?" Doctors and nurses have no occasion to ask this question with other forms of child abuse as they have not been placed in the role of being the means by which a parent harmed their child.

Multidisciplinary Team

The treatment of MCA, as with other forms of child abuse, is best done in conjunction with an active child protection multidisciplinary team. Attempting to conduct child abuse evaluation and treatment for a medical child abuse case on the serious end of the spectrum, without the use of a multidisciplinary team (MDT), is almost impossible. Often, it is the nurse, pediatric intern, social worker, or speech therapist who has more consistent, close interaction with the abuser during a child's hospitalization and raises the initial suspicion (Bursch et al., 2008). While other professionals may note suspicions and concerning behaviors, medical child abuse remains a pediatric condition and it is the physician who makes the final medical diagnosis.

Child protection and law enforcement professionals can add valuable collateral information from interviews with school officials and community members involved with the family, as well as gather evidence of drugs or medical equipment that may be available to the suspected abuser. Having multiple points of view allows for comparison between these accounts and the story derived from the primary caretaker. They can also assist in obtaining medical records from other sources. As some cases may be quite complex, it is prudent to have seasoned, experienced investigators knowledgeable about MCA involved. Mothers who have abused their children in the medical setting can be disarmingly charming and elicit little suspicion for many years. Once a report is made, the authorities should become part of the multidisciplinary team to optimize case management and ensure communication and coordination of interventions.

Treatment

As stated above treatment of MCA follows the general principles involved in treatment of all child abuse. The first step is recognizing that abuse is taking place. The second step involves stopping the abuse. Stopping MCA is somewhat different than stopping physical or sexual abuse. Stopping medical abuse means ending harmful medical treatment. This can happen only when medical personnel in charge of the treatment come to realize that it is based on false information and decide to halt the treatment and repair any damage. Thus, while medical care personnel are necessary for the commission of medical abuse, they are also necessary for bringing it to a halt.

The next step in child abuse treatment involves the provision for the ongoing safety of the child. To provide for the ongoing safety of a child who has been receiving harmful medical care, the medical care delivery team must revise the treatment plan and get the cooperation of caretakers to follow the treatment. This step in medical abuse treatment might be as simple as holding a meeting with parents and announcing the new medical care plan. It might also trigger a realization that the perpetrator of the abuse is unable or unwilling to cooperate with appropriate medical care. It would be at this point that child protective services would most likely become involved.

As soon as the safety of the child can be ensured therapy can begin to assess and treat the physical and psychological consequences of the abuse. These consequences can be mild or devastating. Treatment is tailored to the needs of the individual child. The prognosis of the child victim is dependent on the extent, scope, and length of time the child has endured the abuse. McGuire and Feldman (1989) report a range of psychological problems exhibited by such child victims, including infant feeding disorders, withdrawal, hyperactivity, hysteria, and adoption of Munchausen behavior in the child. Here is a range of potential interventions that correspond to mild to severe presentations of medical child abuse (Table 8.3). The intervention need to be only as powerful as necessary to make sure that treatment can proceed and result in a safe outcome.

Table 8.3 Spectrum of treatments, least to most intrusive.

Counseling in office setting
Refer patients for therapy/medication
Refer for family counseling
Involve outside agencies to monitor care
Refer for partial hospitalization
Inpatient trial of separation from parents
Refer to social services
Remove child from home
Termination of parental rights
A prosecution/incarceration

The final step in child abuse treatment is to attempt to maintain the family's integrity as much as possible while protecting the child (Roesler & Jenny, 2008). In the mild to moderate forms of MCA just as with other forms of child abuse having the child be maintained in the family is often possible. This is usually predicated on the perpetrator understanding the consequences of her actions and entering into a reasonable treatment relationship with those attempting to help. If the perpetrator denies responsibility and is unable to see how her actions have affected her children, then, just as with other abuse victims more significant intervention in the life of the family is necessary. In instances of severe forms of medical child abuse, the child must be separated from the perpetrator to ensure the future safety of the child.

Pediatricians will rarely become involved in the rehabilitation of adult perpetrators of medical abuse just as they are seldom asked to take part in the treatment of sexual perpetrators. However, they are often asked to continue to treat the child with the remaining family unit that may or may not include the person who harmed the child in the first place.

References

Aranibar, H., & Cerda, M. (2005). Hypoglycemic seizure in munchausen-by-proxy syndrome. *Pediatric Emergency Care, 21*(6), 378–379.

Ayoub, C. C., Alexander, R., Beck, D., Bursch, B., Feldman, K. W., Libow, J., et al. (2002). Position paper: Definitional issues in Munchausen by proxy. *Child Maltreat, 7*(2), 105–111.

Bools, C. (2007). *Fabricated or induced illness in a child by a carer: A reader.* Oxford: Radcliffe Publishing.

Bools, C., Neale, B., & Meadow, R. (1994). Munchausen syndrome by proxy: A study of psychopathology. *Child Abuse and Neglect, 18*(9), 773–788.

Bursch, B., Schreier, H. A., Ayoub, C. C., Libow, J. A., Sanders, M. J., & Yorker, B. C. (2008). Further thoughts on "Beyond Munchausen by proxy: Identification and treatment of child abuse in a medical setting". *Pediatrics, 121*(2), 444–445; author reply 445.

Carter, K. E., Izsak, E., & Marlow, J. (2006). Munchausen syndrome by proxy caused by ipecac poisoning. *Pediatric Emergency Care, 22*(9), 655–656.

Denny, S. J., Grant, C. C., & Pinnock, R. (2001). Epidemiology of Munchausen syndrome by proxy in New Zealand. *Journal of Pediatric Child Health, 37*(3), 240–243.

de Ridder, L., & Hoeska, J. H. (2000). Manifestations of munchausen syndrome by proxy in pediatric gastroenterology. *Journal of Pediatric Gastroenterology and Nutrition, 31*(2), 208–211.

Evans, D. (1994). Covert video surveillance in Munchausen's syndrome by proxy. *British Medical Journal, 308*(6924), 341–342.

Evans, D. (1995). The investigation of life-threatening child abuse and Munchausen syndrome by proxy. *Journal of Medical Ethics, 21*(1), 9–13.

Evans, D. (1996). Covert video surveillance – A response to Professor Southall and Dr. Samuels. *Journal of Medical Ethics, 22*(1), 29–31.

Fisher, G. C., & Mitchell, I. (1995). Is Munchausen syndrome by proxy really a syndrome? *Archives of Disease in Childhood, 72*(6), 530–534.

Hall, D. E., Eubanks, L., Meyyazhagan, L. S., Kenney, R. D., & Johnson, S. C. (2000). Evaluation of covert video surveillance in the diagnosis of munchausen syndrome by proxy: Lessons from 41 cases. *Pediatrics, 105*(6), 1305–1312.

Holstege, C. P., & Dobmeier, S. G. (2006). Criminal poisoning: Munchausen by proxy. *Clinics in Laboratory Medicine, 26*(1), 243–253.

Levin, A. V., & Sheridan, M. S. (Eds.). (1995). *Munchausen syndrome by proxy: Issues in diagnosis and treatment.* New York: Lexington Books.

Libow, J. A. (1995). Munchausen by proxy victims in adulthood: A first look. *Child Abuse and Neglect, 19*(9), 1131–1142.

McClure, R. J., Davis, P. M., Meadow, S. R., & Sibert, J. R. (1996). Epidemiology of Munchausen syndrome by proxy, non-accidental poisoning, and non-accidental suffocation. *Archives of Disease in Childhood, 75*(1), 57–61.

McGuire, T. L., & Feldman, K. W. (1989). Psychologic morbidity of children subjected to Munchausen syndrome by proxy. *Pediatrics, 83*(2), 289–292.

Meadow, R. (1977). Munchausen syndrome by proxy. The hinterland of child abuse. *Lancet, 2*(8033), 343–345.

Meadow, R. (2002). Different interpretations of Munchausen syndrome by proxy. *Child Abuse and Neglect, 26*(5), 501–508.

Meadow, R., & Lennert, T. (1984). Munchausen by proxy or Polle syndrome: Which term is correct? *Pediatrics, 74*(4), 554–556.

Mian, M. (1995). A multidisciplinary approach. In A. V. Levin & M. S. Sheridan (Eds.), *Munchausen syndrome by proxy: Issues in diagnosis and treatment* (pp. 271–286). New York: Lexington Books.

Morley, C. J. (1995). Practical concerns about the diagnosis of Munchausen syndrome by proxy. *Archives of Disease in Childhood, 72*(6), 528–529; discussion 529–530.

Raspe, R. E. (1944). *The surprising adventures of Baron Munchausen.* New York: Peter Pauper.

Roesler, T. A., & Jenny, C. (2008). *Medical child abuse: Beyond Munchausen by proxy.* Elk Grove Village: American Academy of Pediatrics Press.

Rosenberg, D. A. (1987). Web of deceit: A literature review of Munchausen syndrome by proxy. *Child Abuse and Neglect, 11*(4), 547–563.

Sanders, M. J., & Bursch, B. (2002). Forensic assessment of illness falsification, Munchausen by proxy, and factitious disorder, NOS. *Child Maltreatment, 7*(2), 112–124.

Schreier, H. (2002). Munchausen by proxy defined. *Pediatrics, 110*(5), 985–988.

Southall, D. P., Plunkett, M. C., Banks, M. W., Falkov, A. F., & Samuels, M. P. (1997). Covert video recordings of life-threatening child abuse: Lessons for child protection. *Pediatrics, 100*(5), 735–760.

Southall, D. P., & Samuels, M. P. (1996). Guidelines for the multi-agency management of patients suspected or at risk of suffering from life-threatening abuse resulting in cyanotic-apnoeic episodes. North Staffordshire Hospital Trust, Staffordshire Social Services and Staffordshire Police. *Journal of Medical Ethics, 22*(1), 16–21.

Southall, D. P., Stebbens, V. A., Rees, S. V., Lang, M. H., Warner, J. O., & Shinebourne, E. A. (1987). Apnoeic episodes induced by smothering: Two cases identified by covert video surveillance. *British Medical Journal (Clinical Research Ed), 294*(6588), 1637–1641.

Stirling, J., Jr. (2007). Beyond Munchausen syndrome by proxy: Identification and treatment of child abuse in a medical setting. *Pediatrics, 119*(5), 1026–1030.

Trent, M. (2008). A horrific case of 'medical child abuse'. *The Prosecutor, 38*, 1–3.

Chapter 9

Other Patterns of Injury and Child Fatality

Vincent J. Palusci, Carl J. Schmidt, and Pamela Wallace Hammel

Introduction

In addition to overt skin, head, and abdominal injuries, there are more subtle ways in which parents and caregivers physically harm their children. These are more insidious injuries to the mouth and teeth through abuse or neglect, or children can be intentionally poisoned with drugs or chemicals. In a small fraction of cases, they die as a result of maltreatment. This chapter discusses a range of injuries found in abused children, some of which are easily identified as inflicted, whereas others are less common and more easily overlooked.

Oral and Dental Trauma

Dentists and physicians have important ethical responsibilities in recognizing inflicted injuries. More than half of child abuse injuries are to the head and neck, clearly visible to the dental team or knowledgeable observers such as teachers, social workers, health care professionals, or law enforcement (Kellogg & The Committee on Child Abuse and Neglect, 2005a). In a review of 300 records of non-accidental injuries at a children's hospital over 5 years, the head, face, neck, and mouth were involved in 67% of the cases (Naidoo, 2000). The face was most attacked (41%), with the cheek being the most common site for injury. Oro-facial injuries included fractures of the skull and facial bones, intracranial injuries, bruises, burns and lacerations. Injuries to the mouth included fractured

A.P. Giardino et al. (eds.), *A Practical Guide to the Evaluation of Child Physical Abuse and Neglect*, DOI 10.1007/978-1-4419-0702-8_9, © Springer Science+Business Media, LLC 1997, 2010

and avulsed teeth, lacerations to the frenum, tongue, and lips, and jaw fractures. The head and face are thought to be frequently attacked because they represent the sense of "self" of the child, the center of communication and nutrition. The mouth is often injured due to the abuser's desire to silence the child's crying. Despite the high incidence of facial injuries in abused children, dentists infrequently report suspected abuse (Needleman, 1986). Likewise, physicians are not always thorough in their examination of the mouth, so that many injuries may go unrecognized. The dentist and physician should consider non-accidental injuries when there are one or more concerning injuries present, particularly in young children (< 2 years) (Table 9.1). Bite marks, discussed elsewhere in this book, are a skin injury that can often be linked forensically to the alleged offender. There is a bimodal age distribution of affected children, with the majority of injuries occurring in the 0- to 4-year age group and another peak occurring during adolescence (da Fonesca, Feigal, & ten Bensel, 1992).

Table 9.1 Oral and dental injuries concerning for abuse.

- Soft tissue bruising, i.e. cheeks, neck
- Pattern injuries such as bite marks, handprints, finger or nail marks, belts; injuries with identifiable shapes from cords, belts, irons, etc.
- Bruises or fingernail marks on the pinna of the ear
- Any facial fracture, including fractured teeth
- Lacerations of the mouth, frena, and injuries to the corners of the mouth due to gags
- Bilateral injuries

The face and mouth examination of the abused child is simple if the child is cooperative and not in a great deal of pain. Important abnormalities are detected by a thorough mouth examination. Examiners should be sure to look for Battle's sign (bruising behind the ears) and soft tissue injuries of the neck and cheeks. Also, examine for partial alopecia due to being picked up/swung by the hair. Begin by examining the face for symmetry and external injuries. If possible, have the child open and close his or her mouth a few times and observe for asymmetry or difficulty; listen for any noises. Palpate along the mandibular borders, zygoma, nasal areas, and around the eyes, searching for areas of tenderness or evidence of fractures. Examine the child's teeth and look for bleeding, missing or injured teeth, malocclusions, and caries. When assessing for tooth mobility, fingers are inaccurate. Use a mouth mirror handle and an explorer (as fingers may compress around the tooth). Have the child bite down and assess for pain. Reflect the lips back individually to examine for frenum lacerations, scars, burns, and abrasions. Sublingual frenum tears (which are often missed) can be indicative of abuse–forced feeding–spoon, nipple, and pacifier. Move the upper teeth back and forth between the fingers to check for maxillary fractures, loose teeth, and instability. Examine the molars for caries and check the buccal mucosa for injuries. Finally, have the child stick out his or her tongue. Check for injuries and lift the tongue to examine the lingual frenum.

The pharynx is a frequent site of sexual abuse in children (Kellogg & The Committee on Child Abuse and Neglect, 2005b; Schlesinger, Borbotsina, & O'Neill, 1975). Most injuries are nonspecific, and the diagnosis of abuse rests on the history or additional physical findings that indicate trauma. Unexplained erythema or palatal petechiae at the junction of the hard and soft palate could indicate forced fellatio. Certain sexually transmitted infections in the mouth or pharynx are pathognomonic of sexual contact. The most common sexually transmitted infection in child abuse is gonorrhea; there may be mucosal or pharyngeal lesions that are generally asymptomatic. Condylomata acuminata (genital warts) and syphilis also manifest with oral lesions. Detection of semen in the oral cavity is possible for several days after exposure, and swabs should be taken from the buccal mucosa and tongue after recent contact.

Abusive peri-oral injuries are widely distributed, the lips and labial frenum being the most common areas injured. There may be contusions of the tongue, buccal mucosa, gingiva, hard and soft palate, and lingual frenum. Fractures of the facial bones, jaws, or teeth are suspicious, as are teeth that are displaced or avulsed. Teeth that are discolored due to pulpal necrosis can indicate previous abuse. Other abusive intra-oral injuries are widely distributed to the lips, gums, tongue, and palate, and fractures are seen with intrusion and extrusion of the dentition, bites, and contusions. Injuries may be inflicted by blunt trauma or with instruments such as eating utensils, feeding bottles, pacifiers, fingers, hot or caustic liquids. Mucosal injuries are rather common and include burns, contusions, and lacerations. Direct blows to the mouth that trap the lip between the teeth and the external object can result in abrasions, contusions, or lacerations. Lacerations may require suturing, which is best done by a plastic or oral surgeon.

Frenum or frenulum tears have been noted to occur during attempts to silence a crying infant or to feed a refusing child if hands, pacifiers, bottles, or eating utensils are forced into a child's mouth. A frenum tear has been thought to be indicative of abuse in young infants and is managed conservatively but may require suturing if the injury is extensive or the alveolar bone is exposed (Needleman, 1986). Thackeray reported three infants with labial or lingual frenulum tears who later returned with manifestations of severe abusive head injury (Thackeray, 2007). It is now thought, however, that labial or lingual frenum tears may result from either accidental or inflicted trauma. Upper frenum tears are common accidental injuries in older infants and young toddlers who are unsteady on their feet, because the child may fall and strike his or her mouth against the ground or other hard objects. Associated abrasions or contusions to the lip or philtrum may be found. Teece and Crawford (2004) have concluded that there "seems to be no evidence for the sensitivity/specificity of torn frenum in the investigation of non-accidental injury." A recent systematic review of these injuries found nine studies documenting torn labial frenula in young children and abuse fatalities (McGuire et al., 2007). Most children were less than 5 years, but many were fatally abused. Only a direct blow was substantiated as a mechanism of injury. One might therefore conclude that while a frenum injury represents trauma, the exact nature of that injury, abusive or accidental, is more difficult to determine.

Injuries to the teeth of children are very common accidental injuries; none is pathognomonic for abuse. Da Fonesca et al. (1992) report that of more than 1,200 cases of child maltreatment reviewed, only five tooth injuries were reported. It is not known whether this is an underrepresentation of the actual number of inflicted tooth injuries. The management of loose teeth is dependent on the age of the child. Direct blows to the mouth may result in loosening of a tooth or teeth. Severe blows to the incisal edge of the teeth may cause tooth intrusion into the alveolar bone. Intruded teeth may appear shorter than the surrounding teeth, and those completely intruded may appear to be missing. In this case, radiographs identify the location of the tooth. A severe blow to the mouth that results in avulsion, or removal, of the teeth more commonly occurs to the permanent teeth. Immediate dental referral is arranged when permanent teeth are avulsed because the tooth needs to be placed back in the socket as soon as possible to salvage it. Fractures to the anterior teeth occur from direct blows, commonly with falls. Finally, dental color changes resulting from previous pulpal injuries may be seen in accidental injury or abuse. All children with tooth injuries should be referred to a dentist for definitive evaluation and treatment.

Facial fractures are relatively uncommon abusive injuries, representing less than 5% of facial injuries (Becker, Needleman, & Kotelchuck, 1978). The most commonly reported injury is to the mandible, although the nasal bone, mandible, zygoma, or maxilla may be fractured. Mandibular fractures are usually bilateral, can be missed on skeletal survey, and are better detected clinically. There may be contusions over the fracture. Palpation of the mandibular condyles will elicit pain, and jaw opening may be difficult. All children with mandibular fractures should be referred to an oral surgeon for full evaluation (including radiographic evaluation) and treatment.

Dental neglect is the chronic failure of a parent or guardian to provide a child under the age of eighteen with basic dental care. The definition of dental neglect varies by state, institution, and individual, and is imprecise. There are numerous factors that contribute to the neglect of oral health, including parental ignorance, family isolation, financial restraints, and lack of perceived value of oral health (AAP Committee on Early Childhood, Adoption and Dependent Care, 1986). As defined by the American Academy of Pediatric Dentistry (2003), dental neglect is "the willful failure of a parent or guardian to seek and follow through with treatment necessary to ensure a level of oral health essential for adequate function and freedom from pain and infection." Most often physical and dental neglect occur simultaneously, therefore the oral cavity of the neglected child should be examined by a dentist when there are concerns of other neglect. Dental neglect affects the child's ability to perform basic functions of attending school, playing, or working. Dental infections can cause chronic pain, life-threatening abscesses, retard a child's growth and development, and make routine eating difficult or impossible. The health care professional should educate the family regarding the effects of dental neglect, and if attempts to improve oral health fail or the child's oral health has been adversely affected, a report to the child protective services is indicated.

Abuse by Poisoning

There are over 1.2 million ingestions of potentially poisonous substances annually among children under 6 years of age in the US (AAP Committee on Injury, Poisoning and Violence Prevention, 2003). There are also 250,000 outpatient prescription medicine errors annually which are unintentional; one in six children will experience a medication error (Institute of Medicine, 2007). Historically, common scenarios for accidental poisoning included toddlers visiting grandparents who had one or more prescription medications without proper safety provisions or supervision for the child. Marked decreases have been noted overall in poisonings due to child resistant containers, safer products, anticipatory guidance given to families, general public education about medication storage, and establishment of a national network of poison control centers (Paschall, 2005). Fortunately, there are relatively few deaths, with only 25 fatalities recorded in 1997. Because of this low fatality rate and the potential dangers of its use, ipecac, an over-the-counter agent administered to induce vomiting after poisoning, is no longer recommended. However, poisoning as a pattern of abuse remains a poorly understood and underreported form of child maltreatment (Dine & McGovern, 1982; Fazen, Lovejoy, & Crone, 1986; Rogers & Bentovim, 1981; Sibert & Murphy, 1980). The American Association of Poison Control Centers has reported that intentional poisoning is noted in 0.5% of reported exposures, with subsequent increased risk of subsequent physical abuse and death as compared to accidental poisoning cases (AAP Committee on Injury, Violence and Poisoning Prevention, 2003).

Intentional or abusive poisoning is more deadly than accidental poisoning, with higher fatality estimates due to, in the example of acetaminophen, delays in seeking medical care and nonspecific symptoms on presentation for medical care (Alander, Dowd, Bratton, & Kearnes, 2000). The peak age for accidental poisoning is 2 years of age. Infants and teens are more likely to have been intentionally poisoned (Bays, 1994). Intentional poisoning with sedatives may be used to control a child's behavior, but other prescription medications or over-the-counter items such as iron or caffeine are also very common and potentially deadly, given inaccurate or absent medical history being given to medical providers (Black & Zenel, 2003; Perez, Scribano, & Perry, 2004; Rivenes, Bakerman, & Miller, 1997). Commonly used poisons in reported cases of abuse include iron, alcohol, caffeine, benzodiazepines, glutethimide, insulin, ipecac, laxatives, marijuana, oral hypoglycemics, pepper, salt, and a variety of other prescription and illicit substances (Bays, 1994). In addition, the health care provider must consider substances used in complementary or alternative medical practices. Dine and McGovern (1982) and Bays (1994) report that approximately 20% of their respective samples of abusive poisoning cases also had evidence of additional physical abuse.

Fischler (1983) as modified by Perez et al. (2004) organizes intentional poisoning into seven patterns: (a) impulsive parental acts related to stress (e.g., use of sedatives, alcohol, antihistamines, or paregoric to quiet a child); (b) neglect (e.g., unsupervised child ingests medications or alcohol, or repeated ingestions); (c) bizarre parenting practices (e.g., using toxic doses of vitamins, minerals, or herbs, and water or salt intoxication); (d) punitive acts to control child behavior; (e) when the caretaker gets child "high" as form of entertainment; (f) to dispose of child by premeditated act; (g) Munchausen by Proxy (e.g., medication or chemical given to create a fictitious illness). However, the clinical presentations of intentional and accidental poisoning overlap. Common symptoms include altered states of consciousness, cardiorespiratory depression or excitation, gastrointestinal symptoms, seizures, and other challenging and unexplained symptom complexes (Wiley, 1991). A detailed review of poison presentations and treatments is beyond the scope of this text, and the reader is referred to one of several available texts.

Intentionally poisoned children may be presented for medical care with a history of "accidental" ingestion, signs of poisoning without history, recurrent unexplained illnesses, apparent life-threatening event, or unexpected sudden death, and a thorough evaluation is needed (Bays, 1994). History to be obtained to assist in determining whether a poisoning is accidental or intentional includes a complete list of drugs in the child's environment, including transdermal patches, herbal remedies, and over-the-counter preparations. Information should be sought regarding the quantity and storage of these items as well as safety measures employed. A developmental history of the child's abilities is important to aid in the assessment of access to these potential poisons, and formal testing may be needed when disparities arise. The degree of parental supervision and stresses in the home should also be reviewed, particularly when recurrent poisoning is being considered, as such family stresses are correlated with repeated ingestions. Historical factors that raise the concern for intentional poisoning include: (a) previous poisoning in child or sibling, (b) implausible history, (c) changing history, (d) history discordant with child's development, (e) child or sibling blamed, (f) excessive delay in seeking treatment, (g) infancy, and (h) unexplained symptoms (such as an apparent life-threatening event) that resolve when the child is not in the care of a suspected perpetrator (Perez et al., 2004; Pitetti, Whitman, & Zaylor, 2008). A summary of potential clinical indicators is listed in Table 9.2.

Laboratory assessment plays an important role in identifying the poison in many cases (Wiley, 1991). However, the yield in infants remains relatively low despite improvements in testing and detection. Cocaine and its metabolites are most readily identified as are alcohol and other drugs of abuse. Testing procedures may not be able to differentiate toxic levels vs. mere presence, and care should be taken to set detection limits as low as possible for non-therapeutic agents. Wiley (1991) reports limitations and wide variability in the accuracy of toxicological testing. Laboratories frequently receive inadequate specimens, mostly because of a common misperception that a blood sample alone is sufficient. Proper toxicological screening requires both blood and urine; gastric contents can be a useful addition if available. The urine sample allows for qualitative determinations of substances, whereas the blood sample allows for specific quantitative analysis. In addition, not all drugs and chemical compounds can be identified by standard laboratory processes used for toxicological screens. The most comprehensive screens available

Table 9.2 Potential clinical indicators of intentional poisoning.[a]

• Infancy
• History inconsistent with child's development or non-existent
• Prior poisoning in this child or family
• Poisoning inconsistent with medications in home, safety procedures, or physical environment
• Sibling blamed
• Delay in seeking medical care
• Other signs of abuse or neglect
• Bizarre drugs or substances of abuse
• Multiple agents
• Unexplained seizures
• Apparent life-threatening events (ALTEs)
• Sudden, unexpected, or unexplained infant or child death
• Chronic unexplained symptoms that resolved when removed from caretaker and/or placed in safe environment

[a] Adapted from Bayes (1994) and Paschall (2005).

detect only about 90 compounds (Wiley, 1991). There are wide local and regional variations in which drugs and substances are screened for on "drugs of abuse" screens. Substances such as ipecac, ammonia, clonidine, chloral hydrate, cyanide, insulin, petroleum distillates, gamma-hydroxybutyric acid (GHB), and sodium sulfate (found in shampoo) are best identified when specific testing is requested (Fazen et al., 1986; Wiley, 1991). Therefore, the health care provider is encouraged to contact the reference laboratory used at his or her own institution to obtain a list of what the screen tests, which screens need a special request, and what is not available, and what needs to be sent to a reference laboratory.

Death of the Abused Child

Epidemiology

It is estimated that 1,530 children were the victims of fatal child abuse in the US in 2006, but an exact number is difficult to assess given that the accurate identification and collection of child abuse and neglect deaths depends on a variety of agencies and the child welfare system (US DHHS, 2008). This rate of 2.04 per 100,000 has remained fairly constant over the last 10 years in data collected by NCANDS (the National Child Abuse and neglect Reporting System administered by the US government) and has not changed despite repeated national outcries for system improvement and prevention (US Advisory Board, 1995). However, the actual total number of child abuse and neglect deaths is thought to be higher. Fatal maltreatment is underestimated because of both underascertainment of child homicides and inaccurate classification of pediatric fatalities in official reports, and child homicides were often misclassified as occurring from accidents, drowning, falls, natural illness, or undetermined causes (Ewigman, Kivlahan, & Land, 1993; Overpeck et al., 2002). McClain, Sacks, Froehlke, and Ewigman (1993) estimated that between 15 and 30% of official death records are properly coded to identify the fatality as due to child abuse and neglect. Homicide, the legally determined death of a person at the hands of another, includes maltreatment deaths and those from non-familial persons. For example, the National Violent Death Reporting System noted that the 2003 homicide rate for children 0 – 4 years of age was 3.0 per 100,000, with African Americans 4.2 times more likely as Whites to be victims of homicide. The vast majority of deaths is at the hands of parents and caretakers, however, and used weapons including household objects and direct blows (King, Kiesel, & Simon, 2006; Bennett, Hall, Frazier, Patel, & Shaw, 2006). Among US infants, a unique pattern of homicide has emerged with the first week of life posing the greatest risk (Paulozzi, 2002). Death rates due to abuse also vary geographically, with the highest rates reported in the South and West of the US and the lowest rates in the Northeast (McClain et al., 1994).

Consistent patterns emerge in child maltreatment deaths. More than three-quarters (78%) of these deaths were in children under 4 years of age and 44% were among infants in 2006 (US DHHS, 2008). There were more boys than girls and infant boys had the highest rate (18.5 per 100,000). Younger children are thought to be more vulnerable to fatal maltreatment because of their small size, their inability to communicate verbally, and because they live a relatively isolated existence, out of contact with adults other than their caregivers (AAP Committee on Child Abuse, 1999). Many (43%) were White, but 29% were African American and 17% were Hispanic. This agrees with data over time which shows higher mortality for all causes of fatal injuries in African American, Native American, and Alaskan Native children in the US (Pressley, Barlow, Kendig, & Paneth-Pollak, 2007). In addition to race, increased intentional injury deaths have also been noted among children in poorer social classes (Roberts, Li, & Barker, 1998).

Interestingly, neglect was the leading reason (41%) for maltreatment deaths in the US, followed by abuse and neglect (31.4%) and abuse alone (22.4%) (US DHHS, 2008). A 25-year retrospective review of neglect deaths identified that starvation and dehydration were the most common causes, followed by "accidental" ingestions, exposure to the elements, delayed medical care, electrocution, and drowning/aspiration (Knight & Collins, 2005). In general, while most maltreatment deaths (75.9%) are caused by one or more parents and 27.4% are caused by the mother alone (US DHHS), Schnitzer and Ewigman (2005) noted that children residing in households with unrelated adults were nearly 50 times more likely to die of inflicted injuries than were children living with two biological parents. In their sample, most perpetrators were the child's father or the boyfriend of the mother (Schnitzer & Ewigman, 2005). Overall, children known to child protective services agencies have increased risk of death from all causes, including child maltreatment (Sabotta & Davis, 1992). In one study, however, a prior referral to child protective services did not increase the risk that their infant's death was caused by inflicted injuries

(Krous et al., 2006). Some children (13.7%) who died from child abuse or neglect had received services from child protective services agencies within 5 years, and a small number (2.3%) had been in foster care and had been returned home to their parents (US DHHS, 2008). Many children have evidence of prior injury at the time of death, and some have findings that could have allowed for protective actions to prevent fatality (Brewster et al., 1998; Jenny, Hymel, Ritzen, Reinert, & Hay, 1999).

Patterns of Fatal Injury

Perhaps the most important and disconcerting diagnostic issue in fatal child abuse is that there may not be a distinct pattern of injury. A child can be injured fatally without any external signs of trauma.

Head injury is the most common cause of fatal child abuse. This can happen without any external evidence of injury, whether by shaking or blunt trauma to the head (Gilliland & Folberg, 1996). Although violent shaking of the child's head is controversial, it is likely that it happens at least some of the time. Confessions have been collected and documented in the literature (Starling et al., 2004). It is also possible that a child's head impacts a softer surface, such as a mattress or a firm pillow that partially molds itself around the infant's head, thus distributing the impact over a larger surface area, blurring any evidence of impact (Case, 2007). Be that as it may, catastrophic head injuries, whether or not they result in the child's death, don't occur spontaneously and, as with most trauma, the extent of the injury reflects the magnitude of the energy that impacted on the child's head (Duhaime, Christian, Rorke, & Zimmerman, 1998). Photo 9.1 shows the skull of a 13-month-old child that died with extensive bilateral subdural hemorrhage and swelling of the brain so intense that it caused diastatic separation of the sagittal and coronal sutures. The gap

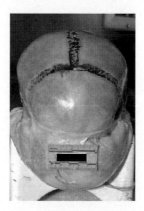

Photo 9.1   Skull of a 13-month-old child who died with extensive bilateral subdural hemorrhage and swelling of the brain that caused diastatic separation of the sagittal and coronal sutures.

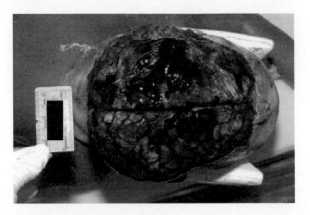

Photo 9.2 The brain after removal of the calvarium.

between the bony plates is evident in the picture. There is no discrete impact site. Photo 9.2 shows the brain after removal of the calvarium. The dura over the right hemisphere is reflected upward, showing the extent of the subdural hemorrhage, which was similar on the left hemisphere.

More commonly, impact sites are present on the scalp and on the skull. Typical cortical cerebral hemispheric contusions may be evident, as will contrecoup contusions if the head was moving and stopped suddenly by striking a firm surface. Because the head is shaped partially like a sphere, diffuse hemorrhagic infiltration of the scalp indicates that the head suffered multiple impacts whose individual signatures became blurred by the confluence of the bleeding.

Fractures of the skull are not always present because the elasticity of bones in children allows some deformation of the skull to occur before the bone fails. Fatal head injury often occurs without a skull fracture (Itabashi, Andrews, Tomiyasu, Erlich, & Sathyavagiswaran, 2007). However, fractures suffered from a simple fall tend to be linear and often occur in the parietal region; the context in which the child is brought for treatment will generally confirm the mechanism of injury. Fractures due to abuse tend to be multiple, often radiating from a central defect if the head was struck by an object with a narrow profile, and tend to cross the midline or traverse a suture. If there are multiple fractures, each one tends to correspond to an individual impact, which is useful for documentation when there is confluent hemorrhagic infiltration of the scalp due to multiple blows. Photo 9.3 shows the reflected scalp of a child that suffered numerous, confluent impacts to the scalp. Although impact sites are often present on the skin, the definitive way to document them is to reflect the scalp.

Other useful markers of abusive head trauma are perioptic nerve sheath hemorrhage and retinal hemorrhage, especially as markers of the severity of injury (Case et al., 2001). The former is shown in Photo 9.4 and retinal hemorrhage in Photo 9.5. This picture shows hemorrhagic infiltration near the ora serrata. More anterior distribution of hemorrhage in the retina is associated with

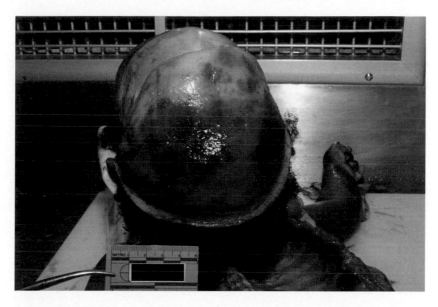

Photo 9.3 The reflected scalp of a child who suffered numerous, confluent impacts to the scalp.

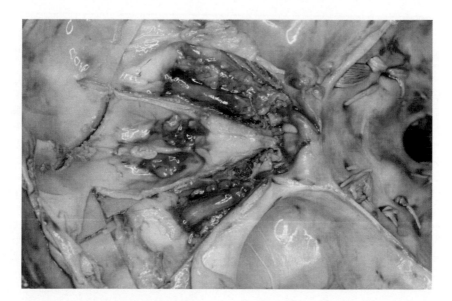

Photo 9.4 Perioptic nerve sheath hemorrhage on a gross specimen of a child who suffered from severe abusive head trauma.

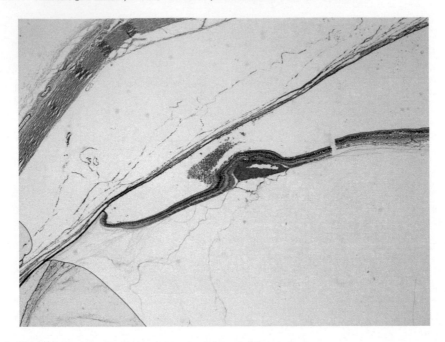

Photo 9.5 Microscopic examination showing retina hemorrhage.

abusive head trauma. Often, useful signs are present in the mouth. Photo 9.6 shows a 2-year-old child whose upper lip is hemorrhagic due to tearing of the mucosa by the teeth at the moment the child was slapped, and traumatic rupture of the frenum. The healing scabbed lesions on the face were due to chicken pox.

The lack of a pattern of injury is even more likely to occur in the chest and abdomen. This is because of the absence of a firm bony surface, unlike the skin over the skull, and the skin's inherent elasticity. The extent of trauma that a child can suffer without evidence of impact is impressive. Photo 9.7 shows the back of an infant's body with some barely visible ecchymoses. Photo 9.8 shows the hemorrhagic infiltration of the skin. The width of the area of hemorrhage and its sharply demarcated upper and lower boundaries helped associate it to the causal object, a metal rectangular bed post. In this case, there were no rib fractures but there were hemorrhagic contusions on the pleural surfaces of the lungs. Sometimes, if the chest is struck at end-diastole, rupture of the heart can occur.

In abdominal trauma, the magnitude of injury can be astounding (Dolinak, Matshes, & Lew, 2005). Photo 9.9 shows multiple tears of the right lobe of the liver. The hint of a semicircular outline to the tears is due to the imprint of the ribs on the liver. Depending on the rate of bleeding, these children can survive for hours after the injury happened. Photo 9.10 shows the posterior surface of the organ block from a 3-month-old infant. There is profuse hemorrhage in the right retroperitoneum that

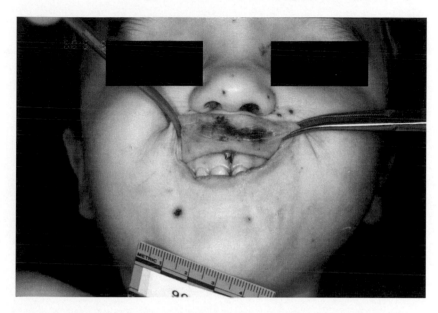

Photo 9.6 A 2-year-old child whose upper lip is hemorrhagic due to tearing of the mucosa by the teeth at the moment the child was slapped; traumatic rupture of the labial frenum is also noted.

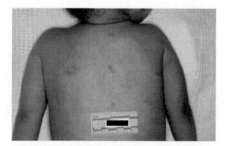

Photo 9.7 The back of an infant's body with some barely visible ecchymoses.

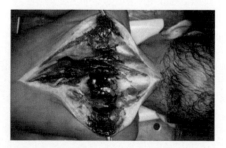

Photo 9.8 The hemorrhagic infiltration of the skin which shows the extent of the injury despite barely visible superficial bruises.

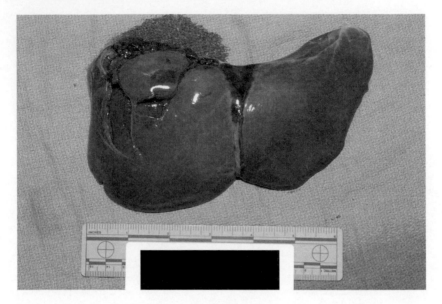

Photo 9.9 Multiple tears of the *right lobe* of the liver.

completely surrounds the right kidney and split the right adrenal gland in half. Hemorrhages in such anatomically protected areas implicitly point to the extent of the force inflicted on a child.

Sometimes injuries are caused by an object whose profile is not hard to define, as when a child is struck by a belt, hair curler, or some other portable object. The left panel on Photo 9.11 shows the head of a child that was struck multiple times by the belt buckle shown on the right panel. The numerous circular and semicircular scars and the erosion in the center of the head indicate abuse that took place over a period of time. Photo 9.12 shows another child in a similar circumstance, but the inset shows the looped electrical cord with which he was beaten. These kinds of injuries have other implications aside from the time span in which these children suffered. These children are often kept sequestered at home or some similar environment so that the abuse is not detected. An injury pattern should prompt the search for the object that caused the lesion. The location of some injuries also aids in determining what caused them. Photo 9.13 shows tears in the pharynx of an infant. This was caused by the forceful insertion of a curling iron in the child's mouth. A feature of child abuse that is not appreciated as widely as it should be is its association with mental illness (Mullick, Miller, & Jacobsen, 2001). This can lead to some of the more horrific instances of child abuse. Photo 9.14 shows an infant whose airway was stuffed with gauze, and then packed with a towel. The mouth was then sealed with tape and the child was placed in a plastic bag for disposal. The perpetrator complained of being afraid of the infant's secretions and was acutely psychotic.

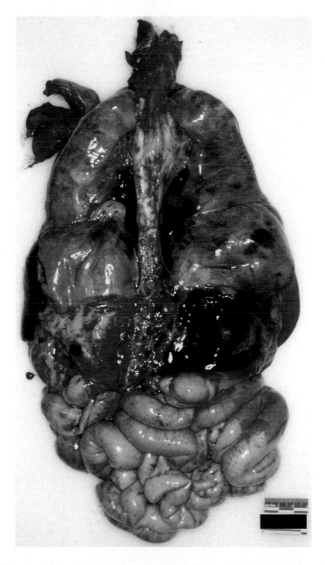

Photo 9.10 The posterior surface of the organ block from a 3-month-old infant which demonstrates profuse hemorrhage surrounding the *right kidney*.

Distinguishing Fatal Child Abuse from Accident and Sudden Infant Death Syndrome

Sudden infant death syndrome (SIDS) is defined as the sudden and unexpected death of an infant under 1 year of age that remains unexplained after a thorough case investigation, including performance of a complete autopsy, examination of the death scene, and review of the clinical history (AAP Task Force on SIDS, 2005). SIDS is rare during the first month of life, peaks at 2 – 4 months

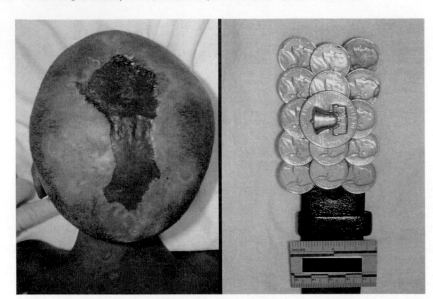

Photo 9.11 The head of a child who was struck multiple times by the belt buckle shown on the *right panel*.

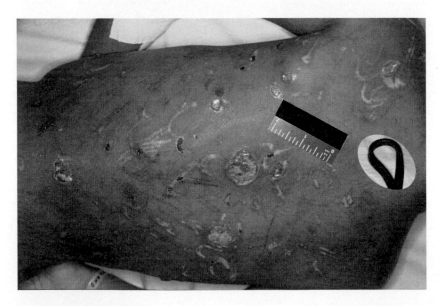

Photo 9.12 The back of a child who was struck multiple times with the looped electrical cord shown in the inset photo.

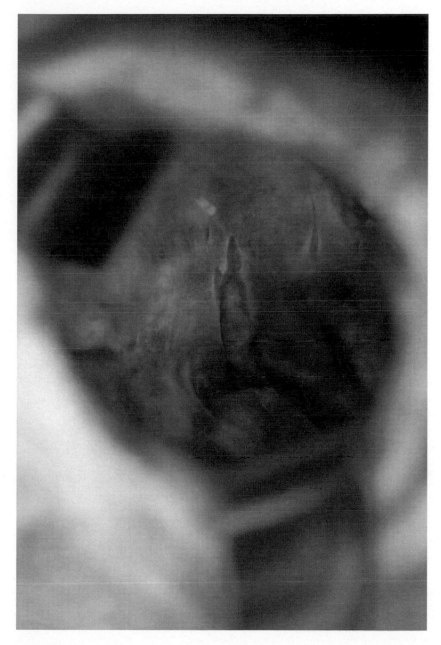

Photo 9.13 Tears in the pharynx of an infant caused by the forceful insertion of a curling iron into the child's mouth and throat.

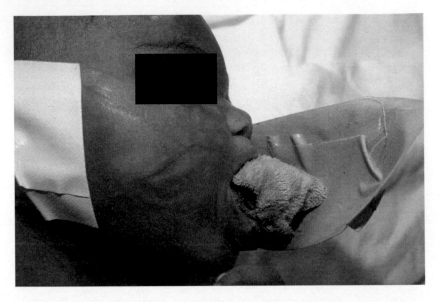

Photo 9.14 Infant whose airway was stuffed with gauze and then packed with a towel and whose mouth was sealed with tape.

of age, and then declines. SIDS accounts for more than 5,000 deaths in the United States each year (0.5–0.6 per 1,000) and is the leading cause of infant death between 1 week and 1 year of age. Rates were twice as high before "Back to Sleep" campaigns were begun to address unsafe prone and side-sleeping positions. Other epidemiological factors consistently identified in multiple studies include sleeping on a soft surface, maternal smoking during pregnancy and after the birth, preterm birth, low birth weight, overheating, and late or no prenatal care. Higher rates are found in African American and American Indian/Alaskan Native children. None of these factors is proven to cause SIDS, and it is presently impossible to predict which infants will ultimately die of SIDS.

Recent research has highlighted additional potential risk factors and the increasing incidence of identified positional asphyxia. The typical history of a SIDS death is as follows: A previously healthy infant is put down for a nap or for the night. Some infants have a history of recent upper respiratory infection but are otherwise healthy. Some time later, the baby is found dead. No struggle or crying was heard. At times, some pink, frothy discharge may be found at the nose, at the mouth, or on the sheets, and postmortem lividity may be present. The caregiver immediately calls for emergency help and the infant is brought to the nearest hospital or pronounced dead at the scene. Pacifiers and head covering have been linked with increases in SIDS, and fan use is associated with an 80% or more reduction (Mitchell et al., 2008; Coleman-Phox, Odouli, & Li, 2008). With more thorough investigations, many infants are found in situations which, while previously labeled as SIDS, are actually more consistent with overlay or other unintentional suffocation. Bed sharing with an adult can place the infant at increased risk for overlay under certain conditions, but this is controversial. Confounders include parental smoking, substance abuse, and alcohol ingestion. The risk is even higher with multiple bed sharers or when the bed sharer is overtired. The most protective sleep setting for infants is thought to be on their backs in a crib in the parent's room. Home monitoring has not been found to prevent SIDS (AAP Committee of the Fetus and Newborn, 2003).

There have been numerous theories that attempt to explain the biologic etiology of SIDS, but the cause with the most scientific support appears to be related to local carbon dioxide buildup and rebreathing. Abnormalities in the arcuate nucleus in the brainstems of some SIDS victims suggest a role of poor arousal or cardiorespiratory control (Hymel, 2006). A respiratory cause is supported by seasonal variations in SIDS deaths, the frequent association of upper respiratory infection shortly before death, and the characteristic intrathoracic petechiae found on postmortem examination (Culbertson, Krous, & Bendell, 1988). Fifteen percent or more of unexpected infant deaths are discovered to have a known cause by postmortem examination (Keens & Davidson Ward, 1993). Congenital and cardiac anomalies, metabolic diseases, infection, tumors, and accidental or inflicted trauma may all cause sudden and unexpected death that is not identified until autopsy (Emery, Chandra, & Gilbert-Barness, 1988). Death scene investigation may also identify environmental factors that contributed to death (Bass, Kravath, & Glass, 1986; Holton et al., 1991).

The possibility of child abuse is sometimes raised when an infant dies suddenly and unexpectedly. Many of the risk factors reported for infant mortality overlap with risk factors for abuse, causing further concern. In reality, only a small percentage of SIDS deaths are attributable to fatal child abuse, and the investigator's and health care provider's approach to families of SIDS fatalities should be supportive and not accusatory throughout the investigation (Smialek & Lambros, 1988; Hymel, 2006). A comprehensive approach has been recommended by the National Association of Medical Examiners which includes a detailed scene investigation, review of the child and family history, and certain autopsy procedures (Corey, Hanzlick, Howard, Nelson, & Krous, 2007). There are also standards for reporting SIDS on death certificates. Although differences may identify some children who are intentionally suffocated, differentiating fatal abuse by suffocation from SIDS remains difficult (Hymel, 2006). The findings on postmortem examination in cases of SIDS and suffocation can be indistinguishable (Smialek & Lambros, 1988) and the death scene investigation can therefore contribute much more to the investigation. This is why SIDS is a term used to describe infants who die suddenly and unexpectedly and whose cause of death remains unknown after a full postmortem evaluation, including death scene investigation, and clinical review of all information. SIDS remains a diagnosis of exclusion, and there must be a full investigation of the cause of death in all infants and children before the death is labeled SIDS.

Child Death Reviews

Since differentiating fatal abuse from natural and accidental causes of death may be difficult, some have suggested that active surveillance by review teams at the time of death offers an opportunity to more accurately collect identification and improve investigation, but it is costly (Schloesser, Pierpont, & Poetner, 1992). Differentiating SIDS, metabolic diseases, accidental suffocation, and other natural causes of death from homicide requires a careful, complete investigation. Few jurisdictions in the United States have the resources—both money and properly trained personnel—to conduct an immediate, thorough investigation into each childhood death (AAP Committee on Child Abuse, 1999). Retrospective reviews at the state level using multiple data sources have improved identification of maltreatment deaths, but these reviews occurred 1–3 years after the death (Schnitzer, Covington, Wirtz, Verhoek-Oftedahl, & Palusci, 2008).

To address this, most states and many jurisdictions have developed child death review teams to proactively identify and understand the causes of childhood deaths (Durfee, Gellert, & Tilton-Durfee, 1992). Child death review teams were initially established to review suspicious childhood deaths, although many jurisdictions now review all pediatric deaths. Members of the review team vary by jurisdiction but are generally composed of professionals from specific disciplines. Standard team members include coroners and/or medical examiners, law enforcement agents, prosecuting attorneys, CPS workers, pediatricians, and public health professionals. Additional representatives can come from mental health agencies, schools, fire departments, and prevention agencies. Child death review teams provide an important method for systematic review of the factors contributing to pediatric deaths which can lead to preventing further fatalities. Multidisciplinary reviews are more complete than are single agency reviews, can more easily identify suspicious deaths, and can provide the opportunity to review protocols within and among participating agencies (Durfee et al., 1992). Implementation of death review teams may also improve the quality of death investigations at the local level, identify barriers to death investigations, allow for better allocation of limited resources, and improve the understanding of the causes of child death (AAP Committee on Child Abuse, 1999).

Most child death review teams in the country have been developed during the past 5–10 years, and national outcome data are limited. It is hoped that death investigations will improve prevention strategies, hold more adults responsible, and better protect siblings of murdered children from future harm. Improvements have been made in death certificate identification, and new International Classification of Disease coding has been developed to more completely identify the maltreatment nature of some deaths. Many states, like Missouri, now mandate review of all child deaths, and most have adopted prevention as the primary focus of the child death review program and are inadequately funded (Webster, Schnitzer, Jenny, Ewigman, & Alario, 2003). In Arizona, the state review team was able to identify and correct an incorrect cause of death in 13% of death certificates and suggested that 38% of all child deaths after the first month of life could be prevented. Several areas for work to prevent childhood deaths from a variety of accidental and intentional causes were identified (Rimsza, Schackner, Bowen, & Marshall, 2002). Internationally, reviews have produced policy changes and the identification of system themes in effective prevention, including assessment, interagency communication, responsibility, the number of professionals involved, the role of general practitioners, training, and parental choice (Sanders, Colton, & Roberts, 1999).

In a separate but related development, case reviews of children in the child welfare system have been mandated by the US government in an effort to improve outcomes in the child protective, adoption, and foster care systems. These "citizen review panels" or CRPs were first required in 1996 for US states as part of re-authorization of the Child Abuse Prevention and Treatment Act (CAPTA), and many states have instituted CRPs to review child maltreatment fatalities (US Department of Health and Human Services, 1998). CRPs are ideally made up of a representative sample of the community, meet at least quarterly, and fulfill a broad mandate which includes ensuring that the state is in compliance with CAPTA, Title IV-E programs, and child fatality review requirements (Jones, Litzelfelner, & Ford, 2003). CRPs have had some impact on child welfare policies, although several obstacles have been noted to their effectiveness (Bryan, Jones, Allen, & Collin-Camargo, 2007). Regardless of the process involved, physicians and pediatricians have an important role to play in reviewing child deaths and assisting the community in its efforts to prevent future fatality (AAP, 1999).

In Brief

- There is a high incidence of facial injuries in abused children that go unreported by dentists and physicians.
- Oro-facial injuries are common in abused children, and dental neglect affects large numbers of US children.
- Most oral injuries that result from physical abuse are nonspecific, and the diagnosis of abuse rests on the history or additional physical findings.
- Infant frenum tears occur when hands, pacifiers, bottles, or eating utensils are forced into a child's mouth in an attempt to silence a crying infant or feed a refusing child. They can also occur accidentally.
- Cases of accidental poisoning can appear to be similar to cases of abuse, and a comprehensive psychosocial assessment can help in determining the underlying cause.
- 1,530 children were confirmed victims of fatal abuse in the United States in 2006, but this is an underestimation because of both under-identification of child homicides and inaccurate classification of pediatric fatalities in official reports.
- Approximately 40% of fatal abuse occurs among infants and 75% occurs to children less than 5 years of age.
- Child abuse deaths may have few or no external signs, and a comprehensive autopsy can reveal certain patterns of head and other organ injury which allow accurate determination of the abusive nature of the death.

- Death review teams that review suspicious childhood deaths may improve the quality of death investigations, identify barriers, allow for better allocation of limited resources, improve the understanding of the causes of child death, and help in designing prevention activities to reduce further death.
- A small percentage of SIDS deaths are attributable to fatal child abuse but investigators and physicians should take a supportive and not accusatory approach during the investigation of a sudden, unexpected infant death.
- A comprehensive investigation including scene investigation, autopsy, and review of clinical history is needed to make a diagnosis of SIDS.

References

Alander, S. W., Dowd, D., Bratton, S. L., & Kearnes, G. L. (2000). Pediatric acetaminophen overdose: Risk factors associated with hepatocellular injury. *Archives of Pediatrics and Adolescent Medicine, 154*, 346–350.

American Academy of Pediatric Dentistry. (2003). Definition of dental neglect. *Pediatric Dentistry, 25,* 7.

AAP Committee on Child Abuse and Neglect and Committee on Community Health Services. (1999). Investigation and review of unexpected infant and child deaths. *Pediatrics, 104*, 1158–1160.

AAP Committee on Early Childhood, Adoption and Dependent Care. (1986). Oral and dental aspects of child abuse and neglect. *Pediatrics, 78*, 537–539.

AAP Committee on Fetus and Newborn. (2003). Apnea, sudden infant death syndrome, and home monitoring. *Pediatrics, 111*(4), 914–917.

AAP Committee on Injury, Violence and Poison Prevention. (2003). Poison treatment in the home. *Pediatrics, 112*, 1182–1185.

AAP Task Force on Sudden Infant Death Syndrome. (2005). The changing concept of sudden infant death syndrome: Diagnostic coding shifts, controversies regarding the sleeping environment, and new variables to consider in reducing risk. *Pediatrics, 116*(5), 1245–1255.

Bass, M., Kravath, R. E., & Glass, L. (1986). Death-scene investigation in sudden infant death. *The New England Journal of Medicine, 315*, 100–105.

Bays, J. (1994). Child abuse by poisoning. In R. M. Reece (Ed.), *Child abuse: Medical diagnosis and management* (pp. 69–106). Philadelphia: Lea & Febiger.

Becker, D. B., Needleman, H. L., & Kotelchuck, M. (1978). Child abuse and dentistry: Orofacial trauma and its recognition by dentists. *Journal of the American Dental Association, 97,* 24–28.

Bennett, M. D., Hall, J., Frazier, L., Patel, N., & Shaw, K. (2006). Homicide of children aged 0–4 years, 2003–04: Results from the National Violent Death Reporting System. *Injury Prevention, 12*(S2), ii39–ii42.

Black, J., & Zenel, J. A. (2003). Child abuse by intentional iron poisoning presenting as shock and persistent academia. *Pediatrics, 111*, 197–199.

Brewster, A. L., Nelson, J. P., Hymel, K. P., Lucas, D. R., McCanne, T. R., & Milner, J. S. (1998). Victim, perpetrator, family and incident characteristics of 32 infant maltreatment deaths in the United States Air Force. *Child Abuse and Neglect, 22*, 91–101.

Bryan, V., Jones, B., Allen, E., & Collin-Camargo, C. (2007). Civic engagement or token participation? Perceived impact of the citizen panel review initiative. *Children and Youth Services Review, 29*, 1286–1300.

Case, M. E. (2007). Abusive head injuries in infants and young children. *Legal Medicine (Tokyo), 9*(2), 83–87.

Case, M. E., Graham, M. A., Handy, T. C., Jentzen, J. M., Monteleone, J. A., & National Association of Medical Examiners Ad Hoc Committee on Shaken Baby Syndrome. (2001). Position paper on fatal abusive head injuries in infants and young children. *American Journal of Forensic Medicine and Pathology, 22*(2), 112–122.

Coleman-Phox, K., Odouli, R., & Li, D. K. (2008). Use of a fan during sleep and the risk of sudden infant death syndrome. *Archives of Pediatrics and Adolescent Medicine, 162*(10), 963–968.

Corey, T. S., Hanzlick, R., Howard, J., Nelson, C., & Krous, H. (2007). A functional approach to sudden unexplained infant deaths. *American Journal of Forensic Medicine and Pathology, 128*(3), 271–277.

Culbertson, J. L., Krous, H. F., & Bendell, R. D. (1988). *Sudden infant death syndrome: Medical aspects and psychological management.* Baltimore, MD: Johns Hopkins University Press.

da Fonesca, M. A., Feigal, R. J., & ten Bensel, R. W. (1992). Dental aspects of 1248 cases of child maltreatment on file at a major county hospital. *Pediatric Dentistry, 14*(3), 152–157.

Dine, M. S., & McGovern, M. E. (1982). Intentional poisoning of children – An overlooked category of child abuse: Report of seven cases and review of literature. *Pediatrics, 70*, 32–35.

Dolinak, D., Matshes, E. W., & Lew, E. (2005). *Forensic pathology: Principles and practice.* Burlington: Elsevier.

Duhaime, A. C., Christian, C. W., Rorke, L. B., & Zimmerman, R. A. (1998). Nonaccidental head injury in infants – The "shaken-baby syndrome." *New England Journal of Medicine, 338*(25), 1822–1829.

Durfee, M. J., Gellert, G. A., & Tilton-Durfee, D. (1992). Origins and clinical relevance of child death review teams. *The Journal of the American Medical Association, 267*, 172–175.

Emery, J. L., Chandra, S., & Gilbert-Barness, E. F. (1988). Findings in child deaths registered as sudden infant death syndrome (SIDS) in Madison, Wisconsin. *Pediatric Pathology, 8*, 171–178.

Ewigman, B., Kivlahan, C., & Land, G. (1993). The Missouri child fatality study: Underreporting of maltreatment fatalities among children younger than five years of age, 1983 through 1986. *Pediatrics, 91*, 330–337.

Fazen, L. E., Lovejoy, F. H., & Crone, R. K. (1986). Acute poisoning in a children's hospital: A 2-year experience. *Pediatrics, 77*, 144–151.

Fischler, R. S. (1983). Poisoning: A syndrome of child abuse. *American Family Physician, 28*(6), 103–108.

Gilliland, M. G., & Folberg, R. (1996). Shaken babies – Some have no impact injuries. *Journal of Forensic Sciences, 41*(1), 114–116.

Holton, J., Allen, J., Green, C., et al. (1991). Inherited metabolic diseases in the sudden infant death syndrome. *Archives of Disease in Childhood, 66*, 1315–1317.

Hymel, K. P., & The Committee on Child Abuse and Neglect. (2006). Distinguishing sudden infant death syndrome from child abuse fatalities. *Pediatrics, 118*(1), 421–427.

Institute of Medicine, Committee on Identifying and Preventing Medication Errors, Board on Health Care Services, & Aspden, P., Wolcott, J. A., Lyle Bootman, J., Cronenwett, L. R. (Eds.). (2007). *Preventing medication errors.* Washington, DC: The National Academies Press.

Itabashi, H. H., Andrews, J. M., Tomiyasu, U., Erlich, S. S., & Sathyavagiswaran, L. (Eds.). (2007). *Forensic neuropathology: A practical review of the fundamentals*. Burlington, MA: Elsevier Academic Press.

Jenny, C., Hymel, K. P., Ritzen, A., Reinert, S. E., & Hay, T. C. (1999). Analysis of missed cases of abusive head trauma. *The Journal of the American Medical Association, 281*(7), 621–626.

Jones, B., Litzelfelner, P., & Ford, J. (2003). The value and role of Citizen Review Panels in child welfare: Perceptions of citizen review panel members and child protection workers. *Child Abuse and Neglect, 27*, 699–704.

Keens, T. G., & Davidson Ward, S. L. (1993). Apnea spells, sudden death, and the role of the apnea monitor. *Pediatric Clinics of North America, 40*, 897–911.

Kellogg, N. D., & The Committee on Child Abuse and Neglect. (2005a). Oral and dental aspects of child abuse and neglect. *Pediatrics, 116*, 1565–1568.

Kellogg, N. D., & The Committee on Child Abuse and Neglect. (2005b). The evaluation of sexual abuse in children. *Pediatrics, 116*, 506–512.

King, W. K., Kiesel, E. L., & Simon, H. K. (2006). Child abuse fatalities: Are we missing opportunities for intervention? *Pediatric Emergency Care, 22*(4), 211–214.

Knight, L. D., & Collins, K. A. (2005). A 25-year retrospective review of deaths due to pediatric neglect. *American Journal of Forensic Medicine and Pathology, 26*(3), 221–228.

Krous, H. F., Haas, E. A., Manning, J. M., Deeds, A., Silva, P. D., Chadwick, A. E., et al. (2006). Child protective services referrals in cases of sudden infant death: A 10-year, population-based analysis in San Diego County, California. *Child Maltreatment, 11*(3), 247–256.

McClain, P. W., Sacks, J. J., Ewigman, B. G., Smith, S. M., Mercy, J. A., & Sniezek, J. E. (1994). Geographic patterns of fatal abuse or neglect in children younger than 5 years old, United States, 1979–1988. *Archives of Pediatric and Adolescent Medicine, 148*, 82–86.

McClain, P. W., Sacks, J. J., Froehlke, R. G., & Ewigman, B. G. (1993). Estimates of fatal child abuse and neglect, United States, 1979 through 1988. *Pediatrics, 91*, 338–343.

McGuire, S, Hunter, B., Hunter, L., Sibert, J. R., Mann, M., Kemp, A. M., et al. (2007). Diagnosing abuse: A systemic review of torn frenum and intra-oral injuries. *Archives of Disease in Childhood, 92*, 1113–1117; Published online 27 April 2007, doi: 1136/adc 2006.113001.

Mitchell, E. A., Thompson, J. M. D., Beocroft, D. M. O., Bajanowski, T., Brinkman, B., Happe, A., et al. (2008). Head covering and the risk of SIDS: Findings from the New Zealand and German SIDS case-control studies. *Pediatrics, 121*, e1478–e1483.

Mullick, M., Miller, L. J., & Jacobsen, T. (2001). Insight into mental illness and child maltreatment risk among mothers with major psychiatric disorders. *Psychiatric Services, 52*(4), 488–492.

Naidoo, S. (2000). A profile of the oro-facial injuries in child physical abuse at a children's hospital. *Child Abuse and Neglect, 24*, 521–534.

Needleman, H. L. (1986). Orofacial trauma in child abuse: Types, prevalence, management, and the dental profession's involvement. *Pediatric Dentistry, 8*, 71–79.

Overpeck, M. D., Brenner, R. A., Cosgrove, C., Trumble, A. C., Kochanek, K., & MacDorman, M. (2002). National underascertainment of sudden unexpected infant deaths associated with deaths of unknown cause. *Pediatrics, 109*(2), 274–283.

Paschall, R. (2005). The chemically abused child. In A. Giardino & R. Alexander (Eds.), *Child maltreatment: A clinical guide and reference*, 3rd edn. Saint Louis, MO: GW Medical Publishing, Inc.

Paulozzi, L. (2002). Variation in homicide risk during infancy – United States, 1989–1998. *Mortality and Morbidity Weekly Report, 51*(9), 187–189.

Perez, A., Scribano, P. V., & Perry, H. (2004). An intentional opiate intoxication of an infant: When medical toxicology and child maltreatment services merge. *Pediatric Emergency Care, 20*, 769–772.

Pitetti, R. D., Whitman, E., & Zaylor, A. (2008). Accidental and non-accidental poisonings as a cause of ALTEs in infants. *Pediatrics, 122*, e359–e362.

Pressley, J. C., Barlow, B., Kendig, T., & Paneth-Pollak, R. (2007). Twenty year trends in fatal injuries to very young children: The persistence of racial disparities. *Pediatrics, 119*(4), e875.

Rimsza, M. E., Schackner, R. A., Bowen, K. A., & Marshall, W. (2002). Can child deaths be prevented? The Arizona Child Fatality Review Program experience. *Pediatrics, 110*(1), e11.

Rivenes, S. M., Bakerman, P. R., & Miller, M. B. (1997). Intentional caffeine poisoning in an infant. *Pediatrics, 99*, 736–738.

Roberts, I., Li, L., & Barker, M. (1998). Trends in intentional injury deaths in children and teenagers (1980–1995). *Journal of Public Health Medicine, 20*(4), 463–466.

Rogers, D. W., & Bentovim, A. (1981). Nonaccidental poisoning: The elusive diagnosis. *Archives of Disease in Childhood, 56*, 156–157.

Sabotta, E. E., & Davis, R. L. (1992). Fatality after report to a child abuse registry in Washington state, 1973–1986. *Child Abuse and Neglect, 16*, 627–635.

Sanders, R., Colton, M., & Roberts, S. (1999). Child abuse fatalities and cases of extreme concern: Lessons from reviews. *Child Abuse and Neglect, 23*, 257–268.

Schlesinger, S. L., Borbotsina, J., & O'Neill, L. (1975). Petechial hemorrhages of the soft palate secondary to fellatio. *Oral Surgery, Oral Medicine and Oral Pathology, 40*, 376–378.

Schloesser, P., Pierpont, J., & Poetner, J. (1992). Active surveillance of child abuse fatalities. *Child Abuse and Neglect, 16*, 3–10.

Schnitzer, P. G., Covington, T. M., Wirtz, S. J., Verhoek-Oftedahl, W., & Palusci, V. J. (2008). Public health surveillance of fatal child maltreatment: Summary of three state programs. *American Journal of Public Health, 98*(2), 296–303; Published online May 30, 2007, doi: 10.2105/AJPH.2006.087783.

Schnitzer, P. G., & Ewigman, B. G. (2005). Child deaths resulting from inflicted injuries: Household risk factors and perpetrator characteristics. *Pediatrics, 116*(5), e687–e693.

Sibert, J. R., & Murphy, J. F. (1980). Child poisoning and child abuse. *Archives of Disease in Childhood, 55*, 822.

Smialek, J. E., & Lambros, Z. (1988). Investigation of sudden infant deaths. *Pediatrician, 15*(4), 191–197.

Starling, S. P., Patel, S., Burke, B. L., Sirotnak, A. P., Stronks, S., & Rosquist, P. (2004). Analysis of perpetrator admissions to inflicted traumatic brain injury in children. *Archives of Pediatrics and Adolescent Medicine, 158*(5), 454–458.

Teece, S., & Crawford, I. (2004). Torn frenulum and non-accidental injury in children. *Emergency Medicine Journal, 22*, 125.

Thackeray, J. D. (2007). Frena tears and abusive head injury. *Pediatric Emergency Care, 23*, 735–737.

U.S. Advisory Board on Child Abuse and Neglect. (1995). *A Nation's shame: Fatal child abuse and neglect in the United States.* Washington, DC: US Department of Health and Human Services.

U.S. Department of Human Services, Administration on Children, Youth and Families. (2008). *Child maltreatment 2006*(pp. 65–74). Washington, DC: U.S. Government Printing Office.

U.S. Department of Health and Human Services. (1998). *Establishment of the citizen review panel requirement under the child abuse prevention and treatment act* (No. ACYF-PI-CB-98-01). Washington, DC: U.S. Government Printing Office.

Webster, R., Schnitzer, P. G., Jenny, C., Ewigman, B. G., & Alario, A. J. (2003). Child death review: The state of the nation. *American Journal of Preventive Medicine, 25,* 58–64.

Wiley, J. F. (1991). Difficult diagnoses in toxicology: Poisons not detected by comprehensive drug screen. *Pediatric Clinics of North America, 38,* 725–737.

Part III

Related Issues

Chapter 10

Maltreatment of Children and Youth with Special Healthcare Needs

Patricia M. Sullivan, John F. Knutson, and Eleanor J. Ashford

Introduction

Children with special healthcare needs have an increased risk for child abuse and neglect (Sullivan & Knutson, 1998; Sullivan & Knutson, 2000). The maltreatment of these children and youth is frequently unidentified and unrecognized in health-care settings. Consequently, efforts are needed to inform healthcare providers about the risk factors for child maltreatment among children with special healthcare needs. This requires that healthcare providers be vigilant in their medical assessments of these children for both maltreatment and disability status. This chapter presents maltreatment risk factors, perpetrator characteristics, and maltreatment characteristics of children with special healthcare needs that have been identified through research in healthcare settings. These risk factors and maltreatment characteristics have diagnostic and treatment implications for medical professionals. Practical guidelines for pediatricians in identifying maltreatment among children with special healthcare needs are presented with special emphasis on the abuse potential of restraint used in both medical and behavioral hospital settings. Guidelines for working with the families of children with special healthcare needs are presented. Case study examples of neglect, physical abuse, and sexual abuse of children with special healthcare needs are also given.

The maltreatment of children with special healthcare needs is a significant public health issue facing medical professionals. Violence, in any form, is a leading health indicator in Healthy People 2010, and children with disabilities were included for the first time in our nation's health agenda as a specific subpopulation since the

335

A.P. Giardino et al. (eds.), *A Practical Guide to the Evaluation of Child Physical Abuse and Neglect*, DOI 10.1007/978-1-4419-0702-8_10, © Springer Science+Business Media, LLC 1997, 2010

inception of the national health promotion and disease prevention agenda in 1979 (Sullivan, 2003). Children with special healthcare needs (CSHCN) are defined by the US Department of Health and Human Services, Health Resources and Services Administration (HERSA), Maternal and Child Health Bureau (MCHB) as

...those who have or are at increased risk for a chronic physical, developmental, behavioral, or emotional condition and who also require health and related services of a type or amount beyond that required by children generally. (U.S. Department of Health and Human Services, 2008)

This definition is broad and inclusive in emphasizing the common character- istics of children with a wide range of medical diagnoses. The National Sur- vey of Children with Special Healthcare Needs (NS-CSHCN) is a compendium of state and national data on the epidemiology of children with special health- care needs. This survey is sponsored by the Maternal and Child Health Bureau (MCHB) and conducted by the National Center for Health Statistics within the Centers for Disease Control and Prevention. It provides detailed information on prevalence, demographic characteristics, types of medical services needed, as well as access to and satisfaction with the services received. No data are gathered on child maltreatment. Children are identified due to the need for public assistance to fund healthcare services. Accordingly, their numbers are defined by socioeco- nomic parameters that do not include children from all socioeconomic strata. The 2005/2006 survey found almost 14% of children in the US have special health- care needs and 22% of households with children have at least one child with a special healthcare need. Moreover, the National Mental Health Information Cen- ter identified 2.9 million children with special mental health needs that include emotional, behavioral, or developmental disorders that require treatment (US Department of Health and Human Services, 2008). Thus, children with special healthcare needs are a significant group of children in the US. It should be noted that this chapter covers children in medical settings with diagnosed health con- ditions for which they receive medical interventions and require public assistance in funding that treatment. Although many of these children receive special educa- tion services, they are not commensurate with children receiving special education services under the Individuals with Disabilities Education Act (IDEA). These chil- dren have medical, not educational disabilities. This distinction is made given that the focus of this book is children with health related disabilities. Thus, the terms special healthcare or medical disability are used interchangeably throughout the chapter.

Research on Maltreatment of Children with Special Healthcare Needs

There is a growing body of research conducted in medical settings on the mal- treatment of children with special healthcare needs. Early work looked at samples of children from medical settings and reported the incidence of maltreated children within those samples. This research was criticized for subject selection biases because medical settings typically have large numbers of abused individuals seeking treatment. Sullivan and colleagues (1991) found that sexual abuse or a combination of sexual and physical abuse perpetrated by family members were the most common forms of maltreatment in a sample of 482 consecutively referred maltreated children with medical disabilities in a specialty hospital setting. The children's special healthcare needs encompassed communication disorders including speech and/or hearing impairments, learning disabilities, and cleft lip and/or palate. Males had high rates of sexual abuse and placement in a residential school was identified as a major risk factor for sexual abuse among deaf and hard-of-hearing children. In a 5-year retrospective study of 4,340 child patients in a pediatric hospital, the majority (68%) were victims of sexual abuse while 32% were victims of physical abuse perpetrated by family members (Willging, Bower, & Cotton, 1992).

Researchers in Norway mailed questionnaires to 26 pediatric hospitals requesting information on the incidence of children receiving medical services for suspected sexual abuse including their demographic characteristics of disability type, age, gender, and the determination of the abuse allegations (Kvam, 2000). There were 1,293 children ranging in age from infancy to 16 years seen in these hospitals because of suspected sexual assault between 1994 and 1996. Data obtained through medical record reviews identified 54 girls and 29 boys with medical disabilities accounting for 6.4% of the total sample. Identified medical disabilities included mental retardation, cerebral palsy/physical disabilities, and deafness. These children were at increased risk for sexual abuse and this risk increased with the severity of the disability. Children with behavior disorders, mental retardation, and physical disabilities were the most susceptible to sexual abuse and boys were more susceptible than girls. These results support earlier findings that sexual abuse is a major form of maltreatment found among disabled children accessing healthcare services.

In the US, Giardino and colleagues (2003) conducted an archival study of the medical records of consecutive referrals to a hospital-based healthcare team conducting medical evaluations for suspected child maltreatment in children with special healthcare needs. The medical records of 60 children ranging in age from 3 to 16 years were examined. Identified special healthcare needs included ADHD, autism, blindness, cerebral palsy, developmental delay, hearing impairment, mental retardation, and speech/language delays. Some 31% of the children were victims of maltreatment, the majority of it sexual.

Sullivan and Knutson (1998) conducted a population-based study of the maltreatment incidence and characteristics of all children seen at the Boys Town National Research Hospital (BTNRH) from 1982 to 1992. The names of these children and youth were merged with the Nebraska Department of Social Service Central Registry, the Nebraska Foster Care Review Board database, and five regional law enforcement agencies to identify cases of intrafamilial and extrafamilial maltreatment. The completed study comprised of the merger of over 39,000 hospital records with these databases, resulted in over 6,000 maltreatment incident matches and a hospital-wide maltreatment prevalence rate of 15%. A similar merger was conducted in 2000 with over 165,000 hospital records and the same 15% prevalence rate was identified. This base rate warrants routine screenings for both maltreatment and disabilities by pediatricians and other healthcare professionals in hospital settings.

Characteristics of Maltreated Children with Special Healthcare Needs

The following maltreatment characteristics and risk factors among children with special healthcare needs have been identified in the research studies summarized above. They are presented here categorically to assist pediatricians in their maltreatment evaluations of children with special healthcare needs by delineating risk factors and characteristics that are germane to diagnosis and treatment.

Types of Maltreatment. The most frequent forms of maltreatment experienced by children with special healthcare needs, in descending order of magnitude, are neglect, followed by physical abuse, sexual abuse, and emotional abuse. Many children are victims of multiple types of maltreatment.

Gender of Victims. A higher percent of boys (56%) than girls (44%) was identified for all types of maltreatment in the Sullivan and Knutson (1998) hospital-based study. The higher percentage of boys likely reflects the higher base rate of most disabilities among boys than girls. However, it also reflects that large cohorts of boy victims are consistently appearing in epidemiological studies of maltreatment among children with special healthcare needs.

Type of Disability. High rates of disabilities were also found among the subjects in the Sullivan and Knutson (1998) hospital-based study. Some 73% of the abused sample had one or more disabilities in contrast to 32% of the nonabused control sample. Among the abused children, behavior disorders, speech and language disorders, mental retardation, and hearing impairments were the most common types of disabilities. The inclusion of a nonabused control group in the research provided the opportunity for comparisons between abused and nonabused children with special healthcare needs. Maltreated children were 2.2 times more likely to have a medical disability than nonabused children. Furthermore, the children with special healthcare needs were 1.8 times more likely to be victims of neglect, 1.6 times more likely to be physically abused, and 2.2 times more likely to be sexually abused than nondisabled children. Abused children are 2.2 times more likely to have multiple disabilities than nonabused disabled children.

Disability/Abuse Associations. Certain types of medical disabilities are at greater risk for certain types of abuse (Sullivan & Knutson, 1998). Children with behavior disorders, speech and language disorders, and mental retardation are at increased risk for neglect. Behavior disorders, hearing impairment, and mental retardation are high-risk disabilities for physical abuse. Children with Attention Deficit/Hyperactivity Disorder (Without Conduct Disorder), behavior disorders, learning disabilities, and mental retardation appear to be at increased risk for sexual abuse. Children with behavior disorders and mental retardation are at increased risk for all three forms of maltreatment.

Age at First Maltreatment. A little more than half (53%) of the abused children in the Sullivan and Knutson (1998) study were maltreated at 4 years of age or younger. This indicates that children with medical disabilities tend to be maltreated at very young ages and underscores the need for early intervention and support services for families with young children, including infants, toddlers, and preschoolers with medical disabilities.

Severity of Maltreatment. Children with medical disabilities tend to endure the highest severity levels of neglect and sexual abuse which include life-threatening neglect and oral, anal, and/or vaginal intercourse, respectively (Sullivan & Knutson, 1998). For physical abuse, slightly lower severity levels were identified and included potentially injurious events and tissue damaging injuries requiring medical or dental attention. Children with multiple disabilities experienced the most severe forms of maltreatment.

Duration of Maltreatment. Most children with medical disabilities who are abused tend to experience abusive episodes for long periods of time (Sullivan & Knutson, 1998). Half of the sexually abused children were abused for periods of one year or more while the other half were found to experience one episode of sexual abuse. For physical abuse, two-thirds of the children were abused for one year or longer. Neglect of children with disabilities tends to occur for long periods of time with 98% neglected for longer than one year's time. Children with multiple disabilities had significantly longer durations of neglect, physical abuse, and sexual abuse than children with a single disability.

Perpetrators. Children with disabilities tend to be maltreated by individuals they know and trust. The overwhelming majority of perpetrators of children with special healthcare needs are parents who account for 95% of neglect perpetrators, 76% of physical abuse perpetrators, and 39% of sexual abuse perpetrators (Sullivan & Knutson, 1998). The majority of the remaining physical abuse and neglect is interfamilial and perpetrated by extended and other family members. Extrafamilial abuse accounts for a large portion (40%) of sexual abuse of children with special healthcare needs. Stranger abuse accounts for 7% of this extrafamilial abuse. The remaining sexual abuse is perpetrated by extended family members. Since these extrafamilial assaults are typically archived in police databases, epidemiological studies involving children with disabilities must include law enforcement databases. Female perpetrators account for almost 70% of neglect, 51% of physical abuse, and 18% of sexual abuse of children with health related disabilities.

Chronic Illness or Disability. Almost 20% of maltreated children with special healthcare needs have a parent with a chronic illness or disability compared to 10% of parents of nondisabled maltreated children. Maltreatment by a chronically ill or disabled parent is associated with all types of maltreatment (i.e., neglect, physical abuse, emotional abuse, and sexual abuse) (Sullivan & Knutson, 1998). Children without a disability, who have a disabled or chronically ill parent, were victims of neglect, physical abuse, and emotional abuse. Professionals need to be aware of the presence of disabilities in parents of maltreated children and make prevention and intervention efforts that target both the child and parent.

Single Parent Families. Significantly more children (61.8%) with medical disabilities who were victims of neglect, emotional abuse, and sexual abuse were from single-parent families than any other type of family constellation (Sullivan & Knutson, 1998).

Site of Abuse. The majority of children with disabilities are abused in their own homes or in homes of their perpetrators (Sullivan & Knutson, 1998). A variety of other sites were found which also have implications for prevention programs for children with disabilities. Children with special healthcare needs are at risk to be abused in public restrooms, public transportation systems, hospitals, detention centers, and in shopping malls.

Family Stress Factors

Family stress factors have been associated as correlates in the maltreatment of children with special healthcare needs and are deserving of attention in the medical evaluation of potential maltreatment. Substantially more family stress factors were present in the families of maltreated children with disabilities than in those of maltreated, nondisabled children. Significant associations between family stress factors and disability groups were identified in the Sullivan and Knutson (1998) hospital-based research. The Sullivan and Knutson (1998) hospital epidemiological study also found that family stress factors were associated with specific types of maltreatment (See Table 10.1).

In addition to these factors, depending on the special healthcare needs of the child, there may be other sources of stress in the family:

- New communication demands
- Emotional demands
- Extra laundry and cleaning
- Additional lifting and dressing
- Sleep deprivation in one or both parents

Healthcare professionals can help families address these stressful challenges in a number of constructive ways that offer support and help families develop insight into what is causing the increased family stress. The goal for the healthcare professional is to empower the family in a manner that helps them to function well and provide appropriate care to their children (See Table 10.2).

Restraints

Children with special healthcare needs are often in out-of-home placements in which restraint is used as a behavioral intervention. Healthcare professionals must be cognizant of the abusive potential inherent in this type of treatment. Condoned physical interventions dispensed under the guise of therapeutic interventions with children with special healthcare needs in hospitals and residential treatment centers

Table 10.1 Significant associations between family stress factors and disability groups.

Disability groups	Description of family stress factors
Behavior disabilities	Associated with mental/emotional problems in parent, parent/child conflict, disabled child in family, child delinquency, and child alcohol and/or drug dependency
Communication disorders	Associated with inadequate parenting, inadequate housing, financial problems, pregnancy/birth of newborn, mental/emotional problems in parent, social isolation, and fetal alcohol syndrome
Health related disabilities	Associated with inadequate housing, financial problems, pregnancy/birth of newborn, parent ill/disabled, mental/emotional problems in parent, social isolation, disabled child in family, and fetal alcohol syndrome
Mental disabilities	Associated with inadequate parenting, inadequate housing, financial problems, parent ill/disabled, mental/emotional problems in parent, social isolation, disabled child in family, and fetal alcohol syndrome
Multiple disabilities	Associated with pregnancy/birth of newborn and disabled child in family
Maltreatment type	Description of family stress factors
Neglect	Associated with inadequate parenting, inadequate housing, financial problems, mental/emotional problems in parent, social isolation, and involvement with the legal system
Physical abuse	Associated with inadequate parenting and involvement with the legal system
Sexual abuse	Associated with mental/emotional problems in parent, alcohol/drug problem in parent, social isolation, and involvement with the legal system
Emotional abuse	Associated with inadequate parenting, inadequate housing, financial problems, pregnancy/birth of newborn, parent ill/disabled, mental/emotional problems in parent, alcohol/drug problem in parent, social isolation, and involvement with the legal system

can escalate to abuse (Sullivan, 2006). The use and misuse of restraints can become an added complication when identifying maltreatment concerns. Furthermore, physical devices can be used to exert inappropriate control and power with children with special healthcare needs and add potential psychological maltreatment. Methods of restraint are also frequently seen in both psychiatric and group home settings and can easily escalate to abuse and/or physical injury of the child or youth. Care must be undertaken to ensure that the restraint is undertaken to modify the behavior of the child, not for the convenience of the parent or staff member implementing the procedure. Because physical restraint remains a controversial intervention and can cause physical injuries, appropriate condition must guide those who are using them. Caveats and cautions in the use of restraints are summarized in Table 10.3.

Table 10.2 Suggestions for working with families.

Help the parents to	• Focus on the child rather than on his/her disability • Understand disability facts and issues, in order to work with their child constructively • Acknowledge and respond to their feelings regarding the disability • Accept the disability without devaluing the child • Assist the child in developing individual and family potentials, together and independently • Connect with local resources which would benefit the child and family members
Determine what the family knows about	• Their child's disability, including his/her medical prognoses • Educational implications and programs for their child • Assistive devices for their child • Available support groups for parents and their child
Enlist the father's participation since it provides	• Paternal support, involvement and commitment to the child, mother, and other family members • Gender balance, strengthening the family bond, and lessening the risk of spouse abuse
Doctor – parent communication should be relevant to the parents'	• Intellectual ability, language, communication methods, culture, and lifestyle • Model effective communication and problem-solving skills • Discuss and interpret available information • Clarify problems and goals • Facilitate problem resolution through collaboration • Encourage boundary setting
Abuse prevention	• Improve parental awareness and encourage proactive behavior across settings and situations • Gain the cooperation and involvement of the parents in abuse prevention • Build upon parents' love and commitment to their child • Encourage parents to use the effective parenting skills they possess and to develop new skills as needed • Provide guidelines to assist parents with selecting safe caregivers using personal references, state license, credential checks, police checks, and unannounced visits to care center

Adapted from Sullivan (1996).

The presence of "restraint injuries" over padded body surfaces such as the buttocks, upper arm, thigh, back of calf and covetous area, such as the abdomen and cheeks, should raise suspicion of inappropriate restraint and/or poor monitoring and supervision of the restraint intervention by parent or staff.

Areas most commonly affected in lying positions are

- Hips
- Heels
- Shoulder blades
- Sacrum
- Elbows

Table 10.3 Caveats and cautions in the use of physical restraints in children with special healthcare needs.

Too much pressure caused by physical restraint can result in	• Ischemia • Edema • Paresthesia
Too little pressure can result in	• Friction injuries from loose or rubbing straps • Shear injuries
Signs of skin damage due to restraint	• Red areas that do not disappear. (Difficult to determine in children of color) • Raw, open lesions, blisters, rashes, or abraded areas • Bruising and swelling • Blue, red, purple, or black skin color • Depressions in the flesh that do not go away overnight • Complaints of pain; or, in children with limited verbal communication skills, changes in behavior, irritability, restlessness, crying, and vomiting

Adapted from Steinberg and Hylton (1998, pp. 207–209) (used with permission).

Areas most commonly affected in sitting positions are

- Ischial tuberosities
- Elbows
- Spinous processes
- Ribs
- Anterior superior iliac spines (ASIS, or front hip bones)

Areas most commonly affected in bracing of the spine are

- Underneath pressure pads
- ASIS
- Sacrum
- Ribs (especially the 10th and 11th)

Areas most commonly affected in bracing of the foot are

- Navicular bones
- Ankle malleoli
- Back of Heel

Children at most risk for being injured by restraints are those who

- Cannot move
- Cannot feel pressure
- Cannot communicate their discomfort
- Are self-destructive
- Are restrained for long periods of time without proper supervision and monitoring
- Are restrained frequently
- Find the restraint reinforcing, pleasurable, and attention getting

American Academy of Pediatrics (AAP) Guidelines

Hibbard and Desch (2007) in consort with the Committee on Child Abuse and Neglect and Council on Children with Disabilities of the American Academy of Pediatrics (AAP) developed guidelines for pediatricians to follow in their evaluations of suspected child abuse in children and adolescents with special healthcare needs and disabilities. These are summarized as follows: (adapted from Hibbard & Desch (2007))

1. Recognize signs and symptoms of maltreatment in all children and youth, especially those with special healthcare needs and disabilities.
2. Be aware that some disabilities can both mimic abuse and are at increased risk of accidental injury that gives the appearance of abuse.
3. Offer emotional support and referral to resources to the parents and family.
4. Evaluate all maltreated children for the presence of a disability.
5. Advocate for and assist families in acquiring a medical home.
6. Participate in both collaborative team evaluations and treatment plans for children with disabilities.
7. Assess a family's strengths and need for resources to help with stress factors faced by the family.
8. Advocate for wrap-around services for children with disabilities within the medical home to include identification, intervention, and prevention of maltreatment.
9. Advocate for the use of positive behavioral interventions and the elimination of aversive interventions, including physical restraints in home, school, and institutional settings for children with special healthcare needs.
10. Advocate for comprehensive healthcare coverage from both private and governmental insurers for children with all types of disabilities (See Table 10.4).

In Brief: Common Case Findings of Abuse and Neglect in Medical Evaluations of Children with Special Healthcare Needs

- Findings of some form of maltreatment
- Primary perpetrators are family members
- Multiple perpetrators of maltreatment are common
- Severe levels of maltreatment
- Long durations of maltreatment
- History of inadequate or inappropriate healthcare
- Frequent failure to meet medical appointments
- Inappropriate use or misuse of prescribed treatments and medications
- Misleading caretaker behavior and statements about child's injury

Table 10.4 Recommended protocol: for health providers' evaluation of suspected child abuse in CSHCN.

---

1. Conduct a thorough physical examination.
2. In so doing, look for signs of maltreatment including neglect, physical and sexual abuse.
3. Is there a disclosure of maltreatment? Yes ___ No ___
   - Does the child's condition fit with the caregiver's explanation?
   - Does the explanation change or vary over time?
   - Is the explanation inconsistent with the child's developmental abilities?
   - Is there a credible disclosure of abuse?
   - Are there physical or historical findings consistent with abuse?
   - Is there evidence of poor physical care, inadequate nutrition, emotional neglect, or physical neglect?
   - Is there failure to follow through on medical recommendations or meet medical appointments?
4. Does the child have a disability or special healthcare need?
5. If yes, how does this disability or medical condition affect this child?
6. Gather collateral information about the child
   (school, family, & medical history)
7. Are there any conditions or syndromes that could be confused with abuse?
   (Monteleone, 1998)
   - Mongolian spots
   - Folk medicine: Vietnamese coining; Cao Gio; Chinese spooning; Russian cupping; Mexican fallen fontanelle
   - Easy bruisability: Hemophilia; Vitamin K deficiency; leukemia; Henoch-Schonlein; erythema multiform; Ehlers-Danlos syndrome
   - Burns and burn-like lesions: Impetigo; car seat burn; frostbite
   - Congenital indifference to pain
   - Osteogenesis imperfects
   - Hair tourniquet
   - Congenital syphilis
   - Copper, Vitamin C or D deficiency
   - Toddler's fracture or fractures from passive exercise
   - Self-inflicted injuries; Cornelia De Lange syndrome; Nesch-Nyhan syndrome; headbanging

---

Recommended for use in agencies, clinics, and services that receive or assess reports alleged child maltreatment among children with special healthcare needs.

- Use of disability to explain the maltreatment or minimize the child's condition
- Blaming injuries or condition on the child
- Professional empathy for caretakers diverts focus and attention on the child
- Concerns and reports of maltreatment ignored by authority figures in institutions
- Multiple contacts with healthcare providers and other professionals, with failure to recognize or respond to maltreatment
- Ignoring, misunderstanding, or misinterpreting signs and symptoms of maltreatment by family and professionals

Case Studies

A total of seven case studies are briefly presented to illustrate the neglect and physical abuse of children with special healthcare needs. One example of sexual abuse is also given.

Case 1: Physical Abuse by Mother

A 33-month-old male with global developmental delay, blindness and seizures presented with erythema, swelling, desquamation, and blistering of the right hand and forearm. At the proximal forearm, was a very distinct demarcation between normal skin and injured skin. His mother indicated that she had placed tube socks around his wrists during the night to keep him from hurting himself. While this boy had documented self-injurious behaviors (i.e., striking at his face and eyes and scratching at his skin), this injury pattern was consistent with an immersion burn, not a restraint injury.

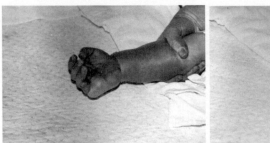 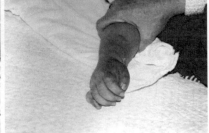

Case 2: Physical Abuse by Classroom Teacher

A 9-year-old girl with mild mental retardation was presented with linear bruising and scratches in the middle of her back. She had temporal lobe seizures and was exhibiting aggressive outbursts in school; subsequently her teacher had pushed her

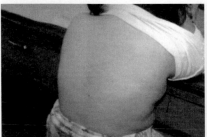 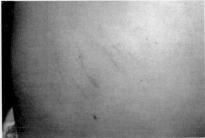

to the floor, pulled her arms behind her, and held her down by pushing his shoe in the middle of her back causing the injuries to her back.

Case 3: Sexual Abuse by Family Member

Abnormal genital examination was found in a 2½-year-old girl with spina bifida. Findings include an extremely dilated vaginal orifice and a very thin rim of stretched out hymenal tissue surrounding the orifice. She had been seen previously with bruising of the posterior fourchette. At that time, her examination was normal other than the bruise and the bruising was assumed to be caused by a urethral catheterization. This subsequent examination was prompted when a sibling disclosed sexual abuse by a family member. Children with spina bifida lack innervation of the genital area. Some laxity of the musculature surrounding the vaginal orifice is to be expected but this degree of dilation and hymenal thinning cannot be explained by the disability or catheterization.

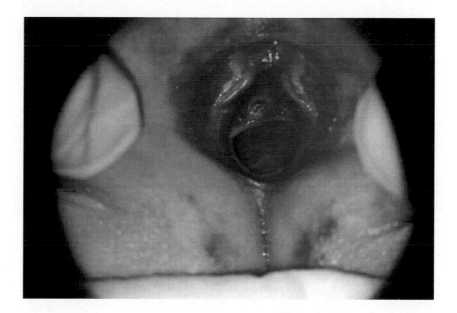

Case 4: Physical Abuse

Deep bruising of the upper arm, upper chest, and abdominal wall was found in this adolescent with mental retardation. Bruising of cavitous areas, such as the abdomen, are especially concerning for inflicted trauma.

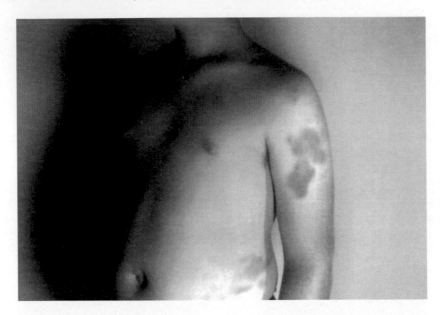

Case 5: Photos A and B Physical Abuse and Neglect

This 4½-year-old boy was taken into protective custody in the aftermath of a violent, domestic altercation between his inebriated parents. In foster care, he was noted to be developmentally delayed, especially in the areas of speech and self-care skills. He was microcephalic and had other physical features consistent with Fetal Alcohol Syndrome. His upper front teeth were carious, and he had deep, old bruising and subcutaneous fat necrosis of the buttocks and outer thigh.

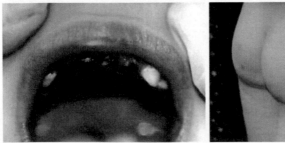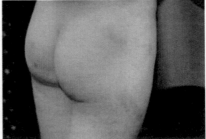

Case 6: Neglect and Physical Abuse

A 16-month-old boy born with global developmental delays and hypotonia had been placed in medical foster care due to allegations of neglect and abandonment. Prior to entering foster care a developmental assessment was performed confirming his diagnoses. At the time of the assessment the child could sit with pelvic support and was beginning to roll over. He had started to finger feed and could hold a bottle by himself. He was alert and social with emerging expressive and receptive language skills. Within days of entering foster care, his condition deteriorated quickly and significantly, including dramatic weight loss, recurrent bruising, broken bones, retinal hemorrhages, and subdural hematomas. He was admitted to the hospital numerous times, each time discharged to his foster mother. The possibility of maltreatment was not initially considered because the foster mother was a nurse. Just prior to his discharge back to foster care after the third hospitalization, the nursing staff consulted the hospital child abuse team. They had long-standing concerns regarding the child's well-being and the foster mother, who exhibited controlling, disruptive, and possessive behavior during each of the child's hospitalizations. Physicians had repeatedly dismissed the nurses' concern. The child abuse team reviewed the child's history and physical examination and recommended a skeletal survey. He was found to have diffuse osteopenia and old fractures of his right proximal femur and left distal femur.

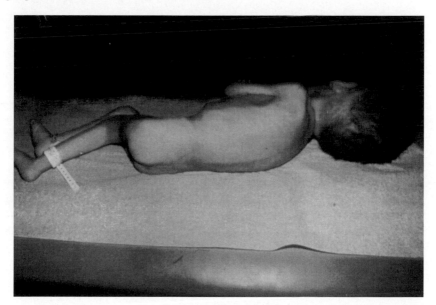

Case 7: Neglect

This 4-year-old was discovered in an extremely deprived environment. He had marked developmental delays, short stature, and abdominal distension. He appeared to be a much younger child than his chronologic age. In foster care, he made significant gains in his development and growth.

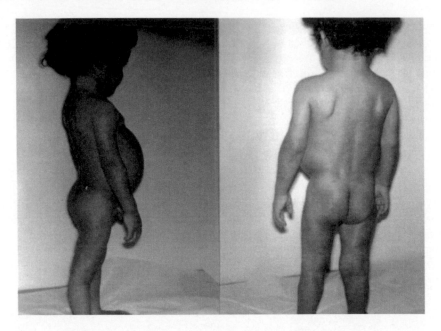

Conclusions

Epidemiological research indicates that healthcare professionals, including physicians, nurses, physical therapists, occupational therapists, dentists, psychologists, and social workers, may expect that some 15% of their child patients will be victims of maltreatment and over half of them will have some type of disability (Sullivan & Knutson, 1998). This suggests that the rate of referral of maltreated children to medical facilities is quite high. It further indicates that child maltreatment is a significant public health issue and should be an integral part of pediatric care, particularly for infants, toddlers, and preschoolers less than 5 years of age. Healthcare professionals need to be aware of the increased incidence of maltreatment among children referred to them for care and treatment and, accordingly, need to screen for histories of maltreatment and be alert for signs and symptoms of abuse and neglect. Given the high percentage of children with disabilities among maltreated children, healthcare professionals also need to routinely screen for disabilities so this information can be available to law enforcement and social service personnel in the conduct of child maltreatment investigations. Medical personnel play a key role in the identification and treatment of maltreated children with special healthcare needs. Pediatricians, in particular, play a significant role in the well-being of children with special healthcare needs. It is critical that they be well-informed on maltreatment risks and characteristics as well as educate parents, caregivers, and other professionals about them. Pediatricians must not only provide a comprehensive medical evaluation but also play the crucial role in advocating for all children in the healthcare arena. In so doing, they impact the child victims, their families, and public health policy.

References

American Academy of Pediatrics. (2001). Assessment of maltreatment of children with disabilities, *Pediatrics, 108*, 508–512.

Giardino, A. P., Hudson, K. M., & Marsh, J. (2003). Providing medical evaluations for possible child maltreatment to children with special healthcare needs. *Child Abuse and Neglect, 27*, 1179–1186.

Hibbard, R. A., Desch, L. W., & The Committee on Child Abuse and Neglect and Council on Children with Disabilities. (2007). Maltreatment of children with disabilities. *Pediatrics, 119*, 1018–1025.

Kvam, M. H. (2000). Is sexual abuse of children with disabilities disclosed? A retrospective analysis of child disability and the likelihood of sexual abuse among those attending Norwegian Hospitals. *Child Abuse and Neglect, 24*(8), 1073–1084.

Monteleone, J. A. (1998). *Quick-reference child abuse for health professionals, social services, and law enforcement.* Saint Louis: GW Publishing.

Steinberg, M. A., & Hylton, J. R. (1998). *Responding to maltreatment of children with disabilities: A trainer's guide* (NCCAN No. 90CA1561). Portland, OR: Child Development and Rehabilitation Center.

Sullivan, P. M. (1996). *Developmental disabilities training project* (pp. 183–184). Boys Town National Research Hospital, Center for Abused Children with Disabilities.

Sullivan, P. M. (2003). Children with Disabilities and Healthy People 2010: A call to action. *HP2010 Chapter 6: Implementing the Vision 2003: First steps.* Atlanta, GA: Centers for Disease Control and Prevention.

Sullivan, P. M. (2006). Children with disabilities exposed to violence: Legal and public policy issues. In M. M. Feerick & G. B. Silverman (Eds.), *Children exposed to violence: Current status, gaps, and research priorities* (pp. 213–237). Baltimore: Brookes Publishing.

Sullivan, P. M., Brookhouser, P. E., Scanlan, J. M., Knutson, J. F., & Schulte, L. E. (1991). Patterns of physical and sexual abuse of communicatively handicapped children. *Annals of Otology, Rhinology, and Laryngology, 100*(3), 188–194.

Sullivan, P. M., & Knutson, J. F. (1998). The association between child maltreatment and disabilities in a hospital-based epidemiological study. *Child Abuse and Neglect, 22*(4), 271–288.

Sullivan, P. M., & Knutson, J. F. (2000). Maltreatment and disabilities: A population-based epidemiological study. *Child Abuse and Neglect, 24*(10), 1257–1274.

U.S. Department of Health and Human Services, Health Resources and Services Administration, Maternal and Child Health Bureau. (2008). *The national survey of children with special healthcare needs chartbook 2005–2006.* Rockville, Maryland: U.S. Department of Health and Human Services.

U.S. Department of Health and Human Services, Substance Abuse and Mental Health Services Administration, Center for Mental Health Services. (2008). *2007 Uniform reporting systems results.* Rockville, Maryland: U.S. Department of Health and Human Services.

Willging, J. P., Bower, C. M., & Cotton, R. T. (1992). Physical abuse of children: A retrospective review and an otolaryngology perspective. *Archives Otolaryngology - Head and Neck Surgery, 118*, 584–590.

Chapter 11

Intimate Partner Violence

Jennifer Jarjosa Tscholl and Philip V. Scribano

Introduction

Intimate partner violence (IPV) is characterized by a pattern of coercive behaviors that may include battering and injury, psychological abuse, sexual assault, progressive social isolation, deprivation, and intimidation. These patterns of abuse are used to maintain power and control within the context of an adult or adolescent intimate relationship. In the literature, IPV is often used interchangeably with the terms domestic violence or family violence, used to describe violence in relationships and distinguished from other types of violent experiences. An intimate relationship is used broadly because domestic violence can take many forms and can include the following: dating and live-in partners, married couples, same sex couples, parents and their adult or teenage children, adults who share a child in common, two adults, related by blood who live together, teenagers who are in a dating relationship, ex-live-in partners, ex-husbands and wives, and ex-girlfriends and boyfriends (Burke, Denison, Gielen, McDonnell, & O'Campo, 2004; Toohey, 2008; Rhatigan, Moore, & Street, 2005).

The Centers for Disease Control and Prevention (CDC) define IPV as a spectrum, which includes four types of behavior:

(1) *Physical abuse*
(2) *Sexual abuse*
(3) *Threats* of physical or sexual abuse (includes any means by which intent to cause harm is conveyed)

A.P. Giardino et al. (eds.), *A Practical Guide to the Evaluation of Child Physical Abuse and Neglect*, DOI 10.1007/978-1-4419-0702-8_11, © Springer Science+Business Media, LLC 1997, 2010

(4) *Emotional abuse* (harming a partner's sense of self-worth, threatening posses-
sions or loved ones, etc.)

Although IPV victimization is not gender-specific, the majority of victims are
women who are perpetrated by male partners. In the most basic conceptual framework, IPV is thought of in terms of one partner exerting power over another via the
behaviors listed above. Figure 11.1 (Power & Control Wheel) demonstrates specific
behaviors by which one partner attempts to exert his/her power and control over
the other. Specifically, that power and control may manifest as physical or sexual
violence, and the means by which this power and control is demonstrated includes
social isolation, as well as threats on self, children and other relationships.

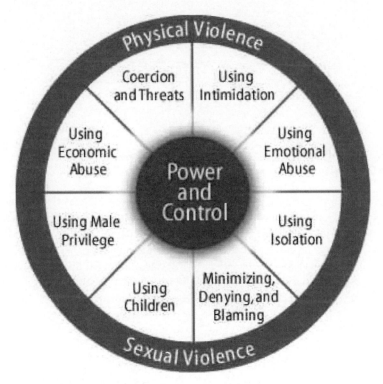

Figure 11.1 Dynamics of IPV – "Power and Control Wheel".
Reproduced with permission from D.A.S.H. (2008).

It is important to recognize that an individual experiencing IPV may not initially
recognize the behavior as unacceptable or as a problem. The transtheoretical model
(also know as the stages of change model) has been proposed as a contextual framework for the process of behavior changes that may occur in women experiencing
IPV (Table 11.1) (Burke et al., 2004). While the proposed stages of change do not
necessarily occur in a sequential fashion, and there is not necessarily always forward movement through the steps, this framework aids clinicians in a better understanding on how to offer assistance, support, and protection for these women and

Table 11.1 Stages of change for intimate partner violence.

Stage of change	Definition
Precontemplation	The victim does not recognize the abusive behavior as a problem and is not interested in change.
Contemplation	The victim recognized the abusive behavior as a problem and has an increasing awareness of the pros and cons of change.
Preparation	The victim recognizes the abusive behavior as a problem, intends to change, and has developed a plan.
Action	The victim is actively engaged in making changes related to ending the abusive behavior.
Maintenance	The abusive behavior has ended, and the victim is taking steps to prevent relapse

Burke et al. (2004) used with permission from PNG Publications, www.ajhb.org

their families. This model makes it apparent that ending IPV, even on an individual basis, is a process which occurs over time. This can be frustrating for some medical providers who may feel uncomfortable with potential decisions a person may make in this context.

Epidemiology

An estimated 2–4 million women are victims of IPV and 3.3–10 million children are exposed to this violence annually in the US. Two million are severely physically assaulted by their male partners, and in-home homicides are correlated with increased risk of homicide from an intimate partner (Novello, Rosenberg, Saltzman, & Shosky, 1992; Berkowitz, 2004; Bair-Merritt, Blackstone, & Feudtner, 2006a; Bair-Merritt, Feudtner, Mollen, Winters, Blackstone, & Fein, 2006b; Newman, Sheehan, & Powell, 2005).

Approximately 33% of homicides of women and 3% of homicides of men were committed by intimate partners (Fox & Zawitz, 2007). Additionally, in these households, 38% of the reported incidents of IPV against women had children residing in those households. Looking at the IPV mortality risks from a slightly different perspective, homicide data from the Federal Bureau of Investigation's Uniform Crime Reporting Program demonstrates that, among female homicide victims for whom their relationships with their offenders were known, 32.9% were murdered by their husbands or boyfriends. These statistics seem to support a need for greater efforts to address this problem, and support the additional evidence that this type of violence exposure incurs great costs of physical/mental health, quality of life, as well as financial costs due to health care needs and lost productivity (i.e. time away from work) (Berkowitz, 2004).

IPV can occur in any household; there is no prototype to guide medical providers. There has been a limited understanding of racial differences regarding IPV. While some research has identified similarities in IPV experiences across racial groups (Short et al., 2000), other studies have reported some differences. Alcohol-related difficulties were more closely associated with IPV for African-American couples compared to Caucasian couples (Cunradi, Caetano, Clark, & Schafer, 1999). In households where child protective services are already involved, a history of caregiver major depressive disorder or drug dependence has been considered a risk factor for recent household IPV (Hazen, Connelly, Kelleher, Landsverk, & Barth, 2004).

The increased prevalence of IPV during pregnancy spans across developed and developing countries, with certain caveats (Campbell, 2002). The prevalence of IPV in pregnant American women ranges from 0.9 to 20.1% (Gazmararian et al., 1996). IPV during pregnancy is less likely to occur in the absence of abuse prior to pregnancy (Martin, Mackie, Kupper, Buescher, & Moracco, 2001). However, most women who were already victims of IPV report either an increase in or steady frequency of abuse during pregnancy (Coker, Sanderson, & Dong, 2004). A considerable amount of research has been dedicated to examining the association of IPV during pregnancy with adverse pregnancy outcomes, especially low birth-weight, preterm delivery, intra-uterine growth restriction, perinatal death, and induced and spontaneous abortion (Coker et al., 2004; Janssen et al., 2003). Adverse outcomes have been postulated to have multifactorial causation, including direct trauma to the fetus, maternal stress, isolation or poor prenatal care related to the abuse, and maternal risky health behaviors related to coping with the abuse (Coker et al., 2004).

Health Consequences of IPV

The acute and chronic health consequences of IPV to women are profound. Acute trauma resulting from IPV is reported as 2–3% in an emergency department setting; however, ED evaluations for non-acute trauma or non-trauma complaints secondary to IPV are 12–17% (Campbell, 2002). An increased risk for health problems (Table 11.2), such as headaches, back pain, anorexia, irritable bowel syndrome, chest pain, hypertension, sexually transmitted diseases, pelvic pain, alcohol and drug abuse, depression, anxiety, and post-traumatic stress disorder, exists in women experiencing IPV. These chronic health problems can cause significant morbidity to women (Campbell, 2002; Coter, Smith, Bethea, Kiny, & McKcown, 2000; Dieneman, Campbell, Wiederhorn, Laughon, & Jordan, 2003). The chronicity of IPV has been recognized within the health care system; however, health care professionals, and the systems they work within, are inconsistent in their identification and intervention for IPV (Campbell, 2002). Additionally, women at highest risk (those who were either murdered or an attempt made on their life by their intimate partner) are much more likely to be seen in the health care system than seek domestic violence victim services prior to the terminal event (Campbell, 2004). Therefore, efforts to reduce IPV mortality may be more greatly impacted through better identification and intervention within the healthcare system than domestic violence service providers at the initial intervention phase.

Table 11.2 Health problems frequently associated with IPV.

Gastrointestinal	Cardiac
• Decreased appetite	• Hypertension
• Eating disorders	• Chest pain
• Chronic irritable bowel syndrome	
	Mental health
Neurologic	• Depression[a]
• Seizures	• Post-traumatic stress disorder[a]
• Fainting	• Anxiety/panic disorders
	• Insomnia
Chronic pain	• Alcohol/drug abuse
• Headaches	• Social dysfunction
• Back pain	
• Fibromyalgia	Other
	• Low birth-weight infants
Gynecologic	• Forced, "elective" abortion
• Pelvic pain	
• Sexually transmitted infections	
• Sexual dysfunction	

[a] Most prominent mental health sequelae

Female victims of IPV generate approximately 92% more costs annually than non-victims, with mental health services accounting for the majority of increased costs (Wisner, Gilmer, Saltzman, & Zink, 1999). The estimated annual healthcare cost of IPV ranged from 2.3 to 8.3 billion dollars (Brown, Finkelstein, & Mercy, 2008; Max, Rice, Finkelstein, Bardwell, & Leadbetter, 2004). These estimates do not necessarily take into account all economic burdens of IPV, which could also include lost work productivity via absenteeism or distraction (Reeves & O'Leary-Kelly, 2007). In addition, the health care costs and utilization for children whose mothers experienced IPV is similarly higher with greater emergency department visits, mental health services, primary care visits, and other ancillary health care utilization, and this increased cost and utilization was present even if the mothers' IPV experiences ended prior to the child being born, compared to mothers who reported no IPV (Rivara et al., 2007).

IPV and Child Maltreatment

While we can understand and recognize the adverse effects of child maltreatment for the child and IPV for the adult, there are risks of adverse effects in children who witness intimate partner violence. Exposure to family violence has significant detrimental effects on the health and well-being of children in these households. Only a fraction of children may be directly injured as a result of an intimate partner violence episode. These injuries may occur in young children being held by the caregiver during an intimate partner violence incident, or in older children attempting to intervene (Christian, Scribano, Seidl, & Pinto-Martin, 1997).

Perhaps more significant is that most children in these home environments are vulnerable to the chronic exposure to maladaptive behaviors resulting in poor mental and physical health (Repetti, Taylor, & Seeman, 2002). IPV-exposed children are shown to have significantly increased rates of both internalizing behaviors, such as anxiety and depression, and externalizing behavior problems, such as aggression, oppositional-defiant, and conduct problems, when compared to non-exposed children. This results in poor social, emotional, and developmental growth (McFarlane, Groff, O'Brien, & Watson, 2003; Bair-Merritt et al., 2006a; Tulman, Edleson, 1999; Mohr 2000; Jaffee, Moffitt, Caspi, Taylor, & Arseneault, 2002; Litrownik et al., 2005; Kernic et al., 2003). Even when adjusting for other risk factors associated with child behavior problems, severe IPV is associated with these maladaptive child behaviors. Harsh parenting (parental psychological aggression and use of corporal punishment) is a significant correlate of children's behavior problems, whereas maternal depression was not found to have a correlation with child behavior problems in this violence-exposed setting (Hazen, Connelly, Kelleher, Barth, & Landsverk, 2006).

With regard to the physical health of children exposed to IPV, when compared to non-IPV exposed children, these children are more likely to experience: poorer overall physical health, failure to thrive, under-immunization, speech pathology referrals, and adolescent risk-taking behaviors such as alcohol and drug use and sexual activity (Bair-Merritt et al., 2006a; Attala & Summers, 1999; Attala & McSweeney, 1997; Kernic et al., 2003; McFarlane et al., 2003; Knapp & Dowd, 1998). Figure 11.2 is a theoretical model linking a risky home milieu to eventual adverse child health outcomes (Bair-Merritt et al., 2006a).

Child and adolescent experiences have been shown to have significant effects into adulthood through the work done in the Adverse Childhood Experiences (ACE) studies, which focuses on how these ACEs relate to health risk factors and morbidity later in life (Felitti et al., 1998; Dong et al., 2004; Dube, Anda, Felitti, Edwards, & Williamson, 2002). From this work, the health outcome paradigm can eventually lead to risky health behaviors, poor health outcomes, and early death (Figure 11.3). The adverse childhood experiences evaluated for by the ACE studies include: emotional, physical, and sexual abuse; emotional and physical neglect; and, household dysfunction defined as: parental separation or divorce, household substance abuse or other criminality, household mental illness, and intimate partner violence.

A challenge to this work is to fully understand the independent effects of IPV exposure in children, since there is a strong inter-relatedness of different adverse childhood experiences. Children who are exposed to IPV are also likely to have had other adverse childhood experiences. Of note, the prevalence of reporting growing up with any of the adverse childhood experiences was 2–4 times higher among persons who reported witnessing IPV compared with persons who had not been exposed to IPV during childhood (Dong et al., 2004). In addition, the most commonly reported co-occurrence with IPV in the household is physical abuse (Dube et al., 2002).

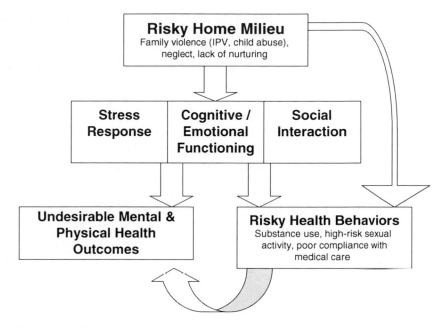

Figure 11.2 Association of environmental (home) violence exposure, response to violence exposure, and negative health behaviors and outcomes.
Adapted from Bair-Merritt et al. (2006a) (Reproduced with permission).

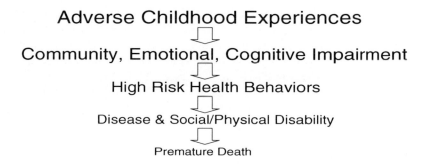

Figure 11.3 Adverse childhood experiences and relationship to risk behaviors, and subsequent health impairment in later life.
Adapted from Felitti et al. (1998).

The co-occurrence of other ACEs with IPV lends itself to a broader definition of child maltreatment, as there may not be a single cause of childhood trauma. Multiple factors at work in the individual, family, community, and culture in which the child and family are embedded determine what is perceived as child maltreatment (Belsky, 1980). If nothing else, if a history of IPV in a household is elicited, this should be a red flag that there are potentially other forms of abuse occurring in the household. It is important to note that exposure to IPV, in and of itself, should not be interpreted as child maltreatment, solely based upon this household exposure, as each child's perception of the trauma they experience may vary. As examples, the perceived trauma can stem from visually observing IPV of a parent or caregiver, hearing IPV, witnessing the aftermath of a physical assault, getting caught in the middle, being separated from a loved one after an IPV event, and/or watching the cycle of violence and manipulation from a father figure. Although there are a multitude of potential negative outcomes from these adverse experiences, there are still many children who survive a childhood of witnessing IPV relatively unaffected, without any evidence of negative developmental outcomes. Further, there are still others who may develop strong coping abilities or resilience through these experiences (Edleson, 1999).

Dating Violence

In the context of IPV relationships, dating violence typically refers to the violence experiences specific to a dating relationship, usually adolescents or young adults. Teens are at risk for all types of dating violence (psychological, physical, and sexual) and are often unaware he/she is experiencing IPV. Additionally, the adolescent may not view the abuse as serious enough to call it IPV, or, due to the bi-directionality of the abuse (physical and emotional), it may not be identified as IPV.

The estimated overall prevalence of teen dating violence is 10–15%. Physical and emotional violence are experienced at similar rates between males and females; however, females are more than twice as likely to experience sexual dating violence (Halpern, Young, Waller, Martin, & Kupper, 2004; Eaton, Davis, Barrios, Brener, & Noonan, 2007; Silverman, Raj, & Clements, 2004). A greater prevalence of substance use, unhealthy weight control, suicidality, pregnancy, and other sexual risks are present in the context of violence in the dating relationship (Silverman et al., 2004; Olshen, McVeigh, Wunsch-Hitzig, & Rickert, 2007).

Adolescents report an understanding that dating violence is a struggle for control and can appreciate the connection between physical abuse and psychological abuse. Feelings of embarrassment can prevent teens from disclosing dating violence; however, they desire the skills to have healthy relationships (Sears, Byers, Whelan, & Saint-Pierre, 2006).

Assessment of IPV in the Clinical Setting

In its summary, the US Preventive Services Task Force (USPSTF) found insufficient evidence to recommend for or against routine screening of women for IPV, as there was no direct evidence from the literature that screening for IPV leads to a reduction in disability and premature death (USPSTF, 2004). However, the American Academy of Pediatrics, the American College of Obstetrics and Gynecology, the American Academy of Family Physicians, and the American Medical Association have all published policy statements which support the use of universal IPV screening and have provided guidelines on how to incorporate such screening into medical practice (ACOG, 2002; Wathen & MacMillan, 2003; AAFP, 2008; USP-STF, 2004; AAP Committee on Child Abuse and Neglect, 1998).

Because of the known detrimental effects IPV has on children, IPV screening has been recognized as an important tool to identify women at risk for abuse, and it has been incorporated into both the pediatric office and pediatric emergency department clinical environments (Siegel, Hill, Henderson, Ernst, & Boat, 1999; Parkinson, Adams, & Emerling, 2001; Newman et al., 2005; Bair-Merritt et al., 2006b). In addition, consensus guidelines have been established to assist clinicians in understanding the approach to evaluating IPV in the pediatric health care encounter and equipping them in this process (Family Violence Prevention Fund, http://endabuse.org/programs/healthcare/files/Pediatric.pdf). Considerable IPV screening research has focused on both the method of screening (i.e. face-to-face interview, paper, computer) (Chuang & Liebschutz, 2002; Anderst, Hill, & Siegel, 2004; MacMillan et al. 2006; Webster & Holt, 2004), as well as the instrument used for screening.

The American Academy of Pediatrics (AAP) recognizes the various adverse effects of childhood exposure to IPV, and has recommended screening for IPV during pediatric health care visits because "the abuse of women is a pediatric issue" (AAP, 1998). In addition, when conducting these assessments, pediatricians should be aware of the dynamics of IPV and the resources available for families struggling with IPV (AAP, 1998). There have been obstacles within the pediatric healthcare community, including lack of training, limited time, not knowing what to do with positive screens, as well as just not appreciating IPV is a pediatric issue (Bair-Merritt, Giardino, Turner, Ganetsky, & Christian, 2004).

The AAP 1998 Policy Statement Recommendations include the following:

(1) Residency training programs and continuing medical education (CME) program leaders incorporate education on family and IPV and its implications for child health into the curricula of pediatricians and pediatric emergency department physicians;
(2) Pediatricians should attempt to recognize evidence of family violence in the office setting;
(3) Pediatricians should intervene in a sensitive and skillful manner that maximizes the safety of women and children victims; and
(4) Pediatricians should support local and national multidisciplinary efforts to recognize, treat, and prevent family and intimate partner violence

While this clinical care approach may seem daunting to some, pediatric health care providers are in a unique position to offer support and interventions for their patients and caregiver. Any assessment and intervention on behalf of women struggling with IPV should include an understanding of the need to respect their autonomy and to be offered in the context of advocating, collaborating, and demonstrating concern for their health and safety (Campbell et al., 2002). When a victim of IPV is motivated to take action to end the abuse in a relationship (whether that includes leaving the relationship or not), this time period can be the most dangerous phase in her relationship, and support for safety and protection becomes paramount (Burke et al., 2004). To be most helpful to victims and their families, it is important to know how to advocate for them and to do so without jeopardizing their safety. Table 11.3 includes a succinct set of clinician skills to provide an adequate foundation for effective support to IPV victims.

Table 11.3 Clinician skills for addressing IPV.

Education: Know the background and the magnitude of the problem of IPV
Definitions: Be able to identify the various forms of IPV
Screening: Initiate routinely and engage all members within your practice to
 recognize IPV as an important family issue to be addressed
Safety: Recognize potential dangers for victims and children. Learn to develop
 effective safety plans with them:
 • Call shelters, know legal options, and find local resources ahead of time
 • Prepare emergency bag (kept in discreet location) ahead of time
 • Have plan of where to go and when
 • Involve friends in developing safety plan, and use code words for help
 • Educate children on how to call for help, if necessary
Legal issues: Find out what types of abuse necessitate mandated reporting
Community resources: Collect list of community resources and be able to
 distribute to patients and families. Integrate efforts with the community. Provide
 education to families

Adapted from Knapp (1998) (Reproduced with permission)

Another unique issue regarding the IPV assessments during a child's health visit is how one documents the results of the assessment. Health care providers should be aware that, if the abuser is also a parent of the pediatric patient, he will have access to the child's medical record and may obtain documentation regarding the abusive relationship that could place the mother at risk. With this safety caveat in mind, documenting the results of IPV screening can be accomplished without disclosing specific details, should the abuser gain access to the medical record. For example, using a standardized documentation for all patient visits such as "Performed screening for IPV, and appropriate handouts provided" enables the health care provider to document the screening and relies upon standard practice regarding the interventions available and offered to families.

IPV mandated reporting laws vary from state to state; therefore, a clinician should be aware of their local laws. If the IPV results in harm to the child and a suspicion of child maltreatment exists, providers in all states are mandated to report abuse or neglect regardless of the IPV mandated reporting laws for adult victims. Specifically, direct physical injury, serious concerns regarding the physical safety of the child, threats to the child, and/or child verbalizing feeling unsafe warrant a report to the child protective services agency.

Methods and Types of IPV Screening Tools Available

It has been demonstrated that women report face-to-face interviewing as a significant barrier to effective screening. In addition, time efficiency has been identified as a barrier for health care providers to screen (Dowd, Kennedy, Knapp, & Stallbaumer-Rouyer, 2002). The use of a short, validated IPV measure, using a self-administered (paper and pencil or computer) interface, appears to provide the optimal detection rates with the greatest preference by women and their providers (Webster & Holt, 2004; MacMillan et al., 2006). When comparing three screening methods (face-to-face interview, written self-report questionnaire, and computer self-report questionnaire), preference for the more anonymous screening methods (written or computer) were most favored by women. In addition, the increasing use of computer technology in health care encounters may be an efficient and anonymous alternative for busy clinical settings to conduct these assessments. This was demonstrated in one study (Rhodes et al., 2006) which found that computer-based screening increased rates of health care provider–patient IPV communication with a subsequent increase in IPV disclosure to the health care provider. As a result, increased opportunity for counseling and/or referrals were notable, positive outcomes of this effort for abused women.

There is an exhaustive listing of instruments that can be used to assess IPV in the clinical setting. An excellent resource from the CDC offers a compendium of these options (Thompson, Basile, Hertz, & Sitterle, 2006). Examples of short, efficient instruments with good detection rates are the Partner Violence Screen (PVS) and Woman Abuse Screening Tool (WAST). These are limited in the types of violence (PVS addresses physical violence only) and may still be longer to administer than is desired. Several of the IPV screening tools and their descriptions are listed in Table 11.4.

Time constraints have been cited by pediatricians as one of the barriers to performing IPV screening in the clinic setting. In fact, the most time-consuming aspect should be the process of development of an effective screening program, as opposed to the process of screening once all the elements have been put into place. Of the utmost importance is gaining support and "buy-in" from the entire clinic staff and administration, so that everyone shares a common goal when instituting a new process. Choosing an appropriate screening instrument, educating all personnel, implementing a clinic protocol, identifying potential challenges, and acquiring the skills are all important aspects of preparing to institute an IPV screening program. Once all clinic members have been assigned a role in the screening process and protocols are in place, the practice itself becomes more streamlined and less time-consuming to the providers.

Safety Interventions and Community Resources

The optimal care for the woman in an abusive relationship depends on the physician's working knowledge of community resources that can provide safety, advocacy, and support (AMA, 1992). While the first step in providing support to those

Table 11.4 Commonly used IPV screening tools.

Tool	Description	Targeted population	References
Revised Conflict Tactics Scales (CTS-2)	78-item scale assesses victimization and perpetration. 39-item victimization scale includes 12-item PA subscale.	Partners in dating, cohabiting, and marital relationships	Straus & Douglas (2004), Straus, Hamby, Boney-McCoy, & Sugarman (1996)
Composite Abuse Scale (CAS)	30-item scale with 4 subscales (severe combined, emotional, physical abuse, and harassment). PA subscale includes 7 items.	Females with current or former intimate partners for >1 month	Hegarty, Fracgp, Bush, & Sheehan (2005a), Hegarty, Bush, & Sheehan (2005b)
Partner Violence Screen (PVS)	3-item questionnaire assesses past PA and current perception of safety.	Females with current or former intimate partners over the past year	Feldhaus et al. (1997)
Abuse Assessment Screen (AAS)	5-item questionnaire assesses past and present PA, SA, and perception of safety.	Pregnant females with current or former intimate partners	Norton, Peipert, Zierler, Lima, & Hume (1995)
Woman Abuse Screening Tool (WAST)	8-item questionnaire assesses relationship tension, PA, and SA.	Females in relationships	Brown, Lent, Schmidt, & Sas (2000), Brown, Lent, Brett, Sas, & Pederson (1996)
Hurt, Insulted, Threatened, Screamed Scale (HITS)	4-item scale that assesses physical and emotional violence and threats	Females in relationships	Sherin, Sinacore, Li, Zitter, & Shakil (1998)

experiencing intimate partner violence is evaluating whether this is present or not in a screening program, providers should be prepared to take appropriate action when confronted with a positive screen (Groves, Augustyn, Lee, & Sawires, 2002). Begin by maintaining a supportive attitude with the IPV victim by expressing concern for safety, avoiding any judgment, and reassuring the victim that he/she is not to blame and does not deserve abusive treatment. Depending on a victim's frame of mind and/or process within the stages of change described earlier, she may or may not be receptive to offers to provide more information or to contact resources; however, attempts should be made to address all these issues. Establish with the victim whether or not she would like the issue of IPV to be discussed with the child patient,

Table 11.5 Basic elements of IPV safety planning.

During an incident of violence:
• Have a safe place to go
• Teach children how to call for help
• Protect self until out of imminent danger

When preparing to leave:
• Prepare emergency bag and keep in discreet location
• Keep copies of important documents and financial savings with emergency bag
• Have a plan of where to go; know local resources
• Involve friends; create code words to indicate imminent danger

When in separate residence:
• Maintain all home safety features (door/window locks, alarms, strong materials)
• Inform neighbors and child caregivers of perpetrator history and potential for recurrence

as parents may feel more or less comfortable doing so with children depending on their ages or developmental abilities. Assess the child and parent victim's immediate and future safety and be prepared to develop a safety plan with them. Elements of a safety plan are described in Table 11.5.

Becoming familiar with local resources will aid in making appropriate referrals for families in need. The National Domestic Violence Hotline (NDVH) is a national resource that is always available and a good starting point for any victim or provider in search of help. The NDVH can be reached online at   www.ndvh.com   or by calling 1-800-799-SAFE (7233).

In addition to providing support to the victim and children, providers should inform the family if there are any indications for mandated reporting, as this intervention can become a safety issue for both child and parent due to the disclosures made that prompted an investigation. Ensuring an appropriate safety plan (as described in Table 11.5) in this setting is paramount.

IPV is a problem with family functioning and can be a significant negative factor in physical and emotional health of the pediatric patient. Understanding the dynamics of IPV, the approach to screening in routine healthcare practice, and the needs for both adult and child can enhance the well-being of both parent and child and improve health.

References

ACOG. (2002). *Guidelines for women's health care*, 2nd ed. Washington, DC: American Coll Obstetricians and Gynecologists.

American Academy of Family Physicians. (2008). *Family violence and abuse*. Accessed 7 November 2008: http://www.aafp.org/x16506.xml on

American Medical Association. (1992). *Diagnostic and treatment guidelines on domestic violence*. Chicago, IL: American Medical Association.

Anderst, J., Hill, T. D., & Siegel, R. M. (2004, January–February). A comparison of domestic violence screening methods in a pediatric office. *Clinical Pediatrics (Philadelphia), 43*(1), 103–105.

Attala, J., & McSweeney, M. (1997, October–December). Preschool children of battered women identified in a community setting. *Issues in Comprehensive Pediatric Nursing, 20*(4), 217–225.

Attala, J., & Summers, S. M. (1999). A comparative study of health, developmental, and behavioral factors in preschool children of battered and nonbattered women. *Child Health Care, 1*(28), 189–200.

Bair-Merritt, M. H., Blackstone, M., & Feudtner, C. (2006a, February). Physical health outcomes of childhood exposure to intimate partner violence: A systematic review. *Pediatrics, 117*(2), e278–e290.

Bair-Merritt, M. H., Feudtner, C., Mollen, C. J., Winters, S., Blackstone, M., & Fein, J. A. (2006b, March). Screening for intimate partner violence using an audiotape questionnaire: A randomized clinical trial in a pediatric emergency department. *Archives of Pediatrics and Adolescent Medicine, 160*(3), 311–316.

Bair-Merritt, M. H., Giardino, A. P., Turner, M., Ganetsky, M., & Christian, C. W. (2004, January–February). Pediatric residency training on domestic violence: A national survey. *Ambulatory Pediatrics, 4*(1), 24–27.

Belsky, J. (1980, April). Child maltreatment: An ecological integration. *American Psychologist, 35*(4), 320–335.

Berkowitz, C. D. (2004, September). Domestic violence: A pediatric concern. *Pediatrics in Review, 25*(9), 306–311.

Brown, J. B., Lent, B., Brett, P., Sas, G., & Pederson, L. (1996). Development of the woman abuse screening tool for use in family practice. *Family Medicine, 28*, 422–428.

Brown, D. S., Finkelstein, E. A., & Mercy, J. A. (2008, February 26). Methods for estimating medical expenditures attributable to intimate partner violence. *Journal of Interpersonal Violence, 23*, 1747–1766.

Brown, J. B., Lent, B., Schmidt, G., & Sas, G. (2000, October). Application of the Woman Abuse Screening Tool (WAST) and WAST-short in the family practice setting. *Journal of Family Practice, 49*(10), 896–903.

Burke, J. G., Denison, J. A., Gielen, A. C., McDonnell, K. A., & O'Campo, P. (2004, March–April). Ending intimate partner violence: An application of the transtheoretical model. *American Journal of Health Behavior, 28*(2), 122–133. www.ajhb.org

Campbell, J., Jones, A. S., Dienemann, J., Kub, J., Schollenberger, J., O'Campo, P., et al. (2002, May 27). Intimate partner violence and physical health consequences. *Archives of International Medicine, 162*(10), 1157–1163.

Campbell, J. C. (2002, April 13). Health consequences of intimate partner violence. *Lancet, 359*(9314), 1331–1336.

Campbell, J. C. (2004, December). Helping women understand their risk in situations of intimate partner violence. *Journal of Interpersonal Violence, 19*(12), 1464–1477.

Christian, C. W., Scribano, P., Seidl, T., & Pinto-Martin, J. A. (1997, February). Pediatric injury resulting from family violence. *Pediatrics, 99*(2), E8

Chuang, C. H., & Liebschutz, J. M. (2002, October). Screening for intimate partner violence in the primary care setting: A critical review. *Journal of Clinical Outcomes Management, 9*(10), 565–571.

Coker, A. L., Sanderson, M., & Dong, B. (2004, July). Partner violence during pregnancy and risk of adverse pregnancy outcomes. *Paediatric and Perinatal Epidemiology, 18*(4), 260–269.

Coker, A. L., Smith, P. H., Bethea, L., King, M. R., & McKeown, R. E. (2000, May). Physical health consequences of physical and psychological intimate partner violence. *Archives of Family Medicine, 9*(5), 451–457.

Committee on Child Abuse and Neglect of the American Academy of Pediatrics. (1998). The role of the pediatrician in recognizing and intervening on behalf of abused women. *Pediatrics, 101,* 1091–1092.

Cunradi, C. B., Caetano, R., Clark, C. L., & Schafer, J. (1999). Alcohol-related problems and intimate partner violence among white, black and hispanic couples in the U.S. *Alcoholism: Clinical and Experimental Research, 23,* 1492–1501.

D.A.S.H. Foundation. (2008). http://www.dashfoundation.net/ on 11 November 2008.

Dienemann, J., Campbell, J., Wiederhorn, N., Laughon, K., & Jordan, E. (2003, September–October). A critical pathway for intimate partner violence across the continuum of care. *Journal of Obstetrics Gynecology, and Neonatal Nursing, 32*(5), 594–603.

Dong, M., Anda, R. F., Felitti, V. J., Dube, S. R., Williamson, D. F., Thompson, T. J., et al. (2004, July). The interrelatedness of multiple forms of childhood abuse, neglect, and household dysfunction. *Child Abuse and Neglect, 28*(7), 771–784.

Dowd, M. D., Kennedy, C., Knapp, J. F., & Stallbaumer-Rouyer, J. (2002, August). Mothers' and health care providers' perspectives on screening for intimate partner violence in a pediatric emergency department. *Archives of Pediatrics and Adolescent Medicine, 156*(8), 794–799.

Dube, S. R., Anda, R. F., Felitti, V. J., Edwards, V. J., & Williamson, D. F. (2002, February). Exposure to abuse, neglect, and household dysfunction among adults who witnessed intimate partner violence as children: Implications for health and social services. *Violence and Victims, 17*(1), 3–17.

Eaton, D. K., Davis, K. S., Barrios, L., Brener, N. D., & Noonan, R. (2007). Associations of dating violence victimization with lifetime participation, co-occurrence, and early initiation of risk behaviors among U.S. high school students. *Journal of Interpersonal Violence, 22,* 585–602

Edleson, J. L. (1999, August). Children's witnessing of adult domestic violence. *Journal of Interpersonal Violence, 14*(8), 839–870.

Feldhaus, K. M., Koziol-McLain, J., Amsbury, H. L., Norton, I. M., Lowenstein, S. R., & Abbott, J. T. (1997, May 7). Accuracy of 3 brief screening questions for detecting partner violence in the emergency department. *The Journal of the American Medical Association, 277*(17), 1357–1361.

Felitti, V. J., Anda, R. F., Nordenberg, D., Williamson, D. F., Spitz, A. M., Edwards, V., et al. (1998, May). Relationship of childhood abuse and household dysfunction to many of the leading causes of death in adults. The Adverse Childhood Experiences (ACE) Study. *American Journal of Preventive Medicine, 14*(4), 245–258.

Fox, J. A., & Zawitz, M. W. (2007). *Homicide trends in the United States.* United States Department of Justice, Bureau of Justice Statistics. http://www.ojp.usdoj.gov/bjs/pub/pdf/htius.pdf

Gazmararian, J. A., Lazorick, S., Spitz, A. M., Ballard, T. J., Saltzman, L. E., & Marks, J. S. (1996, June 26). Prevalence of violence against pregnant women. *The Journal of the American Medical Association, 275*(24), 1915–1920.

Groves, B. M., Augustyn, M., Lee, D., & Sawires, P. (2002, September). *Family identifying and responding to domestic violence: Consensus recommendations for child and adolescent health.* San Francisco, CA: Violence Prevention Fund.

Hegarty, K., Fracgp, Bush, R., & Sheehan, M. (2005a, October). The composite abuse scale: Further development and assessment of reliability and validity of a multidimensional partner abuse measure in clinical settings. *Violence and Victims, 20*(5), 529–547.

Hegarty, K., Bush, R., & Sheehan, M. (2005b, October). The composite abuse scale: Further development and assessment of reliability and validity of a multidimensional partner abuse measure in clinical settings. *Violence and Victims, 20*(5), 529–547.

Hall, D., & Lynch, M. (1998, May 23). Violence begins at home. Domestic strife has lifelong effects on children. *British Medical Journal, 316*(7144), 1551.

Halpern, C. T., Young, M. L., Waller, M. W., Martin, S. L., & Kupper, L. L. (2004). Prevalence of partner violence in same-sex romantic and sexual relationships in a national sample of adolescents. *Journal of Adolescent Health, 35*, 124–131.

Hazen, A. L., Connelly, C. D., Kelleher, K. J., Barth, R. P., & Landsverk, J. A. (2006, January). Female caregivers' experiences with intimate partner violence and behavior problems in children investigated as victims of maltreatment. *Pediatrics, 117*(1), 99–109.

Hazen, A. L., Connelly, C. D., Kelleher, K., Landsverk, J., & Barth, R. (2004, March). Intimate partner violence among female caregivers of children reported for child maltreatment. *Child Abuse and Neglect, 28*(3), 301–319.

Jaffee, S. R., Moffitt, T. E., Caspi, A., Taylor, A., & Arseneault, L. (2002, September). Influence of adult domestic violence on children's internalizing and externalizing problems: An environmentally informative twin study. *Journal of American Academy of Child and Adolescent Psychiatry, 41*(9), 1095–1103.

Janssen, P. A., Holt, V. L., Sugg, N. K., Emanuel, I., Critchlow, C. M., & Henderson, A. D. (2003, May). Intimate partner violence and adverse pregnancy outcomes: A population-based study. American *Journal of Obstetrics and Gynecology, 188*(5), 1341–1347.

Kernic, M. A., Wolf, M. E., Holt, V. L., McKnight, B., Huebner, C. E., & Rivara, F. P. (2003, November). Behavioral problems among children whose mothers are abused by an intimate partner. *Child Abuse and Neglect, 27*(11), 1231–1246.

Knapp, J. F., & Dowd, M. D. (1998, September). Family violence: Implications for the pediatrician. *Pediatrics in Review, 19*(9), 316–321.

Litrownik, A. J., Lau, A., English, D. J., Briggs, E., Newton, R. R., Romney, S., & Dubowitz, H. (2005, May). Measuring the severity of child maltreatment. *Child Abuse and Neglect, 29*(5), 553–573.

MacMillan, H. L., Wathen, C. N., Jamieson, E., Boyle, M., McNutt, L. A., Worster, A., et al. (2006, August 2). McMaster violence against women research group. Approaches to screening for intimate partner violence in health care settings: A randomized trial. *The Journal of the American Medical Association, 296*(5), 530–536.

Martin, S. L., Mackie, L., Kupper, L. L., Buescher, P. A., & Moracco, K. E. (2001, March 28). Physical abuse of women before, during, and after pregnancy. *The Journal of the American Medical Association, 285*(12), 1581–1584.

Max, W., Rice, D. P., Finkelstein, E., Bardwell, R. A., & Leadbetter, S. (2004, June). The economic toll of intimate partner violence against women in the United States. *Violence and Victims, 19*(3), 259–272.

McFarlane, J. M., Groff, J. Y., O'Brien, J. A., & Watson, K. (2003, September). Behaviors of children who are exposed and not exposed to intimate partner violence: An analysis of 330 black, white, and Hispanic children. *Pediatrics, 112*(3 Pt 1), e202–e207.

Mohr, W. K., & Tulman, L. J. (2000, September). Children exposed to violence: Measurement considerations within an ecological framework. *Advances in Nursing Science, 23*(1), 59–68.

Newman, J. D., Sheehan, K. M., & Powell, E. C. (2005, February). Screening for intimate-partner violence in the pediatric emergency department. *Pediatric Emergency Care, 21*(2), 79–83.

Norton, L. B., Peipert, J. F., Zierler, S., Lima, B., & Hume, L. (1995, March). Battering in pregnancy: An assessment of two screening methods. *Obstetrics and Gynecology, 85*(3), 321–325.

Novello, A. C., Rosenberg, M., Saltzman, L., & Shosky, J. (1992, June 17). From the surgeon general, US public health service. *The Journal of the American Medical Association, 267*(23), 3132.

Olshen, E., McVeigh, K. H., Wunsch-Hitzig, R. A., & Rickert, V. I. (2007). Dating violence, sexual assault, and suicide attempts among urban teenagers. *Archives of Pediatrics and Adolescent Medicine, 161*, 539–545.

Parkinson, G. W., Adams, R. C., & Emerling, F. G. (2001, September). Maternal domestic violence screening in an office-based pediatric practice. *Pediatrics, 108*(3), E43.

Reeves, C., & O'Leary-Kelly, A. M. (2007, March). The effects and costs of intimate partner violence for work organizations. *Journal of Interpersonal Violence, 22*(3), 327–344.

Repetti, R. L., Taylor, S. E., & Seeman, T. E. (2002, March). Risky families: Family social environments and the mental and physical health of offspring. *Psychological Bulletin, 128*(2), 330–336.

Rhatigan, D. L., Moore, T. M., & Street, A. E. (2005). Reflections on partner violence 20 years of research and beyond. *Journal of Interpersonal Violence, 20*(5), 82–88.

Rhodes, K. V., Drum, M., Anliker, E., Frankel, R. M., Howes, D. S., & Levinson, W. (2006, May 22). Lowering the threshold for discussions of domestic violence: A randomized controlled trial of computer screening. *Archives of International Medicine, 166*(10), 1107–1114.

Rivara, F. P., Anderson, M. L., Fishman, P., Bonomi, A. E., Reid, R. J., Carrell, D., et al. (2007). Intimate partner violence and health care costs and utilization for children living in the home. *Pediatrics, 120*, 1270–1277.

Sears, H. A., Byers, E. S., Whelan, J. J., & Saint-Pierre, M. (2006). "If it hurts you, then it is not a joke" Adolescents' ideas about girls' and boys' use and experience of abusive behavior in dating relationships. *Journal of Interpersonal Violence, 21*, 1191–1207.

Sherin, K. M., Sinacore, J. M., Li, X. Q., Zitter, R. E., & Shakil, A. (1998). HITS: A short domestic violence screening tool for use in a family practice setting. *Family Medicine, 30*, 508–512.

Short, L. M., McMahon, P. M., Davis-Chervin, D., Shelly, G. A., Lezin, N., Sloop, K. S., et al. (2000). Survivors' identification of protective factors and early warning signs for intimate partner violence. *Violence Against Women, 6*, 272–285.

Siegel, R. M., Hill, T. D., Henderson, V. A., Ernst, H. M., & Boat, B. W. (1999, October). Screening for domestic violence in the community pediatric setting. *Pediatrics, 104*(4 Pt 1), 874–877.

Silverman, J. G., Raj, A., & Clements, K. (2004). Dating violence and associated sexual risk and pregnancy among adolescent girls in the United States. *Pediatrics, 114*, e220–e225.

Straus, M. A., & Douglas, E. M. (2004, October). A short form of the Revised Conflict Tactics Scales, and typologies for severity and mutuality. *Violence and Victims, 19*(5), 507–520.

Straus, M. A., Hamby, S. L., Boney-McCoy, S., & Sugarman, D. B., (1996, May). The revised conflict tactics scales (CTS2): Development and preliminary psychometric data. *Journal of Family Issues, 17*(3), 283–316.

Thompson, M. P., Basile, K. C., Hertz, M. F., & Sitterle, D. (2006). *Measuring intimate partner violence victimization and perpetration: A compendium of assessment tools*. Atlanta, GA: Centers for Disease Control and Prevention, National Center for Injury Prevention and Control. http://www.cdc.gov/ncipc/dvp/Compendium/IPV%20Compendium.pdf

Toohey, J. S. (2008). Domestic violence and rape. *Medical Clinics of North America, 92*, 1239–1252.

U.S. Preventive Services Task Force. (2004, March 2). Screening for family and intimate partner violence: Recommendation statement. *Annals of International Medicine, 140*(5), 382–386.

American Medical Association (Council on Scientific Affairs). (1992, June 17). Violence against women. Relevance for medical practitioners. *The Journal of the American Medical Association, 267*(23), 3184–3189.

Wathen, C. N., & MacMillan, H. L. (2003). Prevention of violence against women: Recommendation statement from the Canadian task force on preventive health care. *CMAJ, 169*, 582–584.

Webster, J., & Holt, V. (2004, February). Screening for partner violence: Direct questioning or self-report? *Obstetrics and Gynecology, 103*(2), 299–303.

Wisner, C. L., Gilmer, T. P., Saltzman, L. E., & Zink, T. M. (1999). Intimate partner violence against women: Do victims cost health plans more? *Journal of Family Practice, 48*, 439–443.

Chapter 12

Prevention of Child Physical Abuse

Christopher S. Greeley

Introduction

In the US over 900,000 children are victims of child maltreatment each year, resulting in physical and non-physical injuries, which can be both acute and long lasting. In over 80% of these cases, the perpetrator is one or both of the child's parents. Theories on the etiology of child abuse have evolved significantly over the past three decades. The causes of child abuse are now appreciated to be a complex interconnected web of influences rather than a single cause—a symptom of a larger disease or diseases of a family or community. The evolution of thought regarding the etiologies of child abuse has been paralleled by changes in theories of child abuse prevention strategies. Conventional interventions strategies in child abuse prevention have included Primary, Secondary, and Tertiary programs. One of the most studied and effective prevention interventions is home visitation by a nurse or paraprofessional. Other child abuse prevention strategies include in-hospital education and community-based family centers. Due to the complexity of the problem of child abuse, it is not surprising that a universal solution remains elusive. Interventions can be either *Ameliorative* (attending to the current problems) or *Transformative* (addressing the underlying social risks). Future directions of child abuse prevention will involve coordinating successful interventions into a larger community context to achieve the correct intervention at the optimal dosage. This will require an increased dependence on data derived from methodologically strong clinical trials to ensure that interventions which are brought to scale are evidence based.

There is little disagreement about the moral outrage inspired by the abuse of a child, yet such abuse continues to occur. Each year, over 900,000 children are victims of child maltreatment in the US, with over 142,000 experiencing physical abuse (US Department of health and Human Services, 2008). In greater than 80% of the

A.P. Giardino et al. (eds.), *A Practical Guide to the Evaluation of Child Physical Abuse and Neglect*, DOI 10.1007/978-1-4419-0702-8_12, © Springer Science+Business Media, LLC 1997, 2010

cases, the perpetrator is either one or both of the child's parents. The effects of child abuse on the child are both physical and non-physical. Child victims may suffer immediate physical injuries, ranging from the relatively minor (bruises and abrasions) to the severe and sometimes fatal. Children with inflicted brain injury are at life-long risk for disability, feeding difficulties, seizures, blindness, and death (Barlow, Thomson, Johnson, & Minns, 2005; Makaroff & Putnam, 2003). Even without overt physical injury, children may still be harmed. Victims often have subtle behavioral and cognitive consequences (Stipanicic et al., 2008). While not the direct victim, a child living in an abusive or neglectful home can itself negatively impact the child (Middlebrooks & Audage, 2008; American Academy of Pediatrics et al., 2008). Children exposed to household abuse have a greater likelihood of receiving a mental health disorder diagnosis in early adulthood (Fergusson, Boden, & Horwood, 2008).

Prevention of child abuse has been the focus of both policymakers and academicians. Despite growing attention to child welfare, there remains disproportion between resources allocated to evaluation, investigation, and prosecution, compared with prevention; with prevention receiving orders of magnitude less (Leventhal, 2005). Child abuse is a tremendous financial and resource burden on society. In 2008, Prevent Child Abuse America estimated the annual monetary cost of child abuse in the United States in 2006 to be greater than US$103 billion (Prevent Child Abuse America, 2008). This estimate includes US$33 billion in direct costs (hospitalization, law enforcement, and child welfare services) and US$70 billion in indirect costs (incarceration, lost productivity, long-term mental and physical health services). Financial burdens are additionally felt by the surviving victims as adults. Women who are self-reported victims of child abuse use medical and mental health resources to a greater degree as an adult than those without such a history (Tang et al., 2006). Women who have been victims of both physical and sexual abuse had nearly twice the annual health care costs for ambulatory services than those without such a history (Bonomi et al., 2008). In the landmark Adverse Childhood Experience (ACE) study (Adverse Childhood studies, 2009), Felitti (1998) reported a dose-dependent relationship between children who are exposed to child abuse and household dysfunction and predictors of early adult death. The ACE study links nine adverse childhood experiences (recurrent physical abuse; recurrent emotional abuse; contact sexual abuse; an alcohol and/or drug abuser in the household, an incarcerated household member; someone who is chronically depressed, mentally ill, institutionalized, or suicidal; a mother who is treated violently; one or no parents; emotional or physical neglect) to adult health indicators. The greater the number of Adverse Childhood Experiences (ACEs) a child had, the poorer the adult health will be; even to the point of shortening their lifespan. Children with significant adverse exposures during childhood had between a 4- and 12-fold increased risk for alcoholism, drug use, and suicide attempts. They also demonstrated a 2-4-fold increase in smoking and sexually transmitted infections (=50 sexual partners) and a 1.4-1.6-fold increase in severe obesity was also demonstrated. These data highlight two important themes regarding child abuse prevention: first, the profound impact that child abuse has on the entire life of the child and second, the complex nature of the relationship between household and community dysfunction and child abuse. Additionally, child abuse, in fact, may be self-perpetuating. An adult who has been a victim of child abuse has an increased risk of themselves perpetrating violence (Fang & Corso, 2007).

One obstacle to effective prevention is the lack of a single, agreed upon definition of what constitutes child abuse (Belsky, 1993; Whitaker, Lutzker, & Shelley, 2005). Differences in orders of magnitude for injury as well as overlap between physical abuse and neglect exist. And while there are obvious examples of the extremes of parental behavior, definitions of abuse often are subject to personal and cultural bias. Further, the circumstances around trivial or minor injuries are different than those around fatal ones. Some abusive parents are also neglectful, some are not. Given the complexity of the problem, it is not surprising that a universal solution remains elusive. As the understanding of the etiology of child abuse has evolved, so have the variety of preventative programmatic responses. What has become clear is that there will be no single "solution" to end child abuse. Rather, it will require a collection of approaches, implemented in a coordinated fashion, at different times of the child's life, in various doses, with the cumulative goal that of universal promotion of child well-being in society at large.

This chapter will examine the current state of knowledge in the prevention of child physical abuse. The chapter will begin with a discussion of the theories of why child abuse occurs, looking at the historic foundations of the etiology of maltreatment and how they have changed over the past three decades. The chapter will then discuss the basics of prevention strategies and how they apply to child physical abuse. Specific models of prevention will be highlighted and the published data which supports them will be presented. The chapter will end with a discussion of the future directions that the field of child abuse prevention will need to take and some of the obstacles which lay before it.

Theories on the Causation of Child Abuse

The combination of causes of phenomena is beyond the grasp of the human intellect. But the impulse to seek causes is innate in the soul of man. And the human intellect with no inkling of the immense variety and complexity of circumstances conditioning a phenomenon, any one of which may be separately conceived as the cause of it, snatches at the first and most easily understood approximation and says here is the cause. (Leo Tolstoy, 1899, War and Peace, Part XIII, Chapter I)

The circumstances which lead to child abuse are very complex. Factors include child, family, community, and cultural forces, as well as the interaction between them. Over the past 3040 years, theories on the causation of child abuse have been developed, expanded, and tested. These theories attempt to distinguish conditions or forces which would increase the risk of child abuse. The ultimate goal of such study is the development of effective prevention approaches to reduce not just the incidence of abuse, but the underlying factors. Theories are fit into a conceptual framework (or paradigms) which allow for testing and subsequent revision. Early theories on child abuse focused on two main paradigms: the *psychodynamic paradigm and the sociological paradigm* (Sidebotham, 2001; Daro, 1993). The psychodynamic theory relies upon identification and description of the psychological parameters of perpetrators as well as the psychological dynamics between the perpetrator and the victim. It takes into account the personal mind-set of the individual (usually the mother) and attempts to define characteristics which might predispose a person to perpetrate child abuse. By defining these characteristics, individuals can be screened for risks and then targeted by interventions in prevention efforts. In contrast, the *Sociological Theory* emphasizes external forces which act upon a person (i.e. unemployment, poverty). Interventions directed toward these external forces then can be targeted in prevention efforts.

The psychodynamic and sociological theories are limiting in that they both oversimplify a very complex set of circumstances and forces which contribute to child abuse. While there may be individual characteristics that may predispose a person to committing child abuse, there are also often complex sociological forces which compound individual weaknesses. The reverse may also be true, in that protective influences may be present as well. For example, poverty may be a significant risk factor for child abuse, but this may have less impact in one individual with protective factors, such as someone with a close social network, than another without.

A third theory, known as the *Environmental Theory*, emphasizes the importance of the context of the child and family in the development of abusive behaviors. The theory proposes that if families had access to more and better resources, they would be less likely to engage in abusive behavior (Daro, 1993). The prior three theories have been expanded in the development of a fourth, the *Ecological Theory* of the etiology of child abuse as outlined separately by Uri Bronfenbrenner (1979) and Jay Belsky (1980). From Bronfenbrenner, the ecological theory of human development "involves the scientific study of the progressive, mutual accommodation between an active, growing human being and the changing properties of the immediate settings in which the developing person lives, as this process is affected by relations between these settings and by the larger contexts in which the settings are embedded" Bronfenbrenner (1979). The *Ecological Theory* of the etiology of child abuse recognizes the complexity of child abuse and incorporates the individual, the family, the community, and the context into a more robust understanding of the forces involved. According to Belsky (1993) "child maltreatment is now widely recognized to be multiply determined by a variety of factors operating through transactional processes at various levels of analysis (i.e., life-course history to immediate–situational to historical–evolutionary) in the broad ecology of parent–child relations." *Individual* (or *child*) risk indicators include age (younger), gender (male), difficult temperament, and being medically fragile or complex. *Family* level risk indicators include household violence (domestic violence, intimate partner violence), family stressors, and family size (rapid repeat pregnancies). *Community* level risk indicators include poverty, crime, violence, and weak community infrastructure.

Belsky (1980) outlines four specific spheres, or domains, of influence on the life of a child: Ontologic Development, Microsystem, Exosystem, and Macrosystem.

- The Ontological Development domain refers to the parents' and family's personal background. Parental level risk indicators include a parent having been raised in an abusive or neglectful family, having poor impulse control, participating in drug or alcohol use, or having psychiatric disorders (depression).
- The Microsystem domain refers to the immediate household members and dynamics; any person with direct contact and interaction with the child.
- The Micosystem domain enlarges as the child grows to include schoolmates, friends, and neighbors.
- The Exosystem includes the larger social network of the family and child. This includes parents' co-workers (if they are employed), neighborhood dynamics, and social contacts.
- The Macrosystem includes cultural and societal forces. These include religious, political, and cultural beliefs, norms, and values.

Bronfenbrenner (1979) also includes the Chronosystem, highlighting that each of these spheres of influence may change over time. The ecological theory can therefore be summarized as the influences affecting the individual child, his or her relationships, the community and the larger society, with these influences changing over time. Each of these spheres of influence can potentially be leveraged in a child abuse prevention strategy. No single prevention approach is effective for all of the potential interactions. Effective child abuse prevention programs need to involve coordination of multiple approaches, influencing multiple factors. The ecological model changes the focus from individual characteristics to interactions between and among people.

Treating the neighborhood as a separate entity (with both its own risk and protective factors) reveals a new sphere of intervention. Neighborhood risk factors may include impoverishment, housing stress, child care burden, unemployment, alcohol and drug availability, family structure, neighborhood density, social support, and immigrant concentration (Freisthler, Gruenewald, Remer, Lery, & Needell, 2006). The neighborhood poverty level is itself a risk factor for child abuse (Coulton, 1995). How poverty places a child at risk for abuse is not completely understood; however, the correlation between poverty and child abuse was strongest with physical abuse and neglect and was independent of the individual family poverty score. There are also likely community level factors, inter-family factors, and family-community interaction factors. Individual risk factors and community risk factors will be explored in more detail.

Individual Level Risk Factors

How an individual person is bonded to his or her local community is often referred to as *Social Capital*. Although there are various definitions of social capital, the term generally refers to community resources which encourage cohesion, and an individual's ability to navigate these resources (Ziersch, 2005). Social capital is a way to quantify how engaged or enmeshed a person is with his or her community, i.e. how connected a person is to others. The greater a person's social capital, the lower their risk of being a neglectful parent and the lower the odds of domestic violence (Zolotor & Runyan, 2006). Deficiency of social capital is also reflected in the lack of connectedness neglectful mothers feel with their community and how a neglectful family views its neighbors. In a study comparing neglectful mothers with their non-neglectful neighbors, differences in how neglectful mothers viewed their neighborhoods were identified. When compared with non-neglectful neighbors, neglectful mothers were more likely to describe their neighborhoods as unfriendly and their neighbors as unhelpful (Polansky, Gaudin, Ammons, & Davis, 1985). Additionally, neglectful mothers were more likely to describe themselves as lonelier than their non-neglectful neighbor mothers. Neglectful mothers were less likely to be affiliated with formal community organizations (i.e. churches) as well. This reflects the lack of connectedness neglectful mothers feel with their community.

Community Level Risk Factors

Various neighborhood level factors have been identified as contributing to an increased aggregate risk of child maltreatment. These include "percentage living in poverty, percentage unemployed, percentage female-headed households, percentage living in overcrowded housing, percentage African-American, percentage Hispanic, percentage affluent (coded negatively), lower median educational attainment, and percentage resident less than 5 years" (Garbarino & Crouter, 1978). In a multiple regression analysis, neighborhood child maltreatment rates involving these 9 characteristics account for 79% of the variance (Garbarino & Crouter, 1978) (i.e. knowing these 9 variables could predict child maltreatment rates with 79% certainty). While social capital applies to a person, *Community Social Organization* applies to the community. *Community Social Organization* refers to "patterns and functions of formal and informal networks and institutions and organizations in a locale" (Coulton, 1995). This translates into a community's ability to provide protection and resources for residents in the community.

Despite neighborhood poverty being a risk factor for child maltreatment, poverty alone does not account for the risks of a neighborhood. Neighborhoods with similar socioeconomic status (SES) can have different child maltreatment rates (Garbarino & Kostelny, 1992). A multiple regression model incorporating SES and demographic variables demonstrated that SES alone accounts for 48% of the variance (Garbarino & Sherman, 1980). In other words, the SES accounts for only half of the factors in the relationship between neighborhood poverty and child abuse rates. This underscores the complexity of interactions that influence child maltreatment rates. Garbarino and Sherman (1980) compared two matched neighborhoods with similar SES but significantly different child maltreatment rates. The authors evaluated non-SES neighborhood factors which might account for the different child maltreatment rates between the two neighborhoods. Neighborhood "expert informants" (community and civic leaders) and random families with children were interviewed extensively. Analysis of the data revealed non-SES factors of "social impoverishment" in the neighborhood with higher rates of abuse. Among the statistically significant ($p < 0.5$) differences identified in the "low risk" low SES neighborhood were fewer "latchkey" children, more neighborhood children as playmates, more people in the child's network (those who have an interest in the child's welfare; i.e. grandparent), more available childcare, and lower rates of self-reported stress (Garbarino & Sherman, 1980). Additionally, families in the "high risk" low SES neighborhood were statistically more likely to describe their own neighborhood as not a good place to raise a child. The authors argue that a neighborhood which is "high risk" for child maltreatment is not simply one with a low SES. A "high risk" neighborhood has additional factors which make its child maltreatment rate higher than would be expected given the low SES. A likely component of a "high risk" community will be resource disparity. The greater the difference between the "haves" and the "have nots", the worse things are for children (Pickett & Wilkinson, 2007). Countries with large Gini Coefficients (a measure of inequality of income distribution; a high Gini Coefficient correlates to large inequalities) have higher rates of infant mortality as well as lower measures of child well-being (Collison, 2007; Pickett & Wilkinson, 2007). The United States has the highest Gini coefficient of all developed nations, indicating a large degree of resource disparity. The United States also has the highest level of children living in poverty among developed nations (UNICEF, 2005). Additionally, independent of household income or characteristics, people in states with greater income inequality have poorer reported health (Kennedy, Kawachi, Glass, & Prothrow-Stith, 1998), including a higher adjusted mortality rates for all causes (Kaplan, Pamuk, Lynch, Cohen, & Balfour, 1996).

Models of Prevention

The extent to which beliefs are based on evidence is very much less than believers suppose. Bertrand Russell, *Skeptical Essays* (1928)

The prevention of illness has been present in the medical writings since ancient times. In *A Regimen for Health* Hippocrates writes in 400 B.C.E. of illness prevention though exercise and diet (Hippocrates, 1983). Commonly, prevention models or interventions are divided into three, and sometimes four, categories. These categories depend upon the target population and are conventionally designated as *Primary*, *Secondary*, and *Tertiary* (and occasionally *Primordial*) prevention (Coles, 2008; Geeraert, van de Noortgate, Grietans, & Onghenea, 2004; Starfield, 2001).

Primary prevention is directed toward unaffected, or pre-affected, populations (i.e. universal intervention). An example of primary prevention which is common in most developed countries is fluoridation of municipal water for the prevention of dental caries. All persons receive the same intervention (fluoride supplementation); there is no decision by the recipient to participate in the intervention.

Secondary prevention is directed toward an at-risk population, it is a targeted intervention. An example of this is the administration of daily penicillin to children with sickle cell disease for the prevention of bacterial sepsis. Only a specified cohort of at-risk children, those with sickle cell disease receive the intervention, and there is voluntary participation in the intervention.

Tertiary prevention is directed toward those already affected. An example would be court-ordered drug treatment programs. Only a well-defined cohort of people (already exposed or victimized) receives the intervention and there is coerced participation by those who receive the intervention. In child abuse prevention, a tertiary prevention strategy would be directed to victims or perpetrators.

Traditionally, prevention efforts have targeted to a child or family with limited attention to the neighborhood or community in which they live. As noted earlier, the neighborhood or community unit itself can be seen as "the client" for prevention efforts. A fourth category, *Primordial* prevention, highlights the importance of the context in which a child, family, or community exists. Primordial prevention is directed at changing social or public policy to reduce not only the disease, but the risk factors for the disease. While not commonly employed, this strategy of prevention aligns well with the ecological model of child abuse and represents a promising future direction. It emphasizes the importance of the context in which a child, family, or community exists.

Evidence-Based Practice

As new strategies for child abuse prevention evolve, there is a growing emphasis both by state and federal funders upon the presumed or demonstrated quality of program evidence that supports a proposed intervention (Chaffin & Frederich, 2004). The term "Evidence Based Practice" (EBP) has been increasingly included as a requirement for funding. Prevention programs are now often expected to have an evaluation and review process which provides a means of assessing the effectiveness of its intervention. The US Preventive Services Task Force (USPSTF) (US Department of Health and Human Services, Agency for Healthcare Research, 2008) uses a grading system to stratify evidence obtained in clinical studies (US Department of Health and Human Services, US Preventative Task Force Procedure Manual, 2008). The evidence levels help inform the strength of a recommendation for a particular intervention (US Department of Health and Human Services, Agency for Healthcare Research, 2008). The levels of evidence and the recommendation categories are outlined in Tables 12.1 and 12.2.

Table 12.1 US preventive services task force levels of evidence.

Evidence level		Minimum source of evidence
I		At least one Randomized-Control Study
II	II-1	well-designed controlled trials without randomization
	II-2	well-designed cohort or case-control analytic studies
	II-3	multiple time series with or without the intervention
III		From respected authorities, based on clinical experience, descriptive studies, or reports of expert committees

Adapted from US Department of Health & Human Services. Agency for Healthcare Research and Quality. US Preventive Services Task Force http://www.ahrq.gov/clinic/uspstf/gradespre.htm#irec

Table 12.2 US preventive services task force recommendation grade.

Grade	Definition
A	The USPSTF recommends the service. There is high certainty that the net benefit is substantial
B	The USPSTF recommends the service. There is high certainty that the net benefit is moderate or there is moderate certainty that the net benefit is moderate to substantial
C	The USPSTF recommends against routinely providing the service. There may be considerations that support providing the service in an individual patient. There is at least moderate certainty that the net benefit is small
D	The USPSTF recommends against the service. There is moderate or high certainty that the service has no net benefit or that the harms outweigh the benefits
I	The USPSTF concludes that the current evidence is insufficient to assess the balance of benefits and harms of the service. Evidence is lacking, of poor quality, or conflicting, and the balance of benefits and harms cannot be determined

US Department of Health & Human Services. Agency for Healthcare and Research Quality. US Preventive Services Task Force http://ahrq.gov/clinic/pocketge08/gcp08app.htm

The strongest level of evidence for an intervention is provided by a *Randomized Controlled Trial* (RCT). Randomized controlled trials are robust, complex processes by which an intervention is compared to a control in a blinded fashion. Randomized controlled trials are complicated and expensive to execute well, and the results are often not available for years. Despite that, well-done RCTs which demonstrate effectiveness are nearly unassailable as strong evidence. There exist other study designs to demonstrate effectiveness which do not involve RCTs, but these methods (case-control trial, pre-post testing) are viewed as providing a weaker level of evidence, subject to bias and criticism.

The increasing emphasis on EBP highlights the lack of national standards in the implementation and quality assurance in prevention practices. This has resulted in states and communities implementing fragmented strategies of variable quality (Chaffin, 2004). The quality and quantity of evidence behind a child abuse prevention program is often weaker than that which would be expected of most conventional medical interventions. Many programs and interventions are developed with good intentions and sound theories but have little reliable data demonstrating a significant decrease in child physical abuse rates. Such programs can be described as "promising" or "evidence-informed" (Chaffin & Frederich, 2004) to highlight the missing strength of evidence.

Obstacles to Evidence

As noted earlier, a common obstacle for prevention studies is the defined end-point. As there is no universal definitive diagnostic test for physical abuse in all cases, there exists much county-to-county, or jurisdiction-to-jurisdiction, variability in the substantiation of a child as a victim of physical abuse. Programs may not be able to generate convincing data as they are unable to compare "apples to apples". Often, prevention strategies use proxy measures (i.e. "parenting skills", "school readiness") instead of the end point (i.e. "child abuse"). While these measures may make it easier to demonstrate success, caution must be used. As noted above, child abuse represents a symptom of a complex family and community disease; it is unlikely that a single intervention, given in a uniform manner, would be effective in preventing all cases of child abuse. Similarly, different interventions are implemented by different people (home visitors, teachers, health care providers), and it is easy to see that the same curriculum or particular model approach may be presented with subtle differences or variations in fidelity to the model. While it is important to rigorously scrutinize all supporting evidence for a program before endorsing it as a successful prevention strategy, care must be taken not to reject promising strategies prematurely simply because they may lack stronger evidence.

Cost Considerations

Increasingly, communities and policymakers examine cost as part of the decision to support prevention programs. Often budgetary constraints are a significant barrier to bringing to scale a program with limited effectiveness data. Many strategies may demonstrate a peak impact only years or decades later, and cost savings of initial outlay of resources may only be truly documentable in the life of the child as an adult. The initial outlays of resources may only result in cost savings 20 years later. Despite the potential for substantial benefit, funders may not give priority of dollars to a program which lacks immediate demonstrable fiscal benefit. If a successful intervention results in lower rates of vandalism or petty crime in 10–15 years, it may be difficult to correlate the absence of that negative directly to the specific program.

An example of the disconnect between financial support and a program with delayed benefits is home visitation. Early evaluation of home visitation as a child abuse prevention approach showed it to be cost effective in various studies (Barnett, 1993). Recent evaluations have likewise shown that home visitation remains a cost effective intervention. This was substantiated in a report by the Washington State Institute for Public Policy (WSIPP) "Evidence-based Programs to Prevent Children from Entering and Remaining in the Child Welfare System: Benefits and Costs for Washington" (Lee, Aos, & Miller, 2008). This report compares different evidence-based programs (from data published in the peer-reviewed literature) and how they impact "likelihood of children entering and remaining in the child welfare system". Of the prevention programs included in the analysis, home visitation, specifically Nurse Family Partnership (NFP) was shown to be cost beneficial with US$3.02 of benefit for every US$1 of cost. The cost analysis in the WSIPP report indicates that NFP cost US$8,931 per participant, a cost which may dissuade a funder from supporting this model. The total benefit (a net Benefit minus Cost of US$18,054 per participant) may not be reaped for many years as manifested as lower expenditures by the community at large.

Another cost metric for the community is the *Willing to Pay* amount. This represents the amount a citizen would be willing to pay in additional taxes for a measurable decrease of a condition, such as a reduction of child abuse by 50% in the community? Another cost metric used is the *Cost Effectiveness* of a program. This describes the outcomes in a way which can be compared to other interventions. If, for every US$100 spent on Prevention A, child maltreatment rates were lowered by 52%, but for every US$100 spent on Prevention B, child abuse rates were lowered by 76%. Prevention B would be more cost effective. Alternatively, Cost Effectiveness can be expressed in costs per episode of child abuse prevented.

Specific Models

We will now look at specific models and approaches to child physical abuse prevention. We will look at the theoretical foundation and the published evidence behind the each strategy. The goal is not to compare each approach to each other, but highlight their strengths and weaknesses.

Home Visitation

One of the best-studied prevention interventions is that of in-home visitation. Visitation of a child and family by a professional in the family's home environment has been part of the medical and community infrastructure for generations. Many developed countries have free home visitation for all infants as part of the national health infrastructure. In Denmark, home visitation has been mandated by law since the late 1930s as a way to lower infant mortality. Home visitation continues to enjoy strong support and indeed there has accumulated much evidence of its benefit in improvement of maternal and neonatal outcomes (Baqui et al., 2008). Home visitation as a specific child abuse prevention strategy was highlighted by C. Henry Kempe in the 1970s (Gray et al., 1966; Kempe, 1976; Kempe, 1978). It has since been endorsed by the American Academy of Pediatrics (1998). In 1977, the first issue of the seminal journal *Child Abuse and Neglect* contained the first RCT of home visitation for the prevention and identification of child abuse and neglect (Gray, Cutler, Dean, & Kempe, 1977). In the United States, although home visitation by nurses has been shown to improve infant outcomes, it is often seen as too costly despite the WSIPP findings (Lee et al., 2008) and support by The Brookings Institute (Issacs, 2008) and The RAND Corporation (Promising Practice Network, 2008).

As noted earlier, first RCT of home visitation involved 100 mothers who were randomized to either an "Intervene" group or a control group (Gray et al., 1977). The intervention was "comprehensive pediatric follow-up with a single physician, a lay health visitor, and/or a public health nurse in the home". After 2 years, 5 children in the control group were hospitalized for injuries "thought to be secondary to abnormal parenting practices" while none of the intervention group were admitted to the hospital. The authors sagely concluded that "The concept of early preventive pediatric and community intervention will, it is hoped, lead to progress in prevention of the harmful effects of child abuse and neglect".

Despite home visitation now having been recognized for three decades as preventing child abuse, little is known about precisely *why* it is successful. There are various models of home visitation, many with common themes. In most, the visits occur in the child's home, the visits are initiated early in the child's life, ideally prenatally, and the visits need to occur with sufficient frequency and duration to make an impact.

Nurse–Family Partnership (NFP) is a rigorous curriculum of nurse engagement with first-time pregnant mothers. The NFP curriculum, described as being both "theory-driven" as well as "research based" (Olds, 2002), involves home visitation by trained nurses. The underlying hypotheses for NFP include the human ecology and the self-efficacy approaches proposed by Bronfenbrenner, and Bandura and Bowlby's human attachment theory. The research base involves multiple published RCTs involving 2,270 mother/baby dyads in three different locations. The NFP nurse visits the pregnant woman before the end of the second trimester and approximately every two weeks while she is pregnant. The nurse then visits the mother and child during the first 2 years of the infant's life averaging over 20 post-natal visits. The NFP nurse curriculum emphasizes three domains: parental education on infant and child development, engaging the mother's social community in the care of the infant, and linking the family to community resources and services (Olds, Henderson, Chamberlin, & Tatelbaum, 1986). In a RCT in 1986, in Elmira, New York the NFP was shown to decrease the rates of child abuse in the target population (Olds et al., 1986). Although the rates did not reach conventional statistical significance ($p = 0.07$), there was compelling impact on the home visited families. Additionally, visited families had fewer visits to the Emergency Room ($p = 0.04$) as well as longer inter-pregnancy intervals than those who were not visited. When the initial Elmira children were followed until adolescence (15 years), they were found to smoke less, drink less alcohol, have fewer lifetime sexual partners, have less drug use, and have fewer arrests (Olds, 2000). Additionally, mothers of these children had longer inter-pregnancy intervals, less drug and alcohol use, fewer arrests and, importantly, had a lower rate of child abuse substantiation ($p < 0.001$) than those who were not visited (Olds, Eckenrode, & Henderson, 1997). It was at this 15-year evaluation that the real child abuse prevention effects became apparent, supporting the argument that one has to view prevention in the long term. When evaluated 15 year after receiving NFP services, participant mothers were identified perpetrators of child abuse at a rate of 0.29 while control mothers had a rate of 0.54 ($p < 0.001$) (Olds et al., 1997). This meets USPSTF level of evidence I.

The NFP model was again replicated in Memphis, Tennessee (Kitzman et al., 1997; Kitzman et al., 2000). The demographics of Memphis are very different from those of Elmira, and notably, the impact of the intervention was less. In the Memphis replication, of the common outcomes being reviewed across sites, benefits to the mother included increased inter-pregnancy intervals and lower poverty levels as measured by fewer on food stamps and more fathers employed. Child abuse rates are not reported. The NFP intervention was again implemented in Denver, Colorado with similar results (Olds et al., 2004). The Denver replication project again showed longer inter-pregnancy intervals as well improved home environments, but the impact on child abuse reduction was not reported. In addition to nurses, the Denver replication included a paraprofessional intervention arm. A paraprofessional was defined as "to have a high school education, no college preparation in the helping professions, and strong people skills". The results of the paraprofessional home visits were comparable to the nurse home visits although the two groups are not explicitly compared. The major criticisms of the NFP model are the dependence upon BSN level nurse visitors and the high costs associated, and the restriction of visitation to first-time mothers. However, these may also account for some of its success.

A common debate regarding home visitation is whether strategies should be universal or targeted. While NFP has a well-defined target population and has been shown to be quite successful, there are data which favor a more universal approach (Guterman, 1999).

Healthy Families America (HFA) is another home visitation intervention which has great acceptance in the United States but is not limited to first-time mothers (Daro & Harding, 1999). Healthy Families America began in the early 1990 s as an expansion of the Hawaii's Healthy Start program. Health Families America has a less rigorous curriculum than NFP and is based upon 12 critical programmatic elements (Healthy Families America, 2008). Healthy Families America uses social worker (paraprofessional) home visitors as contrasted with the nurses used in NFP. While there are promising supporting data regarding family functioning and parenting behaviors, there are limited data with regard to child abuse prevention (Duggan et al., 2007; DuMont, 2008). The availability of HFA to families with multiple children, along with the variability in implementation of the intervention, may contribute to the modest success in prevention of child abuse. This is supported by data showing a protective effect of HFA on child abuse when the selected population matched those visited in the NFP model (DuMont, 2008).

While there are differences between the NFP and HFA home visitation models, as noted earlier, they both have common themes: both endorse a high "dosage" of interventions (frequent and meaningful); both endorse the importance of the rapport between the visitor and the parent as crucial to the therapeutic effect; both endorse the importance of connecting the family to their community; and both endorse curricula with a foundation in effective parenting. Each home visitation model has identified the presence of domestic violence (Intimate Partner Violence) in the household as an obstacle to its successes (Duggan et al., 2004; Eckenrode et al., 2000). Additionally, reports on both NFP and HFA highlight family attrition as a profound problem with a home visitation strategy (Gomby, 2007; Olds et al., 1986). An additional obstacle to implementation of HFA in particular has been fidelity to the original model. Variable model fidelity has contributed to limited published evidence of HFA's decreasing child abuse rates (Duggan et al., 2004; Duggan et al., 2007). Healthy Families America meets USPSTF level of evidence: II-1.

Another home visitation program which shows promising results is the Early Start program from New Zealand (Fergusson, 2005). The Early Start (ES) program is research-based home-visitation service whose critical elements include: "(1) assessment of family needs, issues, challenges, strengths, and resources; (2) development of a positive partnership between the family support worker and client; (3) collaborative problem solving to devise solutions to family challenges; (4) the provision of support, mentoring, and advice to assist client families to mobilize their strengths and resources; and (5) involvement with the family throughout the child's preschool years" (Fergusson, 2005). Each enrolled family receives 36 months of home visitation delivered by either nurses or social workers. Results from a RCT ($n = 443$ families) showed improvements in parental abusive behaviors (improved Conflict Tactic Scale scores) in visited families. Additionally, children who were visited had greater contact with their medical homes, fewer Emergency Department visits and remained in pre-school longer. No difference in child protection agency contacts between the two groups was demonstrated (Fergusson, 2005). This meets USPSFT level of evidence: III. The authors highlight the similarities between the ES and NFP models but do note differences; all delivering families are screened for risks by a nurse within 3 months of birth, enrollment was not restricted to first-time mothers, and services are delivered by both nurses and paraprofessionals.

While most prevention strategies emphasize primary (universal) or secondary (targeted) strategies, tertiary prevention programs (recidivism prevention) present novel challenges. The targets of these interventions have demonstrated a propensity to abuse and are thus likely to have behaviors which would be a challenge to impact. One intervention which has very promising results in child abuse recidivism prevention is *Project SafeCare* (Gershater-Molko, Lutzker, & Wesch, 2002). *Project SafeCare* is an intensive, 24-weeks, in-home parent training program which focuses on three major domains: (1) basic child health, (2) positive parent–child interaction, and (3) home safety. A comparison trial involving 82 families (41 in *Project SafeCare* and 41 receiving Family Preservation services) with substantiated abuse resulted in, at 36 months, the Project *SafeCare* families having a 15% recidivism rate while Family Preservations services (routine CPS response to substantiated abuse) had a recidivism rate of 46% ($p < 0.001$) (Gershater-Molko et al., 2002). This meets USPSTF level of evidence: II-1.

Child–Parent Centers

While home visitation as an intervention has a strong body of supporting literature, there are non-home visitation interventions which also bear consideration. Closely tied with child abuse prevention is school preparedness and educational support. Conditions which hinder development and education are similar to those which are risks for child abuse. The Chicago Longitudinal Study (CLS) (2008) is a federally funded, cohort study, tracking 1,500 low-income children in Chicago. The CLS afforded the opportunity to evaluate the Chicago Child–Parent Centers (CPC) for their impact on child abuse rates. The CPCs are community center-based interventions which tie school preparedness with family strengthening and health monitoring services. Child–Parent Centers provide an environment for parents, mostly single and unemployed, to bring their children for education while they receive support and resources. The program begins at age 3 and continues throughout pre-school up to grade 3. The CPC model has been shown to decrease substantiated reports of child abuse for participant families by 52% (Reynolds, Temple, & Ou, 2003). This meets USPSTF level of evidence: II-2. Additionally, children in participant families had improved scholastic readiness, higher rates of completing high school, and lower rates of juvenile delinquency and arrests, all statistically significant differences from a control matched cohort group. Additionally, the CPC model has been shown to be cost-saving for the community (Lee et al., 2008; Reynolds et al., 2003). The initial costs of US$6,692 per child for 18 months of school resulted in US$47,759 of return per child to society by age 21 years. This translates to a US$7.14 return for each US$1 invested in the CPC.

In-Hospital Parental Education

Another prevention strategy, in-hospital education, has gained support, particularly after a report published by Dias, Backstrom, Falk, and Li (2005). The report was of a regional parental education program administered to all 8 hospitals with maternity services in Western New York State. The parents of all newborns were provided information on the dangers of violent infant shaking, alternatives to soothing a crying infant, and were asked to sign a "commitment statement" after completion. The authors indicate that over 5.5 years, 69% (65,205 of 94,409) of all births in the region had signed commitment statements. They report a 47% decrease in the incidence of an abusive head injury in the catchment area. In the 6 years prior to the intervention, the case rate in the region was 41.5 cases per 100,000 births. In the 5 years after the intervention, the case rate was 22.2 per 100,000 births. While this was not a RCT, the authors report that in the same time interval, the case rate in Pennsylvania, which is geographically proximate, remained unchanged. Such dramatic results are striking, but the intervention has not been duplicated as of yet. This meets USPSTF level of evidence: II-3.

Parental education and intervention surrounding normal infant behaviors remains a very active area of research interest. Two promising programs which, as of yet, have limited child abuse prevention data are "Periods of Purple Crying" (National Center on Shaken Baby Syndrome) and "The Happiest Baby on the Block" (The Happiest Baby).

Community-Based Initiatives

Often missing from many child abuse prevention initiatives is a community engagement component. DePanfilis and Dubowitz (2005) describe a community-based intervention implemented in Baltimore to combat child neglect called *Family Connections*. Family Connections (FC) "is a multifaceted, community-based service program that works with families in their homes and in the context of their neighborhoods to help them meet the basic needs of their children and reduce the risk of child neglect" (DePanfilis & Dubowitz, 2005). Families referred for FC were offered 4 core components: emergency assistance, home-based family intervention, referral services coordination, and supportive recreational activities. Emergency assistance addressed immediate food, shelter, and safety needs. Home-based family intervention consisted of in-home assessments and tailored service plans. Service coordination provided integration of various social services involved with a family to maximize benefit. Multi-family supportive recreational activities were free-of-charge quarterly outings (i.e. museums, boat rides...) for families. Despite poor compliance in the program by enrolled families, a 3-month intervention resulted in improved protective factors and diminished risk factors for participant families. Although, substantiated child abuse rates were unchanged in the participant families, FC remains a promising adjunct intervention (California Evidence-Based Clearing House for Child Welfare 2008). This meets USPSTF level of evidence: III.

Another promising community-based intervention is the Positive Parenting Programmme ("The Triple P") (Sanders, Cann, & Markie-Dadds, 2003). The Triple P is a tiered, population-based intervention with the goals of enhancing parenting skills, promoting healthy environments for children to grow up in, and promoting children's development through positive parenting practices. This is done through a tiered approach based upon the specific family strengths and risks (Prinz, Sanders, Shapiro, Whitaker, & Lutzker, 2009). The first tier (Level 1), *Universal Triple P*, is a media campaign involving radio, television, direct mailings, and Internet sources. The information pertains to positive parenting strategies in an attempt to de-stigmatize seeking assistance for parenting challenges. The second tier (Level 2), *Selected Triple P*, consists of individual parental consultations and group parenting seminars. The content is general parental education and anticipatory guidance. The third tier (Level 3), *Primary Care Triple P*, consists of enhanced parental consultations around specific behavioral management difficulties. The fourth tier (Level 4), *Standard and Group Triple P*, consists of delivery of specific skills training to parents, either in individual or group settings. The fifth tier (Level 5), *Enhanced Triple P*, consists of intensive individualized child–parent intervention and can include other interpersonal management domains (stress, partner communication). The Triple P has shown positive child behavioral and family functioning data (California Evidence-Based Clearing House for Child Welfare and University of Queensland) demonstrating improved parenting practices to recipients. The Triple P does not have data showing participant families having lower child abuse rates than nonparticipant families, but in a novel approach, Prinz et al. (2009) randomized matched counties to receive either The Triple P or routine care. The authors found that in their RCT, counties that received Triple P had lower rates of substantiated child maltreatment, lower rates of child out-of-home placements, and fewer hospitalizations or ER visits for child abuse injuries. In treating the county as the target for their intervention, that authors cannot show specific families having a lower risk of child abuse, but that in aggregate, communities as a whole, having a lower risk. The "Triple P" meets USPSTF level of evidence: I.

Other promising community-based interventions are the Sure Start Local Programmes (SSLP) (Melhuish, Belsy, Leyland, & Barnes, 2008). Sure Start Local Programmes (or "Sure Start") (2009) are regional programs in the United Kingdom which are "area based" and target the lowest 20% of the most deprived regions in England. The services offered at local centers include early education and child care, parenting support, child and family health and medical services, and job training for parents. There are currently over 2,500 centers in the UK offering services to 2.3 million children and families (Sure Start, 2009). A recent study of the SSLPs, which compared similarly deprived regions without a SSLP revealed modest improvements in parenting behaviors, improved home learning environment and improved social development in the children (Melhuish et al., 2008). While not directly a child abuse prevention initiative, the Sure Start model is an example of broad ranging services which are imbedded in communities, with a stated goal to increase "the availability of childcare for all children", to improve "health and emotional development for young children" and support "parents as parents and in their aspirations toward employment" (Sure Start, 2009).

Other Strategies

While the pediatrician's office would seem to be a natural site for prevention services, financial and time constraints have made office-based strategies impractical. The Safe Environment for Every Kid (*SEEK*) model of in-office parent support and abuse prevention (Dubowitz, Feigelman, Lane, & Kim, 2009) has generated some promising preliminary data. The *SEEK* model involves specific physician training, dedicated parental resources, a screening questionnaire, and a dedicated *SEEK* social worker. In a cluster RCT in a pediatric resident continuity clinic, the *SEEK* model resulted in fewer CPS reports involving participant families ($p = 0.03$) (Dubowitz et al., 2009). While this is promising, given the relatively artificial nature of a clinic for pediatric trainees, duplication in a primary care clinic would be required before the *SEEK* model should be considered for wider dissemination.

Another commonly utilized prevention strategy is group-based intervention. This model is common in medical practice as new parent classes or support groups for people with a specific condition or disease. Such interventions are typically offered to prospective or current parents as a prevention strategy to ensure parents have the skills to care for their children. Group-based interventions include parenting classes focusing on discipline techniques and anger management classes. These are often court mandated or part of a constellation of services offered to at-risk parents. There are limited data on the efficacy of group-based child abuse prevention strategies. While they may be part of a larger strategy, their effectiveness as a unique intervention is only speculative.

Often, prevention strategies include a public awareness component. There is little evidence that public awareness initiatives prevent abuse in and of themselves (Daro & McCurdy, 2007), but they can be quite effective as part of a larger community or regional effort (as shown in The Triple P, above). Internet, radio and television commercials emphasizing "Don't Shake Your Baby" may be ineffective, but when tied to a larger educational initiative including, medical, educational, and civic threads could provide a platform for discussions in neighborhoods, supermarkets, schools, community centers, and medical provider offices. A large parental education program ($n = 15,708$) which disseminated educational materials to new mothers in a maternity ward on the dangers of shaking infants had a 21% (3,293) response rate (Showers, 1992). Forty-nine percent of respondents indicated that they were less likely to shake their babies after reviewing the materials. While this shows that large-scale, population education is feasible, whether this alone translates into sustained, altered parental behavior is unknown.

Expanding the Current Models and Theories

Child abuse prevention now has over three decades of study and practice and as past theories and strategies have undergone evolution, our current theories and practices will undoubtedly look different in another three decades. This section will discuss how the current models and theories will likely be expanded beyond child physical abuse, into a more including child well-being approach.

Most child abuse prevention efforts are "program centered". This term highlights the fact that a specific program, curriculum, or intervention is used toward a specific target, usually a child or family. While Primary, Secondary, and Tertiary structure is a simple means to communicate about the target(s) of a specific program, the models of the etiology of child abuse have evolved and thus so have the prevention strategies. Efforts in prevention traditionally have been limited in scope (i.e. a specific age range or time of life), are either universal or targeted (i.e. first time mothers), and are focused on changing a specific person's behaviors or attitudes (i.e. regarding spanking). The evolution of prevention has seen the movement away from site-specific programs toward expansion of community-based collaborations. The designations of Primary, Secondary, and Tertiary can now seem artificial in practice. A child abuse prevention strategy can touch more than one domain or may be primary or secondary depending upon the target or the time in their life. To move beyond the current *"primary, secondary, tertiary"* convention is to make the theory or models of prevention more fluid. An alternative paradigm for child abuse prevention would be to place an intervention along the continuum of timing of abuse. In this way, interventions can be seen as either "proactive" or "reactive" to child abuse. This horizontal intervention axis can be vertically expanded by incorporating the target; starting at the individual level and expanding to encompass an entire community. Prevention can than be thought of along a continuum of individual to community and proactive to reactive (Prilleltensky, 2005). Figure 12.1 gives one example of how an alternative paradigm of prevention could be represented.

Complexity in the causes of child abuse necessitates flexibility in approaches to prevention. A comprehensive prevention effort needs to include components addressing the child, the family, the community and society at large, in various ways, at various stages of the child's life, for various durations. Simply "buying" a program

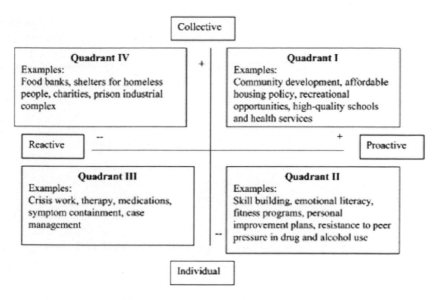

Figure 12.1 Representation of alternative prevention paradigm. Taken with permission Prilleltensky (2005).

(no matter how effective) to roll out in a uniform manner may show short-term gains, but substantial and sustained improvements in child well-being will likely be lacking. For example, implementing an effective home visitation program may touch the lives of those visited children and families, but it is likely to leave the community as a whole unaffected. Similarly, global early-education and pre-K support impacts those who attend, but those who don't remain untouched. Implementing prevention requires integrating programs into a "strategies" or an "approaches". Taking a more expansive view of child abuse prevention allows for inclusion of interventions or strategies which impact child abuse rates but are not conventionally viewed as child abuse prevention. This is best expressed with some of the concepts and language of *Community Psychology*.

Understanding the ecology of a neighborhood is often integral to understanding an individual child's risk for maltreatment. A "sick" neighborhood is a risk to a child and family and manifests its "illness" in a variety of ways. An example is the *Broken Window* theory. Initially described by Wilson and Kelling (1982), the Broken Window theory describes the manifestation of social disorder or dysfunction. Broken windows are included in a list of other manifestations of social strife, gangs, loitering, street violence, and petty crime. Social dysfunction is manifest in the physical structure of a community in the form of potholes in the roads, broken down cars, litter and broken windows. A regression study of 177 census tracts for Cleveland, Ohio identified 3 independent variables which explained 78% of the variance in child maltreatment rates (Coulton, 1995). These three factors were *impoverishment* (poverty rate, unemployment rate, vacant housing rate, and population loss), *child care burden* (ratio of children to adults, ratio of males to females, and percent population that is elderly), and *instability* (proportion of residents who have changed houses within 5 years, proportion of households who have lived in their current home over 10 years and percent of households who have lived in their current household less than 1 year). The *impoverishment* variable had the greatest effect (coefficient $= 11.52$, $p = 0.00$) followed by *child care burden* (4.21, $p = 0.00$), then *instability* (2.76, $p = 0.03$).

Re-conceptualizing Child Maltreatment and Community Intervention

Re-conceptualizing child maltreatment as a manifestation of community despair again requires thinking of it not as a disease in itself but as a symptom. To cure the illness requires focus on the underlying disease and not the symptoms alone. In this way, for example, a strategy to improve access to affordable child care could easily be incorporated into a child abuse prevention initiative. Sustainable child abuse prevention requires engagement with a community or neighborhood to create a new social norm, to change "how things are done."

Community intervention can be seen as either *Ameliorative* or as *Transformative*. Ameliorative interventions aim to promote immediate well-being while Transformative interventions strive to fundamentally change the power structures in a community (to "change the culture") (Nelson & Prilleltensky, 2005; I. Prilleltensky, personal communication, August, 2008; Prilleltensky & Prilleltensky, 2006). Ameliorative interventions address technical and operational processes. They address practical immediate needs. The emphasis is on enhancing protective, strengths-based factors in a community. Transformative interventions address power dynamics and inequalities. The emphasis is on reduction of risk factors in a community ("treat the disease") (Nelson & Prilleltensky, 2005). Both Ameliorative and Transformative community interventions are often necessary. For example, in addressing the problem of homelessness in a community, it is vital to house and clothe those who live on the street, but it is also important to combat the forces that resulted in their homelessness. In response to child abuse, Ameliorative interventions would, for example, provide parenting classes or psychosocial counseling and support with the goal of improved parenting competence and enhanced psychological stability. Transformative prevention interventions, on the other hand, might address parental poverty and social connectedness with the goal of reduction in resource disparity and social isolation. An example of the blending of Ameliorative and Transformative prevention themes into a combined approach is the *Strong Communities for Children* initiative based in Greenville, South Carolina (USA) (Clemson University, 2008a; Kimbrough-Melton & Campbell, 2008). This effort is directed by the US Advisory Board on Child Abuse and Neglect and engages churches, businesses, volunteer groups, and community and civic organizations, bringing together 4,500 volunteers to provide universal assistance to all families of young children in their community (Clemson University, 2008b). The services provided range from simple neighborly check-ins to parenting classes and financial counseling. The goal of these ameliorative activities is to affect a larger transformative community change in how children are valued. The *Strong Communities for Children* initiative required substantial initial outlay of resources, with yearly support by The Duke Endowment of US$1.65 million per year, with the ultimate goal of integration into a permanent change in the day-to-day life in the community. While theory-based, and likely improving child wellbeing, there are no published data on the *Strong Communities for Children* initiatives' impact on child abuse rates specifically.

Modifications of the physical environment are another way for a community to participate in child abuse prevention (Mair & Mair, 2003). One of the best example of the impact of environmental modifications on public health impact is the case of Dr. John Snow and the London Cholera epidemic of 1854 (McLeod, 2000). Dr. Snow, a physician in the Soho District of London, noted a proximal relationship between the Broad Street water pump and clustering of infected patients during a cholera outbreak. Even prior to the recognition of *Vibrio cholerae* as the causative agent, the pump handle was removed and the cases of cholera plummeted. Thus, a modification to the environment, removal of a tainted water source resulted in a cessation of disease. In this way, an intervention can reduce the opportunity for child abuse without directly affecting the motivation.

The *Crime Pattern Theory* describes how routine activities can expose opportunity for crimes. Changing that pattern of activity could result in lower crime due to fewer passive crimes. An example of this is designing subway stations with high-arched ceilings, few support columns, and no public restrooms in order to limit loitering and places to hide. This is called *Situational Crime Prevention* (Clarke, 1997). An analogous example is the relationship between neighborhood alcohol outlets and child abuse. Neighborhood data show that the rates of both reported and substantiated CPS referrals in a neighborhood are correlated to the number of alcohol outlet in the zip code (Freisthler, 2007). By targeting alcohol outlets, specifically off-premise outlets (i.e. liquor stores) the prevention strategy affects the physical environment as a way to prevent child abuse. While this could be viewed as being primary prevention, it is more appropriate to see this as changing the context in which the child and family lives (or *proactive/collective*, Figure 1). *Situational Crime Prevention* and *Broken Window Theory* both address the same underlying cause, a cycle of community disengagement by the residents. People who live in a community in chaos are less likely to engage in the daily life of the community (sit outside in the summer, go for a walk around the block), the absence of community eyes allows passive vandalism to occur and worsen (broken windows, graffiti), crime and dysfunction increases (gangs, muggings), and increasing crime keeps people inside their houses. Community environmental interventions can include redirecting the flow of traffic, improved street lights, increased personal home-ownership, streets which blend housing and businesses thus increasing foot traffic, and redesigned public transportation facilities (Mair & Mair, 2003).

Critical for the success of any comprehensive prevention strategy is its direct integration into existing community and public policy structures. All babies born in a hospital have contact with a medical provider. This provides a tremendous opportunity to either intervene or aid a family which may have needs in caring for the newborn baby. Teachers represent the most common reporter of child abuse in the US (US Department of Health and Human Services, 2008). With the advent of mandated education in 1903, nearly all children in the US have a teacher in their lives. Doctors and teachers are two of the many people who have an interest in the child's well-being; both can be a critical protective factor (Garbarino & Sherman, 1980). A larger community-wide prevention strategy should involve a variety of approaches (primary, secondary, tertiary; proactive, reactive, individual, universal) with various levels of evidence for their success.

The ACE study (www.acestudy.org) noted earlier supports the notion that the context in which a child lives has a long-lasting impact on society. Children exposed to violence (either as victims or witnesses) have a greater risk of negative health behaviors as an adult, including an increased risk of alcoholism, drug use, early teen pregnancy, suicide attempts, and sexually transmitted infections (Middlebrooks & Audage, 2008). The notion of child abuse prevention as a single intervention or program constrains the need for substantive, meaningful improvement in childhood well-being. What is viewed as child abuse prevention should be expanded to include the basics of a healthy childhood. This includes access to healthcare, mental health services (for both the child and the family), education, job training, and financial services, to name a few. The Institute of Medicine (IOM) report *Children's Health a Nation's Wealth* defines children's health broadly as including not just health conditions, but child functioning and the health potential as well (National Research Council and Institute of Medicine, 2004). The report highlights the importance of impacting the trajectory of a child's life by cultivating multiple difference domains: policy, services, social environment, biology, behavior, and physical environment.

Emphasis on the long view is imperative. While policymakers, pundits, and apologists may focus on programs and interventions, the long view is to seek and accomplish progress and evolution. And, while programs and interventions may contribute to a greater evolution of our communities and society, we have to be prepared as a society to accept that they may often lack immediate pay-off. The effects of various programs and interventions, when taken as a whole, may bear fruit in decades in the demonstrable with improvement in the lives of children. This is best seen with the Nurse Family Partnership 15-year review of the Elmira, NY trial (Olds et al., 1997). While the initial, 2-year evaluation was promising, after 15 years the results were quite striking. If decisions to embrace NFP were made solely after the 2-year results, the model may not have been as strongly endorsed.

Future Directions

... it is difficult to imagine that major strides can be made in the battle to prevent, much less remediate, child maltreatment so long as impoverished women, particularly those who are young, are rearing multiple and closely spaced offspring on their own, without sufficient social supports, or both. This observation suggests that fertility planning, education, employment, and economic assistance will be required if serious progress is to be made in the battle to prevent child maltreatment. (Belsky, 1993)

The future of child abuse prevention efforts will depend upon development of crucial infrastructure throughout all levels of human interface. This will include better data collection and management, more rigorous evaluation of interventions, improved collaboration between governmental agencies as well as between governmental and community agencies, and better understanding of how a person or family functions in a community.

The public health model of prevention (universal, prior to "outbreak") has demonstrated enormous improvements in population health (i.e. sanitation, vaccination). That same model of prevention—getting at the root cause—is likely to result in the most sustainable advances for child abuse prevention as well (O'Donnell, Scott, & Stanley, 2008). As noted earlier, a major obstacle in child abuse prevention research has been the differing definitions of child abuse which researchers and agencies use (Whitaker et al., 2005). An additional obstacle is the limited regional or national communication infrastructure for prevention activities. Currently, the National Child Abuse and Neglect Data System (NCANDS) collects data from state's Children Protective Services. These data are used mainly for tracking purposes. There exists no similar national tracking system for prevention efforts. An important step toward understanding the complexity of child abuse prevention is an increase in regional and national collection coordination. To compliment a more rigorous data collection effort, a systematic distribution process needs to be created. The current dissemination system involves data publication in peer-reviewed journals. While our matrix of prevention efforts expands to include other well-being indicators, other local data (pollution, crime, sanitation, food security, and poverty) should like-wise be tracked. Prevention initiatives, when brought to scale, are going to be confronted with the complex nature of the forces in a child life. These initiatives are going to have to be tailored to the child or community. If communities are seen as organisms themselves, tailored interventions can be prescribed to address specific needs. As the community's health improves, then the lives of all its constituents, and thus those of children, in that community will improve.

Despite great enthusiasm for home visitation, NFP in particular, caution should precede whole-sale endorsement. There is still much unknown about home visitation. What is the optimal dose? What is the optimal curriculum? Who are the optimal targets? Most importantly, we need to know why does it work? Home visitation is not a silver bullet for child abuse, not simply "the" answer, and therefore is best part of a larger strategy. Unrestrained support for home visitation has resulted in variable success. This unchecked implementation was seen in the 1990 s with the dissemination of HFA programs in the US. Currently, while HFA is a very valuable prevention program, with programs in over 35 states (Healthy Families America, 2008), there is no central infrastructure for data collection or dissemination. Much could have been learned about HFA, and home visitation in general, if a national strategy for implementation had been in place at the outset.

How individual or family risk factors interface with community strengths and weaknesses remains mostly unknown. As seen in the NFP replication in Memphis, the population chosen was fairly similar (young, mostly single, first-time mothers) but the impact of NFP was much different in this population. The reason behind this is unclear. Rigorous study of the process of home visitation will contribute to a better understanding of the dynamics between children, families, and their communities.

Another future goal is the improvement in understanding how to move theory into practice and to translate effective pilot programs into effective community interventions. There currently is a large gap in the understanding of how to interface effectively with communities (Ohmer & Korr, 2006). Future initiatives may have to look very different than they currently do. Likely, the future will include dynamic collaborations between academia, state or local governments, and community and not-for-profit stakeholders. An example of how this could be constructed is the Saskatchewan Population Health and Evaluation Research Unit (SPHERU) (Mahajarine, Vu, & Labonte, 2006). The SPHERU framework blends public policy and research to evaluate interventions and policies which affect child well-being. The two central concepts are (1) interactions of people in communities can produce measurable health outcomes and (2) these outcomes are affected by overlapping hierarchies of global, state, neighborhood, family, and individual forces. The framework for the SPHERU model includes (1) research based on various study models and data sources and (2) that the research is nested in and engages the community.

Lastly, child abuse prevention services are often located in a single governmental department. The complexity of the causes of child abuse no longer can be constrained to the purview of a single departmental domain. For future success, governmental agencies will require greater coordination to effectively address child abuse. This recently was highlighted in the United Kingdom with the publication of the *Every Child Matters Green Paper* (Every Child Matters, 2003a). One of the cornerstones of the *Every Child Matters Green Paper* is "child protection cannot be separated from policies to improve children's lives as a whole. We need to focus both on the universal services which every child uses, and on more targeted services for those with additional needs" (Every Child Matters, 2003b). The *Every Child Matters Green Paper* was commissioned by then Prime Minister Tony Blair and published in response to the abuse and murder of 8-year-old Victoria Climbie' (Wikipedia, 2008). The public and political discussion resulted in the Children Act 2004. This Act requires local authorities to develop integrated multi-agency Children's Trusts which function under the "duty to cooperate". The "duty to cooperate" provided the legal support for overcoming any inter-agency barriers.

Summary

As the understanding of the etiology of child abuse improves, its complexity increases as well. No longer is it simply bad, sick, or evil people beating their children. Now there is a complex web of influences which protect a child from, or place them a risk of, abuse. These influences range from the child, through the family, into the community, and reach society at large. Each of these spheres of influence change over the life of the child. The changing understanding of why child abuse occurs has been mirrored in a change in approaches to its prevention.

Child abuse prevention began as the identification of "bad" parents and simply watching them more closely. The current themes in child abuse prevention involve mental health, community psychology, social marketing, and public policy. As the "targets" of child abuse prevention are now varied (infants, parents, neighborhoods), there is an increasing emphasis on cohesive, broad strategies as opposed to monolithic program implementation. One of the cornerstones to successful child abuse prevention strategies is the reliance of methodologically sound evidence for support. Many programs may "sound" like they should work, but without rigorous programmatic and process evaluation, they may in fact be dangerous by inhibiting true progress. We cannot spend our time tilting at windmills. There are real giants to joust.

References

Adverse Childhood Studies. (2009). Accessed January 19, 2009: http://www.acestudy.org/

American Academy of Pediatrics. (1998). The role of home-visitation in improving health outcomes for children and families. *Pediatrics, 101*(3), 486–489.

American Academy of Pediatrics, Stirling, J., Jr., and the Committee on Child Abuse and Neglect and Section on Adoption and Foster Care, American Academy of Child and Adolescent Psychiatry, Amaya-Jackson, L., National Center for Child Traumatic Stress, Amaya-Jackson, L. (2008). Understanding the behavioral and emotional consequences of child abuse. *Pediatrics, 122*, 667–673.

Baqui, A. H., El-Arifeen, S., Darmstadt, G. L., Ahmed, S., Williams, E. K., Seraji, H. R., et al. (2008). Effect of community-based newborn care intervention package implemented through two service-delivery strategies in Sylhet district, Bangladesh: A cluster-randomized controlled trial. *The Lancet, 371*, 1936–1944.

Barlow, K. M., Thomson, E., Johnson, D., & Minns, R. A. (2005). Late neurologic and cognitive sequelae of inflicted traumatic brain injury in infancy. *Pediatrics, 116*, e174–e185.

Barnett, W. S. (1993). Economic evaluation of home visiting programs. *The Future of Children, 3*(3), 93–112.

Belsky, J. (1980). Child maltreatment: An ecological integration. *American Psychologist, 35*, 320–335.

Belsky, J. (1993). Etiology of child maltreatment: A developmental-ecological analysis. *Psychological Bulletin, 114*(3), 413–434.

Bonomi, A. E., Anderson, M. L., Rivara, F. P., Cannon, E. A., Fishman, P., Carrell, D., et al. (2008). Health care utilization and costs associated with childhood abuse. *Journal of General Internal Medicine, 23*(3), 294–299.

Bronfenbrenner, U. (1979). *The ecology of human development.* Cambridge, MA: Harvard University Press.

California Evidence-Based Clearing House for Child Welfare. http://www.cachildwelfareclearinghouse.org/program/8

California Evidence-Based Clearing House for Child Welfare. (2008). Accessed October 2008: http://www.cachildwelfareclearinghouse.org/program/92

Chaffin, M. (2004). Is it time to rethink healthy start/healthy families? *Child Abuse and Neglect, 28*, 589–595.

Chaffin, M., & Friedrich, B. (2004). Evidence-based treatments in child abuse and neglect. *Children and Youth Services Review, 26*, 1097–1113.

Chicago Longitudinal Study. (2008).   http://www.waisman.wisc.edu/cls /

Clarke, R. V. (Ed.). (1997). *Situational crime prevention: Successful case studies* (2nd ed.). Guilderland, NY: Harrow & Heston.

Clemson University. Strong Communities. (2008a). Accessed August 2008: http://www.clemson.edu/strongcommunities /

Clemson University. Strong Communities. (2008b). Accessed August 2008: http://www.clemson.edu/strongcommunities/about.html#one

Coles, L. (2008). Prevention of physical child abuse: Concept, evidence and practice. *Community Practioner, 81*(6), 18–22.

Collison, D. (2007). Income inequality and child mortality in wealthy nations. *Journal of Public Health, 29*(2), 114–117.

Coulton, C. J. (1995). Community level factors and child maltreatment rates. *Child Development, 66*, 1262–1276.

Daro, D. (1993). Child maltreatment research: Implications for program design. In D. Cicchetti & S. Toth (Eds.), *Child abuse, child development, and social policy* (pp. 331–367). Norwood, NJ: Ablex Publishing Corporation.

Daro, D., & Harding, K. (1999). Healthy families america: Using research to enhance practice. *The Future of Children, 9*(1), 152–176.

Daro, D., & McCurdy, K. (2007). Interventions to prevent child maltreatment. In L. Doll, S. Bonzo, D. Sleet, J. Mercy, & E. Hass (Eds.), *Handbook of injury and violence prevention* (pp. 137–156). New York: Springer.

DePanfilis, D., & Dubowitz, H. (2005). Family connections: A program for preventing child neglect. *Child Maltreatment, 10*(2), 108–123.

Dias, M. S., Backstrom, J., Falk, M., & Li, V. (2005). Preventing abusive head trauma among infants and young children: A hospital-based, parent education program. *Pediatrics, 115*(4), e470–e477.

Dubowitz, H., Feigelman, S., Lane, W., & Kim, J., (2009). Pediatric primary care to help prevent child maltreatment: The safe environment for every kid (SEEK) model. *Pediatrics, 123*(3), 858–864 (doi:10.1542/peds.2008-1376).

Duggan, A., Caldera, D., Rodriguez, K., Burrell, L., Rohde, C., & Crowne, S. S. (2007). Impact of a statewide home visiting program to prevent child abuse. *Child Abuse and Neglect, 31*, 801–827.

Duggan, A., Fuddy, L., Burrell, L., Higman, S. M., McFarlane, E., Windham, A., et al. (2004). Randomized trial of a statewide home visiting program to prevent child abuse: Impact in preventing child abuse and neglect. *Child Abuse and Neglect, 28*, 597–622.

DuMont, K. (2008). Healthy Families New York (HFNY) randomized trial: Effects on early child abuse and neglect. *Child Abuse and Neglect, 32*, 295–315.

Eckenrode, J., Ganzel, B., Henderson, C. R., Smith, E., Olds, D. L., Powers, J., et al. (2000). Preventing child abuse and neglect with a program of nurse home visitation: The limiting effects of domestic violence. *The Journal of the American Medical Association, 284*, 1385–1391.

Every Child Matters. (2003a). http://www.everychildmatters.gov.uk/aims/background/

Every Child Matters. (2003b). *Chief secretary to the treasury.* Norwich, UK: Stationary Office, p. 5. http://www.everychildmatters.gov.uk/_files/EBE7EEAC 90382663E0D5BBF24C99A7AC.pdf

Fang, X., & Corso, P. (2007). Child maltreatment, youth violence, and intimate partner violence developmental relationships. *American Journal of Preventive Medicine, 33*(4), 281–290.

Feletti, V. (1998). Relationship of childhood abuse and household dysfunction to many of the leading causes of death in adults: The adverse childhood experiences (ace) study. *American Journal of Preventive Medicine, 14*(4), 245–258.

Felitti, V., et al. (1998). Relationship of childhood abuse and household dysfunction to many of the leading causes of death in adults: The adverse childhood experiences (ACE) study. *American Journal of Preventive Medicine 14*(4): 245–258.

Fergusson, D. M. (2005). Randomized trial of the early start program of home visitation. *Pediatrics, 116*, e803–e809.

Fergusson, D., Boden, J., & Horwood, (2008). Exposure to childhood sexual and physical abuse and adjustment in early adulthood. *Child Abuse & Neglect, 32*(6), 607–619.

Freisthler, B. (2007). Exploring the spatial dynamics of alcohol outlets and child protective services referrals, substantiations, and foster care entries. *Child Maltreatment, 12*(2), 114–124.

Freisthler, B., Gruenewald, P. J., Remer, L. G., Lery, B., & Needell, B. (2006). Understanding the ecology of child maltreatment: A review of the literature and direction for future research. *Child Maltreatment, 11*, 263–280.

Garbarino, J., & Crouter, A. (1978). Defining the community context for parent-child relations: The correlates of child maltreatment. *Child Development, 49*, 604–616.

Garbarino, J., & Kostelny, A. (1992). Child maltreatment as a community problem. *Child Abuse and Neglect, 16*, 455–464.

Garbarino, J., & Sherman, D. (1980). High-risk neighborhoods and high-risk families: The human ecology of child maltreatment. *Child Development, 51*, 188–198.

Geeraert, L., van de Noortgate, W., Grietans, H., & Onghenea, P. (2004). The effects of early prevention programs for families with young children at risk for physical child abuse and neglect: A meta-analysis. *Child Maltreatment, 9*(3), 277–291.

Gershater-Molko, R., Lutzker, J., & Wesch, D. (2002). Using recidivism to evaluate project safecare: Teaching bonding, safety, and health care skills to parents. *Child Maltreatment, 7*, 277–285.

Gomby, D. (2007). The promise and limitations of home visiting: Implementing effective programs. *Child Abuse and Neglect, 31*, 793–799.

Gray, J., Cutler, C., Dean, J., & Kempe, C. H. (1977). Prediction and prevention of child abuse and neglect. *Child Abuse and Neglect, 1*, 45–58.

Guterman, N. (1999). Enrollment strategies in early home visitation to prevent physical child abuse and neglect and the "universal versus targeted" debate: A meta-analysis of population-based and screening-based programs. *Child Abuse and Neglect, 23*(9), 863–890.

Healthy Families America. Prevent Child Abuse America.   http://www.healthyfamilies america.org/about_us/faq.shtml

Healthy Families America. (2008). Prevent Child Abuse America.   http://www. healthyfamiliesamerica.org/downloads/critical_elements_rationale.pdf

Hippocrates. (1983). *Hippocratic writings* (G. E. R. Lloyd, Ed., J. Chadwick & W. T. Mann, Trans.). London: Penguin Books.

Issacs, J. (2008, September). *Impacts of early childhood programs.* Washington, DC: The Brookings Institute, http://www.brookings.edu/papers/2008/09_early_ programs_isaacs.aspx

Kaplan, G. A., Pamuk, E. R., Lynch, J. W., Cohen, R. D., & Balfour, J. L. (1996). Inequality in income and mortality in the United States: Analysis of mortality and potential pathways. *British Medical Journal, 312*, 999–1003.

Kempe, C. H. (1976). Approaches to preventing child abuse: The health visitors concept. *American Journal of Diseases of Children, 130*, 941–947.

Kempe, C. H. (1978). Child abuse: The pediatrician's role in child advocacy and preventive pediatrics. *American Journal of Diseases of Children, 132*, 255–260.

Kennedy, B. P., Kawachi, I., Glass, R., & Prothrow-Stith, D. (1998). Income distribution, socioeconomic status, and self rated health in the United States: Multilevel analysis. *British Medical Journal, 317*, 917–921.

Kimbrough-Melton, R., & Campbell, D. (2008). Strong communities for children: A community-wide approach to prevention of child abuse and neglect. *Family and Community Health, 31*(2),100–112.

Kitzman, H., Olds, D. L., Henderson, C. R., Hanks, C., Cole, R., Tatelbaum, R., et al. (1997). Effect of prenatal and infancy home visitation by nurses on pregnancy outcomes, childhood injuries, and repeated childbearing: A randomized controlled trial. *The Journal of the American Medical Association, 278*(8), 644–652.

Kitzman, H., Olds, D. L., Sidora, K., Henderson, C. R., Hanks, C., Cole, R., et al. (2000). Enduring effects of nurse home visitation on maternal life course: A 3-year follow-up of a randomized trial. *The Journal of the American Medical Association, 283*, 1983–1989.

Leventhal, J. (2005). Getting prevention right: Maintaining the status quo is not an option. *Child Abuse and Neglect, 29*, 209–213.

Lee, S., Aos, S., & Miller, M. (2008). *Evidence-based programs to prevent children from entering and remaining in the child welfare system: Benefits and costs for Washington.* Olympia: Washington State Institute for Public Policy, Document No. 08-07-3901.

McLeod, K. (2000). Our sense of snow: The myth of John snow in medical geography. *Social Science & Medicine, 50*, 923–935.

Mair, J. S., & Mair, M. (2003). Violence prevention and control through environmental modifications. *Annual Review of Public Health, 24*, 20–225.

Makaroff, K., & Putnam, F. (2003). Outcomes of infants and children with inflicted traumatic brain injury. *Developmental Medicine & Child Neurology, 45*, 497–502.

Melhuish, E., Belsy, J., Leyland, A. H., & Barnes, J. (2008). Effects of fully-established sure start local programmes on children and their families living in England: A quasi-experimental observational study. *Lancet, 372*(9652), 1641–1647.

Middlebrooks, J. S., & Audage, N. C. (2008). *The effects of childhood stress on health across the lifespan.* Atlanta, GA: Centers for Disease Control and Prevention, National Center for Injury Prevention and Control.

Muhajarine, N., Vu, L., & Labonte, R. (2006). Social contexts and children's health outcomes: Researching across the boundaries. *Critical Public Health, 169*(3), 205–218.

National Center on Shaken Baby Syndrome. http://www.dontshake.org

National Research Council and Institute of Medicine. (2004). *Children's health, the National's wealth: Assessing and improving child health.* Committee on evaluation of Children's health. Board on children, youth and families, division of behavioral and social sciences and education. Washington, DC: The National Academies Press.

Nelson, G., & Prilleltensky, I. (2005). *Community psychology; in pursuit of liberation and well-being.* New York: Palgrave, Macmillan.

O'Donnell, M., Scott, D., & Stanley, F. (2008). Child abuse and neglect—is it time for a public health approach? *Australian and New Zealand Journal of Public Health, 32*(4), 325–330.

Ohmer, M. L., & Korr, W. S. (2006). The effectiveness of community practice interventions: A review of the literature. *Research on Social Work Practice, 16*(2), 132–145.

Olds, D. (2002). Prenatal and infancy home visiting by nurses: From randomized trials to community replication. *Prevention Science, 3*(3), 153–172.

Olds, D. L., Henderson, C. R., Chamberlin, R., & Tatelbaum, R. (1986). Preventing child abuse and neglect: A randomized trial of nurse home visitation. *Pediatrics, 78*(1), 65–78.

Olds, D., Eckenrode, J., & Henderson, C. (1997). Long-term effects of home visitation on maternal life course and child abuse and neglect. Fifteen-year follow-up of a randomized trial. *The Journal of the American Medical Association, 278*(8), 637–643.

Olds, D. (2000). Long-term effects of nurse home visitation on children's criminal and anti-social behavior: 15-year follow-up of a randomized controlled trial. *The Journal of the American Medical Association, 280*(14), 1238–1244.

Olds, D. L., Robinson, J., O'Brien, R., Luckey, D. W., Pettitt, L. M., Henderson, C. R., et al. (2004). Effects of home visits by paraprofessionals and by nurses: Age 4 follow-up results of a randomized trial. *Pediatrics, 114*(6), 1560–1568.

Pickett, K. E., & Wilkinson, R. G. (2007). Child wellbeing and income inequality in rich societies: Ecological cross sectional study. *British Medical Journal, 335*, 1080.

Polansky, N. A., Gaudin, J. M., Ammons, P. W., & Davis, K. B. (1985). The psychological ecology of the neglectful mother. *Child Abuse and Neglect, 9*, 265–275.

Prevent Child Abuse America. (2008, January). Accessed at: http://www.preventchild abuse.org/about_us/media_releases/national_press_release_final.pdf

Prilleltensky, I. (2005). Promoting well-being: Time for a paradigm shift in health and human services. *Scandinavian Journal of Public Health, 33*(Suppl. 66), 53–60.

Prilleltensky, I., & Prilleltensky, O. (2006). *Promoting well-being: Linking personal, organizational, and community change.* New York: John Wiley & Sons, Inc.

Prinz, R. J., Sanders, M. R., Shapiro, C. J., Whitaker, D. J., & Lutzker, J. R. (2009). Population-based prevention of child maltreatment: The US triple P population trial. *Prevention Sciences, 109*(1),1–12.

Promising Practice Network on Children, Family and Communities. http://www.promisingpractices.net/programs_topic_list.asp?topicid=16

Reynolds, A. J., Temple, J. A., & Ou, S. R. (2003). School-based early intervention and child well-being in the Chicago longitudinal study. *Child Welfare, 82*(5), 633–656.

Russell, B. (1928). *Skeptical essays.* Reprinted 1999. New York: Routledge.

Sanders, M., Cann, W., & Markie-Dadds, C. (2003). The triple P-positive parenting programme: A universal population-level approach to the prevention of child abuse. *Child Abuse Reviews, 12*, 155–171.

Showers, J. (1992). "Don't Shake the Baby": The effectiveness of a prevention program. *Child Abuse and Neglect, 16*, 11–18.

Sidebotham, P. (2001). An ecological approach to child abuse: A creative use of scientific models in research and practice. *Child Abuse Review, 10*, 97–112.

Starfield, B. (2001). Basic concepts in population health and health care. *Journal of Epidemiol Community Health, 55*, 452–454.

Stipanicic, A., Nolan, P., Fortin, G., Gobeil, M. F., et al. (2008). Comparative study of the cognitive sequelae of school-aged victims of Shaken Baby syndrome. *Child Abuse and Neglect, 32*(3), 415–428.

Sure Start.   http://www.surestart.gov.uk

Tang, B., Jamieson, E., Boyle, M. H., Libby, A. M., Gafni, A., & MacMillan, H. L. (2006). The influence of child abuse on the pattern of expenditures in women's adult health service utilization in Ontario, Canada. *Social Science & Medicine, 63*(7), 1711–1719.

The Happiest Baby. http://www.thehappiestbaby.com/

The University of Queensland. http://www.pfsc.uq.edu.au/publications/evidence_base.html

Tolstoy, L. (1899). *War and peace*, Part XIII. New York: Thomas Y. Crowell & Co.

US Department of Health and Human Services, Administration on Children, Youth and Families (2008) *Child maltreatment 2006.* Washington, DC: US Government Printing Office, 2008.

US Department of Health & Human Services. Agency for Healthcare Research and Quality. US Preventive Services Task Force   http://www.ahrq.gov/clinic/uspstf/gradespre.htm#irec

US Department of Health and Human Services. Agency for Healthcare Research and Quality. http://www.ahrq.gov/clinic/uspstfab.htm

US Department of Health and Human Services. Agency for Healthcare Research and Quality. http://www.ahrq.gov/clinic/uspstf/grades.htm

US Department of Health and Human Services. US Preventive Services Task Force. Accessed March 26, 2009: http://ahrq.gov/clinic/pocketge08/gcp08app.htm

US Department of Health and Human Services. US Preventive Services Task Force (USPSTF) Procedure Manual, Section 4: Evidence Report Development, subsection 4.3: Assessing Evidence at the Individual Study Level. Accessed at: http://www.ahrq.gov/clinic/uspstf08/methods/procmanual4.htm

UNICEF. (2005). *Child poverty in rich countries*. Florence, Italy: UNICEF Innnocenti Research Centre.

Whitaker, D. J., Lutzker, J. R., & Shelley, G. A. (2005). Child maltreatment prevention priorities at the centers for disease control and prevention. *Child Maltreatment, 10*(3), 245–259.

Wikipedia.   http://en.wikipedia.org/wiki/Victoria_Climbié ;

Wilson, J., & Kelling, G. (1982, March). Broken windows. *Atlantic Monthly*, 29–38.

Ziersch, T. (2005). Neighbourhood life and social capital: The implications for health. *Social Science & Medicine, 60*(1), 71–86.

Zolotor, A., & Runyan, D. (2006). Social capital, family violence, and neglect. *Pediatrics, 117*(6), e1124–e1131.

Part IV
Teamwork

Chapter 13

Multidisciplinary Teams

Maria D. McColgan and Allan DeJong

3 more with DHS files die: the commissioner pointed to added urgency for change
Philadelphia Inquirer, 6-2-07

Infant dies in family under DC supervision
Washington Post, January 19, 2001

Lifting the Veil of Secrecy: Following the deaths of several abused kids in Tucson,
lawmakers aim to reform Child Protective Services
Tucson Weekly, March 20, 2008

Introduction

Cases of child abuse that reach the media are often cases in which child protective service systems are being blamed for allowing children to die in their care. Despite current efforts, an Internet search of child fatalities reveals thousands of headlines of recent deaths of children who were under child protective service (CPS) agency supervision. A thorough, effective investigation of child abuse and neglect can have tremendous effect on the outcome of a case. These stories highlight the breakdowns of the investigations and tend to place blame on those involved. While it is horrifying that cases under investigation can result in such dismal outcomes, the reality is that child maltreatment investigations are complex and difficult. The goal of the investigation is to help create a safe environment that fosters the child's health and development while simultaneously holding accountable the person or persons who put the child in harms way. However, the high volume of child abuse and neglect cases often strains agencies. Child abuse cases are multi-faceted, as cases of child abuse involve social, medical legal, psychological, and other issues. These complexities are beyond the scope of what any one professional can tackle. These inflammatory, high profile cases underscore the need for multidisciplinary cooperation and the

403

A.P. Giardino et al. (eds.), *A Practical Guide to the Evaluation of Child Physical Abuse and Neglect*, DOI 10.1007/978-1-4419-0702-8_13, © Springer Science+Business Media, LLC 1997, 2010

development of ad hoc task forces. They also highlight the failure of legal, medical, or social agencies that are involved in the evaluation of the cases. Therefore, multidisciplinary teams (MDT) were created to foster communication and collaboration between each of these groups and thereby improve the outcome of the investigation and plan for the ultimate well-being of the child and to avoid bad outcomes as in the cases above.

A community response is often stirred up when the media draws attention to a particular case. Political and legal action may occur in response to these situations establishing multidisciplinary oversight in the form of task forces or commissions to identify the failures in the system and lack of appropriate function that led to the poor outcome. For example, failures by social, law enforcement, and medical agencies to recognize ongoing episodes of abuse, eventually, led to the death of a 4-year-old boy in Delaware from a fatal alcohol overdose at the hand of his father's girlfreind. His death prompted the state of Delaware to create the Child Protection Accountability Commission.

Further evidence for the need for improved coordination and communication in child abuse investigations lies in the fact that the efforts of the CPS system often has not been successful in preventing subsequent victimization. In 2006, 13.7% of child fatalities were in families who had received family preservation services in the past 5 years. Only 23 states met the current national standard for a maximal maltreatment recurrence of 5.4% within a 6-month period (Child Maltreatment, 2006). In some states attention to these cases has led to improved state wide funding, increased development of MDTs, and the development of consistency in state wide and regional protocols.

The goal of this chapter is to define a multidisciplinary team (MDT), address the role of an MDT, and discuss the settings in which an MDT can be used to improve the investigation and therefore the medical, legal, and social outcome in cases of child abuse and neglect.

What Is an MDT?

The US Department of Justice defines an MDT as "a group of professionals who work together in a coordinated and collaborative manner to ensure an effective response to reports of child abuse and neglect" (Ells, 2000). The Child Abuse Prevention and Treatment and Adoption Reform Act (CAPTA)(Child Abuse Prevention and Treatment and Adoption Reform, 2003) further defines the professional unit as having representatives from health, social service, law enforcement, and legal service agencies to coordinate the assistance needed to handle cases of child abuse. It further states that a multidisciplinary child abuse team shall be used when it is feasible and that "the court and the attorney for the Government shall consult with the multidisciplinary child abuse team as appropriate." Services that should be provided for a child by the MDT team include

(A) medical diagnoses and evaluation services, including provision or interpretation of x-rays, laboratory tests, and related services, as needed, and documentation of findings;
(B) telephone consultation services in emergencies and in other situations;

(C) medical evaluations related to abuse or neglect;

(D) psychological and psychiatric diagnoses and evaluation services for the child, parent or parents, guardian or guardians, or other caregivers, or any other individual involved in a child victim or child witness case;

(E) expert medical, psychological, and related professional testimony;

(F) case service coordination and assistance, including the location of services available from public and private agencies in the community; and

(G) training services for judges, litigators, court officers and others that are involved in child victim and child witness cases, in handling child victims and child witnesses (Child Abuse Prevention and Treatment and Adoption Reform).

The first known MDTs were created in the 1950 s in Pittsburgh, Los Angeles, and Denver in the hospital setting (Lashley, 2005; National Children's Alliance; Strong, 1997). Community-based MDTs emerged shortly thereafter. Federal funds to develop multidisciplinary task forces became available in 1986. There are now thousands of MDTs with most states having legislative mandates for ongoing MDTs. MDT investigation are recommended by many organizations including the American Academy of Pediatrics, The National District Attorney's Association (NDAA), National Children's Alliance (Shaken baby article), National Children's Advocacy Center, National Association of Children's Hospitals and related Institutions (NACHRI) (Children's Advocacy Center Definitions, 2005; Kellogg, 2007; NACHRI, 2005; National Children's Alliance Standards for Accredited Members; Wilsey, 2004).

Teams can vary based on settings, function, composition, sponsorship, and other characteristics (National Children's Alliance, 2005). An MDT may focus on investigations; policy issues; treatment of victims, their families, and perpetrators; or a combination of these functions (Ells, 2000). An MDT can take the form of a formal team that meets at regularly scheduled intervals, a team that works together on a daily basis, or an informal team that communicates on an as need basis.

The goal of forming an MDT is to provide communication and checks and balances. The benefits of an MDT have been well established and include benefits to the patient and their family, agency staff, investigators, and the community.

There are many benefits to the MDT approach, including (Ells, 2000; Dinsmore, 1993; Giardino & Ludwig, 2002; Kolbo & Strong, 1997)

- Reduction in the number of interviews from the child;
- Decreased trauma to children and families from the investigation;
- Improved communication, coordination and collaboration between agencies;
- Better quality assessments, including more accurate investigations and more appropriate interventions;
- A broader range of viewpoints;
- Reduction in the number of people involved in cases;
- Reduction in duplication of services, and thereby more efficient use of agency resources;
- Otherwise unknown resources identified;

- Enhanced evidence quality for both criminal and civil proceedings;
- Decreased conflicts between various agencies involved;
- Better trained, more capable professionals;
- More cases reviewed and less cases missed;
- More respect in the community and less burnout among child abuse professionals.

MDTs are not without challenges, however. Some reported challenges include difficulty collaborating, with some participants bring hesitant or resisting participation, confusion about leadership roles, unclear ownership of the case, and perceived scrutiny of individual's work. Some participants felt that, at least at first, interdisciplinary decision making was more time consuming than traditional approaches (Kilbo, 1997; Lalayants & Epstein, 2005).

Settings/Types of Teams

While formal MDTs are often used in state and county investigative teams, the MDT model can be applied in a variety of settings. The focus of an MDT may be investigative, treatment of the victims, family, or the perpetrator, or a combination of these functions (Ells, 2000). An MDT may be formed by government agencies, law enforcement and child protective services, medical care organizations, and community advocacy centers. This approach can be used by any agency that deals with or investigates cases of child abuse or treats victims of and their families.

Legal and CPS Investigative Teams

States requesting funding through CAPTA (Child Abuse Prevention and Treatment and Adoption Reform, 2006) are required to establish and maintain a "State multidisciplinary task force on children's justice composed of professionals with knowledge and experience relating to the criminal justice system and issues of child physical abuse, child neglect, child sexual abuse and exploitation, and child maltreatment related fatalities." The bill states that the State task force shall include—

(A) individuals representing the law enforcement community;
(B) judges and attorneys involved in both civil and criminal court proceedings related to child abuse and neglect (including individuals involved with the defense as well as the prosecution of such cases);
(C) child advocates, including both attorneys for children and, where such programs are in operation, court-appointed special advocates;
(D) health and mental health professionals;
(E) individuals representing child protective service agencies;
(F) individuals experienced in working with children with disabilities;
(G) parents; and
(H) representatives of parents' groups (Child Abuse Prevention and Treatment and Adoption Reform 2006).

A summary of each state's legislation mandating multidisciplinary teams can be found at http://www.ndaa.org/pdf/ncpca_statute_multidisciplinary_july_06.pdf.

The National District Attorney's Association (NDAA) recommends a multidisciplinary team consisting of the prosecutor, police, and social services for the investigation and prosecution of cases where a child is alleged to be a victim or witness to abuse in order to reduce the number of times that a child is called upon to recite the events involved in the case as well as to create a feeling of trust and confidence in the child. They further recommend that members of the team receive specialized training in the investigation and prosecution of cases involving child abuse and that the same prosecutor should be assigned to handle all aspects of a case (Wilsey, 2004). In 2000, the Office of Juvenile Justice and Delinquency Prevention (OJJDP) established a national training program on Child Death Investigation that includes modules on child fatality review teams. The NDAA also recommends a team approach in cases where children are witnesses to domestic violence and that domestic violence advocates should participate in child abuse MDTs (Turkel & Shaw, 2003).

In 1993, CAPTA required states to establish child death review teams. As of 2005, all states but one report having state and local child death review teams. The purpose of a death review team is to review all cases of child fatalities to determine the cause of death and to identify which deaths were preventable in cases of accidental trauma and which are identifiable as inflicted trauma, prevent future child deaths and improve the health and safety of the community. As a result of the determination, cases can be handled in an appropriate manner in regard to legal investigation. In addition, the social investigation can investigate the welfare of other children in the home to prevent both accidental and inflicted injury. Child death review is very time consuming as most jurisdictions have many cases per month and each case is multi-faceted. In addition, in the case of child fatality in a child under Child Protective Services supervision, a more specific case review must occur. This review is more in depth than a typical review and not only evaluates the cause and preventability of the individual child's death, but also investigates the failure of the system to protect the child in its care. In addition, all states except Idaho currently have a child death review team. The National Maternal and Child Health Center for Child Death Review states that the purpose of a child death review team is to "conduct a comprehensive, multidisciplinary review of child deaths, to better understand how and why children die, and use the findings to take action that can prevent other deaths and improve the health and safety of children." They provide guidance and tools for local child death review teams on their Website at http://childdeathreview.org/. Additional information on each state's team can be found on this site.

State commissions or task forces may be appointed by the governor to complete an overview of child protection issues. The task force may be charged with evaluating systematic issues throughout the state that involve the investigation, treatment, and prevention of child abuse and neglect and look to creating the legislation to change laws related protection. How state task forces or commissions function is very variable and depends on the purpose of the commission. Some task forces will have a limited specific task to discuss and solve a particular problem and present a solution. Others will be a standing commission that will continue to assess all of the components of the child protection system and support legislation, policies, and provide quality assurance. The role of such commissions is not only to determine if current legislation is appropriate and effective, but through continuous assessment of the function of the child protection system to suggest changes in policy to promote improvement in the functioning of the system. The task force or commission is typically a group of professionals appointed by the governor. For example, in the state of Delaware, the Child Protection Accountably Commission is an appointed state commission composed of personnel from 15 different disciplines such as lawyers, medical mental health, CPS, foster work, independent SW agencies, and law enforcement. This commission's task is to evaluate all of the issues involved in child protection and has oversight for child protection issues in the state of Delaware. This commission does not review particular cases to determine specifics such as whether or not to prosecute the case. Rather, it is meant to involve all aspects of the month-to-month functioning of the child protection system including, but not limited to, legislation, policy, oversight, accountability, etc., and to make suggestions to improve the function of child protection in the state

Global multidisciplinary team or medico-legal advisory boards are assembled in some states. This is typically a team of physicians, CPS, prosecutors, mental health professionals, and law enforcement that helps prosecution teams around the state evaluate cases to decide if a case should be prosecuted or how to proceed in cases where prosecution is being planned. Advisory boards, such as that created in Pennsylvania, are often assembled though the attorney general office. These teams may not be as formal as a governor appointment team and may not have the same oversight that a state wide commission might have. However, the team may also discuss legislation that affects crime against children, may have input into legal issues that affect the child protection system in the state.

In some states there are task forces called together to solve a particular issue. The goal of a task force is to look at the issue, identify the pitfalls, and present solutions to the problem. This type of MDT is typically disbanded after generating a report presenting the solutions. This type of team does not necessarily carry out the proposed changes and may not have the responsibility for the actual oversight.

The Child Advocacy Center

In response to the fragmented approach to child abuse investigations and evaluation, the first Children's Advocacy Center (CAC) was formed by then District Attorney Bud Cramer in 1985 (National Children's Alliance, 2005). As of December 2005, there were over 600 accredited, associate and developing CACs. There are sites in all 50 states, the District of Columbia, and the Virgin Islands (National Children's Alliance, 2005).

The National Children's Alliance places an effective MDT at the core of their philosophy as a Child Advocacy Center (National Children's Alliance Standards for Accredited Members). Their vision statement is as follows:

Children's Advocacy Centers are community partnerships dedicated to a coordinated team approach by professionals pursuing the truth in child abuse investigations. By bringing together professionals from law enforcement, criminal justice, child protective services, victim advocacy agencies and the medical and mental health communities, CAC's provide comprehensive services for child victims and their families (Children's Advocacy Center Definitions, 2005).

The National Children's Alliance defines minimal requirements for certification as an accredited advocacy center. Minimal components include involvement of law enforcement, CPS, prosecution, mental health professionals, medical professionals, victim advocacy, and child advocacy center personnel. The goal of the CAC model is to improve interagency coordination and cooperation and to provide a child friendly atmosphere to reduce the trauma of the investigation on victims and their families. The child forensic interview is a central component of the CAC model. Therefore, trained forensic interviewers are usually employed to conduct interviews of children.

While the concept of a CAC investigation intuitively makes sense, until recently there was a paucity of research proving the benefits of this model. A study published in 2007 examined four CACs and compared cases evaluated at the CACs with those evaluated in comparison communities without CACs. While centers varied in their approach to coordination efforts, CAC cases were more likely to have police involvement in CPS cases, MDT interviews, case reviews, joint police/CPS investigations, and video/audio taping of interviews. In CAC investigations, 85% of child interviews took place in child-friendly CAC facilities while interviews in comparison cases took place in less child-friendly locations such as CPS offices, police facilities, the child's home, or school (Cross et al., 2007). In another 2007 study, CAC and CPT investigations were associated with improved substantiation rates and investigation efficiency as compared with traditional child protective investigations (Wolfteich & Brittany, 2007). Additionally, a cost analysis of CAC cases found that traditional investigations were 36% more expensive than the CAC investigation (Shadoin, Magnuson, & Overman, 2006). They also found that CAC investigations resulted in perception of higher public benefit. Decreased number of child interviews have also been shown to be a benefit, thereby possibly reducing the trauma to the child and improving the outcome of the investigation by providing a sound child interview (Cross et al., 2007).

Medical/Hospital

The first hospital MDTs were developed in Pittsburgh and Los Angeles in the late 1950s, a concept that quickly caught on. Discussion of hospital MDTs first surfaced in the medical literature in the 1970 s and in 1973, pediatrician Ray Helfer recommended that any hospital that sees 25 or more cases of child abuse or neglects per year should have a well-defined MDT (Helfer, 1973; National Center on Child Abuse and Neglect, 1978). In 2005, the National Association of Children's Hospitals and Related Institutions (NACHRI) sponsored a survey of children's hospitals to identify the availability of child abuse services (NACHRI, 2005a). The survey found that 4% of hospitals had no services, and that 38% had child abuse services but do not have a formal team or program. Seventeen percent had a child abuse team and 37% had a child abuse program. NACHRI defined a team as having a minimum of a physician, a social worker, and an administrative coordinator. In the executive summary of the NACHRI survey, it highlights the complexity of the cases seen by these teams and notes that child abuse admissions are twice as long, have twice the diagnosis, and double the cost of other pediatric admissions. Therefore, they recommend that all children's institutions develop a program that fits the needs of the institution and the children they serve. They outline best practices in child maltreatment = evaluations using a three tiered standard for child maltreatment teams: basic, advanced, and a center of excellence. At the bare minimum, a basic team has an administrator and a physician, with access to social work support. The team's responsibilities are to consult on all child abuse cases, help to guide hospital policies on child maltreatment, facilitate timely reporting to CPS, and foster communication with agencies involved. An advanced program has the features of a basic program plus has 24/7 consultation, utilizes a multidisciplinary approach, and participates in community MDT meetings. A center of excellence has a larger MDT, including mental health and social workers. The team members are involved in local, regional, and national leadership activities related to child maltreatment and conduct research and educational efforts. They further define each tier as to services provided in each of six categories: clinical services, policies, advocacy, prevention, community collaboration, education and training, and research.

The MDT approach has been used in the hospital setting in a variety of ways. Functions performed by Copts included consulting on cases of CAN, functioning as a liaison with child protective services, tracking cases of abuse or neglect providing quality assurance on CAN cases, and filing reports with child protective services. Twenty-four-hour consultative coverage was provided by most CPTs, with 94% providing phone consultation and 81% providing in-person consultation when necessary (Tien, Bauchner, & Reece, 2002). Medical institutions for children with a CPT have been found to provide more comprehensive documentation for child abuse and neglect (CAN) and follow-up of children with suspected child abuse, including referral to law enforcement and a CAN clinic for follow-up.

Another benefit of a hospital MDT approach is decrease in misdiagnosis child abuse. For example, a study by Wallace looked at 99 children under 12 months with fracture who were referred to the hospital-based MDT for the concern for physical abuse. Seven percent of the referrals were not reported to child protective services bases on the findings of the MDT. They concluded that hospital-based MDT evaluation can prevent unnecessary referrals to Child Protective Services (Wallace et al., 2007).

In the ideal situation, all children who are suspected victims of child abuse would be evaluated in a children's hospital with a CPT; however, this does not mean that hospitals that aren't children's hospitals can ignore child abuse. The Joint Commission on Accreditation of Healthcare Organizations guidelines (JCAHO, PC.3.10, 2004) require hospitals to have practices in place to identify child abuse and domestic violence. This requirement is not unique to children's hospitals and must be in place in all health care settings. Therefore all hospitals must have some multidisciplinary response to respond to situations where the concern for child abuse and/or domestic violence becomes evident. JCAHO requires the following:

- criteria to identify those patients who may be victims of physical assault, sexual assault, sexual molestation, domestic abuse, or elder or child abuse and neglect.
- maintenance of a list of private and public community agencies that can provide or arrange for assessment and care to assist with referrals of possible victims of abuse and neglect.
- education of staff about how to recognize signs of possible abuse and neglect and about their roles in follow-up.
- criteria to identify possible victims of abuse and neglect;
- assessment of the patient who meets criteria for possible abuse and neglect or refers the patient to a public or private community agency for assessment (JCAHO, PC.3.10, 2004).

A basic team can be formed with a physician and a social worker that are dedicated to improving the system of care. This "team" then can bring in other professionals to help with individual cases even though they may not be parts of the permanent team. For example, they may interact with the investigative team and work with law enforcement and CPS to foster communication and thereby contribute to a more successful evaluation. In addition, it is important for practitioners that work with children to know what teams and other resources exist in the area where they practice. In most outpatient office settings there is no on-site social worker. These offices must be knowledgeable about where to refer victims of abuse. In addition, team members on local and state MDTs should be sure that community physicians are aware of the team and know when and how to refer a child to the team for further evaluation.

Hospital teams provide a variety of clinical services with 97% providing medical exams, 95% inpatient care, 86% psychosocial assessments, and 85% second opinion consults. Non-clinical services provided by teams included court testimony (88%), training and education (90%) (NACHRI, 2005b). A NACHRI report highlights types of evaluations a hospital team might provide in a particular case (NACHRI, 2003):

Evaluation	Goal
Medical/Forensic Evaluation	Offer a medical diagnosis based on the history and exam as to whether abuse may be occurring and make recommendations for further evaluation and treatment.
Psychosocial/Evidentiary Interview	Provide more in-depth interviews of children, completed by specially trained, master's level professionals and designed to draw out specific information about abuse concerns.
Psychological Evaluation	Assess the psychological impact of abuse and offer treatment recommendations.
Multidisciplinary Team Evaluations	Provide a comprehensive assessment of the child and family.
Treatment Services	To help children cope with the emotional and behavioral effects of abuse including sexual behavior problems.
Emergency Evaluations	Provide immediate evaluation in emergency cases.

Funding a child maltreatment team presents difficult challenges. As many of the services provided by teams are not reimbursable, the majority of children's hospital with a CPT subsidize the program, underwriting an average of $246,000 (NACHRI, 2005b).

Function of an MDT

How a team functions will depend on the goal of the team and the role that the team intends to fill. For example, CAC requirements include having all participants meet regularly, keeping documentation of the meetings, communicate within all of the participants at the meeting, follow-up getting the information back to the person who disseminates the information. MDTs in the hospital setting can be extremely variable. They may meet whenever a case dictates the need for MDT involvement vs. periodic, set meetings, or a combination of case specific meetings and periodic case reviews. In well-developed programs, MDTs may only discuss the specific details of the more difficult cases with the full team, allowing the team to function more efficiently. See Table 13.1 for an outline of team members roles and function.

Forming an MDT

The establishment of an MDT involves several steps: identifying and recruiting members, developing a mission statement, defining goals, drafting policies and

Table 13.1 Team members and their roles.

Discipline	Main role	Comments
Physician/Health Care Provider	• Identification and reporting of suspected abuse or neglect • Completion of accurate medical evaluation, including history, physical examination, and appropriate laboratory/radiologic evaluation • Medical treatment and mental health referral for child and family • Follow-up for high risk clinical situations that do not meet the level of reporting • Prevent the misdiagnosis of abuse through a thorough differential diagnosis and ruling out mimics of abuse • Interpretation of findings and expert testimony regarding diagnosis • Providing community efforts to prevent child abuse • Training of medical and non-medical professionals on the medical aspects of child abuse and neglect	• Appropriate training, knowledge, and experience are essential to adequately manage the medical aspects of child abuse and neglect
Health care social worker	• Role is variable but often involves some level of team coordination • Careful assessment of family strengths and weakness • Facilitation of connections with community services and supports • Liaison to CPS and Law enforcement • Support to other team members	• Knowledge of child development, abuse dynamics, and legal process are essential • Skills at interviewing, doing initial information gathering, and working with all disciplines is necessary
Child Protective Services (CPS) worker	• Gathering of reports • Initial assessment • Liaison to other disciplines in investigation • Provision of protection of child and safety plan • Development of individual service plan • Delivery and coordination of services being provided • Provision of updates to court, if involved • Community activities around awareness and prevention	• Knowledge of regulatory and legal issues essential • Collaboration skills are necessary

Table 13.1 (continued)

Discipline	Main role	Comments
Police officer/Law enforcement	• Initial assessment • Possible immediate intervention and protection of child • Criminal investigation and evidence collection	• Professional training in child abuse investigations is essential • Awareness of other disciplines' contributions is necessary to overall investigation
Prosecutor	• Management of the court proceedings if the case goes to trial • Preparation of the child for court • Facilitation of victim advocacy services • Collaboration with other disciplines around community-based efforts dealing with child abuse	• Experience with criminal and juvenile court proceedings is essential • Decision to file charges and proceed to court rests on the severity of case and ability to prove the case
Child advocate	• Protection of needs and interest of the child in court proceedings • Independent investigation • Determinations of child's treatment needs	• May or may not be an attorney depending on the jurisdiction
Mental health provider	• Identification and reporting of suspected child abuse • Mental health assessment • Provision of treatment • Interpretation of findings, and provision of expert testimony • Possible assessment of caregivers' degree of risk for further abuse, baseline mental health status and treatability	• May include principals, teachers, school counselors, and other school related personnel

Adapted from Medical Evaluation of Child Sexual Abuse (Giardino & Ludwig, 2002) (printed with permission).

protocols, establishing and maintaining good working relationships among team members, and evaluating the team function (Ells, 2000).

The benefits of developing written procedures and policies include formalizing the team, thereby allowing for continued coordination and collaboration beyond the participation of individual team members (Ells, 2000). The USDOJ Portable Guide provides an in-depth overview on forming an MDT and questions to consider when developing an MDT can be found in Table 13.2.

In Georgia, an assessment of MDTs was done via surveying 15 MDTs throughout the state (Lashley, 2005). In this analysis, 16 general qualities were found to be indicative of success:

1. Accountability for the team—assures that the team meets local, regional, and national standards and assures that the team is functioning within their purpose and meeting its goals;

Table 13.2 Questions for developing an MDT protocol from USDOJ Portable File.

Questions to help you create a protocol

The following points should be addressed in any MDT protocol
- What is the purpose of the team? This may be the team's mission statement, but it can be more concrete, such as "to investigate all child abuse reports in Box Butte County."
- Who are the members of the team?
- What kinds of cases will the team investigate? All child abuse? Only child sexual exploitation? Only felony physical abuse? Neglect and abandonment?
- How will investigations be conducted? Who will do what?
- Who will interview victims and who will interrogate suspects? Who will remove children from their home? Who will collect physical evidence? Who will refer victims for physical examinations?
- When will team members perform certain tasks? Within a specified time from receipt of report? After consultation with other team members? In a particular sequence?
- Where will particular events occur? Will interviews be conducted at a certain location? Interrogations at a different location? Will specific locations be prohibited unless there are unusual circumstances?
- How will team members carry out assignments? Jointly?
- Who must be present? How long will others wait? Will child interviews be recorded? On video? Audio? Other? Will nonteam personnel be present? Parents or person *in loco parentis?*
- What information can be shared under what circumstances?
- How will decisions be made? By whom and at what stage?
- When and where will the team meet?
- How will meetings be conducted?
- When (or how frequently) will the protocol and team function be evaluated? How and by whom?

Ells, US Department of Justice (2000).

2. Accountability for team members—each individual member maintain their responsibility to team, including attending meetings, being prepared, and following team policies and procedures;
3. Efforts to prevent team member burnout—team members can provide support to one another to deal with the stress of handling child abuse cases;
4. Celebration of accomplishments—this can be crucial to continued success of the team and preventing burnout;
5. Establishing a clear definition of purpose—as an MDTs purpose may vary from team to team, the purpose of a team must be clearly defined and understood by all members;
6. Having consistent, regular representation of all agencies—in order to work well, team members must know each other and work together regularly. Each agency must be represented to assure all pertinent information is shared;
7. Regular evaluation plans—honest evaluation from members allows the team to assure that the team is meeting it purpose and allows to future planning and improvement;

8. Extended MDT concept—teams are more effective when they work together on a daily basis outside of the formal team meetings;
9. Identification of a meeting leader—ensures that meetings run smoothly and effectively;
10. Knowing other team members roles—this helps each member to understand the decisions made by members of the team and prevents conflicts;
11. Orientation for new members—to understand the purpose and process of the team;
12. Development of written protocols—to clarify each agency's role, address confidentiality issues, and serve as an interagency agreement;
13. Development of procedures for resolving conflict—allows the team to focus on the issues at hand rather than placing blame;
14. Supervisor support—to promote improved interagency communication and relationships;
15. Trust, respect, and commitment—critical to the success of a team;
16. Recognition of weaknesses and mistakes—allows the team to compensate for or correct problems.

These qualities can be generalized to any type of team and should be considered while developing a strong, effective team.

Why Does It Work?

MDTs are effective for many reasons. Every discipline has something to contribute, both on an individual level and a program/institutional level.

In 1998, New York City's child welfare agency, the Administration for Children's Services (ACS), launched the Instant Response Team (IRT) program. The IRT aims to have child protective workers, police, and when appropriate, prosecutors respond to reports of severe child abuse or neglect within 2 h and to conduct joint interviews of victims in child-friendly settings. This program has had many successes, such as reduced numbers of child interviews, better information sharing, stronger working relationships, and more effective and efficient case processing (Ross et al., 2004).

In a survey of MDTs, the majority of respondents felt that the participation in the team helped them to do their job better and more efficiently (Lashley, 2005). MDT members can improve the performance of other members because they can add the information or experience that the other person does not have. Both individuals can apply that information to the current case and then be able to use that knowledge and information in future cases to provide continuous learning. The continuous cross-discipline learning is a true benefit that can develop into a continuous learning cycle which will benefit the investigation in future cases. Individual investigators need to know a certain amount of information from the other disciplines involved to make an association between one's domain and the information from another discipline. For example, an investigator may need to understand basic tenets of the radiographic appearance of healing rib fractures to pinpoint a perpetrator. In addition, this basic knowledge can help investigators to know when to ask for additional help and which questions to ask. There is also improved decision-making capability since as a team you are using the experience from multiple disciplines. The continuing education of the team members should improve each individual member's processing of child maltreatment cases, and therefore improve the outcome of the investigation. While it may be time consuming to form a team, ultimately efficiency is a benefit of the MDT approach, as there is quicker interdisciplinary sharing of information which improves the performance of the individual members. This approach is both time and cost-effective, as delineation of each members role can be outlined, thereby reducing the potential for duplication of services. These benefits help MDT members to promote better protection to children. An example of how an MDT evaluation can improve investigations is outlined in Table 13.3.

Where to Find Help?

There are many resources available to help with the formation of an MDT, training for MDTs members, and maintenance of a healthy functioning MDT. See the list in Table 13.4 of valuable resources for further information.

Table 13.3 True case presentation highlighting the potential benefits of early MDT evaluation.

	Case without MDT evaluation	Possible case with early MDT evaluation
Case: 7-week-old, ex-35-week preemie twin A presents to Emergency Department. Fell off bed while in dad's care, looked pale to mom when she returned home. Noted to have bruising on cheek. Head CT done which showed sub-dural hemorrhage (SDH)	Police and CPS are notified, who present to ED and ask if the injury could possibly be accidental. The physician reports that this could possibly be accident, but unlikely, so no further investigation is done. Twin sibling not evaluated. 2 months later twin B presents to the neurologist for increasing head circumference and seizures. On workup is noted to have acute and chronic sub-dural hemorrhages (SDH) and multiple healing fractures. Twin is evaluated as a result and is found to have increasing head circumference, chronic SDH, and healing fractures.	MDT evaluation is done. • Hospital social worker sees family and reports that Mom is 20-years-old. Dad has a history of prior drug use. Dad was a victim of child abuse in the past. SW communicated this to CPS. • CPS notes that dad is 21, is not currently working, and has a history of placement in a youth detention center. • Police are informed of this and retrieve his list of multiple arrests for violent crimes. • Twin sibling is brought to ED for evaluation and is noted to have healing posterior rib fractures and subacute SDH.

Table 13.3 (continued)

	Case without MDT evaluation	Possible case with early MDT evaluation
Outcome	A state investigation ensues due to the children's injuries despite previous report to CPS. The team determined there was • Inadequate police investigation due to misunderstanding of meaning of "possible but unlikely" mechanisms of injury. • Lack of supervision of new CPS worker who did not have adequate knowledge of known risk factors and risk assessment tools and did not contact the medical providers. • Twin not evaluated at the initial presentation, because a worker had contacted the pediatrician who noted that the child was "fine" at the last visit 3 weeks ago.	• Children are placed in kinship care and services to family are provided. Three months later, children are doing well and growth parameters are within normal limits. Parents are receiving services, including parenting classes. They have regularly scheduled visits with the children, and the goal is for reunification.

Table 13.4 Resources—Adapted from US DOJ portable guides (Ells, 2000).

Organizations
American Professional Society on the Abuse of Children
407 South Dearborn Street, Suite 1300
Chicago, IL 60605
312–554–0166
312–554–0919 (fax)
Internet: www.apsac.org

The American Professional Society on the Abuse of Children (APSAC) is the Nation's only interdisciplinary society for professionals working in the field of child abuse and neglect. It supports research, education, and advocacy that enhance efforts to respond to abused children, those who abuse them, and the conditions associated with their abuse. APSAC's major goal is to promote effective interdisciplinary coordination among professionals who respond to child maltreatment.

Table 13.4 (continued)

Missing and Exploited Children's Training and Technical Assistance Program
Fox Valley Technical College
Criminal Justice Department
P.O. Box 2277
1825 North Bluemound Drive
Appleton, WI 54913–2277
800–648–4966
920–735–4757 (fax)
Internet: www.foxvalley.tec.wi.us/ojjdp

The Missing and Exploited Children's Training Program, sponsored by the
Office of Juvenile Justice and Delinquency Prevention (OJJDP) and Fox
Valley Technical College, offer a variety of courses on investigating child
abuse, including an intensive special training for local investigative teams.
Teams must include representatives from law enforcement, prosecution,
social services, and (optionally) the medical field. Participants take part in
hands-on team activity involving:

- Development of interagency processes and protocols for enhanced enforcement,
  prevention, and intervention in child abuse cases.
- Case preparation and prosecution.
- Development of the team's own interagency implementation plan for improved
  investigation of child abuse.

National Center for Prosecution of Child Abuse
American Prosecutors Research Institute (APRI)
99 Canal Center Plaza, Suite 510
Alexandria, VA 22314
703–739–0321
703–549–6259 (fax)
Internet: www.ndaa.org

The National Center for Prosecution of Child Abuse is a nonprofit and
technical assistance affiliate of APRI. In addition to research and technical
assistance, the Center provides extensive training on the investigation and
prosecution of child abuse and child deaths. The national trainings include
timely information presented by a variety of professionals experienced in
the medical, legal, and investigative aspects of child abuse.

National Clearinghouse on Child Abuse and Neglect Information (NCCAN)
330 C Street NW.
Washington, DC 20447
800–FYI–3366
703–385–7565
703–385–3206 (fax)
Internet: www.calib.com/nccanch

Table 13.4 (continued)

NCCAN provides access to the most extensive, up-to-date collection of information on child abuse and neglect in the world. The Clearinghouse will provide, on request, annotated bibliographies on specific topics or a copy of its data base on CD–ROM. NCCAN also publishes the User Manual Series, which includes several titles related to MDT's: *A Coordinated Response to Child Abuse and Neglect: A Basic Manual* (1992), *The Role of Law Enforcement in the Response to Child Abuse and Neglect* (1992), and *Joint Investigations of Child Abuse: Report of a Symposium* (1993). These publications are available from NCCAN.

National Children's Alliance
1319 F Street NW., Suite 1001
Washington, DC 20004–1106
800–239–9950 or
202–639–0597
202–639–0511 (fax)
Internet: www.nca-online.org
Regional Children's Advocacy Centers (CAC's):

- Midwest Regional Children's Advocacy Center, St. Paul, MN,888–422–2955, 651–220–6750 www.nca-online.org/mrcac.
- Northeast Regional Children's Advocacy Center, Philadelphia, PA, 215–387–9500 www.nca-online.org/nrcac.
- Southern Regional Children's Advocacy Center, Rainbow City, AL, 256–413–3158 www.nca-online.org/srcac.
- Western Regional Children's Advocacy Center, Pueblo, CO, 719–543–0380 www.nca-online.org/wrcac.

OJJDP funds the National Children's Alliance and the four regional CAC's to help communities establish and strengthen CAC and MDT programs. The Alliance does this by promoting national standards for CAC's and providing leadership and advocacy for these programs on a national level. The Alliance also conducts national training events and provides grants for CAC program development and support. The four regional CAC's provide information, onsite consultation, and intensive training and technical assistance to help establish and strengthen CAC's and facilitate and support coordination among agencies responding to child abuse. The Alliance publishes a number of manuals and handbooks of use to MDT's, including *Handbook on Intake and Forensic Interviewing in* The Alliance publishes a number of manuals and handbooks of use to MDT's, including *Handbook on Intake and Forensic Interviewing in the CAC Setting, Guidelines for Hospital-Collaborative Forensic Investigations of Sexually Abused Children, Organizational Development for Children's Advocacy Centers,* and *Best Practices.*

National Resource Center on Child Maltreatment (NRCCM)
1349 West Peachtree Street NE., Suite 900
Atlanta, GA 30309
404–876–1934
404–876–7949 (fax)
Internet: www.gocwi.org/nrccm/

Table 13.4 (continued)

NRCCM's objectives are to identify, develop, and promote the application
of child protective service models that are responsive to State, tribal, and
community needs. Operated jointly by the Child Welfare Institute and
ACTION for Child Protection, NRCCM offers training, technical
assistance, consultation, and information in response to identified needs
relating to the prevention, identification, intervention, and treatment of
child abuse and neglect.

American Bar Association (ABA)
Center on Children and the Law
Washington, DC
202–662–1720
202–662–1755 (fax)

American Humane Association
Englewood, Colorado
800–227–4645
303–792–9900
303–792–5333 (fax)

American Medical Association (AMA)
Department of Mental Health
Chicago, Illinois
312–464–5066
312–464–5000
(AMA main number)
312–464–4184 (fax)

C. Henry Kempe National
Center for the Prevention and Treatment of Child
Abuse and Neglect
Denver, Colorado
303–864–5250
303–864–5179 (fax)

Federal Bureau of Investigation (FBI)
National Center for the Analysis of Violent Crime
Quantico, Virginia
703–632–4400

Fox Valley Technical College Criminal Justice Department
Appleton, Wisconsin
800–648–4966
920–735–4757 (fax)

Juvenile Justice Clearinghouse (JJC)
Rockville, Maryland
800–638–8736
301–519–5212 (fax)

Table 13.4 (continued)

National Association of Medical Examiners
St. Louis, Missouri
314–577–8298
314–268–5124 (fax)

National Center for Missing and Exploited Children (NCMEC)
Alexandria, Virginia
703–235–3900
703–274–2222 (fax)

National SIDS Resource Center
Vienna, Virginia
703–821–8955, ext. 249
703–821–2098 (fax)

Prevent Child Abuse America
Chicago, Illinois
800–835–2671
312–663–3520
312–939–8962 (fax)

Summary

The trend of multidisciplinary investigation and evaluation is well-established in legal, child protective services, and medical arenas. The major goal of the MDT is to improve the community response to child abuse and neglect, with some MDTs providing assessment of efficacy and policy recommendations regarding systematic issues and others focusing on individual case management. While there are many benefits of evaluations produced by well-functioning MDTs, teams must be careful to avoid common pitfalls that can undermine an effectively functioning team. Care must be taken to ensure quality investigations and maintain the well-being and smooth function of the team. Many local, state, and federal resources are available to develop, train, and maintain an effective team. Many benefits to the MDT evaluation have been documented. An MDT evaluation can help to improve the outcome in individual cases, and thereby help to create stronger, safer communities.

References

Accreditation Program: Office-Based Surgery Provision of Care, Treatment, and Services. (2008). Washington, DC. http://www.jointcommission.org/AccreditationPrograms/Office-BasedSurgery/

Child Maltreatment (2008). U.S. Department of Health and Human Services. Washington, D.C.: U.S. Government Printing Office.

Child Abuse Prevention and Treatment and Adoption Reform in 42 Chapter 67. (2006). http://uscode.house.gov/uscode-cgi/fastweb.exe?getdoc+uscview+t41t42+4725+ 0++()%20%20AND%20((42)%20ADJ%20USC)%3ACITE%20AND%20(USC% 20w%2F10%20(5102))%3ACITE%20%20%20%20%20%20%20%20%20

Children's Advocacy Center Definitions. 2005 (cited 2008 November 11, 2008). Available from: http://www.nca-online.org/pages/page.asp?page_id=4041

Cross, T. P., Jones, L. M., Walsh, W. A., Simone, M., Kolko, D., Szczepanski, J., et al. (2007). Child forensic interviewing in children's advocacy centers: Empirical data on a practice model. *Child Abuse Neglect, 31* (10), 1031–1052.

Dinsmore, J. (1993). Joint investigations of child abuse: Report of a symposium, U.S. Department of Justice and N.I.o.J. Office of Justice Programs, Editors. Washington, DC.

Ells, M. (2000). Forming a Mulitdisciplinary Team to Investigate Child Abuse, Portable Guides to Investigating Child Abuse, O.o.J.P. US Department of Justice, Editor.

Giardino, A. P., & Ludwig, S. (2002). Multidisciplinary teams. In M. A. Finkel & A. P. Giardino (Eds.), *Medical evaluation of child sexual abuse* (2nd ed.). Thousand Oaks, CA: Sage Publications.

Helfer, R. E. (1973). Seven guidelines in child abuse cases. *Resident and Staff Physician, 19* (8), 57–58.

Joint Commission Standard (2008) available at WWW.JOINTCOMMISSION.Org and www.endabuse.org

Kellogg, N. D. (2007). Evaluation of suspected child physical abuse. *Pediatrics, 119* (6), 1232–1241.

Kolbo, J. R., & Strong, E. (1997). Multidisciplinary team approaches to the investigation and resolution of child abuse and neglect: A national survey. *Child Maltreatment, 2* (1), 61–72.

Lalayants, M., & Epstein, I. (2005). Evaluating multidisciplinary child abuse and neglect teams: A research agenda. *Child Welfare, 84* (4), 433–458.

Lashley, J. L. (2005). Indicators of a healthy multidisciplinary team, in half a nation: The newsletter of the State and National Finding Words Courses. The National Child Protection Training Center: Winona, MN, pp. 1–5.

National Children's Alliance. History of NCA and the CAC Movement. (2005). http://www.nca-online.org/pages/page.asp?page_id=4021

National Children's Alliance Standards for Accredited Members.   http://www.nca-online.org/pages/page.asp?page_id=4032

National Association of Children's Hospitals and Related Institutions (NACHRI) A Children's Hospital Profile in Prevention: Using Multidisciplinary Expertise to Detect Child Abuse; Spurwink Child Abuse Program. The Barbara Bush Children's Hospital at Maine Medical Center, in Children's Hospitals at the Frontlines Confronting Child Abuse and Neglect. (2003). Alexandria, VA: National Association of Children's Hospitals and Related Institutions (NACHRI).

National Association of Children's Hospitals and Related Instiutions (NACHRI) Childrens' Hospitals on the Frontlines: Confronting Child Abuse and Neglect. 2004.

National Association of Children's Hospitals and Related Institutions (NACHRI) (2005a). Defining the Children's Hospital Role in Child Maltreatment; Executive Summary. Alexandria, VA.

National Association of Children's Hospitals and Related Institutions. (NACHIR) (2005b). Children's Hospital Child Abuse Services. National Association of children's Hospitals and Related Institutions. Alexandria, VA.

National Center on Child Abuse and Neglect. Multidisciplinary Teams in Child Abuse and Neglect Programs. (1978). A Special Report from the National Center on Child Abuse and Neglect, Roth, RA (Ed). Herner & Co.: Washington, DC. p. 72.

Ross, T., Levy, F., & Hope, R. (2004). Improving responses to allegations of severe child abuse: Results from the Instant Response Team Program, New York City Admin for Children's Services, Editor. Vera Institute of Justice: NY.

Shadoin, A., Magnuson, S., Overman, L. (2006). *Executive summary: Findings from the NCAC cost-benefit analysis of community response to child maltreatment.* Huntsville, AL: National Children's Advocacy Center http://www.nationalcac. org/professionals/research/CBA%20Executive%20Summary.pdf

Strong, J. K. E. (1997). Multidisciplinary team approaches to the investigation and resolution of child abuse and neglect: A national survey. *Child Maltreatment, 2* (1), 61–72.

Tien, I., Bauchner, H., & Reece, R. M. (2002). What is the system of care for abused and neglected children in children's institutions? *Pediatrics, 110* (6), 1226–1231.

Turkel, A., & Shaw, C. (2003). Strategies for handling cases where children witness domestic violence. Update, *American Prosecutors Institute, 16* (2) http://www.ndaa. org/publications/newsletters/update_volume_16_number_2_2003.html

Wallace, G. H., et al. (2007). Hospital-based multidisciplinary teams can prevent unnecessary child abuse reports and out-of-home placements. *Child Abuse Negectl, 31* (6), 623–629.

Wilsey, D. D. (2004). Ethical obligations of child abuse prosecutors and allied professionals: Understanding the interconnection in Update. The National District Attorney's Association.

Wolfteich, P., & Brittany, L. (2007). Evaluation of the children's advocacy center model: Efficiency, legal and revictimization outcomes. *Child and Adolescent Social Work Journal, 24* (4), 333–354.

Chapter 14

Psychosocial Assessment of Alleged Victims of Child Maltreatment

Kelli Connell-Carrick and Maria Scannapieco

Almost one million confirmed victims of child maltreatment were identified in 2006 in the United States, and child abuse and neglect continues to be a major social issue (U.S. Department of Health and Human Services (USDHHS), 2008). Consistently in the United States, the highest rate of maltreatment victimization is for children ages 0–3, and more than 60% of all victims experience neglect (USDHHS, 2008). The youngest children also experience the greatest rate of fatality due to child maltreatment. Children under the age of four account for 87% of maltreatment related fatalities, and 41% of child fatalities are the result of neglect (USDHHS, 2008). Although the youngest children, due to their critical developmental period, are most vulnerable to death, all ages of children are susceptible to child maltreatment and its serious effects, including physical, cognitive, social, and emotional developmental sequalae (Scannapieco & Connell-Carrick, 2005a). It is imperative to identify child maltreatment when it exists in order to make appropriate referrals and provide treatment, and many children are first identified as alleged victims in hospitals, schools, police departments, child care settings, and social service agencies (Scannapieco & Connell-Carrick, 2005a). In a medical-based setting, a social worker performs a psychosocial assessment to determine the needs and well-being of a family. In doing so and often as part of a multidisciplinary team, the social worker may be the first to suspect a child has been maltreated resulting in the legal mandate to report the incident to the state child protection agency for investigation.

The purpose of this chapter is to present the components of a psychosocial assessment that a social worker in a medical-based setting performs. It also discusses key elements social workers use while interviewing caregivers and children, the role of social workers on a multidisciplinary team, and the differences between a clinical social work psychosocial assessment and child protection investigation. Finally, it outlines the steps of the CPS process from investigation to termination of services.

425

A.P. Giardino et al. (eds.), *A Practical Guide to the Evaluation of Child Physical Abuse and Neglect*, DOI 10.1007/978-1-4419-0702-8_14, © Springer Science+Business Media, LLC 1997, 2010

Psychosocial Assessment

Social workers perform psychosocial assessments with their clients to explore over-all functioning and risk, including psychological and developmental histories, and resources and stressors. The social worker in a medical setting should obtain as much information as possible from the patient's chart and physicians in order to pre-pare for conducting an assessment. A psychosocial assessment includes both inter-viewing and observation, and the social worker should build rapport and express genuine concern for patient's well-being. Although each medical setting will have its own forms and set of criteria to guide an assessment, most psychosocial assess-ments will follow a similar format.

While an assessment may share many of the same methods of inquiry and topics of exploration as a child protection investigation, it is separate and distinct. Psy-chosocial assessment explores the psychosocial history of the child and family, as well as the social, environmental, developmental, and the psychological functioning of the child, caregivers, and family. Psychosocial assessment may occur in conjunc-tion with a CPS investigation or alone; it may produce information that warrants a referral to CPS, but its purpose is not to determine whether the family meets legal definitions of abuse or neglect. Rather, that is the job of the state child protection agency that is legally mandated to investigate charges of child abuse and neglect. Once maltreatment is suspected, a report to CPS should be made immediately. A psychosocial assessment will be able to provide information to the CPS agency and assess for other problems within a family. The information gathered during a psychosocial assessment will inform a CPS investigation, stand alone as an assess-ment of a family's current functioning, and may result in the provision of services to a family outside of the formal child welfare system. Different from a psychoso-cial assessment, a CPS investigation will determine areas of risk, protective factors, safety and family well-being, and is guided by the principles of family-centered, strengths-based, and culturally responsive practice. Most importantly, it will deter-mine whether an incident of abuse or neglect meets the legal definition of mal-treatment, and determine the provisions of services offered to the family, which are discussed in more detail later in this chapter.

Identifying suspected child maltreatment. The signs and indicators of physical abuse and neglect have already been discussed elsewhere in this book, and are there-fore not discussed in detail here. However, in conducting a psychosocial assessment it is important to consider some types of maltreatment that are more easily identifi-able than others and may lead a social worker to a different assessment focus. Two circumstances will be discussed here: neglect and shaken baby syndrome.

Neglect, the most predominant form of child maltreatment, is difficult to assess because it often requires one to assess what is absent. Different from physical abuse which leaves a physical indication of abuse, neglect often manifests in delayed development, lack of attachment and apathy; and, the manifestations of neglect present differently depending upon the age of the child (Scannapieco & Connell-Carrick, 2005a). Thus, more time observing the child, parent, and parent–child inter-action may be warranted to determine whether neglect is suspected. In conjunction with other risk factors, developmental delay may be a sign of neglect. Although in medical or forensic environments developmental delay is often considered a soft sign of abuse (Ferrara, 2002), physicians can corroborate the indicators of neglect with hard evidence such as medical documentation or eyewitness for prosecution (Scannapieco & Connell-Carrick, 2005a).

Second, one specific type of child maltreatment that must be diagnosed medically is Shaken Baby Syndrome (SBS)/Abusive Head Trauma (AHT). SBS/AHT is a unique form of physical abuse that occurs primarily in the first 2 years of life and describes a number of signs and symptoms that result in some damage to the head. The degree of brain damage varies by the amount, duration, and force of the shaking (National Center on Shaken Baby Syndrome (NCSBS), 2008), but the baby must be shaken violently back and forth. Shaking most often occurs during a period of stress, with a peak time of SBS/AHT occurring during the 6-week to 4-month age period (Alexander, Levitt, & Smith, 2001). Because infants have weak head and neck muscles, shaking a baby causes the brain to bounce back and forth inside the skull which results in bruising, swelling, and bleeding. SBS/AHT is diagnosed medically, using computed tomography (CT) scan or MRI. Injuries from SBS/AHT can lead to severe and permanent brain damage and even death (National Institute of Neurological Disorders and Stroke (NINDS), 2008). Common symptoms of SBS include irritability, lethargy, poor feeding, vomiting, pale or bluish skin, and convulsions (NINDS, 2008), with major effects including seizures, coma, stupor, and death (NCSBS, 2008). Many children also present with retinal hemorrhages in one or both eyes (NCSBS, 2008). The classic presenting factors for SBS/AHT include subdural hematoma, brain swelling, and retinal hemorrhages, and some, but not all, children also have bruising on some part of the body that was used for holding the baby during shaking. Thus, as with all forms of child maltreatment, when SBS is suspected a report to CPS must be made immediately.

Although observation and the ability to identify indicators of child maltreatment guide the assessment process, the cornerstone of a psychosocial assessment is the interview. Obtaining as much accurate information from an interview requires skill, the expression of genuine concern and the development of rapport with the client. The following section outlines key aspects of interviews including types, the interview process, and interview techniques.

Interviewing Caregivers and Children

Types of Interviews

Generally there are three types of interviews: (a) informational or social history interviews; (b) assessment interviews; and (c) therapeutic interviews. The type of interview the social worker engages in is based on the purpose and the type of information need. The classification of types of interviews helps define the purposes and objectives.

1. Informational or Social History: The social worker encourages the client to share his/her views and feelings about themselves, the problem and goal, and the situation. The purpose is not to learn all there is to know about the person's background, but to seek information enabling the worker to better understand the client so decisions can be made regarding the kinds of services that should be provided. Information will include both objective and subjective feelings and attitudes.
2. Assessment Interviews: These interviews are more focused in purpose than informational interviews. The social worker arrives at an assessment, diagnosis, evaluation, or recommendation. The questions asked in assessment interviews are aimed at making specific decisions involving human services, i.e. should you report suspected child abuse or neglect.
3. Therapeutic Interviews: The social worker affects or helps to affect change. The purpose of therapeutic interviews is to help clients make changes, or to change the social environment to help clients function better, or both.

Interview: Preparatory Phase

In the assessment process, interviewing is the mechanism used for gathering data from clients. Planful execution of the interview will result in obtaining the most reliable and valid information from the client. Social workers should approach the interview in a standard way ensuring quality. The structure of the interview can be divided into three phases: preparatory phase, rapport building and information gathering, and closure phase.

The preparatory phase of the interview is critical for a thorough assessment and entails several steps.

1. Reviewing: This is a skill where the social worker examines and considers the current information available to the worker and medical facility prior to an initial contact. For example, it is important to review previous records. You want to have factual information to reduce the client having to repeat information previously provided. There could also be disadvantages if the prior records present bias or inaccurate information. The worker should approach this with the focus being to further check out unclear or ambiguous information.
2. Consulting: This involves seeking opinions and advice from a supervisor or colleagues concerning an upcoming first visit with the child or caregiver. Frequently the topics addressed involve identifying objectives for an interview or discussing other related practice considerations.
3. Planning: The worker should define the purpose of the interview, to plan what will be asked, what outcomes will be achieved, and what is the workers specific function or role.
4. Documentation: This is often dictated by the medical setting, e.g., computerized intake form, brief notes concerning identifying characteristics of a person and problem situation.

Interview: Rapport Building and Information Gathering Phase

The beginning phase of the interview starts with the first contact and embarks upon the process of exploration with the client. First impressions are important and the initial contact often affects the nature and extent of all future meetings. Social workers' verbal and nonverbal behaviors impact the effectiveness of rapport building and interviewing. The atmosphere the social worker builds during the interview process will influence the degree to which the client will be willing to disclose personal information. An effective interview results when the social worker and client accomplish the purpose for which they first meet. In general during the interview the social worker hopes to:

1. Facilitate an exchange of introductions
2. Establish a tentative direction or purpose of the meeting
3. Outline the general expectations of the clients and client's role
4. Describe the policies and ethical principles that might apply during this and future encounters with the client
5. Ensure that the prospective client understands the conditions under which the interview takes place (Cournoyer, 2007)

To accomplish these, effective communication skills need to be used. Communication skills enable the social worker to let the client know they are being heard and understood, which is particularly important in the next step, information gathering.

Information gathering is facilitated through a variety of questioning methods for eliciting details concerning the problem or situation. Questions are asked to obtain information and to help the client tell her/his story. Open-ended questions are often used because they are less likely to lead the client and are more likely to elicit information. Probing questions are used by social workers to help the client elaborate on the specific details of their concerns and circumstances. It is important for the social worker to use neutral wording and not use loaded or suggestive questions. A loaded question may be, "when did you last hit your child" versus a neutral question being, "have you ever hit your child." The tone of the questioning should indicate caring and understanding and convey respect.

Interview: Closure Phase

Closing an interview is not always easy. There are a number of strategies recommended for use during closing. The social worker should note when the allotted time is almost up and ensure the caregiver or child is emotionally at ease. Ask the client to summarize decisions arrived at during the interview. Restate the way both the social worker and the client agreed to proceed. Explain to the caregiver or child what will happen next if the caregiver or child is reluctant to end the interview. Confront this situation directly. Since in a medical setting the social worker may not have a follow-up interview, referrals should be made by the social worker if the situation warrants. Other strategies may include switching to a neutral topic. The social worker may want to ask the client what they will be doing next, signaling the end of the interview.

Interview Techniques

In addition to the phases and guiding principles of the interview, there are specific techniques the social worker can use to build rapport and gather information. The following is by no means and exhaustive list of techniques used in interviewing but are presented as fundamental to the process. The techniques needed in an assessment interview are

- Active Listening: The social worker uses verbal cues (e.g. "and then. ...") or repeats part of the client statement in a way that encourages the client to explain in more detail. The social worker reflects or mirrors client content by paraphrasing or summarizing, using words the client uses in what is said back to them, and reflects client feelings in an accurate manner by observing and noting client nonverbal and verbal behaviors.
- Attending Behavior: Some examples are the social worker faces the client directly; has a relaxed but attentive posture; use of eye contact in culturally and age-appropriate ways; verbal and nonverbal behaviors are consistent with one another; voice volume is clearly audible, and voice rate is at an average pace or slower; uses verbal following—stays with flow of interview.
- Empathy and Warmth: This technique involves communicating warmth and using reflective listening. The social worker uses voice tone to express caring for the client, is able to respond to the client statements of feelings with accurate reflections, and uses facial expressions to express caring for the client (i.e. warm smile).
- Genuineness: The social worker is consistent in her/his communication; non-defensive, and authentic; communicates honestly; communicates difficult information to the client; describes the client problem/situation without judgment or discounting the worth of the client because of their circumstances.
- Supporting Self-Efficacy: The social worker recognizes the strengths of the client and their ability to carry out specific tasks and succeed.
- Exploring Techniques: The social worker lets the client know she/he wants to understand their view of the problem/situation. Probes are used to elicit from the client knowledge, ideas, and feelings concerning the person, problem, situation, and potential means for resolution of the difficulties are identified. The social worker seeks clarification to respond to an unclear, subtle, indirect, unfinished, or nonverbal expression; and uses skills such as partialzing—breaking down the issues, paraphrasing, open and close-ended questions, focusing, and summarizing.

Documentation of Information Gained in the Interview

Documentation was briefly mentioned in the preparation phase of the interview but needs more attention given the nature of child abuse and neglect and the need for support in making allegations as a mandatory reporter. All case records are professional documents and should be completed in a timely manner with confidentiality respected at all times. The medical-based setting will dictate in what form this takes, but all records should be in a place that ensures the security of the file. Other guidelines for social workers in documenting interviews are

- Maintain only information that is relevant for the medical-based setting
- Facts should be recorded and distinguished from opinions
- Do not record personal information about the client, e.g. religious or political
- Document as much information as possible on direct communication with the caregiver or child
- Retain and update records to assure accuracy, relevancy, timeliness, and completeness (DePanfilis & Corey, 2003).
- Follow any relevant HIPPA regulations based on the medical-based setting protocol

Working as Part of a Multidisciplinary Team

Given the wealth of information in the areas of specialized child development issues, victim and offender dynamics, diagnostic imaging, traumatic memory, forensic pathology, and brain development, pooling the resources of a group of medical professionals is more advantageous than an individual social worker making a decision alone. In a medical-based setting the social worker often is part of a multidisciplinary team (MDT) with representation from the physician staff, nursing staff, administration, and social services. It is important to remember that the psychosocial assessment, although often an individual interview with a child and family, occurs within the context of the important information available from the multidisciplinary team. Given the complexity of child maltreatment, MDTs serve as a mechanism for team decision-making. Team decision-making requires the full participation and collaboration of team members, who share their knowledge, skills, and abilities in deciding whether a report of child abuse and neglect should be filed with CPS.

Some key components of successful MDTs are

- Committed members who have support of their departments
- An initial meeting during which each member's role is discussed
- The development of a mission statement that clearly sets forth the purpose of the team, scope of activities, and authority
- Confidentiality policies that accord with the medical-setting policies and professional practices
- Periodic self-analysis (Department of Justice, 2000).

MDTs serve as a tremendous asset to medical-based social workers who can seek the expertise of other professionals to determine whether a child is suspected of maltreatment. The wealth of information that can be obtained from a team approach comprised of different groups of individuals who each plays a different role in the care of the patient can lead to a more thorough understanding of the patient's presenting problems and any further action that may need to be taken. Although the MDT model is not unique to medical settings, its utility in identifying maltreatment in this setting is noteworthy.

Good interviewing skills are integral to the success of a psychosocial assessment. In addition, the role of the social worker on an MDT and the use of professional documentation are critical elements in deciding to make a report of alleged maltreatment. Professional documentation provides a sound basis for the report, and the multidisciplinary perspective and access to information from the MDT provides the social worker with a range of information that is unavailable in many settings. These key elements of professional social work practice within a medical setting help identify families in need of assistance and enable the social worker to make appropriate referrals and provide services to families, in addition to upholding one's legal duty as a mandatory reporter of suspected maltreatment.

Conducting a Psychosocial Assessment

In a medical setting, the social worker completes the psychosocial assessment and is often the person who makes a report to CPS when maltreatment is suspected. A psychosocial assessment focuses on areas of a child and family's overall functioning. It includes interviews and observation of the child, parent, and family. It also explores housing and employment, social support, history of prior injuries, substance use/abuse, and domestic violence concerns within the family system. The following are common questions and areas of exploration when conducting a psychosocial assessment.

Child. A psychosocial assessment includes interviewing the alleged victim and observation of the child. The developmental level of the child and the child's verbal ability are important considerations during the assessment process and may require changes to the way the following information is obtained. Assessment of the child focuses on (Scannapieco & Connell-Carrick, 2005a)

- Physical and behavioral indicators of maltreatment
- Developmental indicators of maltreatment, including low weight, developmental delays, and other clinical signs of deprivation
- Child's description of the injury/problem, if child is verbal
- Past injuries the child has experienced, including old and new injuries
- Does the child go to school? If so, what grade?
- Does the child have friends?

Parent. Interviewing the parent(s) is necessary when performing a psychosocial assessment that involves minor children. In cases of suspected maltreatment, a parent's explanation and reactions to the alleged maltreatment must be viewed in combination with what the child is presenting (Scannapieco & Connell-Carrick, 2005a). Some questions that guide parental assessment explore both facts about the parent as well their perceptions of the child, injury, and allegation. Questions for assessment include (Scannapieco & Connell-Carrick, 2005a)

- Parental age
- Parental description of the injury
- Caregiver behavior and appearance. Does the caregiver seem concerned about the child's injury?
- Parental history of past injuries to the child
- Exploring why the child was brought in for care now. What factors precipitated the visit?
- Who is the primary caregiver for the child?
- Caregiver mental health, developmental level, and use of drugs and/or alcohol
- Parental cultural background
- Parental knowledge of child's development, including the ability to articulate when developmental milestones were achieved or any special needs the child may have
- Does the caregiver enjoy being a parent?
- Is the parent satisfied with her/his child?
- Can the caregiver understand her/his role as a parent?
- Does the parent express concern about the child or interest in the child's injuries?
- Does the parent attempt to comfort the child?

With a parental assessment, information is sought not only for the immediate presenting problem, but also the parent's reaction and explanation to the injury. As with the child, it is important to combine interviewing with observation of the parent and parent–child relationship. Because developmental periods require different parenting activities, it is also important to ask age-specific questions. For example, if the child is an infant, parental assessment should also address who feeds the child and what the child eats. The assessment should be tailored to each specific family and take into consideration the age of the child and her/his developmental level.

Family. Family structural and relational characteristics have been shown related to overall family functioning and are essential areas to explore in assessment. Although families may have many risk factors for child maltreatment based on family characteristics, they must be understood within the context of the psychosocial assessment and presenting problem. Some questions that may be useful in assessment of family characteristics and functioning include (Scannapieco & Connell-Carrick, 2005a):

- What is the household composition?
- What is the housing arrangement in which the family lives?
- Who lives in the home?
- With whom does the child spend the most time?
- What is the family routine? What is a typical day like?
- Is the family living in poverty?
- Is there domestic violence in the family?
- Where does the child sleep?
- Who is involved in the child's care?
- What is the parent's current employment and what is the work history?
- Has CPS been involved with the family in the past or present? If so, why?

Social environment. The social environment of the family encompasses larger social structures including work, neighborhood, school, formal and informal support networks, socioeconomic status, and social services. Questions to guide the assessment of the social environment include (Scannapieco & Connell-Carrick, 2005a):

- Is the parent or her/his partner employed?
- Does the caregiver have extended family in the area? How often in the contact?
- When needed, who helps the parent/caregiver with the children? Close friends? Family?
- Does extended family help with resources (emotional or material)?
- Does the family belong to any social or religious organization?
- With what other social service agencies is the family involved?

Overall, all family systems—child, parent, family, social environment, employment, violence, and current problems and stressors—need to be explored in a psychosocial assessment. The assessment should help the social worker identify family functioning, but should also help determine whether child maltreatment is suspected so an appropriate report can be made.

The psychosocial assessment does not have to be complete prior to making a report to CPS when maltreatment is suspected. Once maltreatment is suspected, a report should be made immediately. The information the social worker gathers during her/his assessment can assist the CPS worker obtain information, and provide corroborating medical evidence to inform the CPS investigation.

Child Protective Services

The goal of the child welfare system is to promote the safety, permanency, and well-being of children and families (Child Welfare Information Gateway, 2008), and this overall purpose often differs from the missions of other agencies that interface with CPS. Child protection work is guided by three underlying philosophical principles: (1) family-centered practice; (2) strengths-based; and (3) cultural responsiveness, and is embedded within an ecological theoretical context (Pecora, Whittaker, Maluccio, & Barth, 2000; Scannapieco & Connell-Carrick, 2005a). The three guiding principles will be presented, followed by a brief discussion of the ecological model of child maltreatment.

First, within the child welfare system, the family is considered essential for understanding how child maltreatment occurs. This philosophy maintains individuals are best understood within the context of their family and within the reciprocal relationships that exist within the family (Scannapieco & Connell-Carrick, 2005a). The family-centered practice principle maintains that services should be tailored to a family's specific needs because of the uniqueness of each family and their specific situation.

A second guiding principle of child welfare practice is the strengths-based principle, which sets forth a philosophy that individuals have the ability and motivation to grow and achieve competence (Pecora et al., 2000). Families and individuals within families have the ability to change, grow, and have numerous existing resources and strengths that are incorporated into treatment from which the family grows into a healthier-functioning unit. This perspective emphasizes family capability and strength, rather than family deficits (Scannapieco & Connell-Carrick, 2005a). Family and individual strengths are operationalized into protective factors (Kirby & Fraser, 1997), which are factors at each level of the ecological model that help the family and child ameliorate the risk of child maltreatment or its effects (Scannapieco & Connell-Carrick, 2005a) and will be discussed in more detail below.

The third guiding principle of child welfare practice is cultural responsiveness. The practitioner must possess the knowledge, skill (Lum, 1999), and appreciation for different cultures to be effective in working with multicultural families. The effects of and societal attitudes toward those of different races, socioeconomic statuses, and cultures have profound impacts on families and how they experience the world. Because minority children are overrepresented in the child welfare system and the foster care system (Church, Gross, & Baldwin, 2005; Fluke, Yuan, Hedderson, & Curtis, 2003), understanding this principle and continually striving toward greater cultural competence underpins all child protection work.

In addition to these guiding principles, the overall theoretical perspective that guides child welfare work is the ecological/transactional theory (Bronfenbrenner, 1979; Belsky, 1980). It is beyond the scope of this chapter to present a comprehensive discussion of this theory, which can be found elsewhere in the literature (Bronfenbrenner, 1979; Belsky, 1980; Cicchetti & Rizley, 1981; Cicchetti & Lynch, 1993; Scannapieco & Connell-Carrick, 2005a), but a brief discussion is presented to provide a framework for CPS practice.

The underlying assumption of the ecological/transactional framework is that children's multiple ecologies influence one another, which affect development (Cicchetti & Lynch, 1993). The combined influence of the individual, community, family, and larger culture shape the probabilistic course of the development outcomes of maltreated children (Cicchetti & Lynch, 1993; Scannapieco & Connell-Carrick, 2005a). Thus, the presence of violence at one level does not sentence children to poor developmental outcomes. Rather, it is the interplay between risk factors and protective factors that either contribute to or protect the child from adverse developmental outcomes (Connell-Carrick, in press; Scannapieco & Connell-Carrick, 2005a). As a result, the assessment of risk and protective factors is a key element of child protection work. It is within this ecological/transactional context that child welfare embraces its three guiding principles into practice that attempts to reduce maltreatment and support families by building upon family resources and strengths. CPS workers investigate and determine whether abuse or neglect has occurred, but also assess current and future safety including risk of future maltreatment and the presence of protective factors that may prevent or ameliorate the effects of maltreatment.

A combination of individual, community, societal and family risk factors contribute to the occurrence of child maltreatment. Although risk factors correlate to child maltreatment, they do not cause it; they only increase the likelihood of a particular event occurring. Protective factors, on the other hand, moderate or buffer the risks and therefore should reduce the likelihood of child maltreatment (Scannapieco & Connell-Carrick, 2005a), and exist at the family, societal, and individual level. Numerous studies have examined the risk and protective factors that influence the occurrence of child maltreatment. A brief discussion of risk and protective factors is presented, and a more thorough discussion can be found in the literature (Brown, Cohen, Johnson, & Salzinger, 1998; Connell-Carrick, in press; Connell-Carrick, 2003; Dubowitz, Black, Kerr, Starr, & Harrington, 2000; Erickson & Egeland, 2002; Scannapieco & Connell-Carrick, 2005a; Wu et al., 2004).

Risk and Protective Factors. Several factors have been identified in the empirical literature to increase the risk of child maltreatment including poverty, young maternal age, low education, and domestic violence (Famularo, Kinscherff, & Fenton, 1992; Hay & Jones, 1994; Stier, Leventhal, Berg, Johnson, & Mezger, 1993, Eckenrode et al., 2000). Children with chronic childhood illness, premature birth, and congenital abnormalities have also been shown to increase the risk of maltreatment (Vig & Kaminer, 2002). In fact, DiScala and colleagues (2002) found that children who were physically abused were seven times more likely to have been born prematurely than children without an intentional injury. Other risk factors include a history of parental maltreatment (Straus, 1994), problems during pregnancy (Barth, 1991), parental perception of parenting as not enjoyable (Trickett, Aber, Carlson, & Cicchetti, 1991; Scannapieco & Connell-Carrick, 2005b), substance abuse (Scannapieco & Connell-Carrick, 2007; Chaffin, Kelleher, & Hollenberg, 1996; Gessner, Moore, Hamilton, & Murthy, 2004), depression (Coohey, 1998), single parenthood (Scannapieco & Connell-Carrick, 2005a; Cadzow, Armstrong, & Frazier, 1999), and parental mental illness (Cadzow, Armstrong, & Frazier, 1999).

In addition to parent and child factors, environmental factors such as lack of social support and poor social environment also increase the risk of child maltreatment (Brayden, Atlemeier, Tucker, Dietrich, & Vietze, 1992; Coohey, 1996; Connell-Carrick & Scannapieco, 2006; Scannapieco & Connell-Carrick, 2005b). Environmental factors that have been correlated with child maltreatment include unemployment (Wolfner & Gelles, 1993) and low social support and low social contact within one's community (Brayden et al., 1992; Coohey, 1996; Connell-Carrick, & Scannapieco, 2006; Corse, Schmid, & Trickett, 1990). Social isolation is more characteristic of parents who neglect their children, while social conflict is indicative of abusive parents (Crittendon, 1985). In neighborhoods with equal socioeconomic disadvantage, neighborhoods with more social resources, such as high neighborhood social support, less drug and alcohol availability (i.e. fewer bars and fewer drug possession incidents) (Freisthler, 2004), and residential stability, experience less child maltreatment than neighborhoods with fewer social resources and less social contact (Belsky, 1978; Freisthler, Merritt, & La Scala, 2006;). In addition, families who lack a connection to their community have fewer opportunities for exposure to child rearing practices that could improve their own parenting skills (Trickett & Sussman, 1988). Without this social filter and opportunities for parental learning, at-risk parents lack a connection to emotional and material support during stressful times which may contribute to maltreatment.

On the other hand, several protective factors can help reduce the chance of child maltreatment occurring. Parents whose pasts are free from violence are less likely to commit child abuse and neglect (Scannapieco & Connell-Carrick, 2005a). An easy temperament of a child and personality/emotional attributes that match well with their caregiver's promotes attachment and can protect a child from abuse, as can a child's intellectual ability and responsiveness to a parent (Luthar & Zigler, 1991) and normal or above average development (Hodges, 1993). In addition, mothers in happy, violent-free relationships and the presence of fathers or father-figures decrease the likelihood of maltreatment (Gaudin & Dubowitz, 1997; Marshall, English, & Stewart, 2001; Scannapieco & Connell-Carrick, 2005b). Families characterized by warm and secure family relationships and extra familial support, such as peers and teacher support, can serve as protective factors of child maltreatment (Heller, Larrieu, DImperio, & Boris, 1999), as do access to health care and social services, adequate housing, employment and supportive family environments (CDC, 2008; Heller et al., 1999). Overall, the community plays a large role in setting and enforcing cultural norms. Risk is reduced when communities support parents and take responsibility for preventing abuse (USDHHS, 2003).

Thus, different from some other social work settings, the child welfare system is guided by a family-centered, strengths-based, and culturally responsive philosophy within an ecological context. The family is assessed not only for the occurrence and risk of maltreatment, but also for the strengths and protective factors that exist within the family. The child welfare system is complex and can be confusing at times even to professionals. As a result, the following section outlines the policy that mandates reporting for professionals, what happens after a report is made, and the process that families experience once an investigation is initiated.

Making a Report to CPS

If child maltreatment is suspected, a referral to the state child protection agency is legally warranted according to the Child Abuse Prevention and Treatment Act which was amended in 1996 (CAPTA) (P.L.104-235). In order to qualify for federal funding under CAPTA, all states require certain professionals and institutions to report suspected maltreatment, including health care providers, mental health workers, teachers and school personnel, social workers, day care providers, law enforcement, and in some states the general public. All states have a hotline for reporting suspected child maltreatment. Thus, in addition to a medical-based psychosocial assessment, the child protection agency will perform its own investigation to determine whether the child meets the legal definitions of abuse or neglect and assess risk and safety. The reporter can submit a report anonymously, but it is recommended and extremely valuable to the CPS agency if contact information is provided so they can follow-up with questions if necessary (Crosson-Towers, 2003; Virginia Department of Social Services (VDSS), 2007). When a report is made, the reporter will be asked to provide relevant information regarding the alleged maltreatment such as (Crosson-Towers, 2003)

- Information on the alleged victim, including name, address, and telephone number of the child, and parents, date of birth or age, sex, and race
- Actions taken by the reporter
- Specific information regarding the allegations, including specific information regarding the nature of the maltreatment, locations of bruises, bite marks, burns, signs of inadequate care, signs of parental provision of inadequate care, and developmental delays;
- When/where the alleged maltreatment occurred
- Reporter's name and contact information (if the reporter chooses to provide this information)

The more specific information that can be given to CPS, the better information they have to determine the priority of the maltreatment which guides the timeline in which an investigation will occur.

In addition, the definitions of child abuse and neglect vary by state, but each state's definition is derived from CAPTA (P.L. 104–235) which defines child maltreatment as

Any recent act or failure to act on the part of he parent or caretaker,
which results in death, serious physical or emotional harm, sexual abuse,
or exploitation, or an act or failure to act which presents an imminent
risk of serious harm.

Although each state derives its own definition of child abuse and neglect, federal legislation sets forth these minimal standards with which states must comply to receive federal funding.

What happens after a report is made. A report to CPS is often made through a hotline, in which pertinent information about the alleged maltreatment is given by the reporter. At this "intake" level, it is determined whether the alleged incident meets the state's statutory and agency guidelines. The agency decides whether to conduct an investigation and the urgency with which an investigation is warranted (Crosson-Towers, 2003). Some reports are screened out and never investigated because the referral does not constitute child maltreatment, according to state definitions, or the reporter has provided so little information that the agency has no way of locating the child or family involved in the report (Tumlin & Green, 2000). After a report has been accepted for investigation, a decision regarding the urgency with which CPS must respond is made (Action for Child Protection, 2004). Criteria that inform the prioritization decision include the present danger to the child and child vulnerability. Prioritization decisions vary by states, but general guidelines fall into 4 categories: 0–2 h; the same day; within 24 h; and within 2–5 days (Action for Child Protection, 2004).

During the investigation, CPS will determine through interviews, observation, corroboration with collaterals, such as the hospital-based social worker, physicians, and law enforcement, and examining the family's past history of maltreatment, whether the child has been maltreated and by whom. The current and future safety of the child and risk of future harm will be assessed. The case will be assigned a case determination. This is typically either *ruled out*, which means that the maltreatment was not able to be substantiated or *substantiated* which indicates that enough evidence exists that the child was maltreated. Following a case determination and after conducting a family assessment that explores not only the risks to the family but also the protective factors and their safety needs, a service plan for the child and family will be developed. This plan outlines the specific outcomes and goals that will reduce the risk of maltreatment (Crosson-Towers, 2003) and includes whether the child will be provided out-of-home services (i.e. foster care) or in home services, such as family preservation or parenting education. Specific timeframes for the completion of services and permanency goals will be established. Once the treatment is complete, it is determined whether goals have been met and risk of further maltreatment reduced. Families may be offered more services, a new plan may be developed or the case will be closed if children in the home are safe and risks of further maltreatment has been reduced.

Conclusion

Social workers in a medical setting are in a unique position to serve as part of teams who have access not only to the information gathered during a psychosocial assessment, but also to the information gathered in the medical setting. Corroboration from physicians, doctors, nurses and social services can help inform the assessment process in cases of suspected child maltreatment. To complete a psychosocial assessment, a social worker in a medical setting may have only one meeting with a family, so she/he must be focused in approaching the assessment, obtain available and relevant background information, use good interviewing skills, and document appropriately. When maltreatment is suspected, federal law mandates a report to the state child protection agency for an investigation be made. The information gathered during the psychosocial assessment will be invaluable to the CPS investigation and protecting the child from further maltreatment.

In Brief

- A psychosocial assessment of the child's family is a critical component of the suspected child abuse and neglect evaluation.
- It is imperative to accurately identify the child's family and speak with the adult(s) who is (are) legally responsible and with those who were present when the child became ill or injured.
- It is essential to make the family aware of staff concerns and the legal mandate that requires reporting and sharing the results of the abuse evaluation.
- A thorough psychosocial assessment explores the structure of the family and the function of its members and includes social history and demographics.
- The psychosocial assessment uncovers information concerning the caregiver's understanding of the child's injury and how the injury occurred.

- The clinical social worker is involved early in the evaluation of suspected child abuse and/or neglect to optimize the evaluation.
- The social worker provides support to both the family and the
- staff.

References

Action for Child Protection (2004, April). Prioritization for Response from Intake: The First Safety Decision. Retrieved 8/29/08 from http://www.actionchildprotection/org/archive/article0404.htm

Alexander R., Levitt C., & Smith, W. (2001). Abusive head trauma. In R. Reece & S. Ludwig (Eds), *Child abuse: medical diagnosis and management* (2nd ed.). Philadelphia, PA: Lippincott Williams & Wilkins.

Barth, R. (1991). An experimental evaluation of in-home child abuse prevention services. *Child Abuse and Neglect, 15*, 363–375.

Belsky, J. (1978). Three theoretical models of child abuse. *Child Abuse and Neglect, 2*(1), 37–49.

Belsky, J. (1980). Child maltreatment: An ecological integration. *American Psychologist, 35*(4), 320–335.

Brayden, R., Atlemeier, W., Tucker, D., Dietrich, M., & Vietze, P. (1992). Antecedents of child neglect in the first 2 years of life. *Journal of Pediatrics, 120*, 426–429.

Bronfenbrenner, U. (1979). *The ecology of human development: Experiments by nature and design.* Cambridge, MA: Harvard University Press.

Brown, J., Cohen, P., Johnson, J., & Salzinger, S. (1998). A longitudinal analysis of risk factors for child maltreatment: Findings of a 17 year prospective study of officially recorded and self reported child abuse and neglect. *Child Abuse and Neglect, 22*(11), 1065–1078.

Cadzow, S., Armstrong, K., & Frazier, J. (1999). Stressed parents with infants: Reassessing physical abuse risk factors. *Child Abuse and Neglect, 15*(5), 647–659.

Chaffin, M., Kelleher, K., & Hollenberg, J. (1996). Onset of physical abuse and negelct: Psychiatric, substance abuse, and social risk factors from prospective community data. *Child Abuse and Neglect, 20*(3), 191–203.

Child Abuse Prevention and Treatment Act. (1996). P.L. 104–235.

Child Welfare Information Gateway (2008, April). *How the child welfare system works.* Washington, DC: ACYF.

Church, W., Gross, E., & Baldwin, J. (2005). Maybe ignorance is not always bliss: The disparate treatment of Hispanics within the child welfare system. *Children and Youth Services Review, 27*, 1279–1292.

Cicchetti, D., & Lynch, M. (1993). Toward and ecological/transactional model of community violence and child maltreatment. *Psychiatry, 56*, 96–118.

Cicchetti, D., & Rizley, R. (1981). *Developmental perspective on child maltreatment: New directions for child development.* San Francisco, CA: Jossey-Bass.

Connell-Carrick, K. (2003). A critical review of the empirical literature: Identifying risk factors for child neglect. *Child and Adolescent Social Work, 20*(5), 389–425.

Connell-Carrick K. (in press).,Child abuse and neglect. In T. Wachs & G. Bremner (Eds.). *Blackwell handbook on infant development*, Vol. 2 (2nd ed.). Oxford, UK: Blackwell.

Connell-Carrick, K., & Scannapieco, M. (2006). Ecological correlates of neglect infants and toddlers. *Journal of Interpersonal Violence, 21*(3), 299–316.

Coohey, C. (1996). Child maltreatment: testing the social isolation hypothesis. *Child Abuse Neglect, 29*(3), 241–254.

Coohey, C. (1998). Home alone and other inadequately supervised children. *Child Welfare, 77*(3), 291–201.

Corse, S., Schmid, K., & Trickett, K. (1990). Social network characteristics of mothers in abusing and nonabusing families and their relationships to parenting beliefs. *Journal of Community Psychology, 18*, 44–59.

Cournoyer, B. (2007). *The social work skills workbook.* Belmont, CA: Wadsworth.

Crittendon, P. (1985). Social networds, quality of parenting, and child development. *Child Development, 56*, 1299–1313.

Crosson-Towers, C. (2003). *The role of educators in preventing and responding to child abuse and neglect: ACYF user's manual series.* Washington, DC: U.S. Department of Health and Human Services, Administration on Children Youth and Families.

DePanfilis, D., & Corey, A. (2003). *Child protective services: A guide for caseworkers.* Washington DC: U.S. Department of Health and Human Services, ACYF.

DiScala, C., Sege, R., Li, G., & Reece, R. (2000). Child abuse and unintentional injuries: A 10-year retrospective study. *Archives of Pediatric and Adolescent Medicine, 154*, 16–22.

Dubowitz, H., Black, M., Kerr, M., Starr, R., & Harrington, D. (2000). Fathers and child neglect. *Archives of Pediatric and Adolescent Medicine, 154*, 135–141.

Eckenrode, J., Ganzel, B., Olds, D., Henderson, C., et al. (2000). Preventing child abuse and neglect with a program of nurse home visitation: The limiting effects of domestic violence. *Journal of the American Medical Association, 284*, 1385–1391.

Erickson, M., & Egeland, B. (2002). Child neglect. In J. Myers, L. Berliner, J. Briere, C. Hendrix, C. Jenny, & T. Reid (Eds.). *The APSAC handbook on child maltreatment* (2nd ed., pp. 3–20). Thousand Oaks, CA: Sage.

Famularo, R., Kinscherff, R., & Fenton, T. (1992). Psychiatric diagnoses of abusive mothers. *Journal of Nervous and Mental Disease, 180*, 658–661.

Ferrara, F. F. (2002). *Childhood sexual abuse: Developmental effects across the lifespan.* Pacific Grove, CA: Brooks/Cole.

Fluke, J., Yuan, J., Hedderson, J., & Curtis, P. (2003). Disproportionate representation of race and ethnicity in child maltreatment: Investigation and victimization. *Child and Youth Services Review, 25*, 359–373.

Freisthler, B. (2004). A spatial analysis of social disorganization, alcohol access and rates of maltreatment in neighborhoods. *Children and Youth Services Review, 26*(9), 307–319.

Freisthler, B., Merritt, D., & La Scala, E. (2006). Understanding the ecology of child maltreatment: A review of the literature and directions for future research. *Child Maltreatment, 11*(3), 263–280.

Gaudin, J. M., & Dubowitz, H. (1997). Family functioning in neglectful families: Recent research. In J. D. Berrick, R. P. Barth & N. Gilbert (Eds.), *Child welfare research review* (Vol. 2, pp. 28–62). New York: Columbia University Press.

Gessner, B., Moore, M., Hamilton, B., & Murthy, P. (2004). The incidence of infant physical abuse in Alaska. *Child Abuse and Neglect, 28*(1), 9–23.

Hay, T., & Jones, L. (1994). Societal interventions to prevention child abuse and neglect. *Child Welfare, 73*, 379–403.

Heller, S., Larrieu, J., D'Imperio, R., & Boris, N. (1999). Research on resilience to child maltreatment: Empirical considerations. *Child Abuse & Neglect, 23*(4), 321–338.

Hodges, V. (1993). Assessing strengths and protective factors in child abuse and neglect: Risk assessment with families of color. In P. Pecora & D. English (Eds.). *Multi-cultural guidelines for assessing family strengths and risk factors in child protective services* (pp. I1–I11). Seattle, WA: University of Washington.

Kirby, L. D., & M. W. Fraser. (1997). Risk and resilience in childhood. In M. W. Fraser (Ed.), *Risk and Resilience in Childhood* (pp. 10–33). Washington, DC: National Association of Social Workers.

Lum, D. (1999). *Culturally competent practice: A framework for growth and action.* Pacific Grove, CA: Brooks/Cole Publishing Company.

Luthar, S., & Zigler, E. (1991). Vulnerability and competence: A review of research on resilience in childhood. *American Journal of Orthopsychiatry, 61,* 6–22.

Marshall, D. B., English, D. J., & Stewart, A. J. (2001). The effect of fathers or father figures on child behavioral problems in families referred to child protective services. *Child Maltreatment, 6*(4), 290–299.

National Center on Shaken Baby Syndrome. (2008). Medical Facts about SBS. Retrieved 1/23/08 at http://www.dontshake.org/Audience.aspx?categoryID=8&PageName=MedicalFactsAnswers.htm

National Institute of Neurological Disorders and Stroke. (2008). NINDS Shaken Baby Syndrome Information Page, Retrieved January 18, 2008. http://www.ninds.nih.gov/disorders/shakenbaby/shakenbaby.htm?css=print

Pecora, P. J., Whittaker, J. K., Maluccio, A. N., & Barth, R. P. (2000). *The Child Welfare Challenge: Policy, Practice, and Research* (2nd ed.). NY: Aldine De Gruyter.

Scannapieco, M., & Connell-Carrick, K. (2005a). *Understanding child maltreatment.* New York: Oxford University Press.

Scannapieco, M., & Connell-Carrick, K. (2005b). Focus on the first years: Correlates of substantiation of child maltreatment for families with children 0 to 4. *Children and Youth Services Review, 27*(12), 1307–1323.

Scannapieco, M., & Connell-Carrick, K. (2007). Assessment of families who have substance abuse issues: Those who maltreat their infants and toddlers and those who do not. *Substance Use and Misuse, 42,* 1545–1553.

Stier, D., Leventhal, J., Berg, A., Johnson, L., & Mezger, J. (1993). Are children born to young mothers at risk of maltreatment? *Pediatrics, 91*(3), 642–648.

Straus, M. (1994). *Beating the devil out of them: Corporal punishment in American families.* San Francisco, CA: Jossey-Bass

Trickett, P., Aber, J., Carlson, V., & Cicchetti, D. (1991). The relationship of socioeconomic status to the etiology and developmental sequalae child physical abuse. *Developmental Psychopathology, 27,* 148–158.

Trickett, P., & Sussman, E. (1988). Parental Perceptions of Child-Rearing Practices in Physically Abusive and Nonabusive Families. *Developmental Psychology, 24*(2), 270–276.

Tumlin, K., & Green, R. (2000). The decision to investigate: Understanding state child welfare screening policies and practices. *New Federalism, Issues and Opinions for States, Series A, 38,* 1–8.

United Stated Department of Health and Human Services. (2008). *Child maltreatment reports from the states 2006.* Washington, DC: Author.

United States Department of Justice. (2000). *Forming a multidisciplinary team to investigate child abuse.* Washington, DC: Department of Justice.

Vig, S., & Kaminer, R. (2002). Maltreatment and developmental disabilities in children. *Journal of Developmental and Physical Disabilities, 14*(4), 371–386.

Virginia Department of Social Services, (2007). *A guide for mandated reporters in recognizing and reporting child abuse and neglect.* Richmond, VA: Author.

Retrieved 8/24/08 from http://www.dss.virginia.gov/files/division/dfs/cps/mandated_reporter_information/mandatedreporterbooklet3-07.pdf

Wolfner, G., & Gelles, R. (1993). A profile of violence toward children: A national study. *Child Abuse and Neglect, 17,* 197–212.

Wu, S., Ma, C.-X., Carter, R., Ariet, M., Feaver, E., Rosnick, M., et al. (2004). Risk factors for infant maltreatment: A population-based study. *Child Abuse and Neglect, 28*(12), 1253–1264.

Chapter 15

Legal Issues and Documentation

Suzanna Tiapula and Angelo P. Giardino

Child abuse leaves a footprint on the heart
Anna Salter (1995)

*If indeed this is true, then we, as professionals handling cases involving child maltreatment,
are left with the inescapable conclusion that our societal heart is truly bloodied and beaten.*

In 2006, 1,530 children died of maltreatment; every day approximately four children die of maltreatment in this country. Children less than 4 years old account for 78.0% of these fatalities. An estimated 3.6 million children were accepted by state and local child protective service agencies for investigation of child maltreatment (a rate of 48.3 per 1,000 children in the United States (US Department of Health and Human Services, 2005). Those who survive face a lifetime of potential emotional, physical, and sexual difficulties directly caused by the abuse including a three times greater likelihood of developing psychiatric disorders or abusing drugs and alcohol (Kendler, Heath, Neale, Kessler, & Eaves, 2000).

The investigation of suspected child abuse is a multidisciplinary effort; police officers, child protective services (CPS) workers, prosecutors, and health care professionals all have vital roles to play in the identification and protection of the abused child. There are tensions inherent in the multidisciplinary approach. Professionals must maintain their distinct roles and perform individual responsibilities while recognizing that their actions have a great impact on the efficacy of the investigative effort. Because physicians, nurses, hospital social workers, and paramedics are often the first professionals to have contact with the abused child and his or her family; health care providers become crucial participants in the gathering of information for the investigation and potential prosecution of the perpetrator. The safety of a child

The authors express their appreciation to Susan Perisls Marx, JD, for her contribution to this chapter in the first edition of this text.

445

A.P. Giardino et al. (eds.), *A Practical Guide to the Evaluation of Child Physical Abuse and Neglect*, DOI 10.1007/978-1-4419-0702-8_15, © Springer Science+Business Media, LLC 1997, 2010

often depends on the health care provider's awareness of the information needed by law enforcement officials and prosecutors to identify and prosecute the perpetrator successfully.

This chapter provides a discussion of the legal aspects of the medical professional's evaluation of suspected physical abuse and neglect. It addresses (a) mandatory reporting requirements for the health care professional, (b) medical record documentation in cases of suspected abuse and neglect, (c) guidelines for preparation and presentation of testimony, and (d) hearsay evidence. The practices suggested in the following pages should be discussed by medical professionals, members of hospital child abuse teams and county multidisciplinary investigative teams, and local prosecutors. Health care professionals are encouraged to adapt these suggested procedures to the law and custom in each specific locality.

Reporting Suspected Child Abuse

The reporting of child abuse and neglect is a central responsibility for all health care providers. By 1967, every state had enacted some form of legislation seeking the accurate reporting of injuries inflicted upon children (Myers et al., 2002). Many reporting laws do the following: (a) specify those professionals obligated to report suspicions of abuse, (b) include suspected neglect in reporting requirements, (c) prescribe procedures for investigation of abuse and neglect cases, (d) call for legal advocates or guardians ad litem for the child involved in abuse and neglect cases, and (e) address issues such as confidentiality of records and public and professional educational programs directed at increasing awareness of child abuse (Myers et al., 2002).

Medical professional communities vary in their responses to the enactment of mandatory reporting laws. Some smaller communities have no reporting guidelines, leaving health care professionals without guidance when faced with a case of suspected child abuse. Some health care professionals form multidisciplinary teams (see Chapter 13) staffed by nurses, doctors, clinical social workers, and others. Teams develop protocols for evaluating, reporting, and treating suspected child abuse victims. The clinical social worker on the team often serves as a liaison between hospital staff and local investigators and prosecutors. In some jurisdictions, health care professionals participate in community-based multidisciplinary teams (MDTs), which may include law enforcement officials, prosecutors, CPS workers, mental health professionals, school personnel, and other involved professionals. The local MDT may provide input for the medical professional in designing protocols for reporting procedures. Finally, some jurisdictions assemble a task force of health care professionals, prosecutors, law enforcement and CPS investigators, and other interested community members to draft protocols for reporting child abuse (Bross, Krugman, Lenherr, Rosenberg, & Schmitt, 1988; Investigation and Prosecution of Child Abuse, 2003).

State statutes dictate procedures that health care professionals must follow when they suspect child abuse or neglect. The American Medical Association strongly recommends that medical professionals become familiar with their state reporting laws (Council on Scientific Affairs, 1985; Warner & Hansen, 1994). Local protocols aid health care professionals in determining who must report abuse, when and to whom reports of suspected abuse and neglect should be made, which cases must be reported, and how reports are documented. Protocols should be clear, delineating step-by-step procedures for the medical professional to follow when evaluating and reporting a case of suspected abuse. Health professionals are encouraged to consult with local prosecutors or hospital attorneys to obtain copies of state reporting laws to comply with current reporting practices.

Mandated Reporting: Who Must Report Child Abuse?

Most state statutes delineate specific professionals who must report cases of suspected child abuse (Myers et al., 2002). These professionals and institutions are often referred to as "mandated reporters." Mandated reporters include hospitals, clinics, health care professionals, teachers, social workers, child care providers, mental health professionals, and law enforcement officials. Some state statutes also define "mandated reporters" to include a broader set of individuals or institutions, such as those called upon to render aid or medical assistance to children or having responsibility for the care and treatment of children. Currently, physicians and nurses are mandated reporters in every state (Mandatory Reports of Child Abuse and Neglect: Summary of State Laws, 2008). In all of these cases, the patient–client privilege is superseded by the duty to report (Myers et al., 2002).

Health care professionals who work in hospitals, multi-physician practices, or other organizations must check state law to determine who is responsible for reporting. Some states specifically allow professionals who work as a team and jointly have knowledge of abuse to designate one individual from their team to make the report (Mandatory Reports of Child Abuse and Neglect: Summary of State Laws, 2008). State statutes may relieve the individual who discovered the abuse from the obligation to report when he or she informs an appropriate superior. The supervisor then takes on the responsibilities of the mandated reporter (Myers & Peters, 1987). State law may compel both the health care professional who uncovered the abuse and his or her superior to report (Myers & Peters, 1987).

Who Is Reporting Child Abuse?

The community of medical and mental health providers has often taken the lead in the effort to increase awareness about child abuse. Dr. C. Henry Kempe led many in the field when he championed the cause of child protection and medical recognition of child abuse; his pioneering research published in 1962 to establish battered child syndrome as a medical diagnosis triggered a corresponding response by legislators and law enforcement/prosecutors. The battered child syndrome occurs when a child, typically young, suffers from serious physically abusive injuries to one or more body systems culminating in serious injury or death (Kempe, Silverman, Steele,

Droegemueller, & Silver, 1962). The history of our institutional responses to child abuse and child protection is rife with examples of the leadership demonstrated by medical providers.

On the issue of gun violence and child health, for example, the public health and the medical community has articulated a link between guns maintained in the home and child injuries. Each year incidents involving unintended firearm discharges kill as many as 400 children and injure almost 3,000 children (Centers for Disease Control and Prevention, 1995; Beaman, Annest, Kresnow, & Pollock, 2000; American Medical Association, 1998). At least one study suggests that the incidence of unintended gun death among children may be six times higher than current data sources suggest (Schaechter, Duran, De Marchena, Lemard, & Villar, 2003). If homicides and suicides are included, more than 20,000 children and youths under 20 are killed or injured by guns. Many leading researchers in the public health community have challenged the legal and political leadership to address these concerns with appropriate legislation (Schaechter et al., 2003).

In another more recent example of leadership by the medical community, Barbara Knox, MD, Medical Director, University of Wisconsin, Child Protection Program, and Suzanne Starling, MD, Medical Director, Child Abuse Program, Children's Hospital of The King's Daughters/Eastern Virginia Medical School are involved in research to identify appropriate medical diagnostic criteria for child torture as a form of child abuse. In their work with children, they have a identified specific elements that suggests that a diagnosis of torture should be made. This is one of many examples where the legal community, which currently charges child torture in only 17 states, has not yet recognized significant child abuse issues identified and defined by the medical community.

The Child Maltreatment 2006 Report stated that more than one-half (56.3%) of professionals (see Figure 15.1), who encountered the alleged victim as part of their occupation, reported child abuse to Children Protective Services (CPS) and 43.7% of nonprofessionals including parents relatives, friends, neighbors, alleged victims, alleged perpetrators, anonymous callers, and "other" sources reported the abuse.

Who Is Not Reporting Child Abuse?

Despite the laws mandating that professionals report suspected abuse, only a fraction of the abuse suspected may actually be reported. Research in 1990 suggested significant underreporting by professionals mandated to report; 40% of maltreatment cases and 35% of the most serious cases known to professionals mandated to report were being reported (Finkelhor, 1990). Ten years later, a study found that only 53% of physicians and 58% of physician's assistants were reporting all cases of suspected child abuse (Delaronde, King, Bendel, & Reece, 2000). The reasons posed by mandated reporters range from being uncertain that abuse has actually occurred to the need to maintain a relationship with patients/clients (Delaronde et al., 2000). Although the laws are for the most part

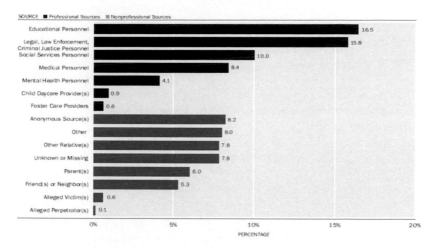

Figure 15.1 Report Sources, 2006. (US Department of Health & Human Services, 2008).

clear, there are a few statutes with some level of ambiguity regarding which injuries are actually reportable. Ambiguity in some mandated reporting statutes may also contribute to underreporting.

Who Receives the Child Abuse Report?

State statutes and local protocols dictate to whom a health care professional reports when he or she suspects that a child has been abused or neglected. Generally, health care professionals are required to call a CPS agency, which investigates allegations of caregiver abuse, or a police department, which investigates all criminal allegations of child abuse. Some jurisdictions require health care providers to determine initially if the suspected perpetrator is a caregiver of the child. If the suspected perpetrator is a caregiver, health care professionals must contact the local CPS agency. In all other cases, law enforcement officials are notified. Some jurisdictions require that the medical professional contact both CPS and law enforcement agencies, regardless of the relationship of the suspected perpetrator to the child. Again, the clinical social worker of a hospital's multidisciplinary team, a team member of the community's multidisciplinary investigative team, or the local prosecutor may be most aware of step-by-step protocols and legal requirements and can provide assistance.

Medical professionals may use local or state telephone hot-lines to make the initial phone report required by most states. It is important to carefully document the telephone call in the medical record, including the name of the agency, individual employee contacted, and the date and time of the report. A follow-up written report of the case is usually required. Hospital emergency departments or local CPS agencies often have a designated form for the reporter to complete.

Time Frame for Reporting Child Abuse: How Quickly Must a Report of Child Abuse Be Made?

State statutes typically require that a telephone report be made *immediately* upon suspicion of abuse (Mandatory Reports of Child Abuse and Neglect: Summary of State Laws, 2008). How quickly a health care provider forms a "suspicion" that a child has been physically abused or neglected varies, depending upon the information available in any given case. After the telephone contact, state law usually specifies a time frame in which written documentation is to be submitted (Making and Screening Report of Child Abuse and Neglect: Summary of State Laws, 2008).

Cases of "Suspected" Child Abuse: When Is a Case "Suspected" Child Abuse?

State law defines such terms as *abuse, neglect, abused child,* and *neglected child.* In general, states mandate reporting when a child's physical or mental health or welfare is harmed, or threatened with harm, by the acts or omissions of a parent or any other person. *Harm,* or an equivalent term in the statute, is often broken into specific subject areas, including, but not limited to, nonaccidental physical injury; mental injury; sexual abuse and exploitation; abandonment; failure to supervise or to supply the child with basic food, clothing, shelter, or health care; and psychosocial (environmental) failure to thrive (Making and Screening Report of Child Abuse and Neglect: Summary of State Laws, 2008). Some states mandate a report when a newborn is physically dependent upon certain drugs or when the mother used a controlled substance during her pregnancy although the ultimate impact on this approach remains in question (Ondersma, Simpson, Brestan, & Ward, 2000). Health care professionals must report suspected nonaccidental physical injury or neglect, even if it purportedly resulted from the caregiver's religious practices (Warner & Hansen, 1994).

Health care providers must report any suspected child abuse. A physician need not diagnose definitively that a condition is the result of abuse in order to trigger the duty to report (Warner & Hansen, 1994). Although the physician participates in the case, it is not his or her responsibility to prove that the case is one of abuse or who the abuser is. The juvenile or criminal court makes these determinations.

When does a medical professional's concern about possible child abuse become a suspicion, triggering the duty to report? In essence, the health care provider must make a report when the provider has evidence that would lead a competent professional to believe abuse or neglect is reasonably likely to have occurred (Myers et al., 2002; Warner & Hansen, 1994). CPS screens the reports to assess which are appropriate for agency intervention. A thorough investigation is conducted by CPS and law enforcement officials to determine if abuse has indeed occurred. CPS investigators then determine if the child's safety is in question and take appropriate steps to protect the child and provide supportive services to the child and the child's family. Law enforcement investigators will determine if a crime occurred and if there is

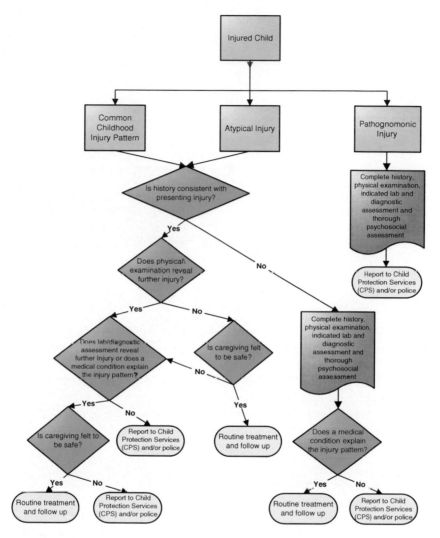

Figure 15.2 Injured Child
Note: Beginning with the injured child, the evaluation progresses differently depending on what is uncovered during the different phases of clinical evaluation.

probable cause to make an arrest. Figure 15.2 provides the health care provider with guidelines for reporting physical abuse when evaluating an injured child.

Liability of the Reporting Health Care Professionals: Will the Reporting Medical Care Professional Be Immune from Liability?

Health care professionals voice concern about professional and personal liability if CPS investigators determine the report to be "unsubstantiated" or "not indicated," or if law enforcement officials do not arrest a perpetrator. (See Chapter 1 for further discussion of substantiation.) Should an angry parent file a lawsuit against the reporter, state statutes provide immunity from civil and criminal liability to all mandated reporters who report suspected abuse in "good faith." This is true even if the report is investigated and determined to be unsubstantiated. Good faith does not include instances when a false report is knowingly made (i.e., the health care provider making the report knew that the report was false) (Myers et al., 2002; Immunity for Reporters of Child Abuse and Neglect: Summary of State Laws, 2008).

Penalties for Failure to Report: Is There a Penalty for Failure to Report a Suspected Case of Child Abuse or Neglect?

It is a criminal violation in most states for a health care professional to fail to report suspected child abuse. Penalties include fines and prison sentences. Some statutes also provide that mandated reporters may be held liable for civil damages caused by a failure to report (Myers et al., 2002; Penalties for Failure to Report and False Reporting of Child Abuse and Neglect: Summary of State Laws, 2007).

Summary

Health care providers fulfill a crucial child advocacy function as central participants in the identification, protection, and treatment of abused and neglected children. Medical communities should be in full compliance with statutes that mandate reporting of suspected child abuse and neglect. It is important that health care providers be familiar with local protocols and community resources, including institutional or local multidisciplinary teams. Should the community lack guidelines and resources, health care professionals can take a lead role in developing protocols and beginning the process of multidisciplinary coordination.

Documentation of Findings

The best interests of abused and neglected children are served when health care professionals provide clear and comprehensive documentation. Entries made in medical records can provide essential clues needed to evaluate the safety of the child's environment. Accurate records that clearly reflect the child's medical history, physical examination, and laboratory findings are often pivotal in the investigation and prosecution of physical abuse and neglect cases. Should the health care professional be called upon to testify, nothing refreshes the provider's memory better than clear, legible, and comprehensive documentation in the medical record. Finally, medical records may be admitted into evidence at trial.

Documentation Guidelines

Statements made by the child, family members, and other caregivers and given to medical professionals before the caregivers have information about the child's actual health care condition may be inconsistent with the degree or type of injury. In addition, the abusing caregiver may give contradictory statements to health care personnel during the initial evaluation and hospitalization, if admission occurs. These statements, coupled with evidence that the child was in the "sole care" or "exclusive custody" of the perpetrator at the time of the injuries, often provide the fulcrum of the prosecution's case. The following sections outline suggested guidelines for documentation of statements and other information relevant to the investigation and prosecution of child neglect and physical abuse.

Documentation of Care: Who Should Document?

All health care professionals, including paramedics or emergency medical technicians, triage nurses, emergency room personnel, attending and consulting medical staff, in-patient care nurses, and social work staff, should document statements and actions of the child, the child's family, and other caregivers during the evaluation of children. Documentation begins as soon as the child arrives at the site of care or the paramedic arrives at the scene. Documentation continues throughout the evaluation, workup, and treatment of the child's injuries. The hospital's multidisciplinary team uses the documentary trail to analyze information, synthesize an impression, and develop an assessment and treatment plan for the particular case. Comprehensive, ongoing documentation allows investigators and prosecutors to evaluate the overall picture that emerges during the child's contact with medical professionals and aids in the identification and prosecution of a perpetrator (Table 15.1 "Verbal evidence checklist") (Myers et al., 2002).

General Documentation Guidelines

The medical record should reflect the statements and interactions of the child and family. The following are entries that should be included in the record:

1. Name of person making the statement or exhibiting the behavior and his or her relationship to the child
2. Date and time of the statement/behavior
3. Questions or actions of the health care professional that immediately preceded the statement/behavior
4. Exact words of the statement, using quotation marks where appropriate, and/or a detailed description of the behavior exhibited
5. Demeanor of the person making the statement or exhibiting the behavior
6. Names of those present at the time the statement was made or behavior was observed
7. Name and beeper number or extension of the person making the entry into the hospital chart

Health care providers should avoid documenting personal opinions regarding caregivers even though working with suspected abusive caregivers may elicit a wide range of negative emotional responses. Comments in the record such as "this mother

Table 15.1 Verbal evidence checklist.

Child's Name:	Date:	Your Name:	Case No

— Document your questions. Don't paraphrase.
— Document child's *exact* words. Don't paraphrase.
— Did child tell anyone else? Who? When? Why? What?

All Professionals Document:
— *What happened? According to the child, what happened?*
— *Elapsed time:* How much time elapsed between the event and the child's description? (Be precise; minutes count)
— *Emotional condition:* Child's emotional condition when child described what happened. (Crying? Upset? Calm? Excited? Traumatized?)
— *Physical condition*: Was the child's description spontaneous?
— *Spontaneous?* Was the child's description spontaneous?
— *Consistency:* If child described the even more than once, are there consistencies across descriptions?
— *Developmentally unusual sexual knowledge or conduct:* Document any developmentally unusual sexual knowledge or behavior, including idiosyncratic details (e.g., smells or tastes).
— *Motive to lie:* Does anyone—child or adult—have a motive to lie?
— *Reliability:* Document **anything** that sheds light on the reliability of the child's statement.

Ask Questions About and Document:
— Child's memory for simple events (e.g., Breakfast this morning? What was on TV today?)
— Child's ability to communicate.
— Child's understanding of the difference between the truth and lies. *Don't* ask children under age 9 to define "truth" and "lie." *Don't* ask kids to give examples of truth or lies. *Don't* ask kids to explain the difference between a truth and a lie. *Do* give simple examples of something that is true and something that is a lie. Then ask the child to identify which it is. (e.g., Hold up a blue pen and say "If someone said this is red, would that be the truth or a lie?" Or, "If someone said this is blue, would that be the truth or a lie?")
— Child's understanding of the importance of telling the truth to you.

Clinical Professionals Providing Medical or Psychological Diagnosis or Treatment
— Inform child of your clinical purpose. (e.g., "I'm going to give you a checkup to make sure you are healthy." "My job is talking to kids to help them with their problems.")
— Inform child of the clinical reasons why it is important for the child to tell the truth to you. (e.g., "I need you to tell me only true thing, only things that really happened. I need you to tell me only true things so I can help you.")
— Document anything indicating the child understood your clinical role, the clinical nature of what you did or said, and why it was clinically important for the child to tell the truth to you.
— Document why what the child told you was pertinent to your ability to diagnose or treat the child.
— If child identified the perpetrator, document whay knowing identity was pertinent to your ability to diagnose or treat the child.

Source: Copyright © by John E. B. Myers used with permission (Myers et al., 2002, p. 325).

is a flake" or "dad doesn't have a clue" signify a loss of objectivity and will certainly undermine the credibility of the health care professional, both in the hospital and in the courtroom. The health care professional should document only what was said or observed.

Members of the hospital or community multidisciplinary team may be helpful in determining the format of the written documentation. Some professionals prefer a question and answer format; others may choose to use a summary format. Either method is effective if accurate and complete (Heger, 1991). It is important that all entries are legible.

Finally, preservation of all records is essential. Destruction or loss of documents may call into question the accuracy and impartiality of the health care provider's findings and subsequent testimony.

Interviewing the Child and Documentation Guidelines

Who Should Conduct the In-Depth Interview of the Child?

In the medical evaluation of possible child maltreatment, health care providers initially determine whether the child's age and/or medical condition will delay or bar an interview. Once a determination is made that a child can be interviewed, the health care professional most familiar with child development and most skilled in interviewing children conducts the in-depth interview of the child. In an emergency situation, however, the examining health care provider will often interview the child.

The In-Depth Interview: What Should the Health Care Professional Ask the Child in the In-Depth Interview?

The health care professional's interview of the child is often crucial to any subsequent CPS and criminal investigations. An in-depth interview of the child, rather than a cursory history-taking, is essential in cases of suspected abuse. Improper questioning when a child is first interviewed may taint the rest of the investigation. Health care providers should receive training regarding proper interviewing techniques to enhance the quality of child interviews and the information elicited. Guidelines for approaching this important interview are provided in Chapters 2 and 14.

If the child is verbal and medically stable, it is appropriate for the health care provider to discuss the physical injury with him or her. The following discussion directs the health care professional to subject areas that will provide information needed to distinguish between abusive and accidental injuries, aid investigators and prosecutors in successful identification and prosecution of the perpetrator, and allow all concerned professionals to accurately assess the safety of the child's environment (Investigation and Prosecution of Child Abuse, 2003; Warner & Hansen, 1994). The "interview" continues during the entire evaluation. It begins by asking the child for a narrative about the incident. Direct questions are used to fill in gaps or clear up confusing statements. Questions should cover the following topics:

1. *Circumstances surrounding the most recent injury.* Ask the child how he or she got hurt, who did it, and any "reasons" the child perceived for the assault (i.e., the child dropped his or her peanut butter sandwich; parent was drunk again). Reassure the child that the injuries were not his or her fault.
2. *Instrument used.* Ask the child whether an instrument was used to hurt the child (e.g., shoe, cigarette, lighter, coat hanger, curling iron). If an instrument was used, ask the child to describe it. Have the child draw it if he or she is unable to describe or name the instrument. Date the picture, indicate who drew it, and include the drawing in the medical record.
3. *Current and prior injuries.* Ask the child about current and prior injuries found on examination. Establish who caused the injuries and how. Record each visible injury on a drawing, labeling each, and describing in detail the size, color, and pattern of the injury. Make sure the child's name or chart number appears on each page of the medical record, including the page with the drawing.

Use of Photographs

All visible lesions should be photographed (Ricci & Smistek, 2000).

Photograph all injuries if possible.

Photograph the injury with an anatomic landmark. The inclusion of an elbow, knee, belly button, or other body part identifies the location of the wound.

When photographing, include a card with the child's name or chart number to identify the child.

When photographing, include an American Board of Forensic Odontology (ABFO) 90-degree scale and color balance chart to allow judges and jurors to evaluate the size and color of the injury (see Photo 15.1). If ABFO 90-degree scale is not available, use a centimeter ruler. The ruler should be photographed both parallel and perpendicular to the mark in question.

Photograph the child's injuries periodically throughout the child's hospital stay to show the healing process and to negate a claim that hospital treatment caused the injury.

Use a digital camera or 35 mm camera, take two pictures of every view and angle; one for file and one for court.

Make sure to accompany all photographs, negatives and digital files with meticulous descriptive text and hand-drawn diagrams, because the quality of photographs cannot be guaranteed.

Make sure photographs and negatives are carefully stored and preserved. Loss of medical photographs could hinder an effective prosecution. See Chapter 2 for further discussion.

4. *Perpetrator's statements to child.* Ask the child if the suspected perpetrator said anything to him or her before, during, or after the assault. Statements such as "I'm going to kill you," made by the perpetrator during a violent assault, reported

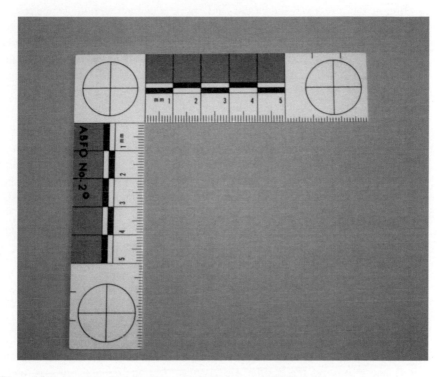

Photo 15.1 American Board of Forensic Odontology (ABFO) ruler

by the child during the evaluation, and documented by the health care provider, may enable the prosecutor to prove that the assault was not accidental.

5. *Report of assault or delay in seeking care.* Determine how the child ended up at the hospital. Did a caregiver bring the child in? Did a teacher notice bruising and report to a CPS worker, who brought the child in for an examination? Failure by the offender to get prompt treatment for an ill child is admissible at trial to show the perpetrator's guilty knowledge and attempt to conceal the injuries.

6. *Injuries to other children.* Find out if the child knows whether any other children in the household were injured. Make sure that a CPS worker or police officer arranges for those children to have a medical evaluation. Document all of the children's statements and injuries. Injuries to other children may be admissible at trial to prove that the perpetrator intended to harm the children and that the injuries were not accidental.

7. *Child's relationship with caregiver(s).* Ask the child about his or her relationships at home. Who is home when he or she gets home from school? What does he or she do after school? With whom does he or she do things? Document the child's appearance: height and weight, developmental level, the condition of his or her clothing, his or her overall cleanliness, whether he or she is hungry, and so on. Carefully note the child's behavior with the caregiver(s) in the hospital

throughout the stay. Does the child avoid physical contact with the caregiver(s)? Does the child look to the caregiver(s) for support? Does the child ask if the caregiver(s) will be coming to visit at the hospital? Include descriptions of the child's demeanor as he or she talks about the caregiver(s). Recognize, however, that there is no "textbook" response or demeanor that an abused child should have toward a perpetrator. Do not make conclusions as to the child's state of mind in the medical record (Investigation and Prosecution of Child Abuse, 2003).

The medical professional documents the following: (a) the child's exact statement about the abuse, even if it is "nothing happened"; and (b) the actions and demeanor of the child (i.e., the child "cried throughout the questioning," "remained silent and stared at the examining table," etc.). The phrase "child denies abuse" should be avoided because it overstates the child's response and may not accurately reflect the medical facts uncovered during the evaluation (Heger, 1991). When appropriate, the medical professional notes that the child's assertion that "nothing happened" is inconsistent with the physical findings.

Interviewing the Caregivers and Documentation Guidelines

What Should the Health Care Provider Ask the Child's Caregiver(s)?

During any medical evaluation, health care providers discuss the child's condition with the child and the child's caregiver(s). Although initial, cursory questions may be asked with all parties present at the triage booth or by a receptionist at a doctor's office, the child and each caregiver should be interviewed separately as soon as a potential abuse situation surfaces. Privacy may encourage each individual to speak openly. Document the following in the medical record: (a) caregiver's answers to questions posed by the health care professional, (b) refusals to answer questions, (c) equivocal responses, and (d) silences when asked questions.

In addition to the formal interview that occurs during the history-taking phase of all medical evaluations, the health care provider should take note of more casual statements made in the emergency room, at the child's bedside, in the hallway, and throughout the child's evaluation and treatment. Documentation of all interactions paints a picture for health care professionals, investigators, and prosecutors that may, in turn, lead to the identification of the perpetrator and safe placement for the child.

Chapters 2 and 14 include detailed descriptions of the interview process. The discussion that follows highlights subject areas that should be included in the caregiver interview:

1. *Time of injury.* The health care provider asks the caregiver when the injury occurred. If the caregiver has difficulty remembering dates or times, some health care professionals encourage the caregiver to draw a timeline in an attempt to fix the time of injury. Have the caregiver sign and date the timeline. Should the caregiver refuse to sign the timeline or should the health care provider feel

uncomfortable requesting a signature, the health care provider may sign the time-line. In this situation, indicate the date, time, and name of the person who drew the timeline. Keep any timelines or drawings in the medical record.

2. *Course of symptoms.* Ask the caregiver to describe the course of the child's symptoms, particularly if the caregiver claims no knowledge of the exact time of the injury. Health care professionals, investigators, and prosecutors can use the detailed description of the course of symptoms to approximate the time of injury or to determine if the caregiver's explanation of the injury makes sense. If needed, have the caregiver draw a timeline.

3. *Exclusive custody.* Ask the caregiver when the injury occurred without revealing the health care professional's estimation of the time of injury. Did the caregiver leave the child with anyone? When? Was the caregiver always watching the child? Was anyone else at home? Any siblings in the home? Ages? Were the siblings left alone with the child? What are the developmental capabilities of the siblings? Identification of the perpetrator becomes much easier should the caregiver admit to having exclusive custody of the child at the time that the injury happened.

4. *Explanations, lack of explanations, and changing explanations.* At the initial interview, ask the caregiver how the injury occurred. Encourage the caregiver to tell all that he or she knows. Record all of the answers in detail. Ask the care-giver to demonstrate explanations using props, and document the demonstration in detail. If, for example, the caregiver admits to shaking the child, have the care-giver use a purse or other object to illustrate the amount of force used in the shaking episode.

The health care professional may not wish to present all that is known about the mechanism of the injury at the beginning of the interview. Later, the inter-viewer may reveal some information should the explanation prove highly implau-sible. Record what information was given and the caregiver's response. For example,

Q: "Tell me what you know about how the child was injured."
A: "Well, I was home alone with the baby. The baby was upstairs in his crib. I was downstairs watching TV. I heard a thud. I ran to the stairway, and the baby was lying at the bottom of the stairs, crying. I guess he fell down the steps."
Q: "Had anything happened to the baby before that?"
A: "No."
Q: "Had you noticed any injuries or odd symptoms before that?"
A: "No."
Q: "This baby has an injury to his abdomen." (Doctor points to the caregiver's abdomen.) "Do you know how he got that?"
A: "Oh yes. I forgot to tell you that he must have hit himself on the table at the bottom of the steps when he landed."
Q: "Can you describe where the table was?"

A: "Well, it's usually off to the side, away from the steps, but I had just moved it in front of the steps to polish it."

The health care professional, as part of a multidisciplinary team or with the investigator and prosecutor, will analyze caregivers' statements in conjunction with the medical findings, photographs of the scene, and other evidence. A caregiver's implausible explanation as to the mechanism of the injury may provide valuable clues as to the identity of the perpetrator.

5. *Self-inflicted injury.* Should the caregiver claim that the child accidentally injured him- or herself, get some details about the developmental capabilities of the child. Also, explore the plausibility of such an injury, given the specifics of the explanation. For example, the caregiver may assert that the child climbed into the bathtub and turned on the hot water spigot. Follow-up questions might include: Where is the bathtub located? Can you show me how tall the bathtub is? What was the water level in the bathtub? Is the child able to walk? How long has the child been walking? When you came into the room, where was the child? Still in the tub? In what position? What was the child doing?

6. *Initial response.* Determine what the caregiver did when he or she noticed injuries or symptoms. Was there a delay in seeking medical care? Did the caregiver attempt home remedies rather than take the child to the hospital? Did the caregiver keep the child home from school for a few days?

7. *Past injuries and illnesses.* A comprehensive history of prior medical problems and treatment is crucial not only to the medical diagnosis but also to the investigation and prosecution of a child abuse case. For example, if the child had actually been examined by a pediatrician 2 days prior to the emergency room visit and was found free from visible injury, the timing of the presenting injury becomes much easier to determine. The identity and intent of the perpetrator may become clearer should the child's medical history reveal neglect by the caregiver, such as failure to obtain immunizations or to bring the child in for well-child care visits. Should a caregiver claim at the emergency room that the child is "accident prone," prior medical records may show old injuries that, in fact, were inconsistent with accidental injury and most likely inflicted. When a caregiver claims that the child falls frequently because of a lifelong problem with recurrent dizziness, the absence of prior complaints regarding that problem is highly significant.

Has the caregiver describe the nature of any prior physical problems? What caused any prior injuries? Where was the child treated? Who treated the child? Any previous hospitalizations? Document the names, addresses, and phone numbers of all prior persons who treated the child, including any medical professionals who provided well-child care. A perpetrator may bring the child to a different doctor each time the child suffers an inflicted injury to avoid suspicion, knowledge, and documenting of repeated injuries by health care providers.

8. *Child's relationship with caregiver.* Have the caregiver describe his or her relationship with the child. Did the child have any disabilities? Special needs? Toilet training difficulties? Was the child on medication for hyperactivity or other condition? Did the caregiver only recently begin caring for the child? With an older child, were there recurrent disciplinary problems? Questions like these will uncover possible "triggers" for an abusive incident.

9. *Caregiver's concerns and demeanor.* Document in the medical chart the concerns voiced by the caregiver. Does the caregiver want to know how long the child will be in the hospital or if the child is in any real danger? Is the caregiver preoccupied with whether the doctor will contact CPS? Does the caregiver show any emotion when discussing the child's condition? Note the demeanor of the caregivers toward each other and toward the child throughout the hospital stay or course of treatment. Does one caregiver forbid another from talking to the medical staff? Does either caregiver visit the child in the hospital or comfort the child? Again, these clues, along with all of the evidence gathered from a myriad of sources during the investigation, add to the investigative picture (Investigation and Prosecution of Child Abuse, 2003; Myers & Carter, 1988).

Documentation of Medical Conclusions

In physical abuse and neglect cases, the circumstances and motivation of the abuser are often significant factors in culpability; these are often difficult to discern (Investigation and Prosecution of Child Abuse, 2003). The exponential increase in medical diagnostic capability has had an effect on the criminal justice response with more cases being charged as our understanding of causation improves. Death review teams have been established in many communities to examine child fatalities with protection of surviving siblings and identifying institutional responses that might have been triggered to save the child before the homicide actually occurred.

Serious child physical abuse and homicide tends to fall into two basic categories: battered child syndrome, with a child presenting with multiple types of injuries in various stages of healing; and, either massive head or abdominal injury resulting from a single explosive incident. As investigators and prosecutors hone their understanding of the medical issues associated with abusive head trauma, these cases are increasingly being litigated in state and local courts throughout the nation.

Medical providers have taken the lead here too with respect to prevention efforts. In one particularly innovative approach, military medical hospitals do not permit parents to take newborn infants home from the hospital until parents have watched an educational video on the injuries associated with rotational forces/abusive head trauma. Given the percentage of babies born in hospitals, this effort represents a comprehensive attempt at grass roots prevention.

Health care professionals routinely record information that they elicit during the history-taking, physical examination, and laboratory assessment stages of clinical evaluation. After the completion of the clinical evaluation, the health care provider formulates a probable diagnosis. In cases of physical abuse, a completely "normal examination" is unlikely because the child's injury is typically what brings the child to the health care provider's attention. When injuries are pathognomonic of abuse, it is certainly appropriate to diagnose child abuse or battered child syndrome. In some cases of suspected physical abuse or neglect, however, the medical evaluation may not yield enough information to diagnose abuse definitively, although the clinician suspects that abuse occurred. In such cases, the most appropriate way to frame the conclusion section of the medical record is to summarize the clinical information from the history, physical examination, and laboratory assessment and state whether the injury is consistent with the history provided. In this way, the conclusion or impression documented at the end of a medical evaluation for physical injury is either injury consistent with history provided, or injury inconsistent with history provided.

Health care professionals may voice concern that CPS workers, law enforcement officers, and prosecutors want more definitive conclusions in the medical records than health care professionals are able to give. Assessment findings that state that there is "no evidence of abuse" or that "evidence confirms abuse" do not allow for the possibility that the CPS worker or police detective may uncover additional information that clearly supports the opposite conclusion.

In cases of suspected neglect with no physical findings on examination, describe the physical examination of each system. Detailed description of a lack of affirmative findings for each system examined can then be compared to prior and subsequent examinations of the child. Avoid use of global statements such as "no evidence of neglect." Investigators and prosecutors may uncover signs of neglect at the home or other locations of which the health care professional was unaware at the time of diagnosis.

Documentation of referrals to CPS and counseling is helpful to those reviewing the chart at a later date. Include the names of the health care professional who made the referral and the CPS intake worker or counselor who accepted the referral (see Tables 15.2 and 15.3).

Health Care Providers in the Courtroom

Health care professionals who treat children, particularly physicians, may be subpoenaed to testify in child abuse cases. In a criminal case, a subpoena directs the health care professional to come to court and provide information to aid a jury or judge in determining the guilt or innocence of a defendant. In a non-criminal case, a subpoena directs the health care professional to come to court and provide information that will aid in a variety of determinations (i.e., whether a child should be removed from the home, offered court-ordered services, or awarded monetary damages for abuse suffered). Subpoenas sometimes order the production of records (subpoena *duces tecum*). Generally, a subpoena *duces tecum* directs that medical records be delivered to the court under seal for review or to the party issuing the subpoena. Upon receipt of a subpoena in a criminal case, the health care provider

Table 15.2 Information documented in the chart.

Who brought child to hospital

Who lives with child

Statements by caregivers and child upon initial contact and throughout hospital
stay (demeanor/actions/statements)

Consent to treat form signed by caregivers (or refusal to sign)

Condition of child when admitted ("critical"; "intensive care")

Caregiver response to medical information/requests for admission or additional
tests

Complete medical examination findings and lab/X-ray results

Description of findings on review of systems

Impression and treatment

Action taken (report to CPS, referral to counseling, etc.)

Caregiver visitation restrictions and compliance

Delivery of child's specimens, clothes, and so on to law enforcement officials

Doctor's name, position, and office and beeper numbers (clearly written)

Table 15.3 Information not included in the chart.

Personal opinions about child, caregivers, and others

Phrases such as "no evidence of abuse" or "no evidence of neglect"

should clarify his or her obligations under that subpoena with the local prosecutor
or hospital counsel.

In a criminal child abuse case, health care professionals may be subpoenaed by
the prosecutor, the defense attorney, or the court. Generally, however, the examining
and treating health care providers are subpoenaed by the prosecutor. The following
discussion will assume that the health care provider has been subpoenaed by the
prosecutor to testify in support of the prosecution's case.

The health care provider should establish protocols with the local prosecutor
to facilitate the process of preparing for and appearing in court. For example, the
name and phone number of the prosecutor handling the case and the name of the
child/patient should be included prominently on each subpoena.

When potentially privileged documents (i.e., psychiatric or psychological
records) are included in the medical record, the medical facility and the prosecutor should develop procedures to ensure judicial scrutiny of the material before the
records are released to the attorneys. The judge will balance the privacy rights of
the child with any legal requirements for disclosure of records. Criminal cases are
often postponed for reasons beyond the control of the prosecutor. Illness of a witness, unavailability of the judge or defense attorney, or failure of the defendant to
appear for trial are some situations that may result in an unscheduled delay in the
trial. Medical professionals often express understandable frustration with repeated
postponements and multiple subpoenas. In some jurisdictions, the prosecutor keeps

the health care provider "on call" during the trial; the medical professional remains at the hospital or clinic until the prosecutor notifies him or her to appear. It is the prosecutor's responsibility to apprise the health care provider as soon as possible that the case has been postponed.

Prior to testifying in court, the health care provider and the prosecutor should schedule a preparatory session. Defense attorneys may also wish to interview or depose the health care professional prior to trial. The health care provider may discuss with the prosecutor the rules that are followed in such a deposition and determine whether the prosecutor will accompany the health care provider to the interview or deposition scheduled by the defense attorney. Interviews or depositions should be held in a neutral, comfortable setting. Preparation prior to any interview, deposition, or trial appearance is essential, and health care providers should know the medical record thoroughly (see Appendix).

The Medical Professional on the Stand: Fact or Expert Witness?

A medical professional may be asked to testify as a "fact" witness, an "expert" witness, or both. A fact witness testifies as to what was observed; an expert witness, because of specialized training, experience, and knowledge, may testify not only to observations but to opinions based on those observations (Cleary, 1983; Myers et al., 2002). The prosecutor and the health care professional discuss the health care professional's level and areas of expertise to determine whether he or she will be called as a fact or expert witness. For example, a pediatric intern, although highly educated and well trained, may not feel him- or herself to be an "expert" in a particular area. On the other hand, many medical professionals underestimate their qualifications and can be readily qualified as experts in court.

Fact Witness

If the prosecutor determines that the health care professional will testify as a fact witness, there is the possibility that a medical expert will augment the testimony of the fact witness. Another physician may testify, for example, regarding causation and the timing of the child's injuries. Whether or not an expert witness will be called, the fact witness should review records during the preparatory session with the prosecutor, explain medical terminology, and review the subject areas for direct testimony. Testimony of the fact witness may include the following:

- Education and experience of witness
- Observations during contact with child (Refer to General Documentation Guidelines section in this chapter.)

  - Who brought child to the hospital or office
  - Child's demeanor, dress, level of cleanliness, and so on child's and caregivers' statements

- Medical findings e.g. bruising, tenderness, X-ray appearance
- Actions taken (reported to CPS hotline, ordered more X-rays)

Expert Witness

A medical expert is often a vital witness in a prosecutor's case because there may be no eyewitnesses to a physical assault, many victims are too young to testify, and most judges and jurors lack knowledge regarding the medical aspects of child abuse (Myers et al., 2002). The expert witness and the prosecutor must have an in-depth preparatory session. The prosecutor should review an updated resume or curriculum vitae of the expert witness. The preparatory session includes subject areas to be covered, limitations in the witness's expertise, and identification of any areas that need to be supplemented with the testimony of an additional expert. The expert witness and the prosecutor together review all of the medical documents that will be used at trial and determine if there are missing medical documents that are vital to the case, such as prior well-child care records, prenatal health care records of the child's mother, X-ray and MRI results, and so on. The medical expert should review all police reports that give accounts of how, when, and where the injuries occurred and prior testimony given by experts in the case (preliminary hearing, grand jury, dependency, or other pretrial hearings). The more information the expert can review, the better grasp he or she will have of the overall picture. Review studies that both support and refute the opinion of the expert. Also discuss diagrams, charts, or models that will be necessary for the trial. Table 15.4 includes subject areas of expert testimony. See Appendix for pointers for expert witnesses.

Testimony in the Courtroom

During testimony in a criminal proceeding, the prosecutor, defense attorney, and judge may ask questions of the witness. In a civil dependency or family court proceeding, the judge and the attorneys for each of the parties, including the attorneys for the parents, the CPS agency, and the child, may ask questions of the witness. "Direct examination" consists of questions put to the witness by the attorney who has subpoenaed him or her to court. "Cross-examination" is questioning by the opposing attorney. Again, the following discussion assumes that the prosecutor subpoenaed the health care provider to court.

Direct Examination

Direct examination should hold no surprises if the witness is adequately prepared. Presumably, after the preparatory session with the prosecutor, the health care provider will know what will be asked of him or her. Consider the following tips:

- While on the witness stand, use medical records to refresh recollection as needed. However, do not rely on the records, be thoroughly familiar with their contents.

Table 15.4 Possible subject areas for expert testimony.

Education and experience (to qualify the witness as an expert)
Condition of child prior to injury
Lack of preexisting illness or condition to account for injury
Clinical course of injury
Timing of injuries
Implausibility of defendant's explanations for the injuries
Nature of paramedic, emergency room, and in-patient care
Implausibility of self-infliction of injury
Implausibility of injury by young sibling
Mechanism of injury
Force necessary to cause injury
Degree of injury
Degree of pain
Medical significance of omissions or misrepresentations made by caregiver
Prior injuries to child
Injuries to other children
Significance of delay in seeking treatment
New explanations for the child's injuries offered by the defense at trial

Source: Investigation and Prosecution of Child Abuse (1993); Myers and Carter (1988).

- If reference to the records is necessary during testimony, fasten notes ("stick-ees") or paper clips to salient pages before you come to court. Fumbling through the medical record while on the stand will create an unfavorable impression and undermine even the most powerful testimony. Prior to trial, consult the prosecutor regarding any obligation to provide the defense attorney with any additional notes made by you during preparation for testimony or any other materials brought to the courtroom.
- Listen carefully to the question. Answer honestly, succinctly, and without equivocation. Avoid "yes" or "no" answers if greater explanation is needed. If there is an objection by either the prosecutor or the defense attorney, do not answer until the judge has indicated that you may do so.
- Use diagrams, tables, and charts to clarify technical points to the jury. Enlargements of photographs and critical pages of the medical record, timelines, medical illustrations with overlays, dolls, and mannequins can be useful.
- If possible, get off the witness stand during direct testimony and draw on a chalkboard or flip chart to better explain concepts. Prior to trial, make arrangements with the prosecutor for the necessary equipment.
- Explain all medical terms, using analogies and examples to clarify medical concepts. Avoid condescending language directed at the jurors or the judge.
- Prosecutors should ask questions on direct examination that elicit any problem areas in the testimony. For example, if there are limits on how exactly the expert witness can date the injuries, explain that limitation on direct examination.

- Acknowledge if there are several possible causes for the injury. Explain to the jury, however, that there is no evidence in the record to support the alternative causes and emphasize that the probability is low that anything other than the mechanism of injury described caused the injury (Investigation and Prosecution of Child Abuse, 2003).

The prosecutor may ask hypothetical questions of the medical expert during direct testimony. The content of the hypothetical question will vary depending upon the medical findings, other evidence gathered by investigators, and the law of the jurisdiction. Attorneys may vary hypothetical questions to include facts that are not part of the medical findings. The following is an example of a hypothetical question:

Q (Prosecutor): "Doctor, assume that Johnny, 10 months old, was watching TV on a sofa, fell asleep, rolled off the sofa onto the floor, and started to cry. Johnny's mother then brought him to the emergency room. At the emergency room, Johnny was found to have pain in his right arm, and an X-ray was taken of the arm. The X-ray revealed a spiral fracture to the upper portion of the arm. In your opinion, to a reasonable degree of medical certainty, is that injury consistent with the history described? Why or why not?"

Prior to trial, review all hypothetical questions with the prosecutor. See Appendix for further information.

Cross-Examination

Cross-examination can be a stress-provoking experience. For the fact witness, cross-examination tends to be narrow in focus, emphasizing discrepancies in the records and the relative lack of experience of the witness. An expert witness may be cross-examined more extensively, first as to qualifications, then as to the opinions given and the bases for those opinions.

Defense attorneys usually cross-examine witnesses to uncover alleged bias. The expert witness should disclose, without any equivocation or apology, any payment received for testimony; in fact, the prosecutor may want to elicit information about any expert witness fee. Reasonable expert witness fees, particularly when a large percentage of the fee goes to the expert's hospital, should be understood by the judge and jurors.

Defense counsel may ask questions concerning the health care provider's role on a hospital or community multidisciplinary team. Explain the function of the team and clarify that not every case consultation results in a finding of abuse or a prosecution. Emphasize that the medical professional's salary does not increase based on the number of cases found to involve abuse. If the defense attorney questions the health care provider about repeated court appearances on behalf of the prosecutor and few, if any, for defense attorneys, point out any prior consultations with defense attorneys on child abuse cases. Although such consultations may not have culminated in courtroom testimony, the willingness to discuss cases with either the prosecutor or defense attorney rebuts claims of bias. Discuss other factors that demonstrate objectivity; the prosecutor should elicit those factors on direct examination (Investigation and Prosecution of Child Abuse, 2003).

Expert witnesses will be cross-examined regarding their opinions and the bases for their opinions. The witness should ask the prosecutor, prior to trial, about the defense attorney's demeanor, familiarity with the literature, questioning style, and other issues of concern. An expert witness should be familiar with the relevant literature because defense attorneys may cite studies without a complete understanding of a study's methodology. Always be patient and polite on the witness stand, even with the most confrontational defense attorney. The expert witness, however, should not allow the attorney to minimize his or her expertise or force opinions in an area outside of his or her expertise.

After testifying, the medical professional may want to discuss the experience with the prosecutor to find out what went well and what steps should be taken to make the testimony more effective in the future (see Appendix).

Hearsay Evidence

Statements made to health care professionals by children and their caregivers are essential to the investigation and prosecution of child abuse cases (see the section on documentation of medical conclusions). The health care provider may be subpoenaed to relate those statements to the jury. The admissibility of such statements at trial depends on the law of hearsay in specific jurisdictions.

Hearsay statements are statements (a) made outside of the courtroom, (b) recounted by the person to whom the statements were made, and (c) offered as evidence of the truth of the statements' contents (Myers et al., 2002). For example, a child may report to an examining physician that "My daddy burned me with an iron." The physician may then be called to the witness stand and asked to tell the judge or the jury what the child said in the hospital. If the testimony is offered as evidence that the father of the child did, in fact, burn the child with the iron, then it is hearsay.

A hearsay statement is inadmissible unless it fits an exception to the hearsay rule. In general, there are certain statements that may be admissible at trial, such as those made by a child, caregiver, or other person when startled or excited by an event ("excited utterances"); statements made by a caregiver against his or her own interest ("statements against interest"); and statements made by a child during the course of a physical examination ("statements made for purposes of medical diagnosis and treatment"). Other out-of-court statements that do not fit traditional hearsay exceptions may be admissible at trial for other reasons. Document all statements carefully, whether or not they appear to fit into a hearsay exception, and check with the local prosecutor regarding the particular nuances of your state's hearsay law. For general reading on the law of hearsay, see Myers (1998).

In Brief

Dos

- Describe medical findings clearly and simply.
- Use diagrams and photographs to supplement written descriptions of injuries.
- Educate yourself regarding proper child interviewing techniques.
- Document thoroughly any statements given by the child or caregiver, using, if possible, the speaker's exact words.
- Document statements throughout contact with the child and the family. Urge the entire clinical staff to do likewise.
- Question caregivers separately from each other and from the child.
- Document speaker's demeanor and behaviors.
- Document caregiver's frequency of visitation and nature of contact with child.
- Note inconsistency of explanations with nature of injury.
- Consult with your local multidisciplinary investigative team and prosecutor.
- Prepare with the prosecutor prior to testifying.
- Listen carefully to all questions put to you by attorneys and judges and answer clearly and truthfully.

Don'ts

- Don't rely on memory; compile a well documented chart to use later to refresh your recollection.
- Don't include personal opinions about the patient or the patient's family in the medical record.
- Don't record preliminary conclusions; wait for all required test and examination results.
- Don't testify without adequate preparation.
- Don't destroy notes or other documentation.
- Don't guess; if you cannot answer with certainty, say so.
- Don't answer a question unless you are sure you understand it.

Appendix Pointers for Expert Witnesses

1. Assume responsibility for ensuring that the lawyer calling you as an expert witness presents you in the best possible light. To accomplish this, you should

    (a) Be prepared. Always know the pertinent facts of the case better than anyone else in the courtroom.

    (b) Demand a pretrial conference with the attorney to learn what s/he wants from you and to educate her/him about the subject matter of your testimony. Review with him/her other cases where you have given similar testimony. Discuss which subjects you will not be permitted to testify about in court.

(c) Avoid using professional jargon. Review your testimony with the attorney and identify the difficult words. Use a thesaurus to find simple and clear alternative words that the judge/jury will understand.

(d) Provide the attorney calling you as a witness with a list of foundation questions. You will be more at ease knowing the questions you will be asked and the attorney will be grateful to you for making her/his job easier.

(e) Provide the lawyer calling you as an expert witness with an up-to-date resume of your professional credentials and educational background.

(f) Dress conservatively.

2. Maintain a ready file of literature pertaining to the specialty area in which you will be offering expert testimony, including mono-graphs, articles, and books. Make these available to the attorney calling you so that s/he will be more educated on your subject. Also, be sure that the attorney is aware of anything you have written pertaining to the subject of your testimony.

3. If you are going to be interviewed by opposing counsel, avoid doing so in your office. By meeting in your personal office you will give the attorney a chance to look around at the various reference books and texts and then challenge you in court with one of your own reference books. A neutral place like a restaurant, conference room, or even the attorney's office is a better place for your meeting.

(a) Avoid sitting for an interview with opposing counsel, or for a deposition, until you are fully prepared, know the facts of your case and the relevant references to the professional literature.

(b) Segregate your personal notes and work product from the case file. Do not disclose them to the opposing counsel without either permission of the attorney calling you as a witness or a court order.

(c) At an interview with opposing counsel or deposition, have a "game plan" to either

   (i) impress the other attorney with the facts supporting your position by "telling all" to encourage settlement, or
   (ii) if litigation is expected, answer questions honestly but narrowly.

4. Always tell the truth and maintain the appearance of being absolutely fair and objective.

5. If you anticipate the advocate for the other side will be calling an expert, suggest to the attorney calling you that you spend time preparing her/him to deal with the adverse expert. You can even sometimes sit with the attorney in court and suggest methods of cross-examination to her/him.

6. Remember, when approaching or inside the courthouse, anyone you pass may be a judge, juror, hostile witness, or opposing attorney. Always conduct yourself accordingly.

7. When you enter the courtroom, do not do anything immediately. Before sitting down, make brief eye contact with the judge and/or jury. Adjust the chair and microphone so that you don't have to lean forward to answer questions.

8. Be aware of spatial positioning and, if possible, use it to your advantage.

    (a) Adversary position—Face to face, squarely in front of the person or group of people.
    (b) Communication position—At an angle to the person or group.
    (c) Cooperation position—Side by side.

9. Before answering each question, control the situation by consciously pausing. This allows the judge/jury to mentally shift from hearing the attorney's question to listening to your answer. For example,

    Q: "State your name and occupation." Three-count pause
    A: "My   name   is_____.   I   am   a   social   worker   for the_____."
    Q: "How long have you been employed?" Three-count pause
    A: "I have been working there for_____years."

10. Answer each question with a declarative statement rather than a word or phrase. The opposing attorney may only want the judge/jury to hear his or her question. By using the three-count pause, the declarative sentence, and spatial positioning you will take psychological control away from the attorney.
11. When answering questions, don't guess. If you don't know, say you don't know, but don't let the cross-examiner get you in the trap of answering question after question with "I don't know."
12. Understand the question before you attempt to give an answer. You can't possibly give a truthful and accurate answer unless you understand the question.
13. Listen and try to avoid asking the lawyer to repeat the question. Keep a sharp lookout for questions with a double meaning and questions that assume you have testified to a fact when you have not done so.
14. Answer the question that is asked and then stop, especially on cross-examination. Don't volunteer information not called for by the question you are asked.
15. Choice of words is very important. Develop your ability to use words that not only depict what happened but also convey the impression you intend.

    Positive "Soft" Words
    mother
    father
    child
    cut
    molest
    bruise

    Negative "Hard" Words
    woman, respondent, abuser
    subject, suspect, defendant
    juvenile, youth

laceration, open wound
rape, sexual assault contusion

16. Talk loudly enough so everyone can hear you, yet softly enough so that you can suddenly raise your voice to emphasize a point.
17. Avoid distracting mannerisms such as eating mints, chewing gum, or fumbling through a file.
18. Give an audible answer so the court reporter can hear it. Don't nod your head yes or no. Remember that the court reporter is writing everything you say for appellate review.
19. Don't look at the lawyer who called you as a witness or at the judge for help when you are on the witness stand.
20. Beware of questions involving distances and time. If you make an estimate, make sure that everyone understands that you are estimating. Think clearly about distances and intervals of time. Be sure your estimates are reasonable.
21. Don't be afraid to look the jurors in the eye. Jurors are naturally sympathetic to witnesses and want to hear what they have to say. Look at them most of the time and speak to them frankly and openly as you would to a friend or neighbor.
22. Don't argue with the lawyer cross-examining you. S/he has every right to question you and the lawyer who called you will object if s/he gets out of bounds. Don't answer a question with a question unless the question you are asked is not clear.
23. Don't lose your temper no matter how hard you are pressed. If you lose your temper, you have played right into the hands of the cross-examiner.
24. Be courteous. Being courteous is one of the best ways to make a good impression on the court and on the jury. Be sure to answer, "Yes, Sir," and "No, Sir," and to address the judge as "Your Honor."
25. If asked whether you have talked to the lawyer calling you as a witness or to an investigator, admit it freely. If you are being paid a fee, admit, without hesitation, that you are receiving compensation.
26. Avoid joking, wisecracks, and condescending comments or inflections. A trial is a serious matter.
27. Most people learn visually. Use blackboards, diagrams, charts, and so on liberally. At the blackboard or easel, turn around and talk to the jury. Almost inevitably, witnesses not following this instruction will get into an inaudible conversation with the blackboard. Remember spatial positioning.
28. Draw in proportion. Before drawing anything—think! Don't start with the old cliche, "Well, I'm not much of an artist." Draw in proportion and never refer to "here" and "there." A reviewing court will not understand what you mean. Describe what you draw orally and number each relevant representation.
29. Never read from notes unless absolutely necessary. If you must, announce the fact that you are doing so and state your reason (i.e., refreshing memory, need for specificity, etc.). The lawyer cross-examining you will most likely have a right to see the notes at that time.

30. Never give an opinion about things you are not trained in, and never give an opinion you cannot support.
31. An opposing attorney may cross-examine you with articles, books, other people's opinions, or things you have said previously. You may be confronted with something that appears contradictory in an effort to show that your opinion is inconsistent with these other sources. Ask to see the book or article the opposing attorney refers to. Read it, compare it, and almost every time you will find that something has been taken out of context or misinterpreted by the attorney. You can then demonstrate not only that you are right, but that the article or book agrees with you.
32. Be familiar with the book Coping with Psychiatric and Psychological Testimony, 5th ed., by J. Zisken, published by Law and Psychology Press, 202 South Rexford Drive, Beverly Hills, California 90212. You can be assured that the lawyer cross-examining you will probably have read this book. If you have not, no matter how competent you are in your field, you may be embarrassed.
33. When you finish testifying, nod to the judge/jury, and say thank you.
34. After each appearance as an expert witness, check with the attorney or others present for a critique of your performance. Use the critique to improve or modify the way you testify.

Copyrightby American Prosecutors Research Institute. National District Attorneys Association (NDAA – APRI).

Note

1. A guardian ad litem is a special guardian, often an attorney, appointed by the court to represent the interests of a child in court proceedings.

References

American Medical Association. (1998). *Physician firearm safety guide*. Chicago, IL: American Medical Association.

American Prosecutors Research Institute. (1993). *Investigation and prosecution of child abuse*. Alexandria, VA: American Prosecutors Research Institute.

American Prosecutors Research Institute. (2003). *Investigation and prosecution of child abuse* (3rd ed.). Alexandria, VA: Sage Publications, Inc.

Beaman, V., Annest, J. L., Kresnow, J. J., & Pollock, D. A. (2000). Lethality of firearm-related injuries in the United States population. *Annals of Emergency Medicine, 35*, 258–266.

Bross, D. C., Krugman, R. D., Lenherr, M. D., Rosenberg, D., & Schmitt, B. (Eds.). (1988). *The new child protection team handbook*. New York: Garland.

Centers for Disease Control and Prevention. (1986–1992). *Firearm mortality and morbidity*, Atlanta, GA: Centers for Disease Control.

Cleary, E. W. (1983). *McCormick's handbook of the law of evidence* (2nd ed.). St. Paul, MN: West.

Council on Scientific Affairs. (1985). AMA Diagnostic and treatment guidelines concerning child abuse and neglect. *The Journal of the American Medical Association, 254,* 796–800.

DeLaronde, S., King, G., Bendel, R., & Reece, R. (2000). Opinions among mandated reporters toward child maltreatment reporting policies. *Child Abuse Neglect,* 901, 905.

Finkelhor, D. (1990, Winter). Is child abuse overreported? *Public Welfare, 48,* 22–29.

Heger, A. H. (1991). Interviewing the child. Child sexual abuse. *Report of the Twenty-second Ross Roundtable in critical approaches to common pediatric problems.* Columbus, OH: Ross Laboratories.

Immunity for Reporters of Child Abuse and Neglect: Summary of State Laws. (2008). Washington, DC: Child Welfare Information Gateway. http://www.childwelfare.gov/systemwide/laws_policies/statutes/immunityall.pdf

Kempe, C. H., Silverman, F. N., Steele, B. F., Droegmueller, W., & Silver, H. K. (1962, July 7). The battered-child syndrome. *The Journal of the American Medical Association, 181,* 17–24.

Kendler, K. S., Heath, A. C., Neale, M. C., Kessler, R. C., & Eaves, L. J. (2000). Medical college of Virginia, Commonwealth University. *Archives of General Psychiatry, 57,* 953–959.

Making and Screening Report of Child Abuse and Neglect: Summary of State Laws. (2008). Washington, DC: Child Welfare Information Gateway. http://www.childwelfare.gov/systemwide/laws_policies/statutes/repprocall.pdf

Mandatory Reports of Child Abuse and Neglect: Summary of State Laws. (2008). Washington, DC: Child Welfare Information Gateway. http://www.childwelfare.gov/systemwide/laws_policies/statutes/mandaall.pdf

Meriwether. M. H. (1986). *Child abuse reporting laws: Time for a change, 20,* Fam. L. Q. 141, 142.

Myers, J. E. B. (1998). *Legal issues in child abuse and neglect practice* (2nd ed.). Thousand Oaks, CA: Sage Publications.

Myers, J. E. B., Berliner, L., Briere, J., Hendrix, C. T., Jenny, C., & Reid, T. A. (Eds.). (2002). *The APSAC handbook on child maltreatment* (2nd ed.). American Professional Society on the Abuse of Children. Thousand Oaks, CA: Sage.

Myers, J. E. B., & Carter, L. E. (1988). Proof of physical child abuse. *Missouri Law Review, 53,* 189–225.

Myers, J. E. B., & Peters, W. D. (1987). *Child abuse reporting in the 1980s.* The American Humane Society, 6–14.

Ondersma, S. J., Simpson, S. M., Brestan, E. V., & Ward, M. (2000). Prenatal drug exposure and social policy: The search for an appropriate response. *Child Maltreatment, 5* (2): 83–108.

Penalties for Failure to Report and False Reporting of Child Abuse and Neglect: Summary of State Laws. (2007). Washington, DC: Child Welfare Information Gateway. http://www.childwelfare.gov/systemwide/laws_policies/statutes/reportall.pdf

Ricci, L. R., & Smistek, B. S. (2000). *Photodocumentation in the investigation of child abuse.* National Institute of Justice. http://www.ncjrs.gov/App/publications/abstract.aspx?ID=160939

Salter, A. C. (1995). *Transforming Trauma: A guide to understanding and treating adult survivors of child sexual abuse.* Thousand Oaks, CA: Sage Publications

Schaechter, J., Duran, I., De Marchena, J., Lemard, G., & Villar, M. (2003). Are accidental gun deaths as rare as they seem? A comparison of medical examiner manner of death coding with an intent-based classification approach. *Pediatrics, 111* (4), 741–744.

Statutory Compilations on Penalties for Failure to Report Child Abuse. (2007).

Statutory Compilations on Immunity for Mandated Reporters. (2008).

US Department of Health and Human Services, Administration on Children, Youth and Families. (2005). *Child maltreatment* (p. 25). Washington, DC: Government Printing Office, 2007.

US Department of Health and Human Services. Administration on Children, Youth and Families. (2008). *Child maltreatment 2006.* Washington, DC: US Government Printing Office.

Warner, J. R., & Hansen, D. J. (1994). The identification and reporting of physical abuse by physicians: A review and implications for research. *Child Abuse Neglect, 18,* 11–25.

Chapter 16

Mental Health Issues: Child Physical Abuse and Neglect

Toi Blakley Harris and Albert J. Sargent III

Introduction

Nationally, child maltreatment is at epidemic proportions. In 2006, the National Child Abuse and Neglect Data System (NCANDS) noted approximately 6.0 million children were referred for alleged maltreatment to child protective services (US Department of Health and Human Services, 2008). Of the 3.3 million that were assessed, 30% of the investigations concluded that at least one child had been victimized (US Department of Health and Human Services, 2008). Although in the last 5 years there has been an increase in the number of investigations by CPS, there is a slight decline in the number of substantiated reports of abuse and or neglect (US Department of Health and Human Services, 2008). Of the 905,000 youth who were documented as being victimized in 2006, the vast majority were found to have been neglected (64.1%), followed by physical abuse (16%), sexual abuse (8.8%), psychological or emotional abuse (6.6%), and medical neglect (2.2%) (US Department of Health and Human Services, 2006). Even with the states' efforts to improve the accuracy of reporting, the literature has shown that these rates underestimate the true number (Crume, DiGuiseppi, Byers, Sirotnak, & Garrett, 2002; Herman-Giddens et al., 1999). The third National Incidence Study of Child Abuse and Neglect noted less than 50% of children screened for maltreatment were actually assessed by child protective services (Sedlack & Broadhurst, 1996; Shaffer, Huston, & Egeland, 2008). Notwithstanding the errors involved with proper identification, the goals of intervention are based upon the physical and emotional well-being of the child or adolescent. Physical and psychological sequelae both can result from child maltreatment. This chapter will focus on psychological symptoms and disorders that develop after childhood physical abuse, psychological abuse and neglect.

A.P. Giardino et al. (eds.), *A Practical Guide to the Evaluation of Child Physical Abuse and Neglect*, DOI 10.1007/978-1-4419-0702-8_16, © Springer Science+Business Media, LLC 1997, 2010

Maltreatment Categories

Four types of child maltreatment are recognized in various iterations by federal and state authorities: neglect, psychological, physical, and sexual abuse. These forms of maltreatment may occur in isolation or in various combinations. They also have differences that are summarized by Glaser in Table 16.1 (2002).

Table 16.1 Forms of Child Maltreatment (Glaser, 2002) (printed with permission).

	Sexual abuse	Physical abuse	Emotional abuse/neglect
Abusive act interaction	Hidden	Hidden or observed	Observable
Identity of abuser	Usually questioned	Sometimes known	Known
Abuser and primary carer	Usually different persons	Same or different persons	Same person
Definition/proof reliant on evidence of	Ill-treatment	Signs of harm to the child	Ill-treatment by caregiver and signs of harm to the child
Immediate protection indicated	Yes	Usually	Rarely

Psychological Maltreatment and Neglect

Psychological and emotional abuse and neglect all occur within "a carer–child relationship" in which there are "harmful interactions, requiring no physical contact with the child" (Glaser, 2002). Glaser wrote that psychological abuse and emotional abuse be considered together "since cognition and emotion are not independent of each other, cognitive appraisal of experiences contributing to the affective experience and vice versa" (2002). Debate in the field occurs about whether to consider "the maltreating behavior or to the consequences for the child, and whether evidence of both is required for its recognition" Glaser (2002) has cited recent reports that "evidence of the ill treatment rather than harm to the child should be sought".

Glaser (2002) developed a definition of psychological abuse which has demonstrated inter-rater reliability. It was deemed to translate internationally; however, cultural norms regarding developmental expectations were reported as factors to consider during evaluation and assessment. Glaser's five categories include (1) emotional unavailability, unresponsiveness, and neglect; (2) negative attributions and misattributions to the child; (3) developmentally inappropriate or inconsistent interactions with the child; (4) failure to recognize or acknowledge the child's individuality and psychological boundary (medical child abuse or factitious disorder by proxy is found in this category); (5) failing to promote the child's social adaptation. These may manifest as categories described by the American Professional Society on the Abuse of Children (APSAC) (1995): spurning, terrorizing, exploiting or corrupting, withholding emotion or affection, isolation, and/or educational, medical, health, and/or psychological neglect. The stratification of this definition is essential to assess the presence and/or absence of psychological maltreatment suggests which types of interventions are needed. For more detailed examination of the relationship between APSAC's and Glaser's frameworks, refer to Glaser (2002).

Physical Abuse

There remains significant controversy about the use of corporal punishment. Within the US, corporal punishment's role in effective parenting and the long-term implications of this type of discipline continue to be debated. The American Academy of Pediatrics and the American Academy of Child and Adolescent Psychiatry caution against the use of physical forms of punishment for the discipline of children and adolescents (American Academy of Pediatrics, 2000; American Academy of Child & Adolescent Psychiatry, 1988). Other professional organizations have cited the link between corporal punishment and physical abuse, where either physical and/or psychological harm to the child occurs when this form of discipline goes away.

There are cultural differences in parenting practices and there appear to be cultural differences in the impact of response to corporal punishment. Horn, Joseph, & Cheng (2004) conducted a systematic review examining longitudinal and cross-sectional data on this issue. Those authors identified either positive or neutral outcomes for African-American children who received non-abusive physical punishment during their childhoods with longitudinal studies. This was in contradistinction to Caucasian youth where less favorable outcomes were more likely.

Authors have explored how the cultural meaning of non-abusive physical discipline mediates developmental outcomes (Whaley 2000; Horn et al., 2004). Durrant's (2008) review of the international data predicts negative longitudinal effects in comparison to fewer studies with positive findings. The studies examined by Durrant's review included diverse ethnic populations of European American, African-American, and Hispanic-American youth. Durrant counters the assertion of culturally accepted discipline strategies. This author reports data that suggests African-American families of working and middle-class backgrounds employ forms of child-centered parenting that involve corporal punishment at lower rates than previously described.

In addition to debates regarding the use, meaning, and impact of physical punishment, there are documented cultural differences in reporting and investigating child maltreatment among various ethnic groups in the US (US Department of Health and Human Services, 2006). Asian Americans are disproportionately less likely to experience child abuse based upon reporting agencies; physical abuse is reported with higher frequency than either neglect sexual abuse (Zhai & Gao, 2008). Despite these findings, some authors offer potential explanations for these differences which include increase value placed on the child's welfare, under-reporting by the child related to family connectedness, and this group's management of disputes and conflicts to the exclusion of outside entities (Zhai & Gao, 2008). Additional study is warranted to better define the role that culture plays in discipline strategies and subsequent longitudinal outcomes.

Psychological Outcomes of Maltreatment

Physical abuse and neglect can be considered as traumatic experiences for children and adolescents. Trauma produces significant psychological effects upon the child's emotional well-being and can influence the child's overall development. Mental health clinicians, child regulatory agencies and researchers have attempted to characterize child maltreatment in terms of frequency or severity, duration, age of abuse and subtype of abuse (English, Graham, Litrownik, Everson, & Bangdiwala, 2005). These parameters have implications for interventions and outcomes.

Pine and Cohen (2002) reviewed the literature and noted that outcomes vary among children depending upon a wide variety of factors and can be affected positively or negatively by a range of responses and interventions. This section will review common responses to trauma for children of different developmental capacities, some variables which influence the nature of psychological responses to trauma, and protective factors which can ameliorate deleterious effects. The chapter will also present data from the literature that discusses long-term implications of childhood maltreatment.

Traumatic stress refers to the physical and emotional responses to events that threaten the life or physical or psychological integrity of the child or someone critically important to the child. Traumatic experiences are unexpected and unpredictable, uncontrollable and terrifying. Emotional responses to traumatic experience are often overwhelming and may include terror, helplessness, and extreme physiologic arousal that do not lead to purposeful and effective reactions. These emotional responses often coincide, leading the child to feel overwhelmed, confused, and out of control. Central nervous system effects of this set of responses can impact later neurophysiologic responses. Hyperarousal and overgeneralization of threat can evolve, leading the child to react in an extreme fashion to events which resemble or remind the child of the original trauma. The degree and frequency of significant arousal responses also reinforces the avoidance of discussion or consideration of traumatic memories. The third common reaction is re-experiencing in the form of flashbacks, nightmares, and intrusive images of the trauma and re-experiencing of traumatic events. Manifestations vary based upon the child's developmental stage. (See assessment for detailed description.)

The individual is always the person who labels an experience as traumatic. It is the responsibility of others (including mental health professionals) to help those who are distressed after frightening and traumatic experiences as defined by them. These traumatic experiences vary in a number of ways: (1) proximal cause, (2) number of experiences, (3) degree of physical effect both immediate and long term, and (4) the occurrence of subsequent disruptive events. Some abuse results in physical injury that requires intensive medical treatment. In those instances, the psychological impact is not only the result of the physical abuse but also effected by the impact of necessary painful medical treatment. The pain and unpredictability of these procedures and any uncertainty in the medical prognosis all heighten the possibility of traumatic stress for children with serious illness or injury. The frequency of developing posttraumatic stress disorder (PTSD), depression, and other significant emotional or behavioral problems varies among these causes but all have the potential to lead to deleterious outcomes (Ethier, Lemelin, & Lacharite, 2004; English et al., 2005). Traumatic stress and PTSD are common following child physical abuse. However, not all children who experience acute stress reactions proceed to develop PTSD. Often psychological recovery accompanies physical recovery and occurs in association with parental support and encouragement for the affected child.

The frequency and total number of traumatic events appears to influence the presence and severity of psychological sequelae. This is also often complicated by further traumatic experiences. Examples of this include subsequent moves among foster homes and CPS (child protective services) placements for children in state custody following abuse and painful surgery and invasive procedures in hospital following a traumatic accidental injury. Death or serious injury of a close relative in the traumatic experience impacts a child in three distinct ways: (1) the child is affected directly by the loss or serious injury, (2) that relative is not available to support the child through his traumatic experience, and (3) there is frequently significant confusion, worry, and sadness in the child's family as the family grieves the deceased loved one or cares for a seriously injured family member, further decreasing support for the affected child.

Children with preexisting mental health problems are frequently more affected by a traumatic experience. This is especially true if the child was previously anxious or fearful or has a slow-to-warm-up temperament. It appears that individuals with significant interpersonal sensitivity and marked emotional reactivity distress to either their own or to other's are also more likely to develop significant traumatic stress. In this light, PTSD can be viewed as a phenomenon occurring as a result of a gene–environment interaction. Witnessing or experiencing traumatic interpersonal violence may lead to traumatic stress in those with high interpersonal sensitivity. Females are twice more likely to develop PTSD than males, while males are more likely to develop conduct disorder, antisocial or criminal behavior following significant violent trauma (Plattner et al., 2007). Shame experienced at the time of the trauma and self-blaming attributions about the cause of the trauma can worsen the psychological outcome. Over time, the overall emotional well-being of the traumatized child is influenced by individual, family, and community factors that will be further explored in this chapter.

Literature Findings

Replicated studies have demonstrated an association between childhood negative life experiences and psychiatric disorders (Saleptsi et al., 2004) (Table 16.2). However, numerous methodological hallenges have hindered the scholarly

Table 16.2 Psychological outcomes of childhood maltreatment: Literature review.

Childhood maltreatment psychiatric disorder(s)	Emotional abuse (EA), neglect (N)	Physical abuse (PA)	Sexual abuse (SA)
Substance related disorders Anxious/depressed schizophrenia	N associated with alcohol related disorders (Saleptsi et al., 2004). N associated with increased rates in patients with schizophrenia and affective disorders; EA associated with increased rates in patients with schizophrenia and personality disorders. (Saleptsi et al., 2004). Chronic N and PA links to anxiety and depression; 49/49 physical and emotional neglect and 25/49 physical abuse (Ethier et al., 2004). N and EA reported with increased frequency in patients with schizophrenia (Saleptsi et al., 2004).	PA associated with alcohol related disorders (Saleptsi et al., 2004). PA predictor of anxiety and depression at age 16 (Lansford et al., 2002). PA endorsed by patients with schizophrenia (Saleptsi et al., 2004).	SA associated with increased rates of affective disorders (Saleptsi et al., 2004). SA associated with increased rates of schizophrenia (Saleptsi et al., 2004).
Aggression/legal history	Chronic N and PA links to aggressive behavior more so than transitory maltreatment or controls (Ethier et al., 2004). N and PA associated with increased arrest rates of violent adult crimes (Widom 1989a, 1989b).	PA in the first 5 years predictive of aggression in adolescence, violent and non-violent delinquency including perpetration of romantic violence (Lansford et al., 2007). PA associated with 2.7 × risk of weapon carrying at age 12 years (Lewis et al., 2007).	SA less predictive of arrests of violent crimes in comparison to PA (Lewis et al., 2007). SA is associated with increased antisocial behavior in comparison to non-maltreated youth (Bergen et al., 2004; Lewis et al., 2007). SA was associated with 4.2 × risk of weapon carrying at age 12 years (Lewis et al., 2007).

Table 16.2 (continued)

Childhood maltreatment psychiatric disorder(s)	Emotional abuse (EA), neglect (N)	Physical abuse (PA)	Sexual abuse (SA)
Personality disorders	EA and N reported with increased frequency in patients with personality disorders (Saleptsi et al., 2004).	PA reported with increased frequency in patients with personality disorders (Saleptsi et al., 2004).	
Somatization		PA has been associated with somatization (Yates. Carlson, & Egeland, 2008).	Sexual abuse has been associated with somatization (Yates, Carlson, & Egeland, 2008).
Suicidal self-harm	Increased rates of intermittent (1–2 incidents) self-injurious behavior (SIB); N occurred with recurrent injurers (Yates, Carlson, & Egeland, 2008).		Sexual abuse with increased frequency in recurrent (3 or more incidents) SIB (Yates, Carlson, & Egeland, 2008).
Work relationships		PA in the first 5 years associated with decreased high school completion rates, increased rates of job failures, and teen parenthood (Lansford et al., 2007).	

Table 16.2 (continued)

Childhood maltreatment psychiatric disorder(s)	Emotional abuse (EA), neglect (N)	Physical abuse (PA)	Sexual abuse (SA)
Neurobiology/cognition post-natal trauma has been associated with deficits in the following: behavior, attention, memory, visual processing, motor functions, language, and abnormalities in the hypothalamic-pituitary-adrenal axis (Henry et al., 2007). Impaired speech development (Coster, Gersten, Beeghly, & Cicchetti, 1989) and decreased communication about affect and physiological states (Cicchetti & Beeghly, 1987; Yates, Carlson, & Egeland, 2008).		PA children are likely to develop "biased patterns of processing social information and misattribute the intentions of others" (Lansford et al., 2007).	

examination of the relationship between childhood adverse life experiences and their impact on child, adolescent and adult functioning which include "definition and identification of maltreatment" (Shaffer et al., 2008). The psychiatric literature documented the relationship between childhood negative life events and subsequent adult psychopathology most successfully when utilizing both retrospective and prospective research strategies (Shaffer et al., 2008). Stressful life events have been documented in the literature to result in a short- and long-term adverse outcomes that cross multiple domains.

The majority of the studies have reported on the effects of sexual abuse with less emphasis on psychological maltreatment and physical abuse. The literature has highlighted previous reports of negative adolescent and adult outcomes of childhood maltreatment: impaired cognitive, language, and neurobiological processes (i.e. hypothalamic-pituitary-adrenal axis), interpersonal difficulties, poor affect regulation, and a wide array of psychiatric disturbances such as posttraumatic stress disorder, recurrent major depression, substance related disorders, suicidality, self-harm and disruptive behaviors, and somatization disorders (Collishaw et al., 2007; Henry, Sloane, & Black-Pond, 2007).

Other researchers have differentiated physical abuse and neglect from other forms of maltreatment and found that these are both related to violent and self-protective behavior later in life (Widom, 1989a, b; Lewis et al., 2007). Lewis et al. (2007) identified an association between early childhood physical and sexual abuse with weapon carrying and the need for "self-protection". Drawing upon data from the Longitudinal Studies of Child Abuse and Neglect (LONGSCAN), they described a sample of 797 youth aged 12 years whose results revealed those who were physically abused were 2.7 times more likely to carry a weapon versus those without. Those youth with a history of sexual maltreatment were 4.2 times more likely to carry a weapon versus those without a history of sexual abuse. Males were 1.7 times more likely than females to carry a weapon with similar maltreatment histories.

In addition to traumatic stress, anxiety, and depressive symptoms, Lansford et al.'s prospective longitudinal study of 574 children followed from the ages 5–21 years (2007) confirmed previous reports that link early childhood physical abuse to adolescent aggression, violent, and non-violent forms of delinquency, teen parenthood, lower high school completion rates, and difficulty maintaining employment. Gender and cultural factors influences were noted. Both genders were at increased risk for being fired from jobs. There was a disproportionate risk of job loss for females who had experienced physical abuse in childhood in comparison to their male counterparts. Moreover, physically abused females were also more likely to become a parent prior to adulthood. African-American males and females in this study were at increased risk of violent and non-violent offenses, failure to graduate from high school, and sustain employment and being a teen parent. The authors emphasized the importance of examining the relationship on race and ethnicity and outcomes of abuse. This scrutiny might identify the role of quality mental health care, unfavorable environmental living conditions for abused youth, and the increased representation in the juvenile and legal systems of minority youth.

Chronicity, severity, and type of maltreatment have a bearing on long-term outcomes. English et al. (2005) conducted a longitudinal study of 519 maltreated children who experienced different forms and severities of trauma over varying periods of time and occurring at different ages. In this study, chronicity was measured in three ways: (1) frequency, (2) calendar definition, and (3) developmental definition. These domains evaluated behavior, adaptation, and trauma. Frequency and age of onset predicted deficits in two out of the three domains.

Chronicity predicted trauma symptoms of posttraumatic stress, depression, externalizing, and total behavior problems. The age at first report was also predictive of subsequent daily living skills; moreover, the older the age of the child, the improved score on the Vineland Daily Living Scale. This data suggests that socialization deficits are related to the *distribution* of insults over time, whereas problematic behaviors (most notably for externalizing symptoms) are associated with the *timing* and quantity of traumatic experiences.

Studies that have examined resilience in adolescence and adulthood following childhood maltreatment have identified essential ingredients to resilience that includes (1) genetic factors, (2) biological factors, (3) cognitive factors, (4) and inter-personal factors (Collishaw et al., 2007). Earlier studies focused on resiliency have noted that individual characteristics such as intelligence, physical attractiveness, and temperament are protective and draw adults to the individual to provide support and care (Masten, Wright, & Garmezy, 1990). More recent studies have identified neurobiological variables. Studies have replicated findings noting that individuals with high levels of monoamine oxidase A have a decreased likelihood of antisocial behavior following maltreatment in childhood (Caspi et al., 2002; Kim-Cohen et al., 2006; Martin & Volkmar, 2007). Other researchers have documented individuals who are homozygous for the long allele of the 5-HTTLPR (serotonin transporter) have less rates of depression than those with either one or two copies of the short allele (Caspi et al., 2003; Kaufman et al., 2004; Eley et al., 2004; Martin & Volkmar, 2007). These studies point to the importance of continued examination of how genes and environmental influences impact development and psychosocial outcomes of maltreated youth.

Several reports have demonstrated that approximately 22–48% were classified as "resilient" when evaluating for adult psychosocial functioning and the absence of psychopathology (antisocial personality disorder, posttraumatic stress disorder, anxiety, depression and 38% without substance related disorder), respectively (Collishaw et al., 2007). Periods without maltreatment also proved to foster resilience among study participants. This finding was consistent with other data in the literature (Cicchetti & Rogosch, 1997; Luthar, Cicchetti & Becker, 2000; English et al., 2005).

Collishaw et al.'s (2007) longitudinal study of maltreated children through adolescence and mid-life also examined resiliency. The resilient dimensions evaluated were similar to other studies: (1) absence of major depressive disorder, recurrent depressive disorder, suicidality, suicide attempt, any anxiety disorder, posttraumatic stress disorder, substance related disorder, (2) personality functioning, (3) relationship stability, (4) legal status, and (5) self-rated health. While controlling for adversity experienced in adolescence, the risk for adult substance related disorders, posttraumatic stress disorder, suicidality, and recurrent depression was increased in the maltreated group in comparison to controls. Despite this increased risk, 44.5% were characterized as resilient. Positively *perceived parental care*, supportive adolescent peer relationships and adult romantic relationships, and personality factors were variables that supported resiliency.

DuMont, Widom, & Czaja's (2007) longitudinal study of maltreated children and age-matched controls through adulthood (an average of 22 years post-maltreatment) revealed 48% manifested resilience in adolescence (61% control group) and 30.2% in adulthood (46% controls). Ethnic, gender, cognitive, and household status variables predicted resiliency differences in adolescence and adulthood. In adolescence, being female, non-White, and residing in a "stable household" promoted resiliency. The literature has documented the protective facets of impoverished African-American, Asian-American, and Hispanic-American communities that include religiosity, extended families and networks (Lim, 2006). Moreover, Jarrett (1993) presented strategies such as "tightening curfews...establishing ties with people who have resources to provide opportunities for success," that have been employed by African-American teens and their families to promote resilience (DuMont et al., 2007).

Female gender continued to predict resiliency in adulthood, but ethnicity and childhood stability did not. By young adulthood, "household stability" and race were no longer predictive. A prominent interaction between intellectual ability and neighborhood advantage was pointed to adulthood resilience. Individuals with increased cognitive abilities who resided in advantaged neighborhoods were resilient approximately three times more so than those from the same type of neighborhoods with lower cognitive abilities. Higher intellect attracts adults and enhances experience of respect admiration and support. Supportive relationships and fewer adverse life events improved an individual's chances of developing or maintaining resilience.

Assessment

In the initial phases of the psychological evaluation process, it is imperative to assess the current level of support received by the victimized youth (Pine & Cohen, 2002). The most important determinant of the degree of psychological distress a child experiences after trauma is the degree of attuned emotional support the child receives from adults important in their lives. Usually, the supportive adults are parents, but they can be others with whom the child has meaningful relationships. This support validates the child's experience and provides an opportunity for the child to feel cared about and understood even when the child is terrified and overwhelmed. For example, the psychological outcome for maltreated children depends a great deal upon the emotional support of the non-offending parent. Many factors affect the degree of emotional support available to the traumatized child (Cohen, Mannarino, & Deblinger, 2006). This child's attachment relationship with his caretakers is very important. The greater the security of attachment, the more the child will trust and rely on the support of others while coping with the arousal associated with trauma. Caretakers' ability to manage their own distress associated with their child's traumatic experience also is an essential element in their ability to be emotionally available to support the child.

The treatment of children who have experienced trauma and have symptoms of traumatic stress begins with a thorough assessment of the child and his or her context. This includes obtaining a history of the child's traumatic experiences throughout his life and gaining an appreciation of the child's strengths and capacities. In gathering this history, one needs to take care not to re-traumatize the child; the use of ancillary historians is essential in this endeavor. Assessment of symptoms, including the psychological symptoms of acute stress reaction, PTSD, and depression as well as behavioral manifestations including aggressiveness, impulsivity, substance use, sexual acting out, and self-harm are essential.

Evaluation of the child's context includes understanding family relationships and individual strengths and deficits. Many individual characteristics have been deemed risk factors for maltreatment and include age (younger children), prematurity, emotional and behavioral disturbances, developmental and physical disabilities, etc. (Hurme, Alanko, Anttila, Juven, & Svedstrom, 2008; US Department of Health and Human Services, 2006). The assessment of the family includes attention to the family's organization, the family members' understanding of the trauma, and the family's capacity to obtain the resources needed for recovery, which may include medical and mental health care. The professional must also report abuse to the child protective system if it is suspected. If child welfare is involved with the child, the clinician can agree to provide support to the child and if feasible support the family's efforts to improve their situation and continue to be connected to their child. The assessment should also include understanding the situations that trigger arousal for the child, which often result in impulsive, aggressive behaviors and recognizing ways that the child calms himself when upset.

Developmental considerations must be applied throughout the evaluation and treatment process. Traumatic experience has varying effects on children of different ages. Preschool children with a history of maltreatment may exhibit problems primarily related to separation (i.e. school refusal, sleeping with a parent or caregiver, difficulty sleeping, nightmares, reactive aggressiveness, and or clinging behavior with parent). However, regressive behaviors such as enuresis and fears may occur. There are similarities with maltreated school age children. They may also experience sleep disturbances, school avoidance, and angry outbursts. Attention and concentration problems, somatic complaints and depression, and withdrawal are other features of abused school age children. During adolescence, maltreatment may manifest as hypervigilance and intrusive thoughts, emotional numbing, avoidance and nightmares along with mood dysregulation and depressive symptoms.

Treatment

Several authors have described approaches to the treatment of children who have experienced trauma and have psychological or behavioral difficulties (Saxe, Ellis, & Kaplow, 2007; Cohen et al., 2006). The National Child Traumatic Stress Network also presents a comprehensive review of Trauma Focused Cognitive Behavior Therapy on its website nctsnet.org. Prior reviews have documented short-term moderate effectiveness in enhancing the psychosocial health and well-being of mothers, infants, toddlers, and older children (Barlow, Coren, & Stewart-Brown, 2002; Barlow & Parsons, 2005; Barlow & Stewart-Brown, 2000). In 2008, the Cochrane Database of Systematic Reviews published findings of a review of randomized controlled trial of short-term parenting programs designed to treat physical child abuse and neglect (Barlow, Johnston, Kendrick, Polnay, & Stewart-Brown, 2008). Seven studies were included in the reviews; however, only three evaluated the affect of the program on measures of child maltreatment. The majority of the results did favor the intervention group, but several failed to produce results that were statistically significant. This was believed to be because of sample size. The use of theoretically based programs such as parent–child interaction therapy and cognitive behavioral therapy was supported to address features of abusive parenting such as "excessive parental anger, misattributions, and poor parent–child interaction."

The goals of treatment are to assist the child's return to safe development and functioning and to build the capacity of the child's context (family and other important adults) to support the child's behavior and development. The process of treatment also assists the child to integrate the memory of the trauma so that the child can remember the trauma, manage his arousal and not need to either avoid or re-experience the traumatic experience. Offering opportunities to voluntarily participate in a debriefing discussion with a trained professional may be helpful for those who freely choose to discuss their traumatic exposure at that time. Treatment is designed to develop and maintain expectations of safety and predictability, reestablish self-control and self-direction, and build the child's capacity for resilience in future experiences of adversity. A final goal of treatment is to reduce the possibility that the child approaches his or her life as a victim with limited self-respect and self-regard.

Sargent (2009) describes the treatment process in a series of eight steps (see Table 16.3). These stages are appropriate in the acute treatment of children after traumatic injury and acute abuse as well as in treatment of children with PTSD and children who have experienced repeated trauma and evidence complex traumatic stress.

Step 1—Safety

The first step involves ensuring the child's safety. In situations of acute danger this involves making sure that the child is physically safe. Compassion and caring involvement of police, rescue workers, health care professionals, and child

Table 16.3 Eight steps in traumatic stress treatment.

(1) Ensuring safety
(2) Ensuring availability of basic needs
(3) Building child and family knowledge about the trauma and its effects
(4) Reinforcing normative behavioral routines
(5) Identifying and supporting the child's emotional states
(6) Supporting those who support the child
(7) Building the child's trauma narrative and helping the child to share the narrative with important others
(8) Building a compassionate and healing response to the trauma (in family, community, and wider society)

Sargent (2009) http://www.psychiatrictimes.com/print/article/10168/1388613?printable=true.

protective workers maximize the likelihood that the child will feel psychologically supported while these professionals are ensuring the child's physical safety.

Clinicians working with traumatized patients should always ensure that these children feel safe in their lives and in the therapist's office. Some victims of child maltreatment do not have an internal sense of safety and may need to learn relaxation techniques as they become more comfortable with their therapist and in participating in therapy. The therapist can then help the patient to associate safety with the experience of calmness and to begin to search out safety and avoid dangerous situations. In some instances the therapist may need to assist parents in assuring safety for children endangered through domestic violence and community violence.

Step 2—Basic Needs

After ensuring the child's safety and supporting the child psychologically, attention to the child's basic needs for food, shelter, sleep, and medical care is necessary. After traumatic injury this may include surgery and hospital care. For children removed from abusive homes, the state is responsible for certifying that foster homes have the resources needed to care for the child. Ensuring adequate nutrition and sleep are often essential aspects of treatment of both acute and chronic traumatic stress.

Psychopharmacology to assist with sleep, severe anxiety, and significant hopelessness and withdrawal is also often useful. Depression is frequently co-morbid with PTSD in children and adolescents. Selective Serotonin Reuptake Inhibitors (SSRIs) are most commonly used with appropriate informed consent and monitoring. Informed consent by parents and consistent monitoring for suicidal ideation in the youth treated with SSRIs is an essential part of treatment. Frequently, there is off-label use of SSRIs in the child and adolescent population based upon FDA (Food and Drug Administration) approval for adult psychiatric disorders and/or pediatric indications for alternate anxiety or mood disturbances (Leslie, Newman, Perrin, & Perrin, 2005). Sertraline, fluvoxamine, and fluoxetine all have FDA pediatric indications for the treatment of obsessive convulsive disorder; however, only fluoxetine is FDA approved for the treatment of pediatric depression (Martin & Volkmar, 2007;

US FDA, 2003a). Although most SSRIs are widely used in the pediatric population for the treatment of posttraumatic stress disorder, only paroxetine and sertraline have FDA indications for adult posttraumatic stress disorder in adults (Lubit, 2008; US FDA, 2003b). Guanfacine and clonidine have been cited as effective in open trial studies for the treatment of PTSD in pediatric populations; however, neither have FDA approval for this treatment (De Bellis & Van Dillen, 2005; Martin & Volkmar, 2007). If a youth has associated psychosis, affective dysregulation, agitation, and dissociation, atypical antipsychotics may be utilized particularly in the acute phases of care (Martin & Volkmar, 2007). In sum, these categories of pharmacological agents have been successful with careful monitoring in conjunction with a multi-modal treatment plan.

Step 3—Knowledge

It is essential that the child and family understand as fully as possible all aspects of trauma recovery. For acute situations, this involves information about treatment, recovery, and expectations for the future. In all instances, the therapist will need to ensure that family and child understand the psychological effects of trauma and how behavioral symptoms may be a response to traumatic experiences. Parents will need to learn the importance of validating their child's emotional experience and to set consistent limits in a firm but caring manner. Parents may also feel guilty about their inability to protect their child physically and/or emotionally. These caregivers might also feel guilty regarding their perpetration of psychological maltreatment, physical abuse or neglect. Accurate information may help them to resolve their guilt and be available to support their child. Providing information is the first step in developing a recovery-oriented therapeutic collaboration with the child and family. By encouraging the family and child to ask questions and to build a thorough understanding of their situation and what can be expected in treatment, the therapist begins the process of empowerment and builds self-control.

Step 4—Resuming Behavioral Routines

An important next step in the psychological recovery process involves the establishment of behavioral competency. This can occur as the child participates in physical therapy after injury. Exercises are taught, the child practices, and the physical therapist praises the child's participation and reinforces the child's role in his own recovery. The same can occur for children who have not been injured and children who are experiencing chronic traumatic stress. Encouraging the child's attendance and achievement at school, their participation in activities, their successful completion of chores at home, anything that the child can be expected to do and praised for builds the child's sense of competency and self-control. The clinician can ensure that the child and family practice relaxation techniques, calming exercises, and deep breathing. The child and his family can use these skills as methods of managing arousal and affective instability. This process further builds the engagement of the child and family in treatment and with the therapist. Parents can also utilize praise for supporting and reinforcing their child's competency.

Step 5—Affect Exploration and Identification

This step encourages the child and family to appreciate that trauma produces an immediate emotional response including fear and powerlessness and subsequent reactions including continued fear, anger, sadness, and possibly shame. These emotions often occur simultaneously and can be confusing for the child and family. By identifying individual emotions and helping the child to understand how each emotion is appropriate and understandable given the situation, the therapist helps the child's emotional experience become predictable and understandable. In this process, the child learns to manage their emotions and the parents have the opportunity to support their child. This also provides the parents with the experience of parenting effectively and builds their sense of control and competency. The child also learns that he doesn't have to suppress emotion or avoid awareness of their experience.

Step 6—Supporting the Supporters

The therapist creates an atmosphere of emotional support for all participants. Being involved with traumatized children can be arousing and upsetting for all involved, including the therapist. Working with traumatized children can be difficult and requires that special understanding and purposeful support be offered and available to parents and relatives. Emotional support is also essential for first responders, hospital staff, child welfare workers, and other staff who work with traumatized children. Supervision or peer support for the therapist is also an important aspect of the therapeutic process.

Step 7—Creating the Trauma Narrative

Organizing traumatic memories into a coherent narrative of the traumatic experience is an essential part of the recovery process. This helps the child appreciate what has happened and ultimately experience mastery over their recollections. The child is helped to attend to his level of arousal and to monitor arousal while creating a step-by-step description of what happened. One method for this process is to help the child develop an emotion thermometer. This allows the child to rate his level of arousal between 0 and 100. This helps the child know, while building his trauma narrative, to recognize when his level of arousal is rising to a distressing level. The therapist can ask the child to stop telling the story and use relaxation skills to calm him. When arousal decreases to an easily tolerable level, the child can begin to elaborate the trauma narrative again. The goal is for the child to be able to tell his story and manage his arousal. Simultaneously, the therapist strongly supports and reinforces this process. Ultimately the child presents the trauma narrative to his parents, who will need the therapist's support in order to be able to hear the story and praise their child for his courage, his persistence, and for his ability to describe his experience. As the child organizes and manages his narrative, the overwhelming nature of the trauma becomes a memory over which the child enjoys increasing control. The parents have a unique opportunity to understand, accept, and to show their love the child. The resiliency of all is apparent and is readily recognized.

Step 8—Making Meaning of the Trauma

There is always the opportunity for those involved in trauma recovery to make unique meaning or significance of the trauma. This can be personal through artistic expression, journal writing, or via volunteer and professional activity. It can also be community wide, through memorialization or volunteer efforts to improve the community through organizations such as the International Society for the Prevention of Child Abuse and Neglect. National and international efforts to enhance social justice or respond to human rights abuses are also important responses to trauma. These efforts provide an opportunity for those who care about those who experience trauma and those who have survived traumatic experiences to grow through the recovery process.

In addition to addressing psychological sequelae secondary to traumatic experiences, clinicians are called to address other problematic sequelae of abuse. These psychiatric conditions include substance misuse disorders, depression, emotion dysregulation, and aggressive acting-out behavior. For youth who do not demonstrate trauma related anxiety and/or depression but meet criteria for an anxiety or mood disorder, cognitive behavioral therapy, and pharmacotherapy with antidepressants and anxiolytics may also be beneficial. An individualized treatment plan will need to focus on decreasing outbursts, setting limits, providing effective supervision, assisting the child with alternative methods of expression and soothing. The engagement of foster parents, adoptive parents, and extended family is an important part of the therapeutic and recovery process.

Conclusion

Traumatic experiences are common during childhood. Psychological sequelae also occur frequently. This is enhanced when the trauma is physical abuse. These can be persistent and can lead to further difficulties, enhanced symptoms, and poor developmental outcome. Some children's intrinsic capacities and the response of their family and context can lead to resilience and growth. By understanding the elements inherent in resilient situations—predictability, self-control, competence, and meaningful emotional support and working to enhance these elements in situations where symptoms of traumatic stress exist, therapists can build resiliency and support the recovery of those children and families experiencing significant traumatic stress.

References

Academy of Child & Adolescent Psychiatry. (1988). *Policy statement: Corporal punishment in schools.* Downloaded December 26, 2008 from   http://www.aacap.org/cs/root/policy_statements/corporal_punishment_in_schools

American Academy of Pediatrics. (2000). American academy of pediatrics: Corporal punishment in schools, committee on school health. *Pediatrics, 106* (2), 343.

APSAC. (1995). Psychosocial evaluation of suspected psychological maltreatment in children and adolescents. Practice guidelines. *American Professional Society on the Abuse of Children.*

Barlow J., Coren, E., & Stewart-Brown, S. (2002). Meta-analysis of parenting programmes in improving maternal psychological health. *British Journal of General Practice, 52*(476), 223–233.

Barlow, J., Johnston, I., Kendrick, D., Polnay, L., & Stewart-Brown, S. (2008). Individual and group-based parenting programmes for the treatment of physical child abuse and neglect (Cochrane Review), *The Cochrane Library 2008*, Issue 4.

Barlow, J., & Parsons, J. (2005). Group-based parent-training programmes for improving emotional and behavioural health adjustment in 0–3 children (Cochrane review). *Cochrane Database of Systematic Reviews 2005*, Issue 3. doi: 10.1002/14651858.CD003680.

Barlow, J., & Stewart-Brown, S. (2000). Review article: Behavior problems and parent-training programs. *Journal of Developmental and Behavioral Pediatrics, 21* (5), 356–370.

Bergen, H. A., Martin, G., Richardson, A. S., Allison, S., & Roeger, L. (2004). Sexual abuse, antisocial behavior and substance use: Gender differences in young community adolescents. *Australian and New Zealand Journal of Psychiatry, 38*, 34–41.

Caspi, A., McClay, J., Moffitt, T. E., Mill, J., Martin, J., Craig, I. W., et al. (2002). Role of genotype in the cycle of violence in maltreated children. *Science, 297*(5582), 851–854.

Caspi, A., Sugden, K., Moffitt, T. E., Taylor, A., Craig, I. W., Harrington, H., et al. (2003). Influence of life stress on depression: Moderation by a polymorphism in the 5-HTT gene. *Science, 301*, 386–389.

Cicchetti, D., & Beeghly, M. (1987). Symbolic development in maltreated youngsters: An organizational perspective. In D. Cicchetti & M. Beeghly (Eds.), *Atypical symbolic development* (pp. 31–45). San Francisco, CA: Jossey-Bass.

Cicchetti, D., & Rogosch, F. A. (1997). The role of self-organization in the promotion of resilience in maltreated children. *Development & Psychopathology, 9* (4), 797–815.

Cohen, J., Mannarino, A., & Deblinger, E. (2006). *Treating Trauma and Traumatic Grief in Children and Adolescents.* New York: Guilford.

Collishaw, S., Pickles, A., Messer, J., Rutter, M., Shearer, C., & Maughan, B. (2007). Resilience to adult psychopathology following childhood maltreatment: Evidence from a community sample. *Child Abuse & Neglect, 31*, 211–229.

Coster, W., Gersten, M., Beeghly, M., & Cicchetti, D. (1989). Communicative functioning in maltreated toddlers. *Developmental Psychology, 25*, 1020–1027.

Crume, T., DiGuiseppi, C., Byers, T., Sirotnak, A., & Garrett, C. (2002). Under-ascertainment of child maltreatment fatalities by death certificates, 1990–1998. *Pediatrics, 110*(2). Downloaded December 1, 2008, from   http://www.childwelfare.gov/pubs/factsheets/fatality.cfm#refer

De Bellis, M. D., & Van Dillen, T. (2005). Childhood post-traumatic stress disorder: An overview. *Child and Adolescent Psychiatric Clinics of North America, 14* (4), 745–1772.

DuMont, K. A., Widom, C. S., & Czaja, S. J. (2007). Predictors of resilience in abused and neglected children grown-up: The role of individual and neighborhood characteristics. *Child Abuse & Neglect, 31*, 255–274.

Durrant, J. E. (2008). Physical punishment, culture, and rights: Current issues for professionals. *Journal of developmental and behavioral pediatrics, 29*, 55–66.

Eley, T. C., Sugden, K., Corsico, A., Gregory, A. M., Sham, P., McGuffin, P., Plomin, R., & Craig, I. W. (2004). Gene-environment interaction analysis of serotonin system markers with adolescent depression. *Molecular Psychiatry, 9*(10), 908–915.

English, D. J., Graham, C. J., Litrownik, A. J., Everson, M., & Bangdiwala, S. I. (2005). Defining maltreatment chronicity: Are there differences in child outcomes? *Child Abuse & Neglect, 29*, 575–595.

Ethier, L. S., Lemelin, J. P., & Lacharite, C. (2004). A longitudinal study on the effects of chronic maltreatment on children's behavioral and emotional problems. *Child Abuse & Neglect, 28*, 1265–1278.

Glaser, D. (2002). Emotional abuse and neglect (psychological maltreatment): a conceptual framework. *Child Abuse & Neglect, 26*, 697–714.

Henry, J., Sloane, M., & Black-Pond, C. (2007). Neurobiology and neurodevelopmental impact of childhood traumatic stress and prenatal alcohol exposure. *Language, Speech and Hearing Services In Schools, 38*, 99–108.

Herman-Giddens, M., Brown, G., Verbiest, S., Carlson, P., Hooten, E., Howell, E., et al. (1999). Underascertainment of child abuse mortality in the United States. *Journal of the American Medical Association, 282*(5), 463–467. Downloaded December 1, 2008, from http://www.childwelfare.gov/pubs/factsheets/fatality.cfm#refer

Horn, I. B., Joseph, J. G., & Cheng, T. L. (2004). Nonabusive physical punishment and child behavior among African-American children: A systematic review. *Journal of the National Medical Association, 96*(9), 1162–1168.

Hurme, T., Alanko, S., Anttila, P., Juven, T., & Svedstrom, E. (2008). Risk factors for physical child abuse in infants and toddlers. *European Journal of Pediatric Surgery, 18*, 387–391.

Jarrett, R. L. (1993). Focus group interviewing with low-income minority populations: A research experience. In D. Morgan (Ed.), *Conducting successful focus groups* (pp. 184–201). Newbury Park, CA: Sage Publications.

Kaufman, J., Yang, B. Z., Douglas-Palumberi, H., Houshyar, S., Lipschitz, D., Krystal, J., & Gelernter, J. (2004). Social supports and serotonin transporter gene moderate depression in maltreated children. *Proceedings of the National Academy of Sciences of the United States of America, 101* (49), 17316–17321.

Kim-Cohen, J., Caspi, A., Taylor, A., Williams, B., Newcombe, R., Craig, I. W., & Moffitt, T. E. (2006, October). MAOA, maltreatment, and gene-environment interaction predicting children's mental health: new evidence and a meta-analysis. *Molecular Psychiatry, 11* (10), 903–913. Epub 2006 June 27.

Lansford, J. E., Dodge, K. A., Pettit, G. S., Bates, J. E., Crozier, J., & Kaplow, J. (2002). A 12-year prospective study of the long-term effects of early child physical maltreatment on psychological, behavioral, and academic problems in adolescence. *Archives of Pediatrics and Adolescent Medicine, 156*, 824–830.

Lansford, J. E., Miller-Johnson, S., Berlin, L. J., Dodge, K. A., Bates, J. E., & Pettit, G. S. (2007). Early physical abuse and later violent delinquency: A prospective longitudinal study. *Child Maltreatment, 12*, 233–245. Downloaded October 16, 2008, from http://cmx.sagepub.com

Leslie, L. K., Newman, T. B., Perrin, J., & Perrin, J. M. (2005). The food and drug administration's deliberations on antidepressant use in pediatric patients. *Pediatrics, 116* (1), 195–204.

Lewis, T., Leeb, R., Kotch, J., Smith, J., Thompson, R., Black, M.M., et al. (2007). Maltreatment history and weapon carrying among early adolescents. *Child Maltreatment, 12*, 259–268. Downloaded October 16, 2008, from http://cmx.sagepub.com

Lim, R. (2006). *Clinical manual of cultural psychiatry.* Arlington, VA: American Psychiatric Publishing, Inc.

Lubit, R. H. (2008). Posttraumatic stress disorder in children. *eMedicine,* updated March 4, 2008. Downloaded December 26, 2008 from http://emedicine.medscape.com/article/918844-overview

Luthar, S. S., Cicchetti, D., & Becker, B. (2000). Research on resilience: Response to commentaries. *Child Development, 71,* 573–575.

Martin, A., & Volkmar, F. R. (2007). *Lewis's child and adolescent psychiatry: A comprehensive textbook* (4th ed.). Philadelphia, PA: Wolters Kluwer, Lippincott Williams & Wilkins.

Masten, A. S., Wright, K. M., & Garmezy, N. (1990). Resilience and development: Contributions from the study of children who overcome adversity. *Development and Psychopathology, 2,* 425–444.

National Child Traumatic Stress Network at nctsnet.org.

Pine, D. S., & Cohen, J. A. (2002). Trauma in children and adolescents: Risk and treatment of psychiatric sequelae. *Biological Psychiatry, 51,* 519–531.

Plattner, B., Karnik, N., Booil, J., Hall, R. E., Schallauer, A., Carrion, V., et al. (2007). State and trait emotions in delinquent adolescents. *Child Psychiatry and Human Development, 38,* 155–169.

Saleptsi, E., Bichescu, D., Rockstroh, B., Neuner, F., Schauer, M., Studer, K., et al. (2004). Negative and positive childhood experiences across developmental periods in psychiatric patients with different diagnoses—an explorative study, *BMC Psychiatry, 4,* 40, doi:10.1186/1471-244X-4-40.

Sargent, A. (2009, March 13). Eight guides to the treatment of traumatic stress in children and adolescents. *Psychiatric Times.* Accessed June 6, 2009: http://www.psychiatrictimes.com/print/article/10168/1388613?printable=true

Saxe, G. N., Ellis, B. H., & Kaplow, J. B. (2007). *Collaborative treatment of traumatized children and teens.* New York: Guilford.

Sedlack, A. J., & Broadhurst, D. D. (1996). *Executive summary of the third National incidence study of child abuse and neglect.* Washington, DC: US Department of Health and Human Services.

Shaffer, A., Huston, L., & Egeland, B. (2008). Identification of child maltreatment using prospective and self-report methodologies: A comparison of maltreatment incidence and relation to later psychopathology. *Child Abuse & Neglect, 32* (7), 682–692.

U.S. Department of Health and Human Services Administration For Children and Families Administration on Children Youth and Families Children's Bureau. (2008). *Child Maltreatment 2006* (pp. 1–194). Downloaded December 1, 2008, from http://www.acf.hhs.gov/programs/cb/pubs/cm06/cm06.pdf

U.S. Food and Drug Administration. (2003a). FDA Approves Prozac for Pediatric Use to Treat Depression and OCD, *FDA Talk Paper*, T03-01. Downloaded December 26, 2008, from http://www.fda.gov/bbs/topics/ANSWERS/2003/ANS01187.html

U.S. Food and Drug Administration. (2003b). FDA Statement Regarding the Anti-Depressant Paxil for Pediatric Population, *FDA Talk Paper*, T03-43. Downloaded December 26, 2008, from http://www.fda.gov/bbs/topics/ANSWERS/2003/ANS01230.html

Whaley, A. L. (2000). Sociocultural differences in the developmental consequences of the use of physical discipline during childhood for African Americans. *Cultural Diversity and Ethnic Minority Psychology, 6*(1), 5–12.

Widom, C. S. (1989a). Child abuse, neglect, and violent criminal behavior. *Criminology, 27*, 251–271.

Widom, C. S. (1989b). Does violence beget violence? A critical examination of the literature. *Psychological Bulletin, 106*, 3–28.

Yates, T. M., Carlson, E. A., & Egeland, B. (2008). A prospective study of child maltreatment and self-injurious behavior in a community sample. *Development and Psychopathology, 20*, 651–671.

Zhai, F., & Gao, Q. (2008). Child maltreatment among Asian Americans characteristics and explanatory framework. *Child Maltreatment,* published on October 29, 2008 as Doi:10.1177/1077559508326286.

Subject Index

A.P. Giardino et al. (eds.), *A Practical Guide to the Evaluation of Child Physical Abuse and
Neglect*, DOI 10.1007/978-1-4419-0702-8, © Springer Science+Business Media, LLC 1997, 2010